HANDBOOK OF PEDIATRIC AND ADOLESCENT HEALTH PSYCHOLOGY

RELATED TITLES

Handbook of Pediatric Psychology and Psychiatry
Volume I
Psychological and Psychiatric Issues in the Pediatric Setting
Robert T. Ammerman and John V. Campo (Editors)
ISBN: 0-205-16560-5

Handbook of Pediatric Psychology and Psychiatry
Volume II
Disease, Injury, and Illness
Robert T. Ammerman and John V. Campo (Editors)
ISBN: 0-205-27601-6

Approaches to Child Treatment: Introduction to Theory, Research, and Practice, Second Edition
James H. Johnson, Wiley C. Rasbury, and Lawrence J. Siegel
ISBN: 0-205-15604-5

The Child Clinician's Handbook
William G. Kronenberger and Robert G. Meyer
ISBN: 0-205-14752-6

The Practice of Child Therapy, Third Edition
Richard J. Morris and Thomas R. Kratochwill (Editors)
ISBN: 0-205-16818-3

Child Neuropsychology: Assessment and Interventions for Neurodevelopmental Disorders
Phyllis Anne Teeter and Margaret Semrud-Clikeman
ISBN: 0-205-16331-9

For more information or to purchase a book, please call
1-800-278-3525.

HANDBOOK OF PEDIATRIC AND ADOLESCENT HEALTH PSYCHOLOGY

Edited by

ANTHONY J. GORECZNY
University of Indianapolis

MICHEL HERSEN
Pacific University

Allyn and Bacon
Boston   London   Toronto   Sydney   Tokyo   Singapore

RJ
47.53
.H367
1999

Series editor: Carla Daves
Series editorial assistant: Susan Hutchinson
Marketing manager: Joyce Nilsen
Manufacturing buyer: Suzanne Lareau

Copyright © 1999 by Allyn & Bacon
A Viacom Company
Needham Heights, MA 02494

Internet: www.abacon.com

All rights reserved. No part of the material protected by this copyright notice may be
reproduced or utilized in any form or by any means, electronic or mechanical,
including photocopying, recording, or by any information storage and retrieval
system, without written permission from the copyright owner.

Chapter 20, entitled "Posttraumatic Stress Disorder," may be reproduced royalty free
for United States governmental purposes.

Library of Congress Cataloging-in-Publication Data

Handbook of pediatric and adolescent health psychology / edited by
  Anthony J. Goreczny and Michel Hersen.
      p.   cm.
    Includes bibliographical references and index.
    ISBN 0-205-15624-X
    1. Health behavior in children.   2. Health behavior in
  adolescents.   3. Clinical health psychology.   I. Goreczny, Anthony
  J.   II. Hersen, Michel.
    RJ47.53.H367   1998   97-36968
    618.92'89--dc21   CIP

ISBN 0-205-15624-X

Printed in the United States of America
10 9 8 7 6 5 4 3 2 1   02 01 00 99 98

37533975

CONTENTS

PREFACE

Medical and psychological sciences have provided many new assessment and intervention efforts during the past few decades. Even more exciting, the interface of these two branches of scientific inquiry has enabled more efficient development of advances than would have been possible without such interdisciplinary cooperation. Thus, the multidisciplinary field of behavioral medicine has witnessed a large growth in the past few decades, spawning development of a division within the American Psychological Association and formation of a multidisciplinary professional association (Society for Behavioral Medicine) specifically for behavioral medicine researchers and clinicians.

Within the field of behavioral medicine, an area of specific focus has been that of pediatric and adolescent health. Although there are many reasons for this specific focus, one factor that is clearly relevant is that despite the many technological advances and the relatively high status of the American medical community, the United States has one of the highest infant mortality rates among the technologically privileged nations. A second factor is that the United States Public Health Department, in the treatise entitled *Healthy People 2000,* established specific goals for reduction of the major health concerns of U.S. citizens by the year 2000. Many of the identified problem areas and corresponding goals relate primarily to children and adolescents.

Finally, the recent spotlight on health care, both in the presidential elections of 1992 and 1996 and in the years that have followed, has propelled health care

to the forefront of the U.S. agenda. However, it is important to remember that the health care debate is not unique to the United States; adequate health care is central to the survival of peoples from every nation, and obtaining the perspectives of people from other countries is essential to understanding the many challenges this nation faces. This is especially important as the barriers between nations continue to erode. Technological advances have made communications and travel between remote parts of the world more viable than was ever possible. Toward a beginning recognition of this fact, we have included a few chapters from individuals in countries other that the United States. We hope that this will encourage an increase in future discourse among professionals from different nations.

Despite the significant increase in the number of clinical researchers in the multidisciplinary area of behavioral medicine, the many advances these researchers have made, and the increased attention to health care, there remains a significant need for continued research regarding illness assessment, prevention, and rehabilitation. Thus, one of the primary purposes of this book is to stimulate research ideas for clinical researchers in the fields of pediatric and adolescent health psychology.

Another primary purpose of this book is to serve as a resource for clinicians treating children and adolescents. This includes not just psychologists but also family practitioners from diverse disciplines. This book consists of five sections organized along various dimensions related to child and adolescent health psychology: general issues, specific diseases and disorders, addiction issues, health promotion, and topics of special interest.

Ultimately, the intended audience for this book includes all who have an interest in learning about recent advances in pediatric and adolescent health psychology. As such, this book could serve as a textbook for coursework, practicum training sites, or internship/residency studies in child health psychology. The authors who wrote the chapters in this book provide excellent overviews of their respective areas, highlight major concerns within those areas, and instill an interest in development of new research initiatives.

Completion of a book this size requires the efforts, hard work, and determination of many individuals. First and foremost, the contributing authors provided excellent chapters that will undoubtedly supply readers with the information they need to deliver ef-

fective treatment to their clients, stimulate original creative research, and accommodate the learning process. Next, Mylan Jaixen and the staff at Allyn and Bacon deserve recognition for their support of this book and the masterful way they have handled its preparation. Our gratitude is also extended to reviewers of the manuscript—Larry L. Mullins (Oklahoma State University) and James R. Rodrigue (University of Florida)—for their helpful comments. We thank our families, most specifically our wives and children, who have nourished our efforts and provided support and understanding during the many hours of preparation. Finally, we thank Eleanor Gil, Carole Londerée, and Maura Sullivan for their technical help.

A. J. G.
M. H.

ABOUT THE EDITORS

Anthony J. Goreczny, Ph.D., received his Ph.D. from Louisiana State University, where he specialized in medical psychology. Goreczny interned at the Brown University Psychology Internship consortium (Behavioral Medicine track). He then served as Coordinator of Behavioral Medicine at the Pittsburgh (Highland Drive) Veterans Affairs Medical Center and as assistant professor at the University of Pittsburgh School of Medicine. He is now the Director of Clinical Training at the University of Indianapolis Department of Psychology. Goreczny has authored or coauthored 20 articles and 10 book chapters and has presented 18 papers at regional and national scientific conventions. He is the editor of the *International Journal of Rehabilitation and Health* and serves on the editorial board of the *Journal of Clinical Geropsychology.* In addition, he has served as ad hoc reviewer for several other journals.

Michel Hersen, Ph.D., is professor and dean, School of Professional Psychology, Pacific University, Forest Grove, Oregon, and is past president of the Association for Advancement of Behavior Therapy. He has coauthored and coedited 111 books, including the *Handbook of Prescriptive Treatments for Adults* and *Single Case Experimental Designs.* He has also published more than 220 scientific journal articles and is coeditor of several psychological journals, including *Behavior Modification, Clinical Psychology Review, Journal of Anxiety Disorders, Journal of Family Violence, Journal of Developmental and Physical Disabilities, Journal of Clinical Geropsychology,* and *Aggression and Violent Behavior: A Review Journal.* With Alan S. Bellack, he is co-editor of the forthcoming 11-volume work entitled *Comprehensive Clinical Psychology.* Hersen has been the recipient of numerous grants from the National Institute of Mental Health, the Department of Education, the National Institute of Disabilities and Rehabilitation Research, and the March of Dimes Birth Defects Foundation. He is a Diplomate of the American Board of Professional Psychology, Distinguished Practitioner and Member of the National Academy of Practice in Psychology, and recipient of the Distinguished Career Achievement Award in 1996 from the American Board of Medical Psychotherapists and Psychodiagnosticians.

ABOUT THE CONTRIBUTORS

Christina Adams, Ph.D., received her doctorate in clinical psychology from Louisiana State University. She completed this project while attending her internship at the University of Mississippi Medical Center/Jackson VA Medical Center Consortium. Currently, she is an assistant professor in the Department of Psychology at West Virginia University.

Dalia Adams, Ph.D., received her doctorate in clinical psychology from Case Western Reserve University in 1997. She completed her predoctoral internship at the James A. Haley Veteran's Hospital in Tampa, Florida. She is currently working in Tampa as Admissions Coordinator and Director of Research and Program Evaluation at The Children's Home, Inc., a residential and after-care treatment center for children and adolescents.

Albert P. Aldenkamp, Ph.D., received his undergraduate degree from the State University of Groningen in the Netherlands and his doctorate from the University of Amsterdam. Formerly, he served as head of the Neuropsychological Department of Meer & Bosch Epilepsy Centre, coordinator of the cluster of specialized epilepsy outpatient departments in the northeast regions of the Netherlands, and professor of pediatric neuropsychology at the State University in Leiden. Currently, Aldenkamp is head of the Psychology Department and head of the Learning Disabilities Project at Meer & Bosch Epilepsy Centre and a member of the Scientific Board of Epilepsy Centre, Kempenhaeghe.

Gregory L. Austin, B.S., graduated from the University of Florida in 1995 with a B.S. in Chemistry. Each year of his undergraduate studies, Austin performed an internship at the University of Tennessee, Memphis, through the Graduate Achievement Program. During the internships, he worked with Dr. Harshfield's research group in the investigation of hypertension and target organ damage. Currently, Austin is attending Yale University Medical School.

Susan E. Barker, M.A., is completing her predoctoral internship in clinical psychology at the Medical University of South Carolina Department of Psychiatry and Behavioral Sciences. She is currently a doctoral candidate at Louisiana State University, where she earned a master's degree in clinical psychology in 1991. Barker has coauthored several articles and chapters on eating disorders and body image.

Gerard T. Barron, Psy.D., is a clinical neuropsychologist and clinical director of the Neurobehavior Program at HealthSouth Lake Erie Institute of Rehabilitation in Erie, Pennsylvania. He completed his doctoral studies at Indiana University of Pennsylvania and a postdoctoral fellowship in neuropsychology at HealthSouth LEIR.

Stuart M. Berman, M.D., is currently chief, Adolescent Activities Unit with the Division of STD Prevention at the Centers for Disease Control and Prevention. He is a board-certified pediatrician, having trained at UCLA and Yale. He was in pediatric private practice for seven years before coming to the CDC in 1983. His responsibilities include integrating, directing, and strengthening the Division's prevention activities, including research, programmatic, and evaluation components, to prevent sexually transmitted diseases and their complications among adolescents.

Timothy C. Blackson, Ph.D., is a staff scientist at the Center for Education and Drug Abuse Research. His area of interest is temperament variation and its relationship to family interaction patterns and alcohol/drug use. He has published approximately 20 papers on this topic.

Ronald L. Blount is an associate professor in the Department of Psychology and a Research Fellow in the Institute for Behavioral Research at the University of Georgia. His research interests are in the areas of pediatric pain assessment and management, children's coping styles and strategies, coping with chronic conditions, and maintenance and generalization of behavior change.

Ronald T. Brown is associate professor of Psychiatry and Pediatrics at Emory University School of Medicine. He has published more than 100 articles in the area of pediatric and clinical child psychology.

Sandra A. Brown, Ph.D., is a licensed clinical psychologist nationally recognized for her research and clinical work in the area of alcohol and drug abuse. She is a professor in the Departments of Psychology and Psychiatry at the University of California, San Diego, and chief of Psychology Service at the VA San Diego Healthcare System. Her publications and national presentations focus on the development and progression of alcohol and drug abuse for both adolescents and adults. Brown is a Fellow in the American Psychological Association (APA), former Chair of the Education and Training Committee of APA Division 50, a leader in the development of the new APA certificate examination for the treatment of alcohol and drug disorders, and is on the editorial board of several journals.

Willard Cates, Jr., M.D., is senior vice president of Biomedical Affairs for Family Health International (FHI), in Research Triangle Park, North. Prior to joining FHI, Cates was with the Centers for Disease Control and Prevention for 20 years, where he directed the Division of STD/HIV Prevention for nearly half that time. His scientific emphasis was on preventing STD/HIV in adolescents and improving the reproductive health of women. Cates has been on the Editorial Board of *Journal of Adolescent Health Care* and has been the J. Roswell Gallagher lecturer for the Society of Adolescent Medicine.

Isobel Contento, Ph.D., is professor and coordinator of the Program in Nutrition Education at Teachers College, Columbia University, in New York City. Her areas of research and teaching include psychosocial determinants of food choice in children and adolescents, behavioral aspects of diet, and nutrition education for school-aged children.

Natalie C. Frank, Ph.D., is assistant professor of psychology at George Washington University. Her research interests involve stress and coping in chronically ill children and their families.

Mary J. Gage, Ph.D., received her doctorate from Bowling Green State University. She is currently a postdoctoral fellow in Health Psychology at Mellen Center, Cleveland Clinic Foundation in Cleveland, Ohio.

Gregory A. Harshfield, Ph.D., received his B.A. from Wittenberg University in Springfield, Ohio, and his doctorate in Experimental Psychology from Miami University in Oxford, Ohio. He has served on the faculty of the Cornell University Medical College in New York and the Charles R. Drew University Medical School in Los Angeles. Harshfield is currently a professor of Pediatrics at the Medical College of Georgia in Augusta, Georgia.

Sharon S. Ishikawa, M.A., is a doctoral student in clinical psychology at the University of California at Los Angeles. Her research interests include the prediction and consequences of interpersonal violence, with a particular interest in the neuropsychological and biological correlates of aggression.

Debbie J. Javorsky, B.S., received her undergraduate degree from Tulane University. She is presently a doctoral student in the University of Rhode Island's Clinical Psychology Program. Her interests include health psychology and neuropsychology, and she has conducted research in the area of children with diabetes.

Elissa Jelalian, Ph.D., is an assistant professor of Psychiatry and Human Behavior at the Brown University School of Medicine. Her primary research interests are nutrition and eating concerns in chronic illness and overweight populations.

Glenn N. Jones, Ph.D., is an associate professor with the Department of Family Medicine, School of Medicine in New Orleans, Louisiana State University Medical Center. He is at the Center for Primary Care Research, Earl K. Long Hospital, in Baton Rouge, Louisiana. His interests are in the field of behavioral medicine, with particular interests in the role of minor stress on exacerbations of chronic illnesses and primary care psychology.

Alice L. Kahle, Ph.D., is a pediatric psychologist at Texas Scottish Rite Hospital for Children in Dallas, Texas. Her clinical and research interests include pediatric psychology, early childhood behavior problems, early intervention, enhancing adherence with medical procedures, and social adjustment in children with disabilities and chronic illnesses.

Michele A. Keffer is a doctoral candidate in the clinical psychology program at the State University of New York at Buffalo. She is in the process of completing her dissertation, which tests a psychological and biological model to predict periodontal disease indicators. She works as a therapist in Pittsburgh.

Kenneth R. Lofland, Ph.D., is director of Pain Studies at the Pain and Rehabilitation Clinic of Chicago. He obtained his Ph.D. in clinical psychology from the Illinois Institute of Technology with a specialization in Behavioral Medicine. His primary research is in chronic pain syndromes, currently focusing on the quality of health care provided to headache sufferers and the validity of the IHS classification criteria for headaches.

Judith A. Lyons, Ph.D., is a graduate of McGill University and Concordia University. Her work focuses on the assessment and treatment of traumatic stress.

She is a clinical psychologist/associate professor of Psychiatry and Human Behavior at the Veterans Affairs/University of Mississippi Medical Centers in Jackson, Mississippi.

Emily P. McGrath, M.A., is a graduate student in clinical psychology at the University of California at Los Angeles. Her research interests are focused on children's perceptions of acute and chronic stressors and long-term mental health outcomes. Her doctoral dissertation research is on children's perceptions of academic and interpersonal stressors and links to depression.

John Michela, Ph.D., is associate professor and head of the doctoral training program in Personnel and Organizational Psychology at the University of Waterloo, Ontario. His research and teaching concern various topics in organizational behavior (e.g., culture, leadership, stress), organization development and change (e.g., for Total Quality), and research methods and statistics.

Lynn Michell is based in the MRC Medical Sociology Unit in Glasgow, Scotland, and is currently funded by The Scottish Office to work on a longitudinal study of the influence of friends and peers on adolescents' smoking behavior and life-styles. Previously, she was funded by the Imperial Cancer Research Fund to write "Growing Up in Smoke," and by the Cancer Research Campaign to survey the smoking behavior of mainstream and special education pupils.

Deborah L. Miller, Ph.D., received a doctorate in clinical psychology from Louisiana State University and is now a pediatric psychologist and assistant professor of pediatrics at the duPont Hospital for Children/Jefferson Medical College.

Jodi A. Mindell, Ph.D., is associate professor of Psychology at St. Joseph's University and Pediatric Clinical Director at the Sleep Disorders Center at MCP-Hahnemann School of Medicine. She specializes in childhood sleep disorders and maintains a broad-scale clinical research program investigating the assessment and treatment of sleep problems in children.

O. G. Mulder, M.D., received his medical degree from Leiden University, the Netherlands, and served in neurology departments at Roozenburg (the Hague Psychiatric Institute); Municipal Hospital (the Hague), where he later served as chief; and Leiden University Hospital. He was also neurologist in the Instituut voor Epilepsiebestrijding (Institute for Epilepsy) in Heemstede. Mulder now serves as consultant for psychogenic, nonepileptic seizures within the Institute.

Patrick Mahlen O'Neil, Ph.D., is professor of Psychiatry and Behavioral Sciences and director of the Weight Management Center at the Medical University of South Carolina. He earned his Ph.D. in clinical psychology at the University of Georgia. He is the author of many papers and presentations in the area of obesity. Besides his professional writing, O'Neil has for seven years authored "Weighing the Choices," a weekly column on weight control in the Charleston Sunday newspaper. He currently also serves on the South Carolina Board of Examiners in Psychology.

James C. Overholser, Ph.D., received his doctorate in clinical psychology from the Ohio State University in 1989. He completed his predoctoral internship and postdoctoral fellowship at the Brown University Program in Medicine. Overholser is currently associate professor in the Department of Psychology at Case Western Reserve University in Cleveland, Ohio, and a staff psychologist at the Laurelwood Counseling Center of University Circle.

Tomlin J. Paul, M.D., is a lecturer in community health in the Department of Community Health and Psychiatry at the University of the West Indies, Mona, Jamaica. He has worked as part of a research team on epidemiology of childhood disability looking at its prevalence in Jamaica and the development of low-cost methods for its identification. He has also been involved in the development of health promotion programs at the University of the West Indies and is a foundation member of the Caribbean Public Health Association.

Thomas J. Payne, Ph.D., is an associate professor of Psychiatry (Psychology) at the University of Missis-

sippi Medical Center and director of Health Behavior Program at the Jackson VA Medical Center. He received his Ph.D. in clinical psychology from State University of New York, Binghamton. His clinical and research interests include coping with chronic illness, cardiovascular risk factor modification, and learning mechanisms in addictions.

John Pierpont, MSW, professor at the School of Social Work at East Carolina University, in Greenville, North Carolina. He has published in the areas of child abuse prevention, children's mental health, and mental health administration.

John Poertner, DSW, is a professor and associate dean in the School of Social Work at the University of Illinois at Urbana-Champagne. Poernter has published extensively in the areas of child welfare, children's mental health, and the design and management of social programs. Currently, he is responsible for reporting outcomes for children and families at the Children & Family Research Center, a collaboration between the Illinois Department of Children and Family Services and the University of Illinois.

Rena Repetti, Ph.D., received her doctorate from Yale University and is currently an associate professor in the Department of Psychology at UCLA. She is actively involved in UCLA's graduate programs in clinical and health psychology. Her research interests focus on stress and coping processes in work, school, and family roles.

Phyllis A. Richey, Ph.D., is an exercise physiologist for the Division of Cardiology Department of Pediatrics, at the University of Tennessee, Memphis. She completed her B.S.Ed. degree in Fitness Management and her M.S. degree in Exercise Physiology at Memphis State University, where she realized her interest in and career goal of cardiovascular physiology research. She began working for the University of Tennessee, running and assisting in several research studies investigating cardiovascular issues, primarily relating to hypertension and target organ damage. With the completion of her Ph.D. in Exercise Science from the University of Mississippi, Richey is currently pursuing her career objective of clinical exercise physiology and cardiovascular research.

James H. Rimmer, is director of the Center on Health Promotion Research for Persons with Disabilities, University of Illinois at Chicago. He is director of the Exercise Gerontology Clinic in DeKalb, Illinois, and has extensive experiences working with children and adults with mental retardation in the area of fitness promotion.

Laurie Ruggiero, Ph.D., received her B.A. from Pennsylvania State University and her Ph.D. from Louisiana State University, and completed her clinical internships and postdoctoral fellowship at Brown University School of Medicine. She is currently an assistant professor in Psychology at the University of Rhode Island and an adjunct assistant professor (Research) of Psychiatry in the Brown University School of Medicine. Her specialty area is health psychology/behavioral medicine with both adults and children.

Suzanne Salzinger, Ph.D., is a research scientist in the Division of Child and Adolescent Psychiatry at the New York State Psychiatric Institute and Columbia University. For the past 15 years, she has conducted research on the effects of physical abuse on school-age children's social development and on adolescent functioning. She is currently conducting a follow-up study on New York City children who had been physically abused in preadolescence. She is also beginning a short-term longitudinal study of the effects of exposure to community violence on sixth- to eighth-grade inner-city children.

Michael Schwabenbauer, Ph.D., is currently director of Neuropsychology at HealthSouth LEIR and HealthSouth Great Lakes rehabilitation hospitals in Erie, Pennsylvania. He is an adjunct faculty member at Pennsylvania State University/Behrend College campus, Gannon University, and the University of Indianapolis. Schwabenbauer completed a postdoctoral fellowship in neuropsychology at Lake Erie Institute of Rehabilitation (LEIR) and is listed with the National Register of Health Service Providers in Psychology.

Adina Smith is a clinical psychology graduate student at the University of Georgia. Her research interests are in the area of pediatric psychology with a primary focus on the adjustment of siblings who have chronic physical and psychological conditions.

Anthony Spirito, Ph.D., received his doctorate in clinical psychology from Virginia Commonwealth University in 1981. He completed his predoctoral internship and postdoctoral fellowship at Children's Hospital in Boston. Spirito is currently an associate professor in the Department of Psychiatry and Human Behavior at the Brown University School of Medicine and director of child psychology at Rhode Island Hospital in Providence.

Lori J. Stark, Ph.D., is an associate professor of Psychiatry and Human Behavior at the Brown University School of Medicine. Her primary research interests are treatment outcome studies with chronic and acutely ill children. Stark has received funding from the Cystic Fibrosis Foundation and the National Institutes of Health for her research on cystic fibrosis and malnutrition.

David G. Stewart is a doctoral candidate in the San Diego State University/University of California, San Diego Joint Doctoral Program in Clinical Psychology and an intern at the University of Washington. He has conducted research with substance-abusing adolescents focusing on co-occuring antisocial behavior and ethnic and cultural factors in addiction.

James M. Sturges, Ph.D., received his Ph.D. in clinical psychology, with a specialization in child psychology, from the University of Alabama. He is presently an assistant professor of Psychiatry (Psychology) and director of the Behavioral Pediatrics Program at the University of Mississippi Medical Center. His clinical and research interests are in pediatric psychology, with emphases on child coping and in promoting positive health-related behaviors of children.

Susan F. Tapert received her B.A. degree in psychology from the University of Washington and pursued research interests in substance abuse prevention and harm reduction at the Addictive Behaviors Research Center at the University of Washington. She is currently enrolled in University of California, San Diego, and San Diego State University's Joint Doctoral Program in Clinical Psychology. Her research interests include neuropsychological factors associated with substance abuse, relapse prevention in adolescents with comorbid psychiatric disorders, adolescent smoking cessation, HIV prevention, and health risk reduction.

Kenneth J. Tarnowski, Ph.D., is professor of Psychology at Florida Gulf Coast University (formerly University of South Florida at Fort Meyers). He has published more than 100 articles in the area of pediatric and clinical child psychology.

Ralph E. Tarter, Ph.D., is professor of Psychiatry and Neurology at the University of Pittsburgh Medical School and Director of the Center for Education and Drug Abuse Research. His research interests in the field of alcohol and drug abuse span diverse topics, including neuropsychology, behavior genetics, and the effects of liver disease on the brain. He has published over 200 articles on topics pertaining to alcohol and drug abuse.

Marigold J. Thorburn, M.D., is director of 3D Projects, a community-based rehabilitation program in Jamaica. She also is an associate lecturer in the Faculty of Medical Sciences at the University of the West Indies. Thorburn is a graduate of Birmingham University Medical School. Her professional career has spanned pathology and cytogenetics, social and preventive medicine, early intervention, and community-based rehabilitation. She has also been involved in the mental retardation movement and program development in childhood disability services throughout the Caribbean region. Her research interests are in developing low-cost technology for early detection, assessment, intervention, and evaluation of childhood disability problems.

Bruce W. Tuckman is professor of Educational Research at Florida State University in Tallahassee. His current textbooks include *Conducting Educational Research* (4th edition) and *Educational Psychology: From Theory to Application.* Tuckman has published in professional journals and popular magazines such as *Runner's World*, primarily on topics in motivation.

Frances Tylavsky received her B.S. in Biological Health from Pennsylvania State University, a M.S. in Clinical Nutrition from Boston University, and a Dr.PH in Nutrition from the University of North Carolina at Chapel Hill. Her current position is assistant professor in the Department of Preventive Medicine at the University of Tennessee where her main role is to develop and conduct nutrition-related research as it relates to the development, occurrence, and progression of chronic diseases.

Carole J. Vogt, Psy.D., is a graduate of the University of Denver, Graduate School of Professional Psychology. She is a licensed clinical psychologist in the state of Colorado and is employed by Kaiser-Permanente. She is affiliated with Weight Choice of Denver and has strong interest in eating disorders.

Patrick West is a senior nonclinical scientist based in the Medical Research Council's Medical Sociology Unit in Glasgow, Scotland. His current research interests include health inequalities, the youth-adult transition, youth culture, and health-related behaviors, particularly smoking. Prior to joining MRC, West worked on the National Child Development Study and various studies of childhood epilepsy.

PART I

GENERAL ISSUES

This first section of the book addresses issues of general relevance to the areas of child and adolescent health psychology. The first chapter briefly discusses some of the challenges that the current state of health care in the country provides. The chapter then goes on to discuss some of the public policy decisions that we must face as we attempt to improve the status of our children's health and reduce their mortality and morbidity rates. Chapter 2 addresses the issue of infant deaths, with a focus on prevention. In this regard, a focus of the chapter is low birth-weight babies. Issues addressed include pre- and perinatal care as well as the importance of parent education. Another primary topic addressed is that of adolescent sexual activity and pregnancy. Finally, the chapter addresses possible policy implications. The third chapter illustrates some of the difficulties of conducting assessments of children in countries that do not have ready access to many of the personnel and technological advances available to others. Chapter 3 also highlights the authors' experiences in dealing with childhood health problems in Jamaica and reviews screening and assessment tools used.

CHAPTER 1

PEDIATRIC AND ADOLESCENT HEALTH PSYCHOLOGY DURING THE HEALTH CARE REVOLUTION: CHALLENGES AND OPPORTUNITIES

Anthony J. Goreczny, UNIVERSITY OF INDIANAPOLIS
Mary Gage, PITTSBURGH (HIGHLAND DRIVE) VA MEDICAL CENTER

The trajectory of health care policy for children and adolescents is currently in a state of flux. Some of the recent changes are positive in that children and adolescents in today's society are now, more than ever, on the forefront of the health care agenda (Knitzer, 1993). Evidence in support of this view includes the increased number of child health care organizations, policy proposals, funded research, and implemented treatment programs at both the state and federal levels (Knitzer, 1993; Melton, 1995). The primary reason for implementing these changes is to combat the growing number of problems associated with childhood and youth, such as the escalation of violence toward and by children (Osofsky, 1995; Richters & Martinez, 1993). However, the current revolution in health care presents challenges for practitioners and policy makers who are struggling with the changing marketplace. The revolution, however, also presents opportunities to influence health care policies and to set the agenda for health care delivery into the twenty-first century. In order to do this, however, practitioners must keep abreast of the main issues driving the current changes and have a clear direction in mind.

There are multiple facets of child and adolescent health psychology that need to be addressed but are beyond the scope of this chapter. The authors of the specific chapters in this volume have effectively elucidated empirical data on their areas of expertise. The primary emphasis of this chapter is to serve as an overview of the area, highlighting particular topics. One purpose of this chapter is to review the limited research on development of health behaviors and habits. Another purpose is to make clear to readers the importance of changing health care policy for today's youth. A third purpose is to present readers with an overview of the changes in child and adolescent health care policy. Finally, a fourth purpose is to highlight for readers the current functioning and potential future trends of health care.

BEHAVIORAL AND
ATTITUDE DEVELOPMENT

Despite the strong emphasis of behavioral medicine and health psychology on use of the scientific method and on observable behaviors and outcomes, it is quite surprising to see there exists very little controlled research specifically on development of health behaviors and habits. There are at least two possible reasons for this. First, the field of behavioral medicine grew from the application of behavioral principles to amelioration of already detected health problems; the emphasis was on treatment of already identified health difficulties and their maintaining factors rather than on theoretical identification of initiating factors. Second, the behavioral principles that guide behavioral medicine have existed for many years; there was no reasoned need to empirically evaluate Hull's (1943) theory of habit and drive or Thorndike's (1911) law of effect or how they relate to health behavior and health behavior habits. It appears this is no longer true.

Almost all of the major killers of people living in technologically advantaged countries today result from, or at least have as major contributing factors, specific health behaviors. Heart disease, cancer, strokes, accidents, and AIDS all result from a combination of factors, with health risk behaviors as one of the major components. Yet, we do not have empirically tested models that have shown how we develop such health risk behaviors as smoking, food choices, exercise habits, seat belt use, alcohol/drug use, unsafe sex practices, and poor coping/stress management practices. Although some research has begun to identify some of the factors involved in habit development (e.g., peer influence in initiation of smoking behavior; see West & Michell, Chapter 13 of this volume), the actual mechanism of action (e.g., modeling, punishment via ridicule, etc.) remains unknown. Given that such life-style factors are major contributors to the current primary health concerns, research into development of these health habits is now essential.

Behavior patterns are formed at an early age, and there are many sources that tend to influence children's development, such as parenting styles and environmental factors (Austin & Nach-Ferguson, 1995). The formation of beliefs and perceptions continues into the adolescent years, a period of transition that can also be a time of new discoveries, including learning positive (e.g., exercising) as well as negative (e.g., smoking) health behaviors (Cohen, Brownell, & Felix, 1990; Stiffman, Dore, Cunningham, & Earls, 1995). Along with behavioral pattern development, children's attitudes also are formed and shaped by multiple daily experiences and the results of their behavior, such as the consequences of their actions and various cultural expectations (Cothern & Collins, 1992).

Thus, although some researchers have recently begun studying prosocial behavioral development, such as examining sharing and playing behavior in children (Hay, 1994; Palenik, 1993), there is relatively minimal research on positive and negative developmental health habits in children and on implementation of treatment and prevention programs that can change or shape behavior (Weiss, 1992). Some recent studies suggest that poor health behaviors develop at an early age and become increasingly prevalent in adulthood (Battjes, Leukefeld, & Pickens, 1992; Groer, Thomas, Droppleman, & Younger, 1994). For example, Groer and colleagues (1994) found that high school students' stress levels increased along with the number and duration of their negative health behaviors, such as smoking and poor dieting, from their freshman year to their senior year. Thus, although learning experiences can be positive and can have a good influence on developing behavior and attitude, in today's society, children and adolescents are exposed to a large number of experiences associated with violence and poor health habits, and these experiences can have an equal, but negative, effect on shaping individual development.

In addition, recent research has started to confirm the belief that health behaviors begun as children and adolescents will continue into adulthood. For example, one recent study revealed that individuals who abused drugs as teenagers were more likely to engage in risk-taking behaviors (e.g., sharing needles,) as adults than were individuals who did not start abusing drugs as teenagers (Battjes et al., 1992). Obviously, there remain questions as to the causality of this process. It may be that adults who engage in risk-taking behaviors sought out these influences as children. Despite uncertainty as to the cause of destructive behavior, the main concern is prevention. Developing ways to prevent children and adolescents from becoming exposed to negative influences, such as drug use and violence, may help to improve their behavior and attitude as adults, thus benefiting everyone.

In addition to overt behaviors, some cognitive processes may also be important in development of health risk behaviors. For example, a recent study found that although teenagers tend to minimize the perceived risk of health-related activities more than their parents do, they tend to be less optimistic than their parents about avoiding self-injury and illness (Cohn, Macfarlane, Yanez, Imai, et al., 1995). The notion that today's youth are more likely than older adults to take risks and to develop risk-taking behaviors and attitudes that continue into adulthood lends support for the need to reach individuals at a young age. Thus, as suggested by Williams (1994), research examining the developmental factors of today's youth is imperative for understanding how to deter societal health problems in the future. One way to effect changes in health behavior is to implement health policies that will shape children's behavior toward health-engendering habits.

THE ROLE OF GOVERNMENT IN HEALTH CARE POLICY

Historically, a notable change in health care policy occurred in the 1970s, which involved an initial shift from state to federal responsibility. Although health care issues were primarily under the direction of state regulators before the middle 1970s, the focus shifted since that time toward a global consensus between state and federal government, with federal authorities taking the primary lead (Melton, 1995). The improved cohesiveness of jurisdiction gradually developed as the result of various co-occurring factors, such as development of consistency among the states' legal systems and the perceived rights of children as individuals by the Supreme Court.

Federal attention toward children's health issues increased in the 1970s, but it was not until the 1980s that federal regulators seriously began to examine public policy. One milestone was the result of a report issued by the Children's Defense Fund (CDF) in 1982 that identified several weaknesses in the mental

health system for children. The summation of their report was that children's mental health issues did not receive adequate attention and that the services provided did not meet the complex needs of the nation's youth. In 1984, Congress implemented the Child and Adolescent Service System Program (CASSP). The CASSP provided incentive to the states by funding mental health programs and research that followed specific regulations to improve the quality of mental health care (Knitzer, 1993). However, these policy changes often failed to produce the desired outcome. As such, despite the changes in government policy during the 1980s, there has continued to be a substantial increase in problems, such as an increase in the number of inpatient admissions to child psychiatric facilities (Kiesler, 1993) and a surge of violence experienced and witnessed by children (Osofsky, 1995; Richters, 1993).

Although the federal government is now more active in health policy issues than it was prior to the 1970s (Melton, 1995), federal officials have also made attempts to shift some of the direct responsibility of health care back to the states and local governments (Austin, Blum, & Murtaza, 1995). Recently, states have worked to directly involve the aid of local governments in implementing and directing health care programs. The changes in responsibility from federal to state and local authority have caused several problems, such as a lack of revenue for programs and decreased patient access to services, that are likely to continue (Austin et al., 1995).

Since the 1980s, the federal government and states have challenged mental health professionals who work with children to focus on the strengths of the familial unit and to direct their efforts toward working with children and adolescents in their home environment rather than placing the children in residential facilities. Additionally, the consensus among policy makers has been the need to provide troubled individuals with more available and integrated community care programs than has been available in the past (Brindis, 1993; Knitzer, 1993). Although these steps suggest momentum, there continues to remain significant room for growth in the mental health system, especially with respect to providing practical services to those who are truly in need (Knitzer, 1993).

VIOLENCE AMONG CHILDREN AND ADOLESCENTS

Over the years, Congress has dealt with a myriad of child and adolescent problems, with the expectation that they need to address health care policies concerning these topics (Melton, 1995). All of these issues are significant and warrant further attention, but the scope of this chapter and the complexity of these problems precludes an adequate descriptive summation of all of these topics. By far, the number-one cause of death of children and adolescents relates to violence. Because of this, the authors focus attention on this health concern. Salzinger (Chapter 28 of this volume) provides an excellent and comprehensive review of the empirical literature on violence and abuse. Therefore, discourse here is concentrated on policy issues related to violence and abuse.

According to Thompson and Wilcox (1995), the nation as a whole has become increasingly aware of the problems associated with child maltreatment. However, the federal government's focus on issues of child abuse seems to have waned, as demonstrated by their lack of research funding given to the National Center on Child Abuse and Neglect (NCCAN) over the past 15 years. On a positive note, the National Research Counsel recently recommended giving the NCCAN an increase in research funding, which would reverse the decreased trend in allocated research funds (Thompson & Wilcox, 1995). Additionally, despite the lack of funding, research on child abuse has still continued. For example, some studies have focused specifically on the effects of child sexual abuse (see Kendall-Tackett, Williams, & Finkelhor, 1993). Although researchers have continued to learn new information, child maltreatment remains prevalent and more studies are needed (Thompson & Wilcox, 1995).

Many youth are victims of firearm casualties, a form of violence that has continued to increase the rate of suicides and homicides among children and adolescents. Yet, there is no clear policy alternative that would control gun use or prevent children from obtaining these weapons. Proposed government policy has included implementation of increased handgun safety devices, educational programs, school security, and the eventual reduction of children's access to handguns. However, research on effectiveness of these methods for preventing and reducing firearm deaths indicates that these methods have had minimal impact at best (O'Donnell, 1995).

Along with being victims of violence, children and adolescents have witnessed an increasing amount of violence directed toward others (Osofsky, 1995; Richters & Martinez, 1995). Research suggests that many children suffer negative consequences, such as having an increase in anxiety and sleep problems, after experiencing or witnessing a traumatic event (Pynoos, 1993). This is consistent with other literature on secondary traumatization (Goreczny et al., 1996) and highlights the need to implement violence prevention programs in an effort to decrease the possibility of our children developing posttraumatic stress disorder secondary to the violence trauma. As with other problem areas, however, there is a definite need to evaluate the effectiveness of prevention and treatment programs for youth exposed to violence. Additionally, facilitation of education and family incentives for reducing community violence may prove to be more effective in curbing the problem than would be large-scale federal policy mandates (Osofsky, 1995). However, strong empirical validation of such techniques remains lacking.

Along with being victims and witnesses to violence, many of today's youth are also perpetrators of violence (Tate, Reppucci, & Mulvey, 1995; Yoshikawa, 1994). Researchers have attempted to identify predictors of delinquency in order to develop prevention and treatment strategies. A review of the research by Yoshikawa (1994) suggested that family support and education given at an early stage in children's lives may help to reduce delinquency problems. However, the author recognized limitations of the research methodology and considered that any conclusions were only preliminary. Furthermore, researchers completed the only longitudinal studies that reported specific effects in this area in the 1970s and, thus, the results may not generalize to the 1990s. In further support of these cautions, Tate and colleagues (1995) reviewed various methodological difficulties among violent youth delinquency studies and concluded that the data are not clearly supportive of any treatment programs. However, these authors did suggest that treatments targeting social skills deficits showed some progress, the results of which need further examination, especially in determining longitudinal effects (Tate et al., 1995). Thus, as the number-one killer of American youth (i.e., violence) continues to rage unabated, we continue to lack a clear treatment program, whether that involves clinical initiatives or policy change initiatives.

INADEQUATE HEALTH CARE FUNDING AND PROGRAMS FOR YOUTH

Another problem that affects youth in the United States has been the lack of adequate health care at a global level. Although the shift toward managed care may eventually improve the general outlook of service provision, this determination remains unsubstantiated. What must first happen is that we must find a way to provide adequate health insurance coverage for all children and adolescents. This becomes even more important in light of a study by Brindis, Kapphahn, McCarter, and Wolfe (1995) on the use of school-based clinics by high school students in California. This study supported the notion that noninsured students are less likely to seek out health care in general than are students with health insurance. Additionally, demographic characteristics, such as socioeconomic status and ethnicity, also appear to influence student health behaviors. Specifically, this study indicated that white, female, depressed students who are older than age 16 and who have a mother who completed college were more likely to utilize services at the school-based clinic than were other students. Although the authors of the study argue that "factors other than financing are important in the adolescents' decision to use available SBC [school-based clinic] services" (p. 23), the availability of insurance certainly eliminates one important barrier to health care access and may increase appropriate utilization of prevention and treatment services.

According to Hein (1993), one out of every seven adolescents remains uninsured and these individuals tend to underuse physicians' services when compared to other patient groups. The Society for Adolescent Medicine (SAM) implemented several health policy proposals, such as suggesting easier access to adolescent services and updated programs to meet adoles-

cents' needs (Hein, 1993). Other propositions have included the need to provide increased basic health guidance for adolescents' questions regarding health care (Elster, 1993). Unfortunately, many of these proposals have never gained acceptance or implementation. Therefore, many adolescents continue to have limited access to health services and are developing and strengthening health behaviors that place them at risk for premature diseases due to unhealthy life-style practices. As mentioned earlier in the chapter, children and adolescents are likely to continue these health care behaviors into adulthood.

In addition to general physical health benefits, children and adolescents often do not have adequate access to mental health services. Health insurances often do not cover mental health services for children and adolescents. Therefore, public programs mandated to help children, such as the child welfare and juvenile system, have primary responsibility of meeting children's mental health care needs even though it is not their main function. In response, the Clinton Administration Health Security Act proposed several health policy suggestions, including integration of various children's services, provision of limited insurance coverage for each child and adolescent, and home-based as well as community-based residential treatment programs (Stroul, Pires, Katz-Leavy, & Goldman, 1994). However, Theut and Bailey (1994) suggested that although the health act proposal evolved from good intentions, it would have been too restrictive in the allotted provision of mental health care services, and they concurred with the rejection of this plan for mental health care by members of Congress. Nonetheless, what remains is a system that does not adequately cover the full array of mental and physical needs of U.S. children and adolescents.

HEALTH POLICY IMPLEMENTATION

The best health policy initiatives are meaningless if they fail to be put into practice, and, unfortunately, implementation of health policies by various services has been a slow process. For example, Salkever (1994) conducted a study to determine if vocational rehabilitation programs were implementing mandated policy regulations. Although federal regulations have mandated that persons with severe developmental disabilities receive priority in the provision of services, results of the Salkever study suggest that some of those individuals who required more assistance than others are still less likely to receive services than those who are higher functioning (Salkever, 1994). Limitations of this study, such as the inability to generalize and lack of explanations for nonuse of services, preclude any definitive findings, but this study does suggest that successful implementation of health policies requires follow-up and monitoring for compliance.

Despite the apparent lack of successful implementation of some programs, others are clearly moving forward with positive outcomes. For example, recent changes in the mental health care systems in North Carolina appear to be successful and provide an example of how to implement revised health care policy. In a review article, Kirkpatrick, Knisley, Shear, and Blum (1995) indicated that Wake County, North Carolina, recently began to reorganize its mental health system, changing from three separate systems to one integrated system that would better serve the needs of all individuals seeking mental health services. Preliminary data suggest that the attempt to increase patient access to a collaboration of community services has been promising for the mental health system of Wake County, North Carolina. This change in policy has yielded specific improvements, including a decrease in inpatient hospitalization and an increase in use of community services. Although the recency of these changes and lack of long-term outcome information does not permit any serious postulation as to the success of this program, it may provide incentive for other states to implement similar projects.

FUTURE GOALS FOR HEALTH CARE

Present and future proposals for children and adolescent health policy continue to include development and implementation of prevention programs targeting children and families at early problem stages (Brindis, 1993; Knitzer, 1993; Petersen, Richmond, & Leffert, 1993; Yoshikawa, 1994). For example, a proposal by Elster (1993) suggested implementing a Head Start program for adolescents as a tool to provide young teenagers with social skills and supportive

programs in order to prevent difficulties that may occur later in adolescence. Along with early prevention efforts, the general consensus among researchers appears to be that any successful interventions require the collaboration of home, school, health delivery systems, and the community (Brindis, 1993; Knitzer, 1993; Osofsky, 1995).

Additionally, regulators continually encourage policy makers to mandate specialized training for professionals to work with the youth (Brindis, 1993; Knitzer, 1993). With respect to managed health care, researchers tend to agree that reform is both necessary and inevitable in the near future (Elster, 1993; Knitzer, 1993). Finally, another slant by some researchers has been to direct additional focus toward solving problems of the social environment rather than blaming societal difficulties on today's youth (Elster, 1993; Hein, 1993).

CONCLUSION

Although there is some progress toward improving children and adolescent health policy, more research and policy changes need to be implemented at a faster and more efficient rate than has previously been the case. A review of the research suggests that there are several problems facing today's youth. The government and states are addressing these issues, but research directed specifically to health policy issues for children and adolescents has been minimal, as have studies depicting the implementation of new health policy programs. This may be due to a combination of factors. One is that there have been very few policy proposals actually implemented or started long enough to study the outcomes. A second factor is that these studies are methodologically challenging to complete and require close scrutiny of programs that are willing to or must participate. A third factor is that researchers have developed few measurements to gauge the success of program outcomes. Despite these challenges, future researchers need to focus on studying effectiveness of policy changes, including short-term and long-term outcomes affecting various programs on children and adolescents, and the overall effect of these changes on the prevalence rates of current problems.

As mentioned earlier, researchers cannot conduct studies when new policy programs are nonexistent. Thus, further work is required to monitor actual implementation of policies approved by federal and state government authority and to improve the rate at which authorities are implementing these changes. Furthermore, research must focus on developing empirical, data-based studies to determine the outcome of policy changes. Presently, a large proportion of current research appears based on subjective measures or the author's opinion rather than on objective measures and empirical data. Therefore, additional effort must focus on developing adequate measures of program outcome. Finally, results must focus on the trajectory of child and adolescent problems to determine if implemented changes in health policy are globally effective. For example, even if policy makers approve proposed changes, these results do not suggest substantial progress unless the lives of today's children and adolescents are greatly improved in both the United States and at an international level. The United States and its western European allies cannot forge ahead without considering the impact on technologically disadvantaged countries, because given the growing interdependence of nations and ready accessibility to previously difficult to reach, remote parts of the world changes in one country now, more than ever, can have significant changes in other countries as well (Goreczny, 1995; Mann, 1991).

As a final comment, the authors recommend that health policies begin to target specific, high-risk problems and monitor progress based on a priori agreed upon indicators. It appears that prior policy initiatives, when implemented, attempted to address a broad range of problems. Such "shot-gun" approaches rarely produce significant impact because of the lack of a clear focus and clear target indicators. What we need is a policy-making body that is capable of both creating and modifying long-range plans while also implementing initiatives to address short-range (i.e., current) and immediate concerns. This group must be able to plan proactively and to react quickly to changes in health care problems. It must target specific health concerns (Winett, 1995) rather than take a "shot-gun" approach and must consider the impact of any policy decisions as a whole, not just on the target problem (see Goreczny & O'Halloran, 1995). Given the current health issues that are affecting our youth, it appears that the most appropriate targets would be violence and tobacco use. With vio-

lence the number-one killer of our youth and smoking of tobacco cigarettes as a primary contributor to many of the major life-style diseases, these seem to be appropriate targets.

REFERENCES

Austin, E. W., & Nach-Ferguson, B. (1995). Sources and influences of young school-aged children's general and brand-specific knowledge about alcohol. *Health Communication, 7,* 1–20.

Austin, M. J., Blum, S. R., & Murtaza, N. (1995). Local-state government relations and the development of public sector managed mental health care systems. Special issue: Public sector planning for managed mental health care. *Administration and Policy in Mental Health, 22,* 203–215.

Battjes, R. J., Leukefeld, C. G., & Pickens, R. W. (1992). Age at first injection and HIV risk among intravenous drug users. *American Journal of Drug and Alcohol Abuse, 18,* 263–273.

Brindis, C. (1993). What it will take: Placing adolescents on the American national agenda for the 1990s. *Journal of Adolescent Health, 14,* 527–530.

Brindis, C., Kapphahn, C., McCarter, V., & Wolfe, A. L. (1995). The impact of health insurance status on adolescents' utilization of school-based clinic services: Implications for health care reform. *Journal of Adolescent Health, 16,* 18–25.

Cohen, R. Y., Brownell, K. D., & Felix, M. R. (1990). Age and sex differences in health habits and beliefs of schoolchildren. *Health Psychology, 9,* 208–224.

Cohn, L. D., Macfarlane, S., Yanez, C., Imai, W. K., et al. (1995). Risk-perception: Differences between adolescents and adults. *Health Psychology, 14,* 217–222.

Corse, S. J., McHugh, M. K., & Gordon, S. M. (1995). Enhancing provider effectiveness in treating pregnant women with addictions. *Journal of Substance Abuse Treatment, 12,* 3–12.

Cothern, N. B., & Collins, M. D. (1992). An exploration: Attitude acquisition and reading instruction. *Reading Research and Instruction, 31,* 84–97.

Elster, A. B. (1993). Confronting the crisis in adolescent health: Visions for change. *Journal of Adolescent Health, 14,* 505–508.

Goreczny, A. J. (1995). Introductory statement—Forging ahead into the 21st century: Issues in rehabilitation. *International Journal of Rehabilitation and Health, 1,* 1–3.

Goreczny, A. J., Dixon, M., Antick, J. R., Ruboylanes, D., Kocijan-Hercigonja, D., Grguric, J., Walter, K., & Cvitkovic, J. (1996). Effects of chronic war-related stressors on physicians and allied health care providers: PTSD symptomatology in Croatia. Manuscript under review.

Goreczny, A. J., & O'Halloran, C. M. (1995). The future of psychology in health care. In A. J. Goreczny (Ed.), *Handbook of health and rehabilitation psychology* (pp. 663–676). New York: Plenum.

Groer, M., Thomas, S., Droppleman, P., & Younger, M. (1994). Longitudinal study of adolescent blood pressures, health habits, stress and anger. *Health Values: The Journal of Health Behavior, Education and Promotion, 18,* 25–33.

Hay, D. F. (1994). Prosocial development. *Journal of Child Psychology & Psychiatry & Allied Disciplines, 35,* 29–71.

Hein, K. (1993). Evolution or revolution: Reforming health care for adolescents in America. *Journal of Adolescent Health, 14,* 520–523.

Hull, C. L. (1943). *Principles of behavior.* New York: Appleton.

Kendall-Tackett, K. A., Williams, L. M., & Finkelhor, D. (1993). Impact of sexual abuse on children: A review and synthesis of recent empirical studies. *Psychological Bulletin, 113,* 164–180.

Kiesler, C. A. (1993). Mental health policy and the psychiatric inpatient care of children. *Applied and Preventive Psychology, 2,* 91–99.

Kirkpatrick, J. W., Knisley, M., Shear, L. L., & Blum, S. R. (1995). State-local government partnership: Development of children's mental health services in Wake county. *Administration and Policy in Mental Health. 22,* 247–259.

Knitzer, J. (1993). Children's mental health policy: Challenging the future. *Journal of Emotional and Behavioral Disorders, 1,* 8–16.

Mann, J. M.(1991). Global AIDS: Critical issues for prevention in the 1990s. *International Journal of Health Sciences, 21,* 553–559.

Melton, G. B. (1995). Bringing psychology to Capitol Hill: Briefings on child and family policy. *American Psychologist, 50,* 766–770.

Miller, S. M. (1991). Policy review and formulation on substance-exposed infants. *Journal of Adolescent Chemical Dependency, 2,* 59–73.

O'Donnell, C. R. (1995). Firearm deaths among children and youth. *American Psychologist. 50,* 771–776.

Osofsky, J. D. (1995). The effects of exposure to violence on young children. *American Psychologist. 50,* 782–788.

Palenik, L. (1993). Determinants of prosocial behavior development. *Studia Psychologica, 35,* 387–389.

Petersen, A. C., Richmond, J. B., & Leffert, N. (1993). Social changes among youth: The United States experience. *Journal of Adolescent Health, 14,* 632–637.

Pynoos, R. S. (1993). Traumatic stress and developmental psychopathology in children and adolescents. In J. M. Oldham, M. B. Riba, & A. Tasman (Eds.), *American Psychiatric Press review of psychiatry* (Vol. 12). Washington, DC: American Psychiatric Press.

Richters, J. E. (1993). Community violence and children's development: Toward a research agenda for the 1990s. *Psychiatry. 56,* 3–6.

Richters, J. E., & Martinez, P. (1993). The NIMH community violence project: I. Children as victims of and witnesses to violence. *Psychiatry. 56,* 7–21.

Salkever, D. S. (1994). Access to vocational rehabilitation services for persons with severe disabilities. *Journal of Disability Policy Studies, 5,* 45–64.

Stiffman, A. R., Dore, P., Cunningham, R. M., & Earls, F. (1995). Person and environment in HIV risk behavior change between adolescence and young adulthood. *Health Education Quarterly, 22,* 211–226.

Stroul, B. A., Pires, S. A., Katz-Leavy, J. W., & Goldman, S. K. (1994). Implications of the Health Security Act for mental health services for children and adolescents. *Hospital and Community Psychiatry, 45,* 877–882.

Tate, D. C., Reppucci, N. D., & Mulvey, E. P. (1995). Violent juvenile delinquents: Treatment effectiveness and implications for future action. *American Psychologist. 50,* 777–781.

Theut, S. K., & Bailey, H. G. (1994). What is the outcome for children's mental health needs in national health care reform? *Journal of the American Academy of Child and Adolescent Psychiatry, 33,* 1219–1220.

Thompson, R. A., & Wilcox, B. L. (1995). Child maltreatment research: Federal support and policy issues. *American Psychologist, 50,* 789–793.

Thorndike, E. L. (1911). *Animal intelligence.* New York: Macmillan.

Weiss, S. M. (1992). Behavioral medicine on the world scene: Toward the year 2000. *Annals of Behavioral Medicine, 14,* 302–306.

Williams, R. (1994). Adolescent/young adult: Overview. In S. J. Blumenthal, K. Matthews, & S. M. Weiss (Eds.), *New research frontiers in behavioral medicine* (pp. 79–86). Washington, DC: U.S. Government Printing Office.

Winett, R. A. (1995). A framework for health promotion and disease prevention programs. *American Psychologist. 50,* 341–350.

Yoshikawa, H. (1994). Prevention as cumulative protection: Effects of early family support and education on chronic delinquency and its risks. *Psychological Bulletin, 115,* 28–54.

CHAPTER 2

PREVENTION OF INFANT DEATHS

John Pierpont, EAST CAROLINA UNIVERSITY
John Poertner, UNIVERSITY OF ILLINOIS AT URBANA-CHAMPAIGN

Presenting an authoritative discussion on any area of prevention is difficult at best. Not only must one consider a seemingly endless string of potentially relevant contributing factors but one must also be willing to acknowledge that there may still be confounding variables, as yet unidentified, that account for a reduction in the outcome(s) of interest. There is also the logical problem of demonstrating that a particular future event will not occur if prevention strategies are implemented. Although advances in medical technology are responsible for much of the recent decrease in neonatal infant deaths, this chapter focuses on environmental conditions and individual behaviors that contribute to infant deaths. The authors identify factors strongly associated with infant death and discuss environmental/societal conditions and individual behaviors that engender or enhance these factors. There are effective medical technologies for prevention of infant death. However, the focus of this chapter is on environmental conditions and individuals because these hold potential for prevention in areas not currently affected by medical technology.

After setting the context for a discussion of preventing infant death, the text begins with a consideration of low birth weight, focusing on societal conditions and individual behaviors, which make it one of the factors most strongly associated with infant death.

Outreach programs to enlarge the number of women receiving prenatal care and the use of organized settings are two promising approaches to reducing the incidence of low birth weight. Next is the discussion of perinatal risk factors, with a brief discussion of sudden infant death syndrome (SIDS). Infant fatalities due to SIDS, accidental injury, and child maltreatment may be reduced through home visitor programs and parent education classes. These are the two most prevalent approaches to reducing infant deaths through perinatal care. Teen pregnancy and parenting present special issues in prenatal and perinatal strategies for preventing infant deaths. A lengthy discussion of teenage sexual activity and teen pregnancy is provided, followed by a model for reducing incidence of teenage childbearing. Finally, recommendations are offered for policies and programs that have potential for impacting on the societal barriers and individual behaviors so strongly associated with infant death.

For two successive years, 1990 and 1991 (the most recent data available), the infant mortality rates of 9.2 and 8.9 deaths per live births, respectively, were the lowest ever recorded in the United States (Children's Defense Fund, 1994). The 1990 rate reflected an impressive 6 percent reduction from the previous year (Center for Disease Control, 1993). Nevertheless, 38,351 infants died that year before completing their first year of life. In addition, "the United States spends more money on health care per person than any other country. Yet an American baby is less likely to reach its first birthday than a baby born in 21 other nations" (Cooper, 1992). Racial differences in patterns of infant mortality are also troubling. Infant mortality rate for white infants was 7.6 deaths per 1,000 live births, whereas the rate for African American infants was 18 per 1,000. The 6 percent decrease in overall infant mortality rate was only 3 percent for African Americans (Center for Disease Control, 1993). So, while overall infant mortality rate decreased, the discrepancy between African American and white rates increased.

Prevention of infant death begins with understanding its leading causes. In 1989, the five leading causes of infant death (in order) were (1) birth defects; (2) low birth weight (LBW), prematurity, and respiratory distress syndrome (RDS); (3) sudden infant death syndrome (SIDS); (4) maternal complications; and (5) accidental injuries (Cooper, 1992). Birth defects represent the leading cause of infant death overall and for white infants (26 percent of Caucasian infant deaths), but short gestation and low birth weight (less than 2,500 grams at birth) is the leading cause of infant mortality among African Americans and accounts for 16 percent of African American infant deaths. Some 21 percent of the discrepancy between African American and white infant death rates is due to short gestation and low birth weight; an additional 12 percent is accounted for by a higher incidence of SIDS deaths; and 8 percent of the discrepancy is attributable to a higher incidence of respiratory distress syndrome (Center for Disease Control, 1993).

The 6 percent decrease that occurred between 1989 and 1990 was due largely to a 24 percent decrease in deaths due to RDS, which in turn is attributable to improved medical management of respiratory distress (Center for Disease Control, 1993). Since respiratory distress syndrome is one part of the second leading cause of infant death, this dramatic decrease is very promising. Clearly, one road to preventing infant deaths is through enhanced availability and use of medical technologies.

Birth defects are the leading cause of infant death, accounting for 20 percent of all such deaths. This includes heart defects, which are the most common abnormality; respiratory defects; and central nervous system defects such as spina bifida and anencephaly (Cooper, 1992). Prevention in this area is likely to accompany use of procedures (e.g., amniocentesis) to detect such problems, vaccines, and other medical technologies.

The leading cause of infant death and recent advances in its prevention raise questions about the relative role of medical technologies and maternal behavior in preventing infant mortality. This is an important and controversial topic. Some believe we can make substantial improvements in outcomes for infants by focusing on mothers, while others believe that a focus on maternal behavior may be little more than victim blaming. Social and environmental conditions often influence individual behavior. For example, it is well known that prenatal care is strongly associated with positive pregnancy outcomes, and every pregnant woman needs to receive adequate primary care throughout pregnancy. However, a singular focus on a woman's need to obtain prenatal care obscures the fact that primary care is often unavailable to poor, uninsured women; or if it is available, access is made difficult through inadequate clinic hours, lack of public transportation, and the stigma of public welfare application procedures. Infant mortality rates tend to be higher in those areas where environmental factors such as poverty, unemployment, and illiteracy are more problematic (Annie E. Casey Foundation, 1994); a higher number of primary care physicians in a community is associated with decreases in infant mortality (Bowman & Schwenk, 1993).

Failure to consider the importance of the societal context of an individual's behavior (e.g., not using prenatal care because it is unavailable or not easily accessible) leads to a skewed view of the problem of infant death and results in a short-sighted vision of possible solutions. Therefore, the focus of this chapter is on environmental factors as well as individual behaviors. Next is a discussion of these factors as they contribute to low birth weight.

LOW BIRTH WEIGHT AND PREMATURE INFANTS

Low birth weight, prematurity, and respiratory distress syndrome accounted for nearly 20 percent of infant deaths in 1989 (Cooper, 1992). Although there are promising medical advances in managing RDS, the same can not be said for LBW. In fact, this condition is worthy of special consideration because "among all infants who die at any time during the first year of life, 60 percent have low birth weight" (Cooper, 1992). In 1991 (the most recent data available), the low birth-weight rate in the United States was 7.1 per 1,000 live births, exactly the same rate as in 1978. Although the low birth-weight rate continued to decline from 1978 until 1984 (6.7 per 1,000 live births), it has steadily risen since then. Between 1969 and 1991, the low birth-weight rate declined 12.3 percent, an average yearly decrease of 0.6 percent; but since 1980, the rate of low birth-weight births has increased 4.4 percent, a yearly average of 0.4 percent (Children's Defense Fund, 1994).

Factors that predict LBW include poverty, poor nutrition, and lack of access to medical care. Maternal smoking is also associated with LBW, though it is difficult to isolate the effect of smoking relative to other maternal behaviors (Cotton, 1994). The more common sexually transmitted diseases such as syphilis, gonorrhea, chlamydia, and genital herpes contribute to LBW, as does age of the mother. Each of these contributing factors suggests one or more prevention strategies, but it is clear that adequate prenatal care is a key strategy.

Prenatal Care

It is well known that women who receive inadequate or no prenatal care are more likely to give birth to low birth-weight babies. Nevertheless, nearly one in four infants in the United States in 1991 was born to a mother who did not receive prenatal care during the first trimester of pregnancy, and these infants were less likely to be born to mothers who received early prenatal care and more likely to be born at low birth weight than in 1980 (Children's Defense Fund, 1994). In 1991, 292,230 or 7.1 percent of all babies were born with a low birth weight, compared to 6.85 percent in 1985 (Annie E. Casey Foundation, 1994). This decrease in the number of mothers receiving prenatal care and the increase in the low birth-weight rate are particularly troubling because they seem to signify decreases in (1) access to adequate health care, and (2) the overall health status of young women (Annie E. Casey Foundation, 1994).

The decrease in this nation's infant mortality rate during the same period has been largely due to improved medical technology. Although technological improvements are a boon to those who can access and use them, it is disappointing that improvements in infant mortality rates can not be attributed to improved primary care. Women who begin prenatal care early in pregnancy give birth to healthier babies, are less likely to have a baby born with a low birth weight, and are less likely to have a child who dies in the neonatal period, the first 28 days following birth (Racine, Joyce, & Grossman, 1992). Women who do not receive early prenatal care are substantially more likely to give birth to low birth-weight babies, which puts babies at greater mortality and morbidity risk. Infants born to mothers who receive late prenatal care or no prenatal care are three times more likely to die before reaching their first birthday (Edelman, 1987). Absence of prenatal care is associated with adverse health behaviors, which constitute risks to healthy deliveries (e.g., smoking, unhealthy diet, and abusing alcohol and drugs). Conversely, research indicates that receiving prenatal care is strongly associated with ameliorating certain factors known to increase the risk of delivering a low birth-weight baby (e.g., smoking) (Olds, Henderson, & Tatelbaum, 1994) and improved diet (Olds, Henderson, Tatelbaum, & Chamberlin, 1986).

While the infant mortality rate in the United States continues to decline, the disparity between the infant mortality rates for African Americans and for whites continues to widen. In 1991, the infant mortality rate among whites was 7.5 per 1,000 live births, compared to 17.6 among African Americans. This difference is linked to the disparity between prenatal care for these two races. In 1969, the percent of babies born to African American women who received late or no prenatal care was 18.2, compared to 6.3 for whites. These figures declined for both races through 1980 when the percent of babies born to women receiving prenatal care were 8.8 and 4.3, respectively. Since 1981, these improvements have seen a general reversal. Between 1980 and 1991, the average annual increase in the number of babies born to African American mothers who received late or no prenatal care was 2.0 percent. The average annual increase for infants born to white women during the same period was only 0.8 percent (Children's Defense Fund, 1994).

In addition to race, there are other factors that appear to present obstacles to receiving timely and adequate prenatal care. Young age at first pregnancy, marital status, poverty, lower educational achievement, lack of health insurance, and living in the inner city or in isolated rural settings are also thought to be key predictors of receiving poor prenatal care. Worthy of consideration here is the notion that none of these factors, taken alone, may be sufficient to determine poor access to or use of prenatal care, and that most often they work in concert, perhaps with other as yet unrecognized factors to impede the use of prenatal care. Nevertheless, some of these factors have a more immediate and powerful role to play in whether a pregnant woman receives prenatal care. Access to and affordability of health insurance is one such factor.

Women who lack health insurance are among the least likely to receive adequate prenatal care. Cooper (1992) observes that of the 40 million Americans without health insurance, 10 million are of childbearing age. The Children's Defense Fund (1994) reports that in 1992 there were 8.3 million children not covered by health insurance. Nearly one-third of all Hispanics and more than one-fifth of all African Americans had no health insurance in 1992 (Annie E. Casey Foundation, 1994). Therefore, improving health coverage through Medicaid expansion is sometimes a popular public policy strategy. However, it is worth noting that pregnant women with Medicaid coverage delay seeking prenatal care longer than do women with private health insurance (Racine et al., 1992). Enrollment in Medicaid and other means-tested public welfare programs is often stigmatizing and time consuming. Other reasons for this delay may include

> the failure of some physicians to accept Medicaid patients, long travel times and clinic waits, and lack of information and unfavorable attitudes concerning prenatal care. These factors underscore the potential value of outreach programs that aim to deliver, as opposed to finance, prenatal care for the poor. (Racine et al., 1992, p. 45)

Prevention

Any discussion of strategies to prevent infant death by increasing access to and utilization of prenatal care must begin by acknowledging the dearth of research into *how prenatal care works.* Authorities in this field agree that prenatal care does work, but they can not explain how. This is due, in part, to the absence of concern about the content of prenatal care; this absence of concern, in turn, has been fed continually by research findings indicating that, whatever the content of prenatal care, it works (Racine et al., 1992).

Access to prenatal care through insurance coverage is certainly a major strategy in preventing infant mortality, and universal health care coverage has the potential to create significant improvements in prenatal care rates. However, absence of political consensus on the importance of this aspect of the current health care debate suggests that universal coverage may be sometime in the distant future. Therefore, expanding Medicaid to cover a larger number of women at risk of delivering infants with low birth weights remains a necessary and viable intervention strategy. One such program that appears to be achieving success is Baby Your Baby, initially conceived and implemented in Utah.

Baby Your Baby Program

After seeing its infant death rate steadily decline for many years and achieving one of the lowest infant death rates in the United States, Utah's infant death rate became stagnant between 1983 and 1987, while improvement in the neonatal death rate slowed and the perinatal death rate and the percent of low birth rates both increased (Van Dyck et al., 1991). The Utah Department of Health initiated a study comparing pregnancy outcomes for women receiving Medicaid benefits with the pregnancy outcomes of women not receiving Medicaid. The results were startling. The low birth-weight rate for Medicaid-financed mothers was nearly twice as high as for non-Medicaid mothers, and they received prenatal care significantly less early and less often. As well, the death rate among infants born to women who were Medicaid recipients was 18 per 1,000 live births compared to a rate of 9.2 in the non-Medicaid population. An additional finding of the study was that only one-half to two-thirds of the women eligible or potentially eligible for Medicaid were actually enrolled in the program. According to surveys conducted by the Utah Department of Health, the significant obstacles to receiving early prenatal care and enrolling in Medicaid were "lack of knowledge about the importance of early prenatal care and how and where to enroll, as well as the fear of the expense of prenatal care and delivery" (Van Dyck et al., 1991).

In response to these findings, the Utah Department of Health initiated a unique campaign to enroll all eligible women in Medicaid and to educate all women in the state, regardless of financial status, about the importance and availability of prenatal care. The Baby Your Baby campaign was creative insofar as it required a unique partnership between private businesses and nonprofit and public agencies; it offered maternity and baby products as incentives for all women to enroll early in prenatal care; and it included a comprehensive statewide multimedia campaign and a free hotline to provide information about the importance of prenatal care and where to go to obtain prenatal care, regardless of location in the state.

Federal and state policy changes played an important part in the success of Baby Your Baby. In 1986, Congress passed PL 99-409 (SOBRA), which allowed states to (1) establish "presumptive eligibility" to allow prenatal care coverage while actual eligibility was being determined; (2) establish an income eligibility level for Medicaid at 100 percent of the poverty level; (3) eliminate the use of an assets test; and (4) allow continuous eligibility during pregnancy and for 60 days following delivery without having to repeat the process of reapplying and being reapproved or rejected. At the state level, Utah increased the tax on cigarettes to pay for enhanced delivery of prenatal care, which consisted of creating 18 public prenatal health clinics across the state, hiring outreach workers, and coordinating prenatal health care statewide. The state also implemented a Baby Your Baby Hotline and offered coupon booklets for pregnant women.

Women generally found out about the coupon booklets from friends or through the multimedia campaign. After calling the hotline, women were sent a postcard, which was to be taken to her physician who would certify that prenatal care began during the first trimester of the pregnancy. The physician would mail the postcard to the Department of Health, which would then enroll the woman in the Baby Your Baby program and send her a coupon booklet. This procedure provided important information about a woman's progress from calling the hotline to seeing her physician, and later enabled the Department of Health to match hotline callers to birth certificates for program evaluation purposes.

Initial results of the Baby Your Baby campaign are quite encouraging. The program target was to reach all pregnant women under 100 percent of the poverty line. By the end of 1989, the number of women enrolled in the Baby Your Baby program equaled the projected figure for all pregnant women under 100 percent of the poverty level in the state, and between 1985 and 1991, the number of deliveries to poor women enrolled in the Baby Your Baby program nearly tripled (Van Dyck et al., 1991). In 1988, one year after the program's inception, the state's public health vital statistics told the story of an impressive success:

> The infant death rate fell from 8.8 to 8.0 per thousand live births. The fetal death ratio fell from 7.1 to 5.2 per thousand live births and the perinatal death rate fell from 11.3 to 9.0. All of these decreases were the largest in Utah history. Continued analysis shows the provisional infant death rate for 1990 to be 7.5 deaths per 1,000 live births—by far the lowest in the State's history. Entrance into early prenatal care continues to increase. (Van Dyck et al., 1991, p. 4)

Organized Settings for Prenatal Care

An estimated 20 percent of women in the United States receive prenatal care from organized settings. *Organized settings* are facilities such as migrant clinics, community health centers, hospital outpatient departments, and public health department clinics (Perloff, 1992). Women served in these settings tend to have low incomes and lack third-party coverage for prenatal care; they also tend to be young, unmarried, and African American or Hispanic (Perloff, 1992). Although data relevant to the availability and use of services in organized settings is not systematically collected or routinely available, it is clear that demand for prenatal care services in organized settings is increasing as availability of care in these settings is decreasing:

> An Institute of Medicine (IOM) review of evidence about capacity in local health departments and hospitals conducted during the mid-1980s found exces-

sively long waiting times to obtain prenatal care appointments and other indicators of inadequate capacity. Comprehensive national and state data about capacity in organized settings are not available, but the IOM report concluded that "in some communities the capacity of the clinic systems relied on by low-income women is so limited that prompt care is not always available and that in some additional areas care is unavailable altogether. (Perloff, 1992, p. 8)

Although the relative impact of hospital closings on access to prenatal care remains unclear, it is significant that a large percentage of the hospitals closed since 1980 have been public hospitals that had been the only source of care for poor, uninsured, nonwhite women.

Perloff (1992) suggests two strategies pertinent to improving the utilization of prenatal care through organized settings. The first is to systematize data collection to describe and assess the effectiveness of maternal and child care in organized settings. With few exceptions, reliable and systematic information about the availability and use of services in these settings is rarely adequate for purposes of planning and implementing public policy. As a result, levels of need and use for any given area cannot be adequately evaluated, and when budgets are cut, funding for organized settings is sometimes diminished without knowing the damage done to a community's or state's most vulnerable citizens.

A more adequate data collection and reporting system would (1) provide greater understanding of who uses prenatal care in organized settings and how much primary care is delivered there and (2) enhance the possibility that federal and state funds would be used more efficiently by enlarging rather than shrinking the services available to poor, uninsured, nonwhite pregnant women.

The second strategy recommended by Perloff entails enlarging the service capacity of organized settings and requires increasing the nation's financial commitment to improving health care for the underserved. In recent years, cutbacks in health programs have made it nearly impossible for organized settings to enlarge their service capacity. The importance of public hospital closings has already been mentioned. During the 1980s, many programs that finance services in organized settings experienced budget cuts,

and Medicaid reimbursements failed to cover rising costs related to health care. The solution to these difficulties, of course, is expanded public funding to enhance Medicaid reimbursement levels and to enlarge the pool of funds available through Health and Human Services (HHS) grants that finance health care delivery in organized settings. Perloff specifically recommends enhancing HHS grants to recruit and retain physicians in organized settings such as migrant and community health centers.

Two things are clear from the preceding discussion: The first is that expanded prenatal care is a necessary condition for improving pregnancy outcomes in the United States. The second is that expanded prenatal care cannot happen without expanded financing. Medicaid expansion is the most promising strategy now in view because its financing mechanism is open ended. Funding for organized settings, on the other hand, appears to be limited to grants provided by discretionary funds. As Perloff (1992) rightly notes, it has become increasingly difficult for these programs to expand:

> The budget rules established by the Budget Enforcement Act of 1990 will make it very difficult to increase funding for the National Health Service Corps, the Maternal and Child Health Block Grant, or community and migrant health centers because these increases will need to be offset by cuts in military, international, or domestic discretionary spending. (p. 92)

Attempts to enhance discretionary funds for organized settings would inevitably generate opposition from those whose funding would be cut. Whether improved delivery of prenatal care and its concomitant decrease in the incidence of infant death are financed through an increase in the cigarette tax as was done in Utah, or through expanded Medicaid coverage nationwide, they will come at a greater cost to the public purse. Unfortunately, like universal health care coverage, this is a political issue and will be decided not so much on the basis of need as on political will. Nevertheless, every pregnant woman who is eligible for Medicaid should have access to prenatal care, and the authors see no reason why individual states cannot enhance efforts to expand the number of Medicaid patients served in organized settings.

Perinatal Care

Sudden Infant Death Syndrome (SIDS) is a term that refers to a puzzling collection of infant deaths—puzzling because the exact cause of death is not known. Frequently, when a death certificate is completed by someone not well trained in pathology and the cause of death is not obviously something else, the conclusion is that it is a SIDS death (Schloesser, Pierpont, & Poertner, 1992; Cooper, 1992). As Barness (1992) observes, the SIDS diagnosis has been applied to deaths due to metabolic disorders, hazardous beds and bedding, overlying, and intentional suffocation or child abuse deaths.

In the last few years, research activity on SIDS has focused on the various sleeping positions. This research, primarily from New Zealand and Scandinavia, suggests that some infants who sleep in the prone position are at higher risk of SIDS. Although this line of research can be traced back to the 1940s and 1950s (Guntheroth & Spiers, 1992), it has now achieved prominence in the United States, with the Academy of Pediatrics in 1992 formally making recommendations to place healthy infants on their sides or backs when putting them to bed (Poets & Southall, 1993). Even with this recommendation, sleeping position is a controversial subject, and many doctors are not convinced that sleeping position is the most critical factor in preventing SIDS. This skepticism seems to be related to (1) the fact that most infants can turn themselves over after 3 or 4 months of age and (2) the lack of physiologic data linking SIDS deaths to sleeping position (Poets & Southall, 1993). Nevertheless, epidemiological data suggest this is an important prevention strategy.

Research consistently shows that a number of infant deaths officially reported as deaths resulting from SIDS, or accidents, are due to maltreatment (McClain et al., 1993; Mitchel, 1987; Christoffel, Zeiserl, & Chiaramonte, 1985). The National Committee to Prevent Child Abuse (NCPCA) 1993 50 State Survey found that 46 percent of child maltreatment fatalities were under the age of 1 (McCurdy & Daro, 1994). Schloesser and associates (1992) reported that in Kansas, 65 percent of child abuse fatalities were under the age of 1. Jacquot and Roberts in Oregon (1988), Jason and Andereck in Georgia (1983), and Thompson and Wilson in Washington (1989) reported similar findings. It is reasonable to presume that between 520 and 1,314 infants were victims of fatal child maltreatment in 1993.

Prevention of infant deaths due to child maltreatment is difficult. Kadushin and Martin (1988) devote several pages to factors thought to contribute to child maltreatment, but most researchers tend to focus on a few predictive factors associated with child maltreatment, which cluster as attributes of perpetrators and attributes of victims, respectively. Among the most commonly cited contributors to child maltreatment is poverty. In the 1993 annual survey of the 50 states conducted by NCPCA, 35 percent of states responding cited poverty or economic stress as a significant problem faced by families on child protective services caseloads (McCurdy & Daro, 1994). Daro (1988) argues that although considerable effort has been expended to portray child maltreatment as classless, there is ample reason to conclude that children in the poorest families may be at greatest risk, and that the great majority of maltreatment-related fatalities may occur among the poorest of the poor. Daro also notes that among perpetrators of child maltreatment, other factors often accompany poverty—namely, more children in the family, higher incidence of marital disruptions, more social isolation from family and friends, less access to community support programs, and a higher incidence of single mothers.

Other factors associated with child maltreatment, including fatal abuse, are substance abuse (Daro, 1988; McCurdy & Daro, 1994); beginning childbearing at an early age (Schloesser et al., 1992; Jacquot & Roberts, 1998; Smith, 1989); inadequate prenatal care and low birth weight (Schorr, 1988; Schloesser et al., 1992) and lower educational achievement (Schloesser et al., 1992). In the 1993 NCPCA 50 State Survey cited earlier, 63 percent of respondents listed substance abuse as one of the top two problems associated with child maltreatment—a finding similar to 1992 survey results. Schloesser and colleagues (1992) and Jason and Andereck (1983) both found that in 73 percent of abuse cases, mothers of abused infants began childbearing before age 20. Adolescent childbearing will be discussed later in this chapter as a special case of problems pertaining to low birth weight. Again, numerous environmental and behavioral factors must be recognized and addressed if progress is to be made in preventing infant death. Although poverty is strongly associated with infant death due to maltreatment, it is impossible to say that poverty is the primary cause of maltreatment-related infant deaths.

Prevention

In addition to medically based prenatal health care programs, interventions for preventing or ameliorating factors that contribute to infant death generally include one or both of two approaches: home visitor programs and parent education classes. Of the two, home visitor programs are the more promising interventions and have enjoyed renewed interest in the past few years. Unfortunately, however, home visitor programs are seldom coordinated with other service programs, and too often they are not designed and implemented in a manner consistent with current research findings (Olds, 1992). Many designs for home visitor programs are currently used, but the more effective programs focus on families with greatest need for services; have nurses begin home visits during pregnancy and continue to follow up with families for at least two years; promote positive infant caregiving and other health-related behaviors; and improve families' social and physical environments by helping families reduce stress (Olds, 1992).

The study by Olds and associates (1986) set the standard for research on home visitor approaches to perinatal care. Subjects consisted of women in Elmira, New York, who were having their first child and who were at risk for poor pregnancy outcomes because they were poor, very young, or unmarried. Of the 400 women in the study, 89 percent were white and all major findings pertain to this group. Participants were randomly assigned to one of four groups: Group 1 services consisted of developmental screening for children at 1 and 2 years of age. Group 2 services included screening provided to members of Group 1, as well as free transportation for prenatal and well-child care. Participants assigned to Group 3 received screening and transportation services, and prenatal home visits approximately once every two weeks during pregnancy. Those assigned to Group 4 received all of the services provided to participants in the other three groups, as well as home visits throughout the child's first two years, Visits to Group 4 fami-

lies were scheduled about once a week during the first six weeks, and then less frequently until participating families received a visit approximately every six weeks by the end of the child's second year.

Visitors were nurses who began meeting with the expectant women (in Groups 3 and 4) as early in the pregnancy as possible. Focusing on the strengths of the mother, family members, and friends, nurses enlisted family members and friends to provide child care and support for the mother, provided parents and other family members with information pertaining to child development, and linked mothers and other family members with available health and social services. Results of the study were striking:

> In contrast to women in the comparison groups... women who received visits by a nurse during pregnancy... reduced the number of cigarettes smoked, improved the quality of their diets, had fewer kidney infections, experienced greater support from family members and friends, and made better use of the Special Supplemental Food Program for Women Infants and Children (WIC).... Smokers visited by a nurse bore 75 percent fewer preterm infants, and young adolescents visited by a nurse bore infants who were 395 g heavier than their counterparts in the comparison group.... Among poor, unmarried teenagers, the incidence of state-verified cases of child abuse and neglect during the first two years after delivery was 19 percent in the comparison group... and 4 percent in the group that received both prenatal and infancy nurse visitation... an 80 percent reduction. (Olds et al., 1986, p. 206)

In addition, children of women in the experimental group had significantly fewer visits to hospital emergency rooms and were more likely to receive appropriate immunizations in a timely manner.

Parent Education

Parent education classes are a popular strategy for preventing or ameliorating behaviors that contribute to infant death. Like home visitor programs, they may begin during the prenatal or perinatal period, or even later. Because parenting classes are often conceived of as neglect and abuse prevention programs and aim at changing behaviors of caregivers involved in severe or fatal child maltreatment, elements of program design as basic as interventions and intended clientele vary widely. For example, Pfannensteil and Seltzer (1989) reported on "Parents as Teachers," which offers first-time parents small-group classes and some home visiting beginning in the third trimester of pregnancy. Hayes (1987) studied the effects of a court-ordered program of classes on infant and toddler development and behavior management for parents who had abused or neglected their children. And Dickie and Gerber (1980) evaluated the effects of parenting classes among middle-class, white parents in the areas of child development, reading behavioral cues, and problem solving.

Despite the popularity of parenting classes as an intervention, research on the effects of parent education programs has generally suffered from many methodological defects, and to date no true experimental studies have demonstrated a clear connection between knowledge gained in parenting classes and changes in health-related behaviors. Nevertheless, parent education programs abound and some have gained a reputation for being effective well beyond the limits suggested by research. A good example is "Parents as Teachers." This program, which began in Missouri and has been replicated in several states, is quite popular and has been widely received as a most promising program for preventing some of the behaviors associated with fatal infant abuse and neglect. Parenting classes and home visits focus on improving the overall environment, understanding child development, and learning behavioral management skills. However, the most significant research findings indicate that children in the experimental group had significantly higher language and intellectual development compared with children in the control group and that these improvements were not correlated with increased parent knowledge as hypothesized. It is interesting that in the absence of a clear connection between the improvements noted in children's language and intellectual development and parents' knowledge gained, the researchers concluded that home visits were responsible for differences between experimental and control group children on these measures (Pfannensteil & Seltzer, 1985).

Despite the paucity of outcome studies on parent education, the popularity of this intervention seems to be growing. Although Olds's (1992) recommenda-

tions for the constitutive elements of successful programs and evaluation pertained to home visitor programs, they apply as well to interventions involving parenting classes. Specifically, programs should target those most in need of services; services should begin as early in a pregnancy as possible and continue for as long as two years following delivery; and the approach should include family members or close friends, stressing strengths or competencies of caregivers and emphasizing positive health-related behaviors for caring for infants. Research on parent education programs should employ an experimental design using experimental and control groups; take into account a broad array of potentially confounding variables such as income, level of educational achievement, age of caregivers, abuse of alcohol and drugs, and so on; and plan to follow subjects for at least a few years following completion of the program.

As already noted, infant deaths are often misclassified; that is, infant deaths due to maltreatment or accidental injury may be classified as SIDS, and SIDS deaths may be erroneously classified as child maltreatment fatalities. Professionals in the health care and social service fields do not yet have a handle on how many infants die each year from maltreatment, and as yet do not have standardized, uniformly accepted protocols that would provide this information (Stewart, 1990). One strategy for avoiding these misclassifications and for gathering information vital to formulating policies and programs to prevent infant deaths is Active Surveillance.

Active Surveillance

Active Surveillance is the term used to describe investigative efforts that go beyond the mere receipt of reports required by law and includes actively searching for data from other sources, such as laboratory results, hospital records, autopsy reports, state agencies, and even newspaper stories. Active Surveillance would provide a broad range of unique information to professionals concerned with all aspects of infant death.

The authors have argued elsewhere for the establishment of an Active Surveillance team in each state to investigate all child deaths (Schloesser et al., 1992).

The first step is the establishment of a policy that each child death be reviewed by a state level group representing the various departments that have access to relevant information. . . . At a minimum the agencies that keep birth and death certificate information, the state child protection agency, the income maintenance agency, the state law enforcement agency, and the state attorney general should all take part in the information gathering and review process. In addition to these team members, Durfee (1989) suggests the addition of a prosecutor, a pediatrician or forensic pathologist, a legislator, a citizen advocate, and representatives from mental health and private child abuse agencies. This implies a series of inter-agency agreements that establishes who is responsible for providing different kinds of information and includes safeguards for confidentiality. (p. 17)

Clearly, the kind of investigation called for in Active Surveillance cannot happen without full inter-agency cooperation. However, it is equally clear that such cooperation will not happen immediately or without effort. It must be clear that the purpose of Active Surveillance is to establish an epidemiological database linking characteristics of children and families to infant death for the purpose of better understanding and preventing infant death, regardless of its cause. The purpose of Active Surveillance is *not* to affix blame or to determine whether a given professional or agency followed standard policies and procedures. As Durfee points out, members of Active Surveillance teams are not looking for evil but for truth (Durfee, 1989).

Riley (1989) suggests that because the Active Surveillance team will involve several agencies and will need logistical and clerical support, a single agency should be designated as the team's sponsoring agency. This agency will receive reports and data on infant deaths, ensure that all infant deaths are reviewed thoroughly, issue reports and make recommendations, and take the necessary steps to safeguard confidentiality. The problem of guaranteeing confidentiality may be especially problematic for some agencies. A shared database and multidisciplinary meetings raise questions about protecting innocent families on the one hand and compromising criminal prosecution on the other. An important step in protecting confidentiality and respecting privacy is a requirement that each member of the Active Surveillance

team be required to sign an agreement prohibiting unauthorized use of information acquired in the review process (Riley, 1989). Issues of confidentiality as they arise in the investigation of infant deaths can be quite thorny, but anxiety about confidentiality must not become an excuse for inaction.

Active Surveillance requires an information management system capable of receiving and processing data from several components of the review team. However, this does not necessarily entail a large or costly computer system. The tasks required by Active Surveillance are more human than electronic, and can be accomplished by a good public health researcher and a desktop computer. As with confidentiality, anxiety about technology must not become an excuse for inaction:

> The major problem is not technology or the need for expensive information systems. The major block rather consistently is attitudinal and the need for professionals to think of team in a larger sense than just their profession or their individual agency. (Durfee, 1989, p. 10)

Use of this information by states is just beginning. However, the possibilities are numerous. States could use Active Surveillance data to target a given neighborhood, city, or county for prevention efforts based on knowledge of rate of infant death, cause of death, age of infant at time of death, and relevant characteristics of parents. Active Surveillance data might be used by state agencies, singly or collectively, to ascertain the degree to which they provide a safety net for vulnerable children and families. And agencies might use new knowledge gained from the Active Surveillance database to modify existing programs that are found to provide less support than was assumed prior to the availability of the Active Surveillance data.

Finally, information acquired through Active Surveillance would make each infant death relatively unambiguous and less likely to be misclassified. This is a necessary step in efforts to remove or impede those factors that contribute to infant death. Policy and program administrators, as well as frontline practitioners, must have a clear picture of the number and causes of infant deaths, attributes of children and families involved, and societal and environmental factors accompanying each infant death. Without infant, family, and environment profiles based on this information, prevention efforts must necessarily be inadequate and reactive rather than proactive. Prevention efforts, if they are to succeed, must be very well planned, and good planning requires a broad, timely information base.

ADOLESCENT PREGNANCY AND CHILDBEARING

Low birth weight and infant death are strongly associated with the mother's age (Cooper, 1992). In 1990, there were 500,000 births to teens (Glazer, 1993), not an insignificant number. Therefore, it is necessary to consider infant mortality prevention strategies that address the special situation of adolescent childbearing. However, it must be remembered that although age of mother is an important variable in predicting low birth weight, it cannot be isolated from other potentially confounding predictor variables such as inadequate prenatal care that accompanies both teen pregnancy and LBW.

Adolescent Sexual Activity

Only a small percentage of sexually active adolescents become pregnant and give birth. Nevertheless, given the debates about sex education, availability of contraception, and abortion, it is important to understand the context of sexual activity among young women. Although one should argue for equal consideration of sexual activity among young men, we focus the discussion on young women because (1) sufficient research has been conducted to provide significant demographic and outcome data (2) it is they who become pregnant and give birth and (3) it is their environment and their behaviors that can be altered favorably to affect the infant death rate.

One strategy for addressing the problem of infant death associated with teenage childbearing is to delay initial onset of sexual activity, defined as first intercourse. Most adolescents in the United States become sexually active by age 19 (Voydanoff & Donnelley, 1990). There are also indications that sexual activity of younger teens has increased significantly. Hayes (1987) reported that 5.4 percent of girls had sexual intercourse before age 15 in 1983, with the percentage for white girls being 4.7 and for African Americans

9.7. In 1987, Hofferth, Kahn, and Baldwin reported that about 15 percent of white females and 20 percent of African American females engaged in sexual activity by the age of 15. Another study found that the increase in sexually experienced 15-year-olds went from 5 percent in 1970 to 26 percent in 1988 (Glazer, 1993). These increases are dramatic. Clearly, a large number of women in the United States are, at an early age, engaging in sexual activity that could lead to pregnancy and birth.

There are many factors believed to explain this increase in sexual activity. Of course, it is not possible to disentangle causes and effects, and causal explanation may be unattainable. However, awareness of these factors provides an important context for consideration of infant death prevention strategies. Certainly, the fact that the average young woman now starts menstruation at 12.5 years of age is a factor (Glazer, 1989). Voydanoff and Donnelly (1990) provide a good review of the literature on adolescent sexual activity and identify several additional factors that shed light on the context for increased sexual activity. They note that there have been significant changes in the transition from childhood to adulthood in American society.

> Thus many adolescents today—when compared with those of earlier decades—experience increased autonomy, greater opportunity for sexual activity, a reduction in some of the costs associated with sexual activity, less negative attitudes toward sex, and increased length of time during which they are asked to be sexually inactive after becoming sexually mature. (p. 24)

These authors provide considerable evidence for parents' socioeconomic status as a cluster of factors related to sexual activity. Adolescents from poorer families tend to engage in sexual activity at an earlier age, as do teens whose parents did not complete high school. Considering the disparity between African American and white mean family income in the United States, these two factors may explain much of the rather dramatic differences in rates of sexual activity between African Americans and whites.

Religiosity seems to be associated with sexual activity, as teenagers who do not regularly attend religious services are more likely to have nonmarital intercourse. Academic performance is inversely related to sexual activity, with those doing more poorly in school more frequently engaging in sexual activity. Most evidence suggests that exposure to sex education programs is not related to sexual activity. Family structure has been associated with sexual activity, as children experiencing divorce, separation, and single parenting are likely to be more sexually active. Parents may influence their children's sexual activity either directly or indirectly, from controlling dating activities to influencing norms and attitudes associated with sexual activity. Finally, peer influences are associated with sexual activity (Card, Peterson, & Greeno, 1992). In a Louis Harris poll reported by Voydanoff and Donnelly (1990), the most common reason given by teens for not delaying intercourse was social pressure.

The extensive review of factors associated with adolescent sexual activity provided by Voydanoff and Donnelly presents a complex context for this behavior. None of these results can be viewed in terms of cause and effect, although it is tempting to do so. What can be derived from this discussion is the not surprising conclusion that the decision to engage in sexual activity occurs in a context that is complex and rapidly changing. Perhaps the best conclusion is that all young women should be viewed as potential mothers at an early age, and so the focus should be on providing them with resources needed to avoid sexual activity at a young age, prevent pregnancy if they do become sexually active, and assure positive outcomes for them and their children if they give birth.

Adolescent Pregnancy

Although it is easy to establish a large increase in sexual activity among young women over the last decade, the teen pregnancy rate has not changed substantially until very recently. Besharov (1993) reports that 11 percent of teens were pregnant in 1980 and in 1988. However, there seems to be a dramatic increase in teen births since 1988 (Children's Defense Fund, 1994). At this point, it is not possible to determine if this is a new trend or even to guess as to its causes. With 500,000 babies born to teens each year, many of whom are vulnerable to inadequate prenatal care and subsequent low birth weight, it is important to examine the context of adolescent pregnancy. Again, Voydanoff and Donnelly (1990)

provide an excellent overview. Once someone decides to become sexually active, a major factor contributing to teenage pregnancy is use or nonuse of contraception. A study by Zelnik and Kantner (1980) of women 15 to 19 years old found that 27 percent of the sexually active women reported no use of contraception, with 62 percent of that group becoming pregnant. Of those sexually active women who were occasional users of contraception (39 percent), 30 percent resulted in pregnancy. The 34 percent who reported they always used contraception became pregnant in 13 percent of these cases. Contraception clearly reduces pregnancy rates among teenagers.

Age at first intercourse is a major factor influencing the decision to use contraceptives (Voydanoff & Donnelly, 1990). This is frequently explained by the cognitive development of adolescents. How well equipped a 13-year-old is to understand the consequences of the decision is an important issue, particularly if the contraceptive method requires advanced thought and planning. Knowledge is another important factor related to the contraceptive decision. Young teens are particularly uninformed and unrealistic about the possibility of getting pregnant. Morrison (1987) found that teenage women with little understanding about sexuality and contraception were less likely to use contraception. However, knowledge alone does not explain the contraceptive decision. Morrison also found that those who were more knowledgeable were also relatively ineffective users of contraception.

Teens' attitudes are important in determining whether to use contraception. Young women's attitude towards sexuality, birth control, and abortion have all been linked to the use of contraception. Young women with more positive attitudes toward their sexuality are more likely to use contraception. Women who see themselves as likely to have an abortion are less likely to use contraception effectively (Voydanoff & Donnelly, 1990). Although the public discussion about African American teen pregnancy suggests that race or other social and demographic factors may be related to teens' use of contraception, a study by Zelnik, Kantner, and Ford (1981) found that white and African American women with higher socioeconomic status, greater family stability, and higher levels of religiosity are more likely to use contraception at first intercourse. Although this study is somewhat dated, it does underscore the need to disentangle the effects of race and poverty. Finally, a young couple's relationship embodies factors related to contraceptive use. Couples whose relationships include open communication about sexual matters are more likely to use contraception regularly (Voydanoff & Donnelly, 1990).

The previous contextual factors were related to the decisions involving use of contraception. Voydanoff and Donnelly (1990) report additional correlates of teen pregnancy. These include socioeconomic status, a single maternal-headed household, low educational aspiration of the teen, frequency of intercourse, and assessment of the consequences of a pregnancy. None of these is surprising.

Prevention

Given the information available on infant mortality, low birth weight, and adolescent pregnancy, any comprehensive prevention strategy will include a focus on teenage women. One prevention strategy might be to focus attention on low birth weight and other pregnancy-related factors among those teens who do become pregnant. Another strategy is to prevent pregnancy once a young women becomes sexually active. Yet another approach might be to delay initiation of sexual activity. In fact, all of these have been the focus of various programs.

Convincing young people to abstain from sexual activity until a later age is a popular approach among many sectors, and particularly within some religious groups. The appeal of this is not unreasonable when one envisions a large number of young people sexually active from age 13. However, aside from one's value preferences, there seems to be little evidence that adults know how to influence young people to delay sexual activity. Initially, there were some hopeful signs in this regard. One of the landmark programs was "The Self Center" in Baltimore, developed at Johns Hopkins University. This was a multifaceted program that included classroom and small group presentations on sexuality and other personal issues, individual counseling, medical services, and contraceptives. A well-designed evaluation found that participating students postponed their first sexual encounter by about seven months compared with non-

participating students from similar backgrounds (Zabin et al., 1988). Unfortunately, these rather hopeful results have not held up over time and across programs.

These findings lead some to suggest that the focus ought to shift to prevention of pregnancy for sexually active adolescents or at least a double message: Delay first intercourse, but if you do become sexually active, use reliable contraceptive methods. The rather dramatic increases in sexual activity of young women has only recently been accompanied by an equal increase in teen pregnancies and births. This and other evidence suggests that many sexually active teens are effective in preventing pregnancy.

"The Self Center" program with its impressive results, including a 30 percent decline in pregnancy rates in participating schools while nonparticipating schools demonstrated a 58 percent increase, suggested that school-based clinics were the answer to the problems associated with teen pregnancy. In fact, by November 1992, there were 475 such clinics nationwide, a 45 percent increase in just three years (Glazer, 1993). Unfortunately, there is little evidence to suggest a reduction in the rate of teen pregnancy because of these clinics. Perhaps the best overall conclusion about the knowledge in this area is provided by Voyandoff and Donnelly (1990):

> Preventive interventions designed to delay sexual activity and increase effective contraception use several overlapping approaches. These include sex and family life education, family planning services, family communication programs, role modeling and mentoring, and media-focused programs. Some programs are designed to improve the capability of adolescents to prevent pregnancy while others focus on increasing motivation and providing alternatives to childbearing. Unfortunately, little is known about the extent to which these goals are achieved. (p. 100)

The fact that little is known should not be reason for despair. Rather, the occasional positive research findings, along with those indicating no differences between treatment groups, suggests that society has a great deal more to learn. The variety of programs in this area, with their differing designs and components, is impressive. One is also struck by what these programs do not address. How does busing or hours of operation affect clinic availability, particularly to poor women who appear to be most vulnerable? Although some programs go beyond targeting young women, few programs include young men, peers, and parents. If one begins by considering young women, and then broadens the focus to include partners, peers, and parents, the community must soon be considered as well. And since poverty is such a ubiquitous confounding factor, employment, job training, and income transfer programs cannot be omitted from the prevention picture.

The teen pregnancy prevention field might take some lessons from the drug abuse prevention field. Although empirical evidence is equally weak in the area of drug abuse prevention, program design is rather sophisticated. Many of these programs are multifaceted. The best programs focus on the individual and then broaden to include groups, such as family and friends; community institutions such as schools, churches, and synagogues; and the broader community as well as relevant local and state policies. For example, many drug abuse prevention programs include individual components focusing on such topics as information, decision-making skills, and skills to handle peer pressure. They then proceed to create nonalcoholic parties and other events in which youth can participate. Creation of formal organizations such as Students Against Drunk Driving (SADD) and Mothers Against Drunk Driving (MADD) is an important element in the program. Addressing school policies on possession and use of alcohol and other drugs is still another feature. Reaching out into the community to create a climate of decreased alcohol use is a program element that might include decreasing or eliminating alcohol sales at community events such as fairs. Influencing policies and practices regarding how drunk driving arrests are handled and the state's definition of "driving under the influence" is another element. The lesson here is clear. With complex problems such as drug abuse and teen pregnancy, complex, multifaceted programs are probably required to obtain the kinds of results the country desires.

Delay of sexual activity and prevention of pregnancy are not the only strategies for preventing infant death among babies born to adolescents. Clearly, there will continue to be teen pregnancies and births to young women. If one thinks of each young woman as a potential childbearer, her health becomes another major focus for preventing the societal conditions associated with infant mortality. Therefore, everything that has been said previously about prenatal and perinatal care strategies must apply to young women as well.

As discussed earlier, health insurance coverage is an important factor in providing prenatal care and thereby reducing the incidence of infant death. However, young women are confronted with more difficulties in acquiring the care they need. The very young woman who becomes sexually active is less likely to seek health care and is more likely to wait until she absolutely has to seek care because she is undeniably pregnant. Therefore, prenatal care is likely to be late. In addition to other risks, if she begins prenatal care late, it may be difficult to determine if a fetus is small because it is early in the pregnancy or because the fetus is not developing typically, The two situations require different medical responses (Cooper, 1992).

The complexity of the problem of adolescent pregnancy and parenting has led people to suggest the necessity of a comprehensive approach to young women in which a team of care providers addresses the complex set of variables that seem to contribute to positive birth outcomes and infant development, Although there have been some apparent successes using this approach, Collins and Chacko (1993) report that evaluations of comprehensive programs are highly variable and frequently report conflicting results.

When focusing on young women as a target population for prevention of infant death, the best prevention may be to view all young women as potential childbearers and provide them with all of the economic, social, educational, health, and medical resources possible. The National Research Council (1987) suggests a four-pronged approach, including economic support; maternal and infant health care; social, emotional, and cognitive development in children of adolescent mothers; and educational and vocational enhancement of adolescent mothers.

SUMMARY

Although the many advances in medical care and technology are laudable, this chapter has concerned those societal barriers and individual behaviors that contribute to the too high infant death rate in the

United States. The quality of medical care and the pace of medical achievements are remarkable, but too many infants die because of preventable individual behaviors and arbitrary environmental factors. Infants and mothers are most at risk when they are subject to a number of factors such as poverty, poor or no access to medical care, lower educational achievement, and young age at beginning childbearing. In fact, entire communities and neighborhoods, and not merely individuals, can be at risk: "Communities where there is a confluence of several problems, such as poverty, unemployment, and illiteracy, tend to have higher infant mortality rates than . . . more advantaged communities" (Annie E. Casey Foundation, 1994). Therefore, solutions to the multifaceted problem known as infant death must occur at individual, community, state, and national levels. We conclude our discussion of preventing infant death with recommendations regarding specific policy and program options.

RECOMMENDATIONS

In his discussion of home visitor programs, Olds (1992) argues that programs should focus on families and communities and not merely on individuals. He also observes that many of these programs are not coordinated with other efforts, nor are they designed and implemented in a manner consistent with available empirical evidence. We agree with both of these observations and broaden them to include most social policies and programs. Yet, it is becoming increasingly evident that to be successful, health care interventions, whether they are aimed at society or at individuals, must be comprehensive, research based, and coordinated with other relevant interventions. Earlier, we recommended that the teen pregnancy prevention field follow the example of drug abuse prevention. In fact, we suggest that this multitier approach presents a good model for interventions generally, and for preventing infant death in particular. Policies and programs should include national, state, city, and neighborhood components; they should be based on the most rigorous research currently available; and they should be consistent with other policies and programs intended to have an impact on societal factors and individual behaviors that contribute to infant death.

The problem of low birth weight and its importance as a contributing factor to infant death offers a good example of how such a comprehensive approach might be organized. At the national level, increased funding for primary care delivered in organized settings and for Medicaid or other health insurance could ensure that no pregnant woman, regardless of age or circumstances, goes without prenatal care. Based on recent research findings indicating that stigma and other factors inhibit the timely use of Medicaid, the emphasis might be placed on providing care in organized settings and on ensuring access to health insurance other than Medicaid.

At the next level, states can enlarge Medicaid and other outreach efforts through such programs as Baby Your Baby and by working with private insurers to provide health insurance to each family that cannot afford health insurance but does not qualify for public welfare programs. States can also ensure that state-operated clinics observe operating hours that allow ample time for nontraditional workers to access services. States and cities can work together to identify and secure sources to provide incentives to begin prenatal care earlier, and cities can make sure that public transportation routes and hours of operation make it possible for consumers to keep doctor appointments and then return to work or home.

Local businesses as well as government employers can provide work-based health education programs and may even offer incentives for improving prenatal health—for example, by successfully completing a smoking cessation clinic. Neighborhood schools can be made available for before- or after-school programs—or might incorporate health curricula—which inform students about sex and sexuality; help them develop decision making and refusal skills; and, should they already be or decide to become sexually active, teach them about the availability and proper use of contraceptives.

There are currently many programs in virtually every city and state that could become effective or be made more effective by working with other pertinent efforts and by modifying them to reflect what has been learned through research. Although significant progress resulting from program improvements based on research is likely to be costly, it is generally agreed that prevention is more cost effective, and certainly more humane, than reacting to problems after they arise. Additionally, it is reasonable to expect that some progress in the form of amplification of services and outcomes can be made with few additional financial expenditures simply through coordinating existing services.

Preventing infant death cannot begin and end in the professional's office, no matter how important the work done in the office may be. It requires practitioners to examine a variety of policy and program options at the national, state, city, and neighborhood levels—that is, in each of the many arenas in which we work and live. For, as Durfee has rightly commented, "Team interventions and prevention will eventually move from professional actions to involvement of extended family and neighbors. The total task is essentially impossible without the community" (Durfee, 1989). Efforts to prevent infant deaths must involve professionals as well as families and neighbors; and they must occur not only in the office but also in homes and in the seats of government. The task is impossible without the whole community.

REFERENCES

Annie E. Casey Foundation. (1994). *Kids count data book: State profiles of child well-being.* Baltimore, MD: Author.

Barness, L. A. (1992). Pediatrics. *JAMA, 268* (3), 399–400.

Besharov, D. J. (January/February 1993). Truth and consequences: Teen sex. *The American Enterprise,* 52–59.

Bowman, M., & Schwenk, T. (1993). Family medicine. *JAMA, 270* (2), 205–206.

Card, J. J., Peterson, J. L., & Greeno, C. G. (1992). Adolescent pregnancy prevention programs: Design, monitoring, and evaluation. In B. C. Miller, J. J. Card, R. L. Paikoff, & J. L. Peterson (Eds.), *Preventing adolescent pregnancy: Model programs and evaluations.* Newbury Park, CA: Sage.

Center for Disease Control. (1990). Division of Reproductive Health, National Center for Chronic Disease Prevention and Health Promotion; Division of Vital Statistics, National Center for Health Statistics (1993). Infant mortality—United States. *JAMA, 269*(13), 1616–1617.

Children's Defense Fund. (1994). *The state of America's children: Yearbook 1994.* Washington, DC: Author.

Christoffel, K., Zeiserl, E., & Chiaramonte, J. (1985). Should child abuse and neglect be considered when a child dies unexpectedly? *American Journal of Diseases of Children, 139,* 876–880.

Collins, K. C., & Chacko, M. R. (1993). Adolescent parenthood: Role of the pediatrician. *Children and Youth Service Review, 15* (4), 295–308.

Cooper, M. H. (1992). Infant mortality. *CQ Researcher, 2* (28), 641–664.

Cotton, P. (1994). Smoking cigarettes may do developing fetus more harm than ingesting cocaine, some experts say. *JAMA, 271* (8), 576–577.

Daro, D. (1988). *Confronting child abuse: Research for effective program design.* New York: The Free Press.

Dickie, J., & Gerber, S. (1980). Training in social competence: The effects on mothers, fathers, and infants. *Child Development, 51,* 1248–1251.

Durfee, M. (1989). Fatal child abuse: Intervention and prevention. *Protecting Children, 6* (1), 9–12.

Edelman, M. W. (1987). *Families in peril.* Cambridge, MA: Harvard University Press.

Glazer, S. (June 23, 1989). Sex education: How well does it work? *Editorial Research Reports,* 338–431.

Glazer, S. (1993). Preventing teen pregnancy. *CQ Researcher, 3* (18), 409–432

Guntheroth, W. G., & Spiers, P. S. (1992). Sleeping position and the risk of sudden infant death syndrome. *JAMA, 267*(17), 2359–2362.

Hayes, C. D. (Ed.). (1987). *Risking the future: Adolescent sexuality, pregnancy, and childbearing.* Washington, DC: National Academy Press.

Hayes, P. (1987). Evaluation of PACES: A parenting program. *Master's Abstracts International, 27/01* (561–141). Unpublished master's thesis, The University of Texas at Arlington.

Hofferth, S. L., Kahn, J. R., & Baldwin, W. (1987). Premarital sexual activity among U.S. teenage women over the past three decades. *Family Planning Perspectives, 19,* 46–53.

Jacquot, C., & Roberts, D. (1988). *Fatal child abuse and neglect in Oregon: 1985–1988.* Salem, OR: State Department of Human Resources, Children's Services Division.

Jason, J., & Andereck, N. (1983). Fatal child abuse in Georgia: The epidemiology of severe physical child abuse. *Child Abuse and Neglect, 7,* 1–9.

Kadushin, A., & Martin, J. A. (1988). *Child welfare service* (9th edition). New York: Macmillan.

McClain, P. W., Sacks, J. J., Froehlke, R. G., & Ewigman, B. G. (1993). Estimates of fatal child abuse and neglect: United States 1979 through 1988. *Pediatrics Fol., 91* (2), 338–343.

McCurdy, K., & Daro, D. (1994). *Current trends in child abuse fatalities: The results of the 1993 annual fifty state survey.* Chicago: The National Center on Child Abuse Prevention Research, The National Committee to Prevent Child Abuse.

Mitchell, L. (1987). Report on fatalities from NCPCA. *Protecting Children, 6* (1), 3–5.

Morrison, D. M. (1987). *Predicting contraception efficacy.* Unpublished manuscript reported in Voydanoff, P., & Donnelly, B. W. (1990). *Adolescent sexuality and pregnancy.* Newbury Park, CA: Sage.

National Research Council. (1987). Risking the future: Adolescent sexuality, pregnancy, and childbearing. Panel on Adolescent Pregnancy and Childbearing, Committee on Child Development Research and Public Policy, Commission on Behavioral and Social Sciences and Education, National research Council. Cheryl D. Hayes, editor. Washington, DC: National Academy Press.

Olds, D. (1992). Home visitation for pregnant women and parents of young children. *American Journal of Diseases of Children, 146,* 704–708.

Olds, D., Henderson, C., & Tatelbaum, R. (1994). Prevention of intellectual impairment in children of women who smoke cigarettes during pregnancy. *Pediatrics, 93* (2), 228–233.

Olds, D., Henderson, C. R., Tatelbaum, R., & Chamberlin, R. (1986). Improving child abuse and neglect: A randomized trial of nurse home visitation. *Pediatrics, 77,* 16–28.

Perloff, J. (1992). Health care resources for children and pregnant women. In Richard E. Behrman (Ed.), *U.S. Health Care for Children, 3* (3), 78–94. Los Altos, CA: Center for the Future of Children, The David and Lucille Packard Foundation.

Pfannensteil, J. C., & Seltzer, D. A. (1985). *Evaluation report: New parents as teachers project.* Jefferson City: Missouri Department of Education and Secondary Education.

Poets, C. F., & Southall, D. P. (1993). Prone sleeping position and sudden infant death, *JAMA, 329* (6), 425–426.

Racine, A., Joyce, T., & Grossman, M. (1992). Effectiveness of health care services for pregnant women and infants. In Richard E. Behrman (Ed.), *U.S. Health Care for Children, 3* (3), 78–94. Los Altos, CA: Center for the Future of Children, The David and Lucille Packard Foundation.

Riley, J. (1989). The child fatalities review process. *Protecting Children, 6* (1), 6–8.

Schloesser, P., Pierpont, J., & Poertner, J. (1992). Active surveillance of child abuse fatalities. *Child Abuse and Neglect, 16* (1), 3–10.

Schorr, L. (1988). *Within our reach: Breaking the cycle of disadvantage.* New York: Doubleday.

Smith, P. (1989). *Child abuse fatalities: A review of the literature.* Paper presented at the Eighth National Conference on Child Abuse and Neglect, Salt Lake City, UT.

Stewart, B. (1990). Issues in developing a research agenda for child abuse. In Douglas J. Besharov (Ed.), *Family violence: Research and public policy issues* (pp. 146–149). Washington, DC: AEI Press.

Thompson, L., & Wilson, D. (1989). *Report on child fatalities related to child abuse and neglect: April 1986–April 1988.* Olympia, WA: State Department of Social and Health Services, Division of Children and Family Services.

Van Dyck, P. C., Nangle, B., McDonald, S. P., Wells, T. J., & Betit, R. (1991). *Baby Your Baby: Utah's program to enhance prenatal care.* Salt Lake City: Utah Department of Health, Family Health Services Division.

Voydanoff, P., & Donnelly, B. W. (1990). *Adolescent sexuality and pregnancy.* Newbury Park, CA: Sage.

Zabin, L. S., Hirsch, M. B., Streett, R., Emerson, M. R., Smith, M., Hardy, J. B., & King, T. M. (1988, July/August). The Baltimore Pregnancy Prevention Program for Urban Teenagers: How did it work? What did it cost? *Family Planning Perspectives, 20,* 169–192.

Zelnik, M., & Kantner, J. F., (1980). Sexual activity, contraception use and pregnancy among metropolitan-area teenagers: 1971–1979. *Family Planning Perspectives, 12,* 230–237.

Zelnik, M., Kantner, J. F., & Ford, K. (1981). *Sex and pregnancy in adolescents.* Beverly Hills: Sage.

CHAPTER 3

ASSESSMENT OF THE PROBLEM OF CHILDHOOD DISABILITY IN A THIRD WORLD COUNTRY: JAMAICA

Marigold J. Thorburn, 3D PROJECTS, JAMAICA
Tomlin J. Paul, UNIVERSITY OF THE WEST INDIES

The search for objective measures of health status of a population is ongoing and in fact a long tradition of public health. Infant mortality and the mean expectation of life at birth are widely accepted measures as valid indicators of health status. Apart from these, the suggestion that disability can be useful as an indicator of health status (Durkin, Zaman, Thorburn, Hasan, & Davidson, 1991) is gaining recognition as survival increases and issues related to quality of life become prominent.

From a functional perspective, disability measurement can reflect the health status of a population, particularly as measures such as infant mortality rates begin to stabilize. In the Jamaican context, progress has occurred with respect to health status as indicated by the infant mortality rate, which is now in the region of 13 per 1,000 live births.

Health gain will continue to be a significant goal, but improvements need to occur not only in terms of mortality and survival but also in terms of quality of life. Thorburn (1991) argues that the increased sur-

vival of children does not coincide with meaningful enough changes in strategies for prevention or rehabilitation of disability. In developed countries, with manifestations of the epidemiological transition, there is a move away from the traditional emphasis on long life to the broad spectrum of "death, disability, discomfort and dissatisfaction" (Siegmann, 1979). Developing countries experiencing these shifts in disease patterns will find it necessary also to examine this spectrum of perspectives on health.

In developing countries, there is a general lack of information and many misconceptions on childhood disability, particularly in the health field, but recent developments have put the acquisition of appropriate and relevant information within reach.

Helander, Mendis, and Nelson that about 90 percent of veloping countries Epidemiological S (IESCD) focused successfully:

1. Lack of suitable instruments and methods for identification and assessment
2. Lack of suitable and standardized criteria
3. Lack of appropriate personnel

After 10 years of experience with early intervention (EI) and community-based rehabilitation (CBR), the authors realized that these problems must be tackled in order for rehabilitation models to gain credibility as being low cost, relevant, and feasible in developing countries and that childhood disability must receive more serious attention in the epidemiological equation for health status assessment than has been the standard until the present.

This chapter will describe the authors' experiences and conclusions, with particular reference to the roles of different levels of personnel, particularly doctors and health workers, and some of the specific tools that they can use in assessment of disability problems in the community. Three aspects will be addressed:

1. Identification of disability-related problems of children.
2. Clinical assessment of these problems so that affected persons can receive assistance in their communities.
3. The epidemiological aspect that seeks to determine the size of the problem in a community in order to plan services.

These aspects must be inseparable, so the strategies need to be coherent. Unfortunately, the first and third often take place without the second. However, epidemiological information is dependent on accurate assessment of individuals as well as the sampling and analysis that validate the quantification and interpretation of data. What still needs attention is evaluation of feasible intervention/rehabilitation models. This could not take place until all the procedures to describe the problem have undergone testing.

SCREENING FOR AND IDENTIFYING ꞌLDHOOD DISABILITY

ꞌent for developmental disabili-
tices in Jamaica for over 20

years (Thorburn, 1991) but, until recently, it has not undergone proper evaluation. Screening and assessment are the first two components of an intervention process that can assist children with disabilities to live a normal life. Screening reduces the number of children requiring the longer and more complex assessment procedures, and assessment must lead to appropriate and individualized intervention.

Until recently, most of the assessment procedures used required personnel with professional qualifications that are scarce in the Third World. Recent research has developed and tested a range of questionnaires and tests that nonprofessionals can use locally with fair reliability.

An important consideration in development of these procedures is the use of consistent and appropriate classifications and criteria. Jamaica adopted the International Classification of Impairments, Disabilities and Handicaps (ICIDH) (WHO, 1980) in 1981 (Thorburn & Chernesky, 1981); the criteria used have received full discussion elsewhere (Thorburn, Desai, & Davidson, 1992).

There are three main aspects that one must consider when evaluating a screening test:

1. The purposes of screening
2. The choice of diseases or conditions for which one is conducting the screening
3. The criteria on which one is to evaluate the test

Purposes of Screening

The two major types of screening discussed here are detection of presymptomatic disease and identification of cases in the population at large.

Detection of Presymptomatic Disease

The purpose of this type of screening is to reduce or eliminate serious sequelae by early detection. An example of this type is the Denver Developmental Screening Test (DDST; Frankenburg & Dodds, 1967), which has been in use for more than 25 years in Jamaica, along with a shorter, Developmental Screening Checklist (Thorburn & Chernesky, 1981). Neither of these has undergone rigorous validation studies in Jamaica because of cost, but long and extensive experience has given them some degree of face validity.

For example, practitioners are aware that motor milestones in infants tend to occur earlier in this population than among others and a "normal" DDST in this age group does not eliminate a motor delay. In another domain, the language items may be difficult for Creole-speaking children.

Identification of Cases in the Population at Large

The purpose here is to identify cases to include in an intervention program and to provide information for planning of services and measuring population morbidity. An example of this type, which has now received extensive testing and validation in Jamaica (Thorburn, Desai, Paul, Malcolm, Durkin, & Davidson, 1992a) and elsewhere in the IESCD (Zaman et al., 1991) is the Ten Questions (TQ), which can be useful in identifying six types of disability in children 2 to 9 years of age with good sensitivity for moderate and severe degrees of disability (see below).

Choice of Diseases for Screening

Criteria for selection of diseases for screening purposes include:

1. High prevalence
2. Seriousness of the disease or its complications
3. Feasibility of follow-up of cases
4. Effectiveness of methods that exist for management of the condition and prevention of adverse outcomes

Childhood disability (CD) is not a homogeneous disease entity, but there is often common symptomatology and etiology between the various categories. CD occurs in 5 to 17 percent of the childhood population worldwide. In Clarendon, Jamaica, in the IESCD (Paul, Desai, & Thorburn, 1992), the prevalence was just under 10 percent. In approximately 2 percent, the disabilities were moderate or severe (serious), and more than 38 percent of the latter had significant handicaps. Therefore, CD fulfills the first two criteria.

Because of recent developments in community-based rehabilitation (CBR) (Thorburn, 1991a), it is now easier to meet the third and fourth criteria than it was previously, although the fourth may still be argu-

able from a medical standpoint. Disability interventions, however, cannot receive proper evaluation from a strict medical model where outcome indicators often lack a functional orientation.

Criteria for Effective Screening Tests

An effective screening test must be:

1. Cheap, quick, and easy to learn and perform
2. Reliable for use by nonprofessionals
3. Acceptable to the target population
4. Acceptable to the professional community
5. Able to identify an acceptable proportion of cases (sensitivity)
6. Able to identify noncases as noncases (specificity)

The TQ as a Screening Test

The validation study of the TQ took place in a defined area of the rural parish of Clarendon, Jamaica, in 1987 to 1988. This yielded 5,461 children aged 2 to 9 years amongst which data collection was complete. Descriptions of the methods and procedures used appear in the published literature extensively described elsewhere (Thorburn, Desai, & Davidson, 1992).

The TQ for Estimating the Disability Problem and in Prioritizing Service Needs. Health and education services both concern themselves with disability, but both have different priorities. Here, the main concern is with health. In the hands of Community Workers (CWs) in Jamaica, the TQ accurately detected serious degrees of six types of disability except cognitive disability. The poor sensitivity of the TQ for all (mild, moderate, and severe) degrees of disability pooled is entirely the result of the low sensitivity for mild cognitive deficits (the most common disability). However, if the TQ misses only 1 percent of moderately retarded children, it is probably because their behavior is not deviant enough to cause concern. The TQ is thus a potentially useful instrument.

However, the main problem with the TQ was a high proportion of false positives (74 percent), meaning that either another level of screening or professional diagnosis would be necessary for all positive cases. This would be unacceptably burdensome b cause the TQ positive rate was 15.6 percent in Jamaica (Thorburn, Desai, Paul, Malcolm, Durkin, & Davidson, 1992b). Also, for true *early* detection (i.e., in the under 2-year-old age group), the TQ would be of no use.

For educational purposes, the TQ would miss a large proportion of children with mild disabilities who might need special assistance, such as classroom placement, guidance, or glasses. However, it may still be appropriate because it picks up those problems that are of concern to families. Because Third World governments are hardly likely to be able to provide for all the needs of all their children, it would seem to be a pragmatic base on which to begin planning to address the needs of concern to families.

The TQ in Community-Based Rehabilitation (CBR). Similar arguments apply here as above. An earlier report (Thorburn, Paul, & Desai, 1992), showed that 29.5 percent of children with disabilities would benefit from CBR and that this would be necessary for proportionately more of the younger children and the more severely disabled. Family concern and participation are essential for CBR to be successful, so if the TQ measures perception of problems, then a few false negatives will not matter very much.

The false positives are again a problem and would require another level of screening or diagnosis to avoid gross overburdening of rehabilitation services. However, this second level can exist within the initial response and evaluation of the CBR team with hopefully marginal costs. Of course, the psychic costs to the family of getting labeled a false positive must also be a consideration factored into the equation.

The TQ in Monitoring Health or Prevention Programs. It is a generally accepted fact that the etiology of mild and serious mental retardation has different origins, the former being mainly of sociocultural origin and the latter of biological origin (Clarke & Clarke, 1974). Preventive measures are therefore different for each group. Furthermore, information on etiology is likely to be more accurate if estimates take place closer to the time of insult causing the problem. Because most serious disabilities in the Jamaican child population probably originate in the pre- and perinatal periods (Thorburn, 1981), cross-sectional studies of prevalence after 2 years of age are not likely

to give good indicators of changing incidence. So the TQ would give only crude information for this purpose.

Meeting the Criteria for Screening Tests

Of the six criteria given earlier, the TQ fulfills all the requirements. It is low cost, easy, and quick to administer; reliable in the hands of community workers; reasonably sensitive and specific for serious disability; and acceptable to the target population. The high rate of false positives (74 percent) for all degrees of disability does reduce its specificity, however. Although the majority (56 percent) had problems that could benefit from professional advice and treatment, "weeding out "the "true normals "would be ideal because professional services are scarce and costly.

Because the majority of false positives were mental, hearing, and visual impairments, many of the "true normals" could be identified by screening for hearing and vision defects. The authors were able to do this in their clinics as part of the assessment phase of the survey by community workers using the Maico screening audiometer and the Landholdt C chart, respectively. The physician made a decision as to whether a child was normal using agreed cut-off points. However, with appropriate training, community workers could easily make those decisions. If the vision, hearing, and developmental screening were part of the community survey, detection capability at the community level would increase significantly.

Thus, the TQ could serve as a low-cost detector, but it needs to be paired with objective measurements to exclude normal children, as recommended by Feinstein (1977). Therefore, TQ should be administered first, with the other screening tests done only in the positive cases. This will considerably reduce screening time. Despite the appeal of this approach, it requires further research to assess its usefulness.

The predictive value of the TQ, like other screening tests, is dependent on the prevalence of the test condition in the community. As the prevalence increases, the positive predictive value increases. So, in fact, the efficiency of the screening program will change depending on the prevalence of the disability in that community. There are implications here for decision making with respect to targeting areas for screening and cost effectiveness of the program.

Other Forms of Screening

The Developmental Screening Checklist (DSC). This is a short version of the Denver Developmental Screening Test (DDST), and it has been useful as a prescreening test in Jamaica. The DSC requires testing of only 8 to 10 items, as opposed to approximately 30 items in the DDST. Community workers in clinics can administer it relatively easily. It reduces the need for the DDST and therefore reduces screening time. It has been a useful tool in clinics for children with disabilities for many years, but no validity data exist for this instrument.

Hearing. Two types of hearing screening are most popular: gross sound stimuli tests and field audiometers. The IESCD used both, depending on the age and understanding of the child. The Maico field audiometer measures tones from 500 to 4,000 Hertz and 5 to 80 decibels. Most children from 3 years upward can complete testing on it successfully. The Down's test, using a variety of carefully graduated toys, can be a useful test for younger children. Both these methods are for screening only, and diagnosis would still require examination by an audiologist.

Vision. There are three types of screening eye charts: the usual Snellen's chart for children who can recognize letters, the illiterate E, and the Landholt Rings. The latter may be more reliable than the E chart for illiterate children. The IESCD used the illiterate E and found it to be acceptable and usable in most children over 3 years of age. Community workers were able to use the E and Landholt C charts after basic training.

In each of the screening tests just described, except the DSC, which was not in the IESCD, no further, more extensive diagnostic work occurred on the children found to have disabilities, so these methods have not undergone adequate validity assessments.

ASSESSMENT

Assessment of children with disabilities has been a normal practice in Jamaica for over 20 years by many different organizations and individuals, but it has not, to any extent, had formal evaluation and acceptance by the professional community. Because rehabilitation has not received recognition as a human service priority, university programs, such as education and

health, that would normally undertake research, have not become established. Most of the instruments used are imports from other countries.

The IESCD developed and tested a range of questionnaires and tests that practitioners can use locally to make preliminary assessments of disability and handicap without highly specialized personnel and with some reliability. This section reviews recent developments in low-cost assessment procedures and gives guidelines for use.

Purposes and Scope of Assessment

The purposes of assessment here consist of two main groups: clinical/individual and administrative. Individual purposes include diagnosis, prediction, placement, and intervention. Administrative purposes include description, needs assessment, categorization, and planning. Collection, analysis, and documentation of individual assessment data can be useful for administrative purposes, so the discussion here is confined to clinical aspects. The authors also believe that it is not proper to assess individuals purely for academic or administrative purposes. Assessments must be of direct benefit to individuals and, in the long term, contribute to the knowledge of the natural history of disability and handicap.

Criteria for Effective Assessment Procedures

From the preceding, one can see that one criterion for effective assessment procedures is that the procedure leads to diagnosis, affords a prognosis, and guides intervention. Two other important criteria for any test are its reliability and validity in the circumstances used. A fourth requirement is the facility of its use by local personnel. In the Third World context, this means persons with limited training in the speciality area.

The concern in Jamaica, therefore, has been the validation of tests that locally available persons, both at the professional and community levels can use. Nurses, teachers, doctors, and community workers must have these techniques and the guidelines to use and act on them.

Based on these four criteria, many tests used in Jamaica, particularly for assessment of intellectual impairment, have been questionable.

Conditions to Assess

An important consideration in development of
assessment procedures is the use of consistent and
appropriate classifications and criteria for the
conditions one is assessing. Although the broad classifications of the ICIDH (WHO, 1980) have been used
in Jamaica since 1981 (Thorburn & Chernesky,
1981), the detail of this classification was too complex
for the IESCD. The main divisions of impairment, disability, and handicap, were retained, but because community workers (CWs) were used to assess disability
and handicap, a simpler and more practical classification relative to the ICIDH was adapted from the World
Health Organization (Helander, Mendis, & Nelson,
1980).

In this approach, the professionals were responsible for measurement of impairment and disability and
the CWs were responsible for identification and assessment of disability and handicap. The disability
criteria were outlined in previous articles (Thorburn,
1991) and are discussed fully elsewhere (Thorburn,
Desai, & Davidson, 1992). Cognitive, motor, speech,
hearing, and visual disabilities and fits were included.
The handicaps assessed by CWs were essentially activities of daily living—failure to reach developmental and social milestones and barriers to learning.
Thus, there were two levels of assessment in the
IESCD: those used by CWs and those used by professionals.

Assessment of Disability and Handicap

Community Worker Assessment

The CWs in the IESCD used two procedures: the Ten
Question screen with probes (TQP) and the Activities
of Daily Living Questionnaire (ADLQ). CWs tested
the TQP in two ways: its ability to determine the specific disability of a child and its accuracy in estimating severity. CWs received guidelines to assist them
in deciding on the category and severity. This procedure was found to be accurate in identifying fits as
well as motor and visual disabilities, but less so with
cognitive, speech, and hearing disabilities (Thorburn,
Desai, Paul, Malcolm, Durkin, & Davidson, 1992a).
Also, although it was effective in reducing false positive cases, there was an unacceptable increase in false
negatives. The TQP was poor in predicting disability

severity (Thorburn, Desai, Paul, Malcolm, Durkin, &
Davidson, 1992b).

The ADLQ was used to assess handicaps. A
modified version, based on evaluation of the one used
in the IESCD, appears in Figure 3.1. Although only 33
percent of children with disabilities had handicaps,
there was a close correlation between frequency of
handicaps and severity of impairment and disability.
The interrater reliability (the ability of a test to give
consistent results with different interviewers) of the
ADLQ was difficult to assess because of the low frequency of handicaps in the test population and problems in the questionnaire structure. Correction of the
latter may improve reliability. From the criterion of
usability by local CWs, the ADLQ has served as a
standard component of assessment in a community-
based rehabilitation program in Jamaica and has
worked very well.

The potential for using CWs in assessment is
only one part of the scope for this level of personnel.
For a more detailed discussion of this, see Thorburn
(1992).

Professional Assessment

The procedures used by the professional team in the
IESCD were the medical assessment form and psychological assessment procedures.:

The Medical Assessment Form. The medical as-
sesssment form included a full medical history, an
Observation of Function (see Figure 3.2), a medical
(including central nervous system) examination, vision and hearing assessment, and a format for a detailed record of impairments, disease diagnoses, severity of disabilities, and summary of general
treatment needs (Durkin, Davidson, Hasan, Khan,
Thorburn, & Zaman, 1990). The authors developed
standard procedures for all these evaluations and the
criteria for severity of the different disabilities and
listed them in detail in a Medical Evaluation Procedure Manual (available from the authors).

Psychological Assessment Procedures. The Jamaican study used a two-tier approach. The DDST was
used in all children aged 2 to 5 years, the Peabody Picture Vocabulary Test in 6- to 9-year-olds, and the
modified Child Disability Questionnaire (Belmont,
1984) in all children in the first stage.

Figure 3.1 Activities of Daily Living Questionare (ADLQ)

Name of Client.. Age ....

Interviewer.. Date ....

INSTRUCTIONS TO INTERVIEWER: Answer the questions below by circling
YES   NO   or   NA = does not apply
The responses in the second column indicates a handicap.

ACTIVITIES		RESPONSES		COMMENTS
	1	2	3	4
1. Gets up from lying without help		NO	YES	....
2. Moves both arms and legs		NO	YES	....
3. Moves both legs		NO	YES	....
4, Moves around house alone		NO	YES	....
5. Eats and drinks without help	NA	NO	YES	....
6. Washes/bathes without help	NA	NO	YES	....
7. Cleans teeth without help	NA	NO	YES	....
8. Uses toilet without help	NA	NO	YES	....
9. Dresses without help	NA	NO	YES	....
10. Understands what you say to him/her	NA	NO	YES	....
11. Expresses thoughts, needs, feelings	NA	NO	YES	....
12. Others understand his/her speech	NA	NO	YES	....
13. Plays like other children his/her age	NA	NO	YES	....
14. Goes/went to school	NA	NO	YES	....
15. Takes part in family activities	NA	NO	YES	....
16. Moves around community alone	NA	NO	YES	....
17. Takes part in community activities	NA	NO	YES	....
18. Does daily household tasks	NA	NO	YES	....
19. Works, has means of support	NA	NO	YES	....

THE FOLLOWING QUESTIONS SHOULD ONLY BE ASKED IF THE PERSON HAS A MOVING DISABILITY

20. Does he/she have aches and pains in the joints ?   YES   NO
21. If he/she has no sensation in the hands or feet,
       does he/she know how to manage this problem?   NO   YES

LOOK AT COLUMN 2 OF THE RESPONSES AND COUNT THE NUMBER OF HANDICAPS (IF ANY) THE
PERSON HAS. IF THERE ARE ANY, COMPLETE THE IPP.

Number of Handicaps .... Was an IPP completed? .... Date..............

Key :   Questions 1–4 = motor, 5–9 = self-help, 10–12 = language,
             13 & 14 = opportunities, 15–18 = social independence

Source: M. J. Thorburn et al., "Recent Developments in Low-Cost Screening and Assessment of Childhood Disabilities in Jamaica.
Part 2: Assessment," *West Indian Medical Journal, 42* (2), 1993, 46–52. Reprinted by permission.

Figure 3.2 Observation of Functions

Child's Name... Reg No...

INSTRUCTIONS
Observe the child carry out the seven tasks listed below.

As the child and guardian come into the room

1. Observe the child walking at least five steps. Look for limp, asymmetry of gait, toe walking, ataxia, involuntary movements, atrophy and contractures.
2. Welcome the child and observe the response. Does he respond, make an appropriate social response, smile, act shy, speak?
3. Invite the child to squat, pick up a small object such as a paper clip (defined size) using each hand. Observe for fisting, asymmetry of grasp, absence of pincer, difficulty in seeing object.
4. Observe the child as he stands up: Does he need to use his hands to get to standing? (Proximal muscle weakness)
5. Elicit speech by asking questions such as: What did you pick up? What is that? (Point to a cup, chair, etc.) What is this called? (Point to nose, mouth, foot, etc.) What is your name? Look for problems in hearing, comprehension and speech.
6. Ask the child to point to body parts (eyes, mouth, etc). Observe for problems in hearing, comprehension.
7. Give the child paper and pencil and ask him to draw something. Scribble (for 2-year-olds) or shapes (for 3-year-olds, square for 4- to 6-year-olds, kite for 7- to 9-year-olds). Observe comprehension and fine motor.

RATE the child in the following, after observing the tasks:

CODE   Gross motor..
Pass = 1
Fail = 2   Fine motor..
Uncertain = 3
No response = 9   Hearing..

                              Vision...

                              Speech (motor)...

                              Speech (language).......................................

                              Comprehension ....

Then complete the physical examination.

Use the following criteria to determine whether the child should have a full CNS examination:

1. If the child fails or scores uncertain in any of the seven areas rated above.
   or
2. If micro, macro, hydro-cephaly or atrophy on the physical exam.
3. If hearing, visual or other impairment is suspected.

PHYSICIAN: Do you think this child may have a nuero-muscular, visual, hearing or cognitive, impairment?

Yes _____   No _____   Not sure _____   Signed _____ Date _____

Source: M. J. Thorburn et al., "Recent Developments in Low-Cost Screening and Assessment of Childhood Disabilities in Jamaica. Part 2: Assessment," *West Indian Medical Journal, 42* (2), 1993, 46–52. Reprinted by permission.

The McCarthy Scales and Woodcock-Johnson Battery were used in the second stage for children 6 years and older. These tests were chosen because psychologists used these instruments widely in Jamaica and there is the belief that these have less cultural bias than other standard psychological tests. Colleagues in the Bangladeshi and Pakistani research studies used the Stanford Binet Test and a locally devised adaptive behavior scale (Zaman, Khan, Islam, Dixit, Shrout, & Durkin, 1991).

If an impairment or disability was found, a Rehabilitation Referral Form was used to set out the previous treatment history and recommended treatment needs. Using these procedures, the medical assessment in the hands of a generalist community physician and the psychological procedure had interrater reliabilities of 100 percent and 95 percent, respectively (Thorburn, Desai, & Davidson, 1992). The simplified Observation of Function had a sensitivity of 94 percent in detecting neurological impairment, when tested against a full neurological examination. So, if the Observation of Function assessment was negative, a CNS examination would be unnecessary. For determining motor disability in children, specific assessment of weakness, hyper- or hypotonicity, and range of motion of joints would all be indicated.

However, the medical assessment forms were much too long for regular use. We recommend retention of the symptom checklist at the beginning of the examination, the Observation of Function, and the diagnostic summary sheet.

Since the IESCD, the authors have modified the summary sheet to give the main features of the case (see Figure 3.3), including problems, treatment, and placement needs. This and the ADLQ were the instruments the authors used in 1992 in a new study of childhood disability in 439 children in care in Jamaica. The Individual Program Plan derived from the ADLQ was very useful in outlining the training and rehabilitation needs of the children. In this study, the medical assessment form of the IESCD was not used. However, the authors learned that a structured CNS guide, as used in the IESCD, is essential if primary physicians or nurse practitioners take part. In any case, medical personnel will need training or orientation to the standardized form of assessment and management aspects proposed.

Given the preceding procedures and following the recommended criteria, the medical assessment can generate good to excellent information on all disabilities except cognitive ones. In the IESCD, the final diagnosis of cognitive disability was the result of a joint decision by the doctor and psychologist. Comparison of an initial medical and final joint assessment of cognitive disability showed good concordance (Paul & Malcolm, 1988).

As with previous experience with psychological tests in Jamaica, the IESCD showed them still to be questionable, mainly because of their cultural biases. Although the tests used had a record of long use, all had their problems. For instance, the Woodcock-Johnson and McCarthy Scales were not useful for children who had not been to school. On the scores alone, the majority of children would have appeared "mentally retarded."

In the assessment, in addition to using scores of tests to arrive at a cognitive diagnosis, the psychologist also included a rating based on her clinical judgment of the child's adaptive behavior skills. If the child could perform age-appropriate skills and tasks of daily living (e.g., carry out errands; substitute for the caregiver in shopping, cooking, etc.), such a child would receive a rating of "normal" in spite of below-normal test scores.

This method of "quantifying" adaptive functioning or behavior is in accordance with the *Diagnostic and Statistical Manual* (1987) of the American Psychiatric Association for diagnosis of mental retardation. Using this process, the psychologist changed her diagnosis in favor of milder or no disability in nearly 50 percent of children who scored in the mentally retarded range.

Meeting the Criteria

The procedures described here meet most of the criteria discussed earlier. The weakest area is the validity of the psychological tests (for the reasons just given). There is a great need for experienced and specialized personnel in this field. Our psychologist had many years of experience in the Jamaican school system and was able to use her judgment about validity. Unfortunately, such professionals are rare in Jamaica and there is, as yet, no training for this profession. There is indeed a dire need for research and development into simpler forms of assessment than are currently available that teachers and guidance counselors could use to assess and manage these problems, because approximately 8 percent of children in the study had cognitive disabilities and many more had impairments.

Other Forms of Assessment

Three other assessment procedures not tested in the IESCD warrant review here. These relate to the comments on the need for simpler tests than are currently available and for detailed assessments on which to

Figure 3.3 3D Projects Clinical Case Record: Front Summary Sheet

Reg. Number .... / .... /..........

Area ....

SURNAME .... First Name ....

GUARDIAN .... First Name ....

ADDRESS...Town .... Parish ....

BIRTHDATE .... / .... /........ /   Date seen .... / .... / ..../   Age .... mos./yrs   Sex...........................

PRESENTING PROBLEM...   [...... /........]

REFERRING AGENT ....[........]   Where seen ....

DIAGNOSIS ....

DISABILITY: No/Yes

    Gross motor impairment   .... / ....Disability   severity.. [............]
        m248   m281
    Fine Motor impairment   .... / ....Disability   severity.. [............]
        m249   m282
    Hearing impairment   .... / ....Disability   severity.. [............]
        m250   m283
    Vision impairment   .... / ....Disability   severity.. [............]
        m251   m284
    Speech impairment   .... / ....Disability   severity.. [............]
        m252   m285
    Seizure   .... / ....Disability   severity.. [............]
        m253   m286

    Cognitive impairment   .... / ....Disability   severity.. [............]
                                                                          m287

    Other..
        m290

DATE   PROBLEMS   RECOMMENDATIONS

....

....

....

....

ACTION: Following up in clinic ( )   Home visiting ( )   Hearing aid ( )
               Integrated educn   ( )   Special educn ( )   Res care   ( )
               Adolescent/adult pro   ( )   Adaptive aids ( )   Other   ( )
               Refer to other   ( )   Glasses   ( )   Close file   ( )

PROGNOSIS...[......]

Doctor...CRW..

Case coordinator:.. Date .... /............/..........

Source: M. J. Thorburn et al., "Recent Developments in Low-Cost Screening and Assessment of Childhood Disabilities in Jamaica. Part 2: Assessment," *West Indian Medical Journal, 42* (2), 1993, 46–52. Reprinted by permission.

base placement and intervention plans. All three scales mentioned here permit administration by trained CWs, and these instruments cover three different age groups.

The Jamaica-Portage Guide to Early Education. This is a modification of the Portage Guide (Bluma et al., 1976). It comprises an assessment checklist with five developmental areas for children aged 0 to 6 years accompanied by a curriculum to design and teach developmental skills. It has a 20-year history of use in Jamaica for assessing severity of developmental delay. However, it is not a standardized form of assessment, and there is a growing belief that it needs revised to be more culturally relevant.

The Educational Assessment Test. This is a simple achievement test designed to find out whether a child between 6 to 9 years of age is meeting primary school targets. It is not diagnostic of any impairment or disability but displays the child's weaknesses in several basic reading, arithmetic, and prewriting skills.

The Global Assessment Scale. This is a checklist, similar to the Portage Guide, that covers four developmental and academic, behavioral, and vocational domains and is useful in assessing the skills of teenagers to indicate areas of weakness and to identify objectives for prevocational skill training. It has been in use since 1978 in Jamaica and has undergone modification to meet local needs. It is prescriptive but not diagnostic. This and the Educational Test were very useful in the study of children in care.

Recommendations for Use and Follow-Up

Action for most children with disabilities falls into one or more of the following categories (the figures in parentheses represent the percentage of 196 children with disabilities in the IESCD who needed this service) (Thorburn, Desai, & Paul, 1992):

- Community-based training and intervention (29.5 percent)—this can occur based on the results of the ADLQ
- Placement in a specialized program, particularly special education (62 percent)

- Referral for specialized assessment (21 percent)—this will often be necessary particularly in sensory disabilities where glasses or hearing aids may be important
- Medical treatment or management, such as seizure control or orthopaedic or ENT treatment (6 percent)

In general, residential care is a recommendation only if the family support system has completely broken down.

COMMUNITY ASSESSMENT OF CHILDHOOD DISABILITY: RESEARCH AND EPIDEMIOLOGICAL CONSIDERATIONS

In the past two decades, an increasing interest has developed in the assessment of the problem of childhood disability in Third World countries. Three conclusions that seem to have emerged are:

1. Rehabilitation and early intervention as practiced in the so-called developed countries, are often, if not usually, inappropriate and unaffordable for Third World countries.
2. There is a serious lack of information on disability, which means that as a health or educational problem, it will not receive as high a priority until "harder data" are available. This, in turn, leads to lack of policies and resource allocation.
3. The methods of collecting information have been inadequate and inappropriate. This is largely due to lack of professional personnel, data-collection mechanisms (PAHO, 1993), inappropriate techniques, and poor management infrastructure.

A review of seven studies of childhood disability in the Caribbean (Thorburn, 1991b) indicated that only one had generated valid, useful, and beneficial results. Some of the reasons for these poor outcomes have been:

- Unclear purposes of the study
- Inconsistent or no definitions of what the authors were surveying

- Unsuitable identification strategies
- Inadequate and unvalidated screening instruments
- Unrepresentative sampling

One common aim, which none had achieved, was a consensus on the estimate of prevalence. Some basic methodological studies were essential to overcome these constraints.

This chapter has so far described the instruments now available for screening and assessment in Jamaica (Thorburn, 1993; Thorburn, Paul, & Malcolm, 1993). This section will focus on methodological issues of the epidemiology of childhood disability and will describe the experience and lessons learned from the two studies already cited—the IESCD (Thorburn & Desai, 1989) and Assessment of Disabled Children in Care (ADCC) (Thorburn, unpublished work)—which profited from modifications made as a result of the IESCD.

Methodology

Six methods of recognizing and quantifying disabilities in the population are available (Thorburn, Desai, & Durkin, 1991). These include monitoring clinic referrals, performing developmental screening on all babies, inserting questions on disability into a census, developing a registry, asking key informants, and doing a house to house screening survey.

In the IESCD, the authors used a two-stage study design (Durkin, Davidson, Hasan, Khan, Thorburn, & Zaman, 1990):

- Stage 1 was a population-based, house-to-house survey of 2- to 9-year-old children that identified disability-type problems using the TQ as the screening instrument.
- Stage 2 was the assessment of all the screen-positive children plus a sample of screen-negative children to assess the sensitivity of the screening instruments (Thorburn, Desai, Paul, Malcolm, Durkin, & Davidson, 1992a, 1992b).

In the Assessment of Disabled Children in Care (ADCC) study, carried out in 1992, the authors assessed 439 children, thought to have disabilities, who were under the care of the Childrens' Services of the Ministry of Local Government, Youth and Sports. No particular sampling was necessary, and the identification and assessment instruments described in the previous sections were used. From these two studies, the authors have drawn the following conclusions.

Purposes of Surveys and Situation Studies

A clear purpose of the study is necessary because different types of surveys are important for different purposes. There must also be a humane philosophy behind the study so that the target group will benefit either in terms of immediate intervention or prevention in the future. If this is absent, the group will simply feel exploited and frustrated and will unlikely want to participate in future studies. There is a real danger that the results will just get filed and shelved without implementation of any intervention. At the very least, surveys should advance scientific thinking and problem solving. Some of the most important purposes include:

- Improving the methodology for assessment or intervention (this was the primary purpose of the IESCD)
- Identifying and describing a population needing services
- Developing new services or improving existing services
- Planning future services by analyzing needs and identifying trends
- Examining prevalence and identifying and quantifying risk factors that will help formulate prevention programs

Simply doing "head counts" to generate or compare numbers is unacceptable. First, this type of survey tends to be counterproductive because the magnitude and costs uncovered just bewilder and daunt administrators. Surveys can absorb a lot of resources in personnel, time, and analysis, often more than anticipated, so if intervention is not part of the overall plan, the survey data may be wasteful. Of the seven surveys in the Caribbean, only one had direct benefits that would not otherwise have been possible without the survey. Second, "head counts" do not generate information on the needs of the target population. In the IESCD, in the 196 children with disabilities identified,

60 percent needed some form of specialized education but only 30 percent needed rehabilitation (Thorburn, Desai, & Paul, 1992). These needs were not solely dependent on the category or severity of disability.

Study Design

Study design is clearly dependent on the purpose of the study and will range from experimental designs to largely descriptive approaches with no intervention component. In the community setting, the use of an experimental design to ascertain etiology is fraught with ethical issues and, at best, one would resort to quasi-experimental approaches. For instance, when investigating the influence of cannabis use on cognitive disability and psychosocial development in Jamaica, researchers can utilize population members who have used the drug as part of their own cultural practices. The experimental method, however, is a powerful approach for testing new interventions at the community level because it allows for comparison or control group validation of outcomes. The evolution of rehabilitation services in Jamaica through the 3D projects saw a phased implementation in different parishes that allowed for ongoing comparisons and cross evaluations.

For development and testing of identification methodologies, a survey similar to the IESCD is recommended (Durkin, Davidson, Hasan, Khan, Thorburn, & Zaman, 1990), with a two-stage design (field identification and professional assessment) and a control group. If the screening instruments have known validity and are sensitive to the problem under investigation, a control group will not be necessary.

Stein, Durkin, Davidson, Hasan, Thorburn, and Zaman (1992) recommend a control group when administering an instrument in any country for the first time because, for example, sensitivity of the Ten Questions is likely to vary from one country to another. Thus, the two-stage design makes economic use of professionals.

For the straight identification of groups of children needing community-based rehabilitation (CBR), researchers can use a similar approach but without the control group. If early intervention is part of the plan, a developmental screening device will be necessary, in addition to the Ten Questions, because the latter has validity data only on children 2 years old and up. Two stages are necessary because not all children will have identified disabilities, and it is important to identify those needing referral services. The actual CBR program could be initiated based on the community workers' assessments (Thorburn et al., 1993) even before completion of the professional assessments because development of individual programs can result from information on the Activities of Daily Living Questionnaire.

For development of new or improved services for a known population, such as in the ADCC survey, the two stages can become consolidated into one; community workers can identify and measure the disabilities and handicaps, and professionals can confirm the impairments, make clinical diagnoses, prescribe medical treatment, and make recommendations regarding referrals and service needs. The actual procedures used can be any of those described earlier in this chapter. In the ADCC study, all the tests were used because the study group included individuals ranging in age from 1 to 20 years.

For planning future services, probably an initial comprehensive survey will be necessary, followed by rapid community assessments using community workers only from time to time and place to place. In these surveys, changes in trends will be important.

Risk Factor Identification

Planning prevention programs requires identification and quantification of risk factors. Use of a cohort approach to assessment of risk, which is valuable in studying chronic diseases, is problematic for childhood disability, particularly from the viewpoint of measurement of the exposure and outcome variables involved. Risk factors for childhood disability are mostly in the perinatal and postneonatal periods and, as such, risk factor quantification becomes very challenging.

If one uses incidence as an indication of risk, then measuring the incidence of disability in relation to the basic epidemiological variables of time, place, and person can be a useful premise for decision making. If one uses disability prevalence, then risk quantification becomes less sensitive because both ongoing and new cases get captured. Because disability tends to be long term and determination of onset tends to be methodologically difficult, prevalence will have to stand as a crude indicator of risk. This does not detract from its use as an indicator of burden.

The cross-sectional community surveys described here have to be large enough to minimize error of the prevalence estimate. Because some of the disabilities are quite rare in the population, prevalence figures have wide confidence limits, indicating poor accuracy. This was the case in the Jamaican survey (Paul, Desai, & Thorburn, 1992) with just under 5,500 children. Researchers can calculate adequate sample size based on an estimate of the lowest prevalence of the target factor and the acceptable confidence limit. However, the decision regarding sample size may also rest on availability of resources.

Nevertheless, the most obvious medical diagnoses are readily recognizable, and it is generally possible to identify the main risk factors if one collects a wide enough spectrum of data so as to include social, economic, and cultural variables. Cross-sectional studies can, however, generate databases that can be useful for assessment of risk through case control approaches (Thorburn & Paul, 1992). The case control study in this respect is reasonably efficient in terms of time when compared with cohort methodology.

Representative Sampling

The size, type, and limits of the sample required for any survey will depend on the purposes. Only where methodological requirements or risk factor analysis are the main purposes is it necessary to have large numbers. In the IESCD, the population-based sample of 5,461 children was adequate for methodological purposes but not really for prevalence and risk factor information (Paul, Desai, & Thorburn, 1992).

If the reason for the survey is to identify cases for a service, the choice of site and its limits for the sample will depend on where the service will be delivered. If the survey is mainly for long-term planning, samples typical of different demographic, geographic, and other important variables that might affect disability prevalence will be necessary. The prevalence measures obtained in the IESCD study are outcomes of a sample of children from a larger population in which case sampling errors must enter into consideration.

Response rate is a factor that will affect size of the eventual sample. Where childhood disability is a stigma and has strong links to cultural and folk beliefs, as it is in parts of rural Jamaica, then a smaller than estimated sample size may be an eventuality, especially if children are to attend for assessment. Accessibility is also an important factor that necessitates expenditure by the study group on transportation and outreach workers.

Definitions of Target Population. This is still an area of controversy and research in disability generally, not only in the Third World. Defining *disability* is a rather complex issue because it involves the outcome of an abnormal process—a process which itself can often become defined in disease terms and used as a label of the disability problem if one is not careful. The risk here is to ignore the functional consequences of the process. Disability definitions are efforts to capture these functional deficiencies and put them in well-structured measurable terms. There are entire journals and newsletters devoted to applications of the ICIDH (WHO, 1980). In the IESCD, the authors followed the ICIDH partially because of its complexity and its use by nonspecialized personnel. In seeking a solution to this problem, a lesser known set of definitions was used from another WHO manual, *Training the Disabled in the Community* (Helander, Mendis, & Nelson, 1980), which dealt mainly with disabilities and handicaps. In considering the taxonomy on disability, the criterion of utility must be paramount. Our experience of this combination of the two WHO approaches was very satisfactory on the whole, and we recommend it (Thorburn, Desai, & Davidson, 1992; Thorburn, 1994, unpublished work).

Does disability prevalence stand up to scrutiny of an appropriate health indicator? Hansluwka (1985) argues that "one of the problems with a disability-based indicator of the health status of the population is the doubts one has to entertain whether disability is a single, one-dimensional phenomenon which can be measured in an objective way across the world." Progress is taking place on this front, though slowly, even in the IESCD where survey instruments for measuring disability were specifically designed to achieve comparability across countries. Disability, therefore, can live up to the scrutiny of international comparisons if researchers clearly agree on and follow methodological issues.

Identification Strategies

In addition to developing instruments for identification, one also needs to consider how to identify cases. Six methods of recognizing and quantifying disabilities in the population are available (Thorburn, Desai, & Durkin, 1991). These include monitoring clinic referrals, performing developmental screening on all babies, inserting questions on disability in a census, developing a registry, asking key informants, and doing a house-to-house screening survey.

In developed countries, there is usually a case identification and management infrastructure from which researchers can obtain and ascertain specific cases. Some communities intermittently practice developmental screenings that identify at-risk children and follow them until a definite diagnosis is available. These services virtually do not exist in the Caribbean, although special clinics may be able to provide some data. One then has a choice of a "key informant" survey, where persons knowledgeable of family problems identify cases that they know, or a house-to-house survey, an expensive and time-consuming strategy. Unfortunately, the key-informant survey is ineffective in Third World countries (Belmont, 1984; Thorburn, Desai, & Durkin, 1991), so the more expensive survey is necessary. The key-informant method is not a suitable alternative to the survey method for the purposes of prevalence assessment because it would grossly underestimate disability prevalence. One would expect, however, that as services become available and known to the community, lay referral of children with disabilities would increase and key informants would become more knowledgeable than they were prior to availability of such services. Clearly, parents themselves are generally good referral agents for disability, although their effectiveness would correlate with level of severity of the disability. Also, cultural beliefs can affect interpretation.

Data Management and Analysis

In all of the preceding five situations, the data-collection, management, and analysis aspects need to be considered. In the IESCD, although the authors extensively planned this aspect, the actual practice in the three participating countries exposed numerous constraints. Each study site (Bangladesh, Pakistan, and Jamaica) had 11 common databases for the various questionnaires of the study. Members of the research team entered and stored data using dBase III+ software. Because of the interest in the assessment aspect, Jamaica had four additional files. This required a full-time research assistant for three years. Painstaking, accurate, and patient detail was necessary for this person to develop and maintain integrity of the databases. Even then, this person was unable to complete cleaning of the data on time, and the analyses proved to be time consuming. Short-term use of a mainframe computer for the handling of the large quantity of data greatly facilitated the data analysis. Five years after completion of the study, various aspects are still being analyzed, and much more remains.

All the sites experienced basic problems. A hurricane and lack of electricity for four months interrupted the Jamaican study, Bangladesh experienced floods, and Pakistan had communal strife. These are realities that researchers cannot easily predict and plan into their schedules. In one case, the computer purchased was very slow in processing data, which led to unacceptable delays at crucial points in time and delay in the final report. Storage capacity for the large files and manipulation of the data required more sophisticated programs and capabilities than were available. The authors became very dependent on North American colleagues for handling aspects of the data. The collaborative arrangements, however, enhanced the operating capability.

So, unless one intends to implement a full program of research with ample staff and time for analysis, one must not undertake a study such as the IESCD without serious consideration. For the ADCC, a survey of 439 children with disabilities, similar questionnaires were used, except that the medical assessment form was smaller in length than that used in the IESCD and the only computerized sheet was the summary sheet. This allowed for inclusion and analysis of all essential data necessary for providing the information needed for individual and overall program planning. If more detailed research information than that provided on the summary sheet is necessary, then we can enter and analyze more data from files already structured for computer analysis.

In reviewing the experience, the use and development of questionnaires and databases has allowed the authors to be more adaptable and flexible for future projects than prior to this experience.

SITUATION ANALYSES

This type of study is often employed by United Nations agencies to describe the current situation of a particular problem or topic in a country or a region. It may or may not include a field survey. The latter has the limitation of analyzing only one aspect of a problem, usually the magnitude. A situation analysis examines attitudes of the population toward the problem, needs of affected persons, existing resources attempting to cope with the problems, and potential resources that one could mobilize. One may use a variety of questionnaires and approaches, but persons conducting the study would mostly aim their questions at service providers and professionals working in the field rather than going out and doing a field study. There is scope for mixing quantitative and qualitative approaches, such as the Delphi and focus group methods. Detailed accounts of how to do situation analyses, given by WHO (Helander, 1984) and ActionAid, India (Murthy and Gopalan, 1992), appear elsewhere for interested readers. Therefore, that information is not given here.

A situation analysis thus looks at potential solutions as well as stating the problems. Because a field survey is not always available, the situation analysis may indicate the need for one. It is thus a useful way of beginning to look at a problem and how others are attempting to address it. It may also prevent unnecessary field work.

CONCLUSIONS

The approaches for screening and assessment of childhood disabilities described here, although not perfect as yet, make maximum use of persons who are willing and able and promote economic use of professionals who can spend their time on doubtful or difficult cases or those in need of professional management. The assessment aspect also brings the possibility of community capability closer together than was the case prior to the intervention. However, changes in professional attitudes and training of medical and nonmedical personnel in the new procedures will be necessary, as will changes in the system similar to those of primary health care, so that community-level persons can become integrated into existing services, whose roles need expanded. Although early intervention and rehabilitation are necessary in the community and there does not have to be a new and specialized administration, strengthening of linkages and lines of referral and support are necessary, as they are in primary health care.

It is hoped that the accounts given in this chapter will be of use to persons in the field contemplating the gathering of information about disability in Third World countries. The Jamaican experience described here has opened up the field of community-based services and allows one to investigate and act independently instead of always having to rely on expertise from more developed countries.

NOTE

This chapter brings together, coherently, research material previously published in papers in the West Indian Medical Journal with additional material previously unpublished. Much of the work reported here received support from grant no. REA-JM-1-87-68 from the Board on Science and Technology for International Development of the National Research Council, the National Academy of Sciences, Washington, DC.

Analysis of the data occurred at the Free University, Amsterdam, Faculty of Human Movement Sciences, with a grant from the Bishop Bekker Institute, Utrecht, the Netherlands.

We are grateful to our colleagues at the Department of Social and Preventive Medicine, University of the West Indies (Mrs. P. Desai), Dhaka University (Drs. S. Zaman and N. Khan), the Jinnah Postgraduate Medical Centre, Karachi (Drs. M. and Z. Hasan), and the Gertrude Sergievsky Center, Columbia University, New York (Drs. L. Belmont, S. Dixit, M. Durkin, P. Shrout, and Z. Stein) for their collaboration and contributions, and to Professors Brian Hopkins and Adri Vermeer and Mr. T. Westra at the Free University for their interest and support in the analysis of the material.

REFERENCES

Belmont, L. (1984). *The international pilot study on severe childhood disability: Final report.* Available from the Gertrude Sergievsky Center, Columbia University, New York.

Bluma, S. M., Shearer, M. S., Frohman, A. M., & Hilliard, J. M. (1976). *The Portage guide to early education: Checklist, curriculum and card file.* Available from CESA 12, P.O. Box 564, Portage, WI.

Clarke, A. D. B., & Clarke, A. M. (1974). Mental retardation and behavioral change. *British Med. Bulletin, 30,* 179–185.

Durkin, M., Davidson, L., Hasan, M., Khan, N., Thorburn, M. J., & Zaman, S. (1990). Screening for childhood disabilities in community settings. In M. J. Thorburn & K. Marfo (Eds.), *Practical approaches to childhood disability in developing countries* (pp. 179–198). Spanish Town, Jamaica: 3D Projects.

Durkin, M., Zaman, S., Thorburn, M. J., Hasan, M., & Davidson, L. (1991). Population-based studies of childhood disability in developing countries. *International Journal of Mental Health, 20,* 47–60.

Feinstein, A. R. (1977). *Clinical biostatistics* (pp. 101–102). St. Louis: C. V. Mosby.

Frankenburg, W., & Dodds, J. (1967). The Denver Developmental Screening Test. *Journal of Pediatrics, 71,* 181–191.

Hansluwka, H. E. (1985). Measuring the health of populations: Indicators and interpretations. *Soc. Sci Medicine, 20,* (12), 1207–1224.

Helander, E. (1984). *Managing community based rehabilitation.* Geneva: WHO, RHB.94.

Helander, E., Mendis, P., & Nelson, G. (1980). *Training the disabled in the community.* Geneva: WHO, RHB80/1.

Helander, E., Mendis P., & Nelson, G. (1983). *Training the disabled in the community, version 3.* Geneva: WHO, RHB 83/1.

Murthy, S. P., & Gopalan, L. (1992). *Workbook on community based rehabilitation services.* Available from Disability Division, ActionAid India, PB 5406, 3 Resthouse Rd., Bangalore 560–001, India, 14–20.

PAHO/WHO. (1994). *A situation analysis of disability and rehabilitation in the English speaking Caribbean.* Available from PAHO Regional Office, Bridgetown, Barbados.

Paul, T. J., Desai, P., & Thorburn, M. J. (1992). The prevalence of childhood disability and related medical diagnoses in Clarendon, Jamaica. *West Indian Medical Journal, 41,* 8–11.

Paul, T. J., & Malcolm, L. M. (1988). Paper presented at the Eighth Congress of the International Association for the Scientific Study of Mental Deficiency, Dublin, Ireland.

Siegmann, A. (1979). A classification of sociomedical health indicators: Perspectives for health administrators and health planners. In J. Elinson & A. Siegmann (Eds.), *Socio-medical health indicators* (pp. 197–213). Farmingdale, NY: Baywood.

Stein, Z., Durkin, M., Davidson, L., Hasan, M., Thorburn, M. J., & Zaman, S. (1992). Guidelines for assessing children with mental retardation in community settings. In *Assessment of People with Mental Retardation* (pp. 28–64). Geneva: WHO, WHO/MNH/PSF/92.3.

Thorburn, M. J. (1981). In Jamaica: Community aides for pre-school disabled children. *Assignment Children, 53/54,* 117–134.

Thorburn, M. J. (1991a). A community approach to helping disabled children in Jamaica. *International Journal of Mental Health, 20,* 61–75.

Thorburn, M. J. (1991b). The disabled child in the Caribbean: A situation analysis. *West Indian Medical Journal, 40,* 172–179.

Thorburn, M. J. (1992). Training community workers in a simplified approach to early detection, assessment and intervention. *Journal of Practical Approaches to Developmental Handicap, 16,* 24–29.

Thorburn, M. J. (1993). Recent developments in low cost screening and assessment in childhood disabilities in Jamaica. Part 1: Screening. *West Indian Medical Journal, 42,* 10–12.

Thorburn, M. J., & Chernesky, B. (1981). *Introduction to developmental disabilities.* Available from 3D Projects, 14 Monk Street, Spanish Town, Jamaica.

Thorburn, M. J., & Desai, P. (1989). *Low cost methods for the identification and assessment of childhood disability in Jamaica: Final Report.* Kingston: Dept. of Social and Preventive Medicine, University of the West Indies.

Thorburn, M. J., Desai, P., & Davidson, L. (1992). Categories, classes, and criteria: Experience from a survey in Jamaica. *Disability and Rehabilitation, 14,* 122–132.

Thorburn, M. J., Desai, P., & Durkin, M. (1991). A comparison of the key informant and community survey methods in the identification of childhood disability. *Ann Epidem, 1,* 255–261.

Thorburn, M. J., Desai, P., Paul, T. J., Malcolm, L. M., Durkin, M., & Davidson, L. (1992a). Identification of childhood disability in Jamaica: The Ten Question Screen. *International Journal of Rehabilitation Research, 15,* 115–127.

Thorburn, M. J., Desai, P., Paul, T. J., Malcolm, L. M., Durkin, M., & Davidson, L. (1992b). Identification of childhood disability in Jamaica: The Ten Question Screen. *International Journal of Rehabilitation Research, 15,* 262–270.

Thorburn, M. J., & Paul, T. J. (1992). A preliminary report of perinatal risk factors in childhood disability in Clarendon, Jamaica. In C. Berchel, E. Papiernik, & F. de Caunes (Eds.), *Perinatal problems of islands in relation to the prevention of handicaps* (pp. 246–253). Editions INSERM, 101 Rue de Tolbiac, 75654 Paris, Cedex 13, France.

Thorburn, M. J., Paul, T. J., & Desai, P. (1992). Service needs of children with disabilities in Jamaica. *International Journal of Rehabilitation Research, 15,* 31–38.

Thorburn, M. J., Paul, T. J., & Malcolm, L. M. (1993). Recent developments in low cost methods of screening and assessment of childhood disabilities in Jamaica. Part 2: Assessment. *West Indian Medical Journal, 42,* 46–52.

World Health Organization. (1980). *International classification of impairments, disabilities and handicaps.* Geneva: Author.

Zaman, S., Khan, N. Z., Islam, S., Dixit, S., Shrout, P., & Durkin, M. (1991). Validity of the "Ten Questions" for screening childhood disability: Results from urban Bangladesh. *International Journal of Epidemiology, 19,* 613–620.

DISEASES AND DISORDERS

Although the diseases and disorders that affect children and adolescents do not generally have the same mortality concerns during childhood and adolescence as they do during adulthood, concerns regarding physical disorders and diseases during these years of growth are important for at least two reasons. First, they can have an adverse impact on self-image (including body image), which can affect children's subsequent mental and physical health. Second, patterns of behavior learned during these developmental years are likely to affect future behavioral patterns as adults. In addition, there are some disorders (e.g., eating disorders) that usually begin during these developmental years.

This section of the book reviews several disorders especially important for children and adolescents. The chapters included here generally address issues of diagnosis and etiology as well as assessment and treatment considerations. In addition, each chapter highlights specific areas of importance for the particular disorder discussed. Chapter 4 stresses the necessity of training self-management skills to children with diabetes. Chapter 5 discusses health risks associated with anorexia and bulimia as well as psychiatric comorbity and possible risk factors for development of the disorders. The authors of Chapter 6 review literature addressing combined pharmacotherapy and biofeedback therapy for headache. Chapter 7 presents information regarding educational and learning problems associated with epilespy as well as the concern of accurately distinguishing seizures from pseudoseizures. Various developmental and psychological factors related to burns and the prevention of burns are focused on in Chapter 8. Chapters 9 and 10 highlight the importance of adaptation to cystic fibrosis and asthma, respectively, and the role of medication adherence as well as problems in these disorders.

CHAPTER 4

DIABETES SELF-MANAGEMENT IN CHILDREN

Laurie Ruggiero, UNIVERSITY OF RHODE ISLAND
Debbie J. Javorsky, UNIVERSITY OF RHODE ISLAND

Diabetes mellitus is one of the most common childhood metabolic diseases. It affects over 127,000 children and adolescents in the United States (ADA, 1996). Diabetes is a chronic disease that results from a failure of the body to effectively metabolize glucose, the primary fuel of the body. In Type 1 (formerly juvenile-onset diabetes) or insulin-dependent diabetes mellitus (IDDM), this occurs because the pancreas ceases production of insulin, a hormone needed to metabolize glucose to fuel the body (Blackard, 1991; Olefsky, 1992; Lernmark, 1991). As a result, accumulation of glucose in the blood results in elevated blood glucose levels or hyperglycemia. Replacement of insulin by daily injections of exogenous insulin are needed for survival. Although Type 1 diabetes can be diagnosed at any age, it is generally diagnosed during childhood or adolescence (Olefsky, 1992; Lernmark, 1991). Therefore, discussion of diabetes in this chapter will be restricted to Type 1 diabetes, since it accounts for the majority of cases of diabetes in children (Cox & Gonder-Frederick, 1992).

Before focusing on Type 1 diabetes, it is important to mention the second primary type of diabetes, Type 2 diabetes, often referred to as non-insulin dependent diabetes mellitus (NIDDM). Although Type 2 diabetes will not be covered in this chapter because

it has been considered rare in youth, it is notable that there is a rapidly increasing prevalence of this condition in adolescence (Pinhas-Hamiel, & Zeitler, 1997; Pinhas-Hamiel, Dolan, Daniels, Standiford, Khoury, & Zeitler, 1996). In general, this condition is associated with obesity coupled with a low activity level in this adolescent population. It is important, therefore, that the possibility of this condition not be overlooked in obese adolescents. As the prevalence rates increase in adolescents, pediatric health psychologists need to become more familiar with this condition and its management.

TYPE 1 DIABETES MELLITUS

Type 1 diabetes mellitus usually has an acute onset, although some children may have residual insulin production for a period of time after onset. With Type 1 diabetes, the body cannot make use of the glucose in the blood for fuel and the body essentially experiences a state of starvation. As a result, glucose accumulates in the blood and several physiological responses are triggered in an attempt to compensate for these problems. These compensatory responses are associated with a number of presenting symptoms including polyphagia (increased appetite), polyuria (excess urination), polydipsia (increased thirst), dry mouth, blurred vision, fatigue, and weight loss despite excessive eating (Olefsky, 1992; Lernmark, 1991).

Type 1 diabetes may also present with acute cognitive changes because the brain is not getting the glucose needed for fuel (Hoffman, Speelman, Hinnen, Conley, Guthrie, & Knapp, 1989; Holmes, Hayford, Gonzalez, & Weydert, 1983; Stevens, McKane, Bell, Bell, King, & Hayes, 1989). The body may metabolize fat to compensate for lack of available fuel from glucose. This process produces ketones, which are by-products of fat metabolism that accumulate in the blood. The accumulation of ketones results in diabetic ketoacidosis (DKA) or ketosis, a serious acute complication. If left untreated, ketoacidosis can lead to coma and ultimately death (Olefsky, 1992; Davidson, Galloway, & Chance, 1991). Additionally, if blood glucose levels drop too low, a condition called hypoglycemia, an insulin reaction can occur. An insulin reaction can rapidly lead to a number of physical and cognitive symptoms, including trembling, fatigue, sweating, pounding heart, cognitive disorientation, and convulsions. Ultimately coma and death may occur if not treated (Davidson, Galloway, & Chance, 1991).

As is clear from this description, diabetes is a serious condition. Effective management of this disease includes a lifelong and complex self-management routine. There is an important role for health psychology in the management of this disorder, especially in children. Thus, the objective of this chapter is to highlight the role of health psychology in the management of diabetes in pediatric populations. Therefore, the chapter will first provide a brief overview of diabetes management, with a particular focus on self-management. The remainder of the chapter will focus on reviewing the research on diabetes self-management adherence and the factors that influence self-management in pediatric populations. A biopsychosocial perspective will be introduced and used as the organizing framework of this chapter. This will include an overview of the biological, psychosocial, environmental, and provider/treatment factors that may have an impact on self-management in pediatric populations. Last, an overview of interventions targeting self-management adherence in children and suggestions for future research will be provided.

DIABETES SELF-MANAGEMENT

Since the body cannot regulate glucose metabolism on its own, this important function must be carefully self-managed by the child with diabetes and his or her parents with the guidance of a medical team. Self-management of blood glucose levels involves replacing the specific functioning of the pancreas. The goal of diabetes self-management is to maintain blood glucose levels in a stable target range that is close to the normal range for individuals who do not have diabetes and thereby avoid high (hyperglycemia) or low (hypoglycemia) blood glucose levels (Betschart, 1997). The specific target range may be individualized and may vary somewhat for children of different ages (see Betschart, 1997 for specific recommendations). It is also important to note that although maintenance of consistent glucose levels in the target range is the ideal goal, glucose levels outside of this range are likely to occur no matter how carefully the diabetes management plan is followed.

The specific day-to-day tasks of diabetes self-management include taking insulin injections to replace the insulin generally produced by the body, as well as carefully following an eating and exercise plan. Generally, multiple insulin injections are taken each day to make sure the child has enough insulin for a 24-hour period. Some individuals with diabetes may receive their insulin through the use of an insulin infusion pump (Albisser, 1991). Insulin infusion pumps more closely mimic normal functioning of the pancreas by providing continuous delivery of insulin. Close monitoring of blood glucose levels is also needed to adjust the insulin dose to fluctuations in the levels. The pump is a small battery-powered mechanical device worn externally. Insulin is infused through a needle inserted under the skin and taped in place. The pump has been shown to improve blood glucose control (Bojsen, Deckert, Kolendorf, & Lorup, 1979; Riley, Silverstein, Rosenbloom, Spillar, & McCallum, 1980; Rosenstock, Strowig, & Raskin, 1985), but it is less often recommended for children for a variety of reasons. For example, it requires more attention and care; it may interfere with certain activities, such as sports; and it requires a high level of motivation and decision making.

Because the child's body does not produce insulin to compensate for foods eaten, the child's eating plan must focus on the timing of meals, along with the type and quantity of food eaten. In addition to the general benefits of exercise, regular exercise is especially important in self-management of diabetes because it can help lower blood glucose levels. The individual with diabetes, however, needs to be sensitive to his or her blood glucose levels when engaging in vigorous exercise. For example, a child should test his or her blood glucose level before exercising and should carry a snack to compensate for possible hypoglycemia. To aid in tracking changes in blood glucose levels and identifying the need for changes in the self-management program, individuals must also self-test their blood glucose levels. The commonly recommended frequency of self-monitoring of blood glucose (SMBG) levels is at least four times each day, usually before meals and before bedtime (ADA, 1995; Younger, Brink, Barnett, Wentworth, Leibovich, & Madden, 1985). The child should test more frequently in special situations, such as when ill or before engaging in vigorous exercise.

Many individuals are also expected to make complex decisions about modifying their self-management program based on changes in their blood glucose levels. That is, changes in any of the key behaviors (eating, exercise, insulin use) can have an impact on blood glucose levels and may require further compensatory behavior to correct excessive increases or decreases. For example, if a child's blood glucose level is greatly elevated because he or she attended a birthday party and overate, a larger dose of insulin may be required. On the other hand, if the child engaged in vigorous exercise, his or her blood glucose level may be low and additional food may be required. As is underscored in this description, self-management of diabetes involves an extremely complex set of daily behaviors, is often inconvenient and unpleasant for a child, and places challenging demands on the child and his or her family.

Importance of Effective Management of Blood Glucose

Diabetes is associated with a number of long-term complications. These primarily include retinopathy (vision impairment), nephropathy (kidney disease), neuropathy (nerve damage), cardiovascular disease, and stroke (Olefsky, 1992; Cox & Gonder-Frederick,

1992; Surwit, Feinglos, & Scovern, 1983). In medical management of diabetes, it was generally believed that maintaining tight control of blood glucose levels would be associated with fewer long-term complications (Cahill, Etzwiler, & Freinkel, 1976). Until relatively recently, however, this assumption had never been adequately empirically tested. Results of a landmark study, the Diabetes Control and Complications Trial (DCCT) (1993), have had a momentous impact on the management of diabetes. This study addressed the question of whether an intensive management program with the goal of maintaining blood glucose concentrations in the normal range could decrease the frequency and severity of long-term complications. The study included 1,441 individuals between the ages of 13 and 39 years from 29 centers throughout the United States and Canada. Participants were randomly assigned to either a conventional diabetes management program or an intensive program. The conventional program involved one or two daily injections of insulin, daily self-monitoring of glucose levels, and education about diet and exercise. This group visited a health care provider every three months. The conventional treatment goals included absence of ketonuria and symptoms attributable to glycosuria or hyperglycemia, freedom from severe or frequent hypoglycemia, and maintenance of normal growth, development, and ideal body weight.

The intensive management program included three or more insulin injections each day (or use of an insulin infusion pump), blood glucose self-monitoring at least four times each day, along with diet and exercise recommendations. The intensive therapy goals included preprandial blood glucose concentrations between 70 and 120 mg/dl, postprandial concentrations of less than 180 mg/dl, a weekly 3:00 A.M. measurement greater than 65 mg/dl, and glycosylated hemoglobin, measured monthly, within the normal range. Additionally, this group self-adjusted daily insulin dose based on glucose self-monitoring results, dietary intake, and exercise. The intensive management group visited a health care provider at least once a month and received frequent phone contact to review and adjust daily regimens.

Participants were followed an average of 6.5 years (range: 3 to 9 years.). Repeated measures of blood glucose control and complications were taken throughout the study. In terms of study adherence, 99 percent of the participants completed the study and more than 95 percent of all scheduled assessments were completed. There were significant differences in blood glucose control between the groups in the expected direction. The intensive management program was associated with tighter glucose control, and, in turn, tighter control was linked to fewer complications of diabetes. In particular, results indicated significant differences in the onset and progression of retinopathy, nephropathy, and neuropathy in favor of the individuals participating in an intensive management program. Further support for the intensive program was garnered by findings that no significant differences occurred in measures of quality of life. That is, the intensive group did not report a reduced quality of life due to the increased demands on them from following the intensive program.

Benefits of this intensive approach did not come without costs. Financial costs of the intensive program compared with the conventional program were about two times greater. Medical costs included an incidence of severe hypoglycemia about three times higher in the intensive management group. Additionally, the intensive management group gained an average of 4.6 kg. more weight than the conventional group at the five-year assessment. Behavioral costs included increased time and behavioral demands on the individual following an intensive program. Although emotional costs have not been explored, it is likely that there may be increased concern or anxiety about following the intensive regimen, especially for parents of children with diabetes, due to the aversive nature of hypoglycemia.

It is important to underscore that the DCCT did not include any prepubertal children and only a small group of adolescents (approximately 20 percent of the total sample) was included (Drash, 1993). The adolescent sample had the same pattern of results as the adult sample (Brink & Moltz, 1997). As highlighted earlier, even the more conventional approach creates tremendous challenges in adherence for individuals, especially youth. Careful consideration is suggested when generalizing the results of the DCCT to children, and application of the findings from the DCCT to children should be done with caution.

Useful advice on the application of the DCCT findings to youth can be found in the following conclusions drawn by Brink and Moltz (1997):

Applying the message of the DCCT, increasing the blood glucose monitoring and feedback, establishing and revising glucose target goals, and *doing so safely* should now be the modus operandi for Type 1 diabetes care. This should apply to infants, toddlers, older children, and teenagers while always striving to minimize or prevent severe episodes of hypoglycemia—and recognizing that it remains impossible to always have perfect blood glucose control. While this goal is not achievable for all, *any improvement in glycemia* translates into reduced risks for long-term complications.

These authors also point out that when applying the results of the DCCT to young children, the following recommendations are useful: continued close parental supervision of the regimen; flexibility in the daily regimen to match the child's eating and activity patterns; continued age-appropriate diabetes education for the child and parents; and sensitivity to the developmentally appropriate needs and issues of the child. (See Brink and Moltz, 1997, for recommendations for age-specific applications of the DCCT results in children.) Continued work needs to be focused on how to generalize from the DCCT results to children and how best to assist individuals in adhering with such an intensive program.

It is also notable that the group chosen to participate in the DCCT was very carefully selected to include the most motivated and adherent individuals. Therefore, the burden will be on behavioral scientists to examine the feasibility of following such an intensive management program with a general population of individuals with diabetes. Furthermore, it will be the role of the health psychologist to develop effective intervention programs to facilitate adherence with the complex self-management behaviors required in an intensive management program.

Self-Management Adherence

Self-management of diabetes is a core component of successful management of this medical disorder. That is, once the diabetes management plan is determined, most of the burden of management is on the child and family to perform the daily behaviors necessary to maintain control of blood glucose levels. Given the complexity and lifelong duration of diabetes self-management, it follows that adherence with such a program would be a challenge for anyone, especially children and adolescents (Haynes, 1979). Indeed, research dating back from the 1960s to the present has suggested that adherence to diabetes self-management is often poor (LaGreca, 1990; Watkins, Williams, Martin, Hogan, & Anderson, 1967). However, as highlighted by Glasgow and colleagues (1991), it is difficult to present specific rates of adherence for diabetes self-management because of the different conceptualizations and measures used to define this construct. In particular, interpretation of reported adherence rates is often difficult because adherence was defined using absolute levels of self-management behaviors (e.g., number of glucose tests conducted) or standardized scores for composite indices of adherence.

Furthermore, many studies have focused on metabolic control as the primary measure of diabetes self-management. No consistent, clinically significant relationships have been found between diabetes self-management adherence and diabetes control (Cox, Taylor, Nowacek, Holly-Wilcox, & Pohl, 1984; Glasgow, McCaul, & Schafer, 1987; Hanson, Henggeler, & Burghen, 1987b; Johnson, Freund, Silverstein, Hansen, & Malone, 1990; Reid & Appleton, 1991). There are a number of reasons why this may be the case. In particular, glucose control is influenced by other important factors unrelated to adherence, such as illness (Travis, 1987) and physiological changes that occur in the developing child (Amiel, Sherwin, Somonson, Lauritano, & Tamborlane, 1986; Drash & Becker, 1978; Hanson & Henggeler, 1984; Johnson et al., 1992). Furthermore, appropriateness of the prescribed regimen, especially the insulin protocol, plays a key role in diabetes control.

Nevertheless, even with challenges faced in defining, measuring, and reporting adherence rates, a number of consistent findings have emerged. In particular, diabetes self-management adherence is not a unitary or global construct (Glasgow et al., 1991; Johnson, Silverstein, Rosenbloom, Carter, & Cunningham, 1986; Johnson, Freund, Silverstein, Hansen, & Malone, 1990; Glasgow, McCaul, & Schafer, 1987). That is, self-management adherence is made up of a combination of behaviors, especially eating behavior, exercise or activity level, medication use, and glucose self-testing. Furthermore, level of adherence for one self-management behavior is not necessarily related to adherence level of other self-management behaviors. In particular, across age groups, individuals generally closely adhere to their insulin recommendations, but have much more difficulty following recommendations requiring greater life-style changes (e.g., diet and exercise) (Glasgow et al., 1987; Orme & Binik, 1989).

Because the variability in the conceptualization and measurement of diabetes self-management adherence across studies makes it difficult to provide general statements about the rates of adherence, the current presentation will focus on a set of studies by Johnson and colleagues (Johnson et al., 1986; Johnson, Tomer, Cunningham, & Henretta, 1990) that carefully examined diabetes self-management in children. These studies were chosen because of the sophisticated measurement of self-management adherence used and the degree of methodological rigor employed by these researchers. The studies involved large groups of children and adolescents with diabetes ($N = 168, 162$). Self-management adherence was assessed on three separate occasions using a sophisticated 24-hour recall interview procedure with both the child and a parent. From the interview data, scores for 13 different self-management adherence behaviors were calculated. These included one for glucose testing and several for each of the following areas: insulin use, eating habits, and exercise/activity habits.

In general, results indicated good to excellent parent/child agreement on adherence. However, child's age influenced the degree of parent/child agreement, with the most consistency occurring in the 10- to 15-year-old group. The authors noted, however, that information provided by both parent and child offers a more comprehensive picture of diabetes self-management adherence than information from either reporter alone. Therefore, final estimates of adherence used by these researchers involved the combination of parent and child data collapsed across the three interview points. Factor analysis procedures performed on the 13 adherence behaviors indicated four independent factors representing the following areas of self-management: exercise, insulin use, diet, and frequency of self-testing/eating. This finding underscores the importance of focusing on individual self-management behaviors rather than a single global construct when examining self-management adherence. The findings further indicated that, in general, older children were less adherent than younger children. The topic of age-related differences in self-management will be further addressed in later sections of this chapter.

ROLE OF THE HEALTH PSYCHOLOGIST IN DIABETES CARE

Effective management of diabetes involves the expertise of a multitude of individuals working together as a cohesive team. At a minimum, the diabetes management team should include a physician, preferably a pediatric diabetologist, a diabetes nurse educator, a dietitian, and a mental health professional to represent the key professional disciplines important to this team. The other key team members include the child and his or her family. The combined efforts of the diabetes team are needed to assist the family in maintaining adequate adherence at home. Each of the team members plays an important role in the successful management of diabetes, and the success of the team depends on cooperation and collaboration.

Health psychologists are the ideal mental health professionals to participate on a diabetes team, since they have the necessary expertise in the important psychosocial and behavioral issues, as well as health issues. The primary role of the health psychologist is to assist the child and family in the successful self-management of this disease. At first, when the initial diagnosis is made, the primary focus of the health psychologist is to help the child and family learn about this disease and its management, cope with the emotional responses to the diagnosis, and adjust to the new demands and stresses associated with this chronic disease. Many negative emotional responses are likely, especially including fear, anger, guilt, and depression (Hauser & Solomon, 1985; Kravitz, Isenberg, Shore, & Barnett, 1971). These responses may be experienced by any family member since diabetes affects the entire family. Research has shown that the initial emotional upheaval begins to resolve itself within about six months and most families return to premorbid levels of functioning within a year after the diagnosis (Hauser & Solomon, 1985; Kovacs, Iyengar, Goldston, Obrosky, Stewart, & Marsh, 1990; Kovacs, Finkelstein, Feinberg, Crouse-Novak, Paulauskas, & Pollock, 1985).

However, another study that compared children with diabetes to peers without diabetes, found that the first two years after diagnosis are challenging periods of adjustment and important times for the involvement of health psychologists (Grey, Cameron, Lipman, & Thurber, 1995). In particular, these researchers concluded that there are two critical periods of time in which children with diabetes experience significantly greater psychosocial problems than peers. Consistent with other research, they found increased difficulties around the time of diagnosis which generally are resolved by one year after diagnosis. They also found, however, that a second period of difficulty occurs between the first and second year after diagnosis.

Recent research (Kovacs, Goldston, Obrosky, & Bonar, 1997a; Kovacs, Obrosky, Goldston, & Drash, 1997b) suggests that health psychologists should be aware of the high risk for psychiatric disorders, especially anxiety, depression, and conduct disorders, in youth with diabetes. In particular, Kovacs and colleagues (1997a) found that major depressive disorder was the most prevalent psychiatric condition in youth with diabetes with a cumulative probability of 27.5 percent by the tenth year of the diagnosis of diabetes. Furthermore, Kovacs and colleagues (1997b) found that young women with diabetes have a nine times greater risk of recurrent depression than young men with diabetes. In another study it was found that approximately 8 percent of families (Kovacs et al., 1990) may have continued difficulties in coping and should be closely followed, provided with support, and offered treatment where appropriate. It is also important to reassess families at different stages in the child's development, especially adolescence, since normal developmental changes may pose additional challenges and stresses for the child and family in coping with and managing diabetes (Hauser et al., 1986; Johnson, 1982; Tarnow & Tomlinson, 1978). See Wolfsdorf, Anderson, and Pasquarello (1994) for an excellent review of how diabetes management and normal childhood developmental tasks impact each other at different age levels. In addition, see Anderson and Rubin (1997) for useful clinical guidelines for working with children and adolescents with diabetes and their families.

After the initial period of adjustment to the diagnosis, issues related to self-management adherence are among the most frequent reasons for referral to a health psychologist. In terms of ongoing diabetes self-management, the health psychologist may be called on to play either a direct or consulting role in the care of a particular child and family. He or she may be asked to work directly with the family in a therapeutic relationship or may be asked to consult with the diabetes team when a psychosocial or behavioral problem occurs that does not require direct involvement.

Since maximizing appropriate diabetes self-management constitutes one of the greatest challenges for the health psychologist in the ongoing care of children with diabetes, the remaining sections of this chapter will focus on self-management adherence and important factors influencing adherence. In general, research reviewed in the remainder of this chapter was chosen because it directly examined self-management adherence and did not rely solely on metabolic control as a proxy for self-care adherence.

THE BIOPSYCHOSOCIAL MODEL OF DIABETES SELF-MANAGEMENT

The DCCT finding that successfully applying an intensive diabetes management program has a positive impact on long-term complications has an important behavioral corollary. That is, adherence with the greater behavioral or self-management demands associated with intensive management has a positive impact on long-term complications. This intensive management program places more burden and responsibility on the individual for day-to-day management of diabetes. Therefore, behavioral scientists need to focus attention on how best to facilitate self-management adherence in individuals with diabetes. It is especially important to focus on children with diabetes since this early intervention may have the most benefit on improving glucose control and reducing long-term complications.

In examining adherence and the factors that influence adherence, it is important to be systematic. One useful approach to help guide the assessment of factors influencing diabetes self-management would be to take a biopsychosocial perspective (adapted from Anderson, 1990, and Glasgow, 1991). As shown in Figure 4.1, the application of this approach involves the examination of a diversity of factors including psychosocial, environmental, provider/treatment, and biological—that may have a direct impact on self-management adherence and are likely interrelated. As underscored by the findings of the DCCT, maintaining blood glucose levels in the target range through the combination of appropriate medical management and close adherence with self-management behaviors directly and positively influences short- and long-term health outcome. Examination of diabetes self-management adherence from a biopsychosocial perspective may facilitate one's understanding of the complexity of factors that affect adherence and may better guide the development of effective interventions designed to improve self-management.

When working with children with diabetes, it is important first to conduct a thorough assessment of important factors impacting self-management (see Figure 4.2). For children, key biopsychosocial factors include child factors, such as psychological adjustment and regimen responsibility; family factors, such as family relationships and psychological adjustment; and provider/treatment factors, such as provider/patient relationship and diabetes knowledge. Although biological and environmental factors, such as age and socioeconomic status, may not be subject to change through intervention, they are still key to understanding the child's risk of nonadherence. Conducting a thorough assessment of the child and family, including the medical context, will guide the choice of the most appropriate intervention approaches for enhancing adherence. Because of the importance of self-management adherence in successful diabetes management, the focus of the remaining sections will be on reviewing the literature on the influence of various biopsychosocial factors on diabetes regimen adherence.

BIOLOGICAL/BACKGROUND VARIABLES

Gender

The evidence concerning the relationship between gender and adherence is confusing and often contradictory. Some studies have found no relationship between gender and adherence (Anderson, Auslander, Jung, Miller, & Santiago, 1990; Jacobson et al.,

Figure 4.1 Biopsychosocial Model of Diabetes in Children

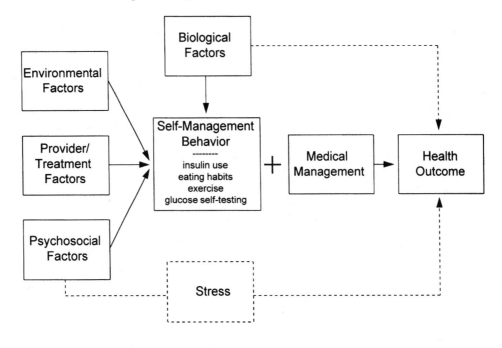

Figure 4.2 Factors Influencing Self-Management Adherence in Children

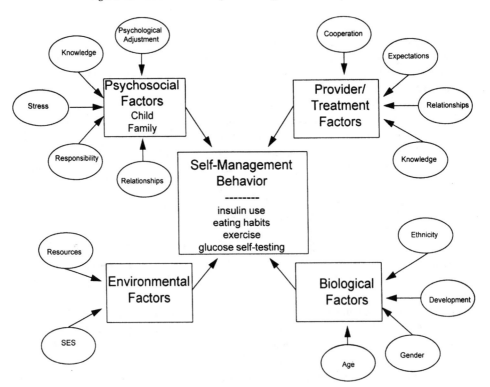

1990; Johnson, Kelly, Henretta, Cunningham, Tomer, & Silverstein, 1992; Kovacs, Goldston, Obrosky, & Iyengar, 1992; Kuttner, Delamater, & Santiago, 1990). Studies that have found a relationship have yielded conflicting results. For instance, Garrison, Biggs, and Williams (1990) found that being male was related to poor diabetes self-management adherence, whereas Littlefield, Craven, Rodin, Daneman, Murray, and Rydall (1992) found that being female was related to being less adherent. Moreover, in line with the multidimensional view of diabetes regimen adherence, gender may be related to adherence only with regard to certain regimen behaviors. For instance, one study found that boys were more adherent than girls only with regard to regularity and frequency of exercise (Johnson, Freund, et al., 1990). To date, it appears that no firm conclusions can be drawn concerning the relationship between gender and adherence.

Age-Related Variables

Age has been found to be an important predictor of diabetes self-management adherence. Many studies have found that older children have lower levels of adherence, both overall (Allen, Tennen, McGrade, Affleck, & Ratzan, 1983; Anderson et al., 1990; Bobrow, AvRuskin, & Siller, 1985; Garrison et al., 1990; Hanson, Harris, Relyea, Cigrang, Carle, & Burghen, 1989; Hanson, Henggeler, & Burghen, 1987a, 1987b; Jacobson et al., 1990; Kovacs et al., 1992) and in specific task areas (Bond, Aiken, & Somerville, 1992; Christensen, Terry, Wyatt, Pichert, & Lorenz, 1983; Johnson et al., 1992; Johnson, Freund et al., 1990; Johnson et al., 1986; LaGreca, Follansbee, & Skyler, 1990). For example, teenagers have been found to eat less frequently, self-test their glucose less frequently, have more variability in insulin injection patterns, and exercise less frequently.

In one study, the average age at which children began to show a pattern of serious and persistent negligence in at least two of three diabetes management areas (insulin administration, glycemic monitoring, and dietary behavior) was 14.8 years (Kovacs et al., 1992). Adolescence appears to be a particularly difficult period for adherence. In their desire for independence, adolescents may become resistant to rules and authority, which may put them at greater risk for self-

management problems. In their attempts to gain peer acceptance, they may try to hide their disease status (Johnson et al., 1986; Simonds, 1979). Peer influences to eat out, especially junk food (Tattersall & Lowe, 1981), and drink alcohol are also common challenges faced by adolescents with diabetes (Glasgow et al., 1991; Tattersall & Lowe, 1981).

In addition to the possible adverse effects due to the adherence problems discussed earlier, the physiological changes that adolescents undergo may have an impact on their metabolic control. For instance, the hormonal changes that accompany the onset and progress of puberty are often associated with increased difficulty in achieving tight metabolic control (Drash & Becker, 1978; Hanson & Henggeler, 1984; Johnson et al., 1992). In many cases, adolescents want to be adherent, but growth hormones physically interfere and make tight glycemic control difficult (see Amiel et al., 1986). For helpful clinical guidelines on working with adolescents with diabetes, see Anderson and Rubin (1996). Other age-related influences on self-management, such as diabetes knowledge and sharing of regimen responsibility, will be discussed in detail in later sections.

Several studies have indicated that a child's knowledge and skill level with regard to diabetes self-management increases in an age-related way (Gilbert, Johnson, Spillar, McCallum, Silverstein, & Rosenbloom, 1982; Harkavy, Johnson, Silverstein, Spillar, McCallum, & Rosenbloom, 1983; Johnson, Pollak et al., 1982). This is consistent with the fact that the cognitive and motor abilities of children, which are important determinants of how much the child can be expected to learn about the management of diabetes, change and become more advanced in age-related stages (Johnson & Rosenbloom, 1982; McKelvey & Borgersen, 1990). Thus, as noted by Johnson (1988b), different aspects of diabetes management should be taught at different ages, and parents and health care providers should be reasonable in their expectations about the skills children of different ages should master. (See Savinetti-Rose, 1994, for recommendations on determining developmentally appropriate diabetes education and self-management tasks.)

Furthermore, it is not sufficient to explain diabetes and its management only once, because children are capable of understanding more complex skills as they progress developmentally, and new questions and concerns arise. Therefore, the child's skills should be assessed on a regular basis and re-education provided where deficits are found (Johnson & Rosenbloom, 1982). Other research has suggested that children who develop diabetes early in life may be at increased risk of cognitive and intellectual deficits (Rovet, Ehrlich, & Hoppe, 1988; Ryan, Vega, Longstreet, & Drash, 1985). These risk factors should be taken into consideration when working with children with diabetes. For example, a child's intellectual and cognitive developmental level should be considered, along with age, when providing informational or skill-based diabetes education.

The relationship between age of diabetes onset and adherence has also been explored. Some studies suggest no relationship (Bobrow et al., 1985; Kovacs et al., 1992); however, one study (Jacobson, Hauser, Lavori, Wolfsdorf, Herskowith, Milley, Bliss, Gelfand, Wertlieb, & Stein, 1990) indicated that children diagnosed at a younger age (less than 13 years) had better self-management adherence over a four-year period than children diagnosed at an older age. Another study (Johnson et al., 1986) found an interaction between age, disease duration, and adherence. In this study, children between 16 and 19 years of age who had diabetes less than five years displayed the most irregular injection times and the most inappropriate meal-injection intervals. As noted by these investigators and others, disease onset during adolescence is an especially critical period. This may be associated with less parental supervision during adolescence and the resultant development of poor habits from the outset (Johnson et al., 1986).

Disease duration in general also appears to be associated with poorer adherence (Garrison et al., 1990; Hanson et al., 1989); that is, adherence apparently deteriorates across time (Glasgow et al., 1987; Jacobson et al., 1987; Jacobson et al., 1990). According to Kovacs and colleagues (1992), there is a 0.45 cumulative probability of nonadherence developing over the first nine years of diagnosis, with the third year being an especially high-risk period. Further research is needed to clarify the interrelationships between time-related variables (e.g., age of diagnosis, duration of diabetes), psychosocial variables (e.g., adjustment, regimen responsibility) and self-management behavior.

Ethnicity

Little research has specifically examined such sociodemographic characteristics as racial and ethnic background with regard to diabetes adherence. The findings of the studies in this area have been mixed (Auslander, Anderson, Bubb, Jung, & Santiago, 1990; Kovacs et al., 1992). More research is needed to determine if particular sociodemographic characteristics place a child at higher risk of nonadherence with diabetes self-management.

PSYCHOSOCIAL VARIABLES

Psychological Adjustment

Child's Adjustment

Although the nature of the relationship between a child's psychological state and adherence is not clear, Johnson (1988a) suggests that psychological disturbances such as anxiety and depression may impede the child's ability to properly manage the disease. One study (Kovacs et al., 1992) found that 60 percent of those children who had been diagnosed as nonadherent, also had a psychiatric disorder, whereas only 19 percent of those free of diabetes management problems had been diagnosed with such a disorder. The psychiatric disorders included major affective disorders (38 percent), conduct or substance use disorders (31 percent), anxiety disorders (19 percent), and other conditions (13 percent). It should be noted, however, that not all studies have replicated these relationships (Kuttner et al., 1990; Nagasawa, Smith, Barnes, & Fincham, 1990). More research is needed in this area to clearly determine the relationship between psychological disorders and adherence.

Another possible psychological influence on adherence involves the perception that negative consequences may occur with close adherence. In particular, close adherence with an intensive management program may lead to increased incidence of hypoglycemia (DCCT, 1993). Fear of the unpleasant and serious symptoms of hypoglycemia have been found to be associated with nonadherence with the prescribed insulin regimen (Cox, Irvine, Gonder-Frederick, Nowacek, & Butterfield, 1987; Weiner & Skipper, 1979).

Additionally, individuals may be more adherent with regard to self-testing their blood glucose levels on days when they have more closely followed their prescribed regimen, compared with days when they have been nonadherent (Cox & Gonder-Frederick, 1992). One explanation is that it is an effort to avoid the negative feedback of obtaining measurements indicating blood glucose levels that are too low or too high. Other studies have identified a relationship between health beliefs and adherence (Bobrow et al., 1985; Bond et al., 1992; Jacobson et al., 1990; LaGreca & Hanna, 1983). In particular, perceived vulnerability, perceived severity of symptoms, and perceived effectiveness of the regimen have been related to adherence.

A growing body of literature has focused on eating disorders in individuals with diabetes. Intensive insulin regimens can lead to weight gain (DCCT, 1993; Jones, 1990), and adolescents, particularly females, may reduce their insulin dosages for the purpose of weight control (LaGreca, Schwarz, & Satin, 1987; Peveler, Fairburn, Boller, & Dunger, 1992). This may be especially true of those individuals who have an eating disorder (Rodin, Craven, Littlefield, Murray, & Daneman, 1991). In some studies (Littlefield et al., 1992; Rodin et al., 1991), adolescents who reported lower adherence tended to report more eating disorders than those with higher adherence scores.

Adolescents with diabetes would seem to be at particular risk for eating disorders because food restriction can increase the likelihood of subsequent bingeing on restricted foods (Polivy & Herman, 1985). Some studies have found a higher prevalence of eating disorders among adolescent and young adult women with diabetes than in the general population (Rodin et al., 1986; Steel et al., 1989). Other studies have shown that children with diabetes are not at a greater risk for eating disorders (Striegel-Moore, Nicholson, & Tamborlane, 1992; Wing, Nowalk, Marcus, Koeske, & Finegold, 1986). Nevertheless, children with diabetes who have an eating disorder face much more severe consequences than do children in the general population, and the subject warrants further investigation.

Stress
Research primarily focused on adults with diabetes has shown stress to play both a direct role in metabolic control (through the release of stress hormones that affect blood glucose levels) (Hanson et al., 1987a;

Surwit & Schneider, 1993; Tarnow & Silverman, 1981–1982) and an indirect role through interference with diabetes self-management (Frenzel, McCaul, Glasgow, & Schafer, 1988; Hanson et al., 1987a; Peyrot & McMurray, 1985). Although more work is needed in this area with children, it is believed that similar patterns of stress responses will be found. Research on coping in children has shown that individual coping skills, including diabetes-related problem solving and overall ability to cope with life, all seem to be related to self-management adherence behaviors (Delamater, Kurtz, Bubb, White, & Santiago, 1987; Hanson et al., 1989; Jacobson et al., 1990). More research is needed to examine specifically the relationship between stress and self-management adherence in children.

Family Adjustment
Having parents with poor coping skills may place a child with diabetes at risk for nonadherence with the treatment regimen, especially in the area of self-monitoring of blood glucose level and insulin injection (Holden, Friend, Gault, Kager, Foltz, & White, 1991). Furthermore, there is evidence that parental anxiety about hypoglycemia in their children with diabetes may lead the parents to encourage maintenance of higher blood glucose levels than recommended. Good social support for family members has been found to be related to better adherence with the medical regimen (Janis, 1983). Unfortunately, in one study (Ferrari, 1986), parents of children with diabetes were shown to perceive themselves as having less social support than parents of "healthy" children. More research needs to be conducted to examine social support in families of children with diabetes and appropriate interventions developed if needed to ensure adequate social support.

Family Relationship Factors

The child's family is an important influence on self-management behaviors. Every member of the family can potentially be affected by the complex regimen (Auslander, Anderson, Bubb, Jung, & Santiago, 1990; Blechman & Delamater, 1993), which requires cooperation and assistance from all family members (Anderson et al., 1990). Family members must share in the responsibility for regimen requirements

(Anderson & Auslander, 1980; Drash, 1981; Drash & Becker, 1978; Wishner & O'Brien, 1978), and parents and children often must alter their life-styles (Horan, Gwynn, & Renzi, 1986). (The topic of regimen responsibility will be covered in detail in a later section.) In particular, the special dietary requirements of diabetes may require restructuring of the family's eating habits (Orr, 1986). Family members may resent the changes (Drash & Becker, 1978), and family conflicts may arise around the treatment regimen (Anderson & Auslander, 1980).

Several studies indicate that there may be an association between various aspects of regimen adherence and positive family relations (Bobrow et al., 1985; Eaton, Mengel, Mengel, Larson, Campbell, & Montague, 1992; Hanson et al., 1987a, 1987b; Hanson, DeGuire, Schinkel, Henggeler, & Burghen, 1992; McCaul, Glasgow, & Schafer 1987; Schafer, Glasgow, McCaul, & Dreher, 1983; Shouval, Ber, & Galatzer, 1982). For purposes of this review, family relations include those factors dealing with how the family functions as a team, such as how they relate to each other on a personal level and their levels of cohesiveness, support, conflict, and organization.

For example, in one study (Bobrow et al., 1985), poorly adhering girls, compared to good adherers, had more difficulty talking with their mothers about their feelings, problems, and concerns, and were more pessimistic about the possibility of their working out issues. On the other hand, good adherers and their mothers were closer, more efficient in negotiation and problem solving, more positive in mood, and more empathic and willing to listen to what the other was saying. Another study found that low levels of anger intensity in regimen-specific discussion may be related to better blood glucose testing adherence in adolescents with diabetes (Kurtz & Delamater, 1984). Additionally, in mother/adolescent pairs, more positive problem-solving skills, more friendliness, and fewer negative problem-solving skills and put-downs were related to better adherence on the adolescents' part.

In another study (Waller, Chipman, Hardy, Hightower, North, Williams, & Babick, 1986) that focused on diabetes-specific family factors, the authors found that for younger children (less than 13 years), greater diabetes-related family guidance and control was re-lated to better metabolic control. Diabetes-specific parental warmth and caring was associated with better metabolic control for both young children and adolescents in this study. The results of a longitudinal study of the family milieu of children with diabetes showed that the child's perception of family conflict in the first year of onset was the best predictor of poor adherence with self-management behaviors at a four year follow-up point (Hauser, Jacobson, Lavori, Wolfsdorf, Herskowitz, Milley, Bliss, Gelfand, Wertbieb, Stein, 1990).

Most studies of the families of children with diabetes have focused on the mother's behavior, because mothers usually take more responsibility for the management of the child's illness and more often attend clinic appointments with their children (Etzwiler & Sines, 1962; Kovacs et al., 1985; Johnson, 1988a; Marrero, Lau, Golden, Kershnar, & Myers, 1982). Some research has been done examining the father's role in diabetes management in children, but the results have been mixed (Hanson, Henggeler, Rodrigue, Burghen, & Murphy, 1988; Shouval et al., 1982). Thus, it appears that further research needs to be conducted in this area to clarify the relationship between parental involvement and children's self-management.

Parenting style, especially with regard to punishment and reward, also may be a critical influence on adherence to treatment. For example, overly critical parents may have a negative impact on their child's adherence (Bobrow et al., 1985; Shouval et al., 1982). This type of parenting approach may result in conflict between parents and their adolescents or in the adolescents' withdrawing from parental interactions (Bobrow et al, 1985).

Evidence concerning the relationship of marital discord to a child's self-management behaviors is equivocal, with some studies finding it to be related to poorer diabetes management (Barkley, 1981; Schafer, Glasgow, & McCaul, 1982), while others found no such relationship (Kovacs et al., 1985; Kovacs, Kass, Schnell, Goldston, & Marsh, 1989). It is likely that marital discord interacts with a variety of other factors, such as the child's age, the degree to which parents assume responsibility for the diabetes regimen, and the degree of support shown for the child. More research is needed in this area to continue to examine the type and degree of relationship between marital and family factors and diabetes management.

Diabetes Regimen Responsibility

Independence in responsibility for diabetes self-management has often been implicated as playing a central role in diabetes management in children and adolescents. As children grow older, they progress from being totally dependent on their parents to being much more independent, and less supervised, in their daily activities (Erickson, 1963). Children may be given varying degrees of responsibility for different regimen tasks (Etzwiler & Sines, 1962; LaGreca et al., 1990). In general, increased age is associated with increased responsibility for self-care (Allen et al., 1983; LaGreca, 1982, 1988; Rubin, Young-Hyman, & Peyrot, 1989). It appears that although adolescents have increased responsibility, they may not actually carry out the tasks as expected by their parents (Anderson et al., 1990; Ingersoll, Orr, Herrold, & Golden, 1986) or may adhere differentially to self-care tasks (Johnson, 1986). In fact, research has suggested that either excessive self-care responsibility or unclear accountability for self-care relative to psychological maturity is associated with high risk of poor treatment adherence, inadequate diabetes control, and more frequent hospitalizations (Wysocki, Taylor, Hough, Linscheid, Yeates, Naglieri, 1996). Parents who directly supervise the treatment regimen may be able to insure that their children assume age-appropriate responsibility for self-care and more closely follow their regimen (Hanson et al., 1987a; Kovacs et al., 1992).

Continued parental involvement in the daily regimen, even during adolescence, has been linked to better overall adherence and metabolic outcomes (Anderson, Ho, Brackett, Finkelstein, & Laffel, 1997; Hanson et al., 1987a; Wysocki et al., 1996). In particular, continued parental involvement in self-testing has been linked to better control in adolescents (Anderson et al., 1997). Additionally, communication about expectations for responsibility must be made clear, especially when the child begins to play an increasing role in self-care (Anderson et al., 1990). Otherwise, a confusing message is sent to the child which may result in uncertainty about who is respon-

sible for regimen tasks (Rabin, Amir, Nardi, & Ovadia, 1986) and this diffusion of responsibility may lead to adherence problems. In sum, regimen responsibility may play a key role in self-management adherence in pediatric groups. Although this complex construct has received much attention from researchers, continued research in this area will help better understand patterns of responsibility across different ages and determine the best age-appropriate balance of responsibility and parental involvement to maximize diabetes control. Continued work will help parents, children, and health professionals apply the best age-appropriate expectations for the assumption of diabetes-regimen-related responsibility and provide the support needed by children and parents in making the decisions and transitions around regimen responsibility.

ENVIRONMENTAL FACTORS

The resources that a family has available can make an impact on the ability to effectively manage a child's diabetes. There is a paucity of research examining these important variables. In general, studies that have examined socioeconomic factors have found no relationship with adherence (Johnson et al., 1992; Kovacs et al., 1992; Kuttner et al., 1990), although one study found a relationship between parents' educational level and the child's adherence (Bobrow et al., 1985). More research needs to be conducted on children and their families to examine the impact of material resources on diabetes self-management.

PROVIDER AND TREATMENT FACTORS

Diabetes Knowledge

Child Knowledge

Without the necessary knowledge and skills, it would be difficult to properly adhere to the daily self-care regimen. Thus, it is not surprising that research supports the notion that greater knowledge about diabetes and key self-care tasks is related to better adherence (LaGreca, 1990). In fact, importance of knowledge to proper adherence is indicated by studies showing that a significant number of children with diabetes make at least one error of a magnitude sufficient enough to result in the self-administration of an incorrect dose of insulin (Harkavy et al., 1983; Johnson, Pollak et al., 1982; Wilson & Endres, 1986). However, although knowledge is the minimum necessary for appropriate self-management, it is not sufficient for achieving good adherence (Johnson, 1984; Wysocki, Hough, Ward, & Green, 1992).

As with other child-related factors that may affect diabetes self-management adherence, it is important to consider the nature and timing of diabetes education. Based on their interpretation of the message of DCCT for children, Brink and Moltz (1997) recommend a diabetes education plan that involves three stages (diagnosis, 1 to 2 months after diagnosis, and then yearly) with different content focus areas. These authors also highlight the importance of continuing assessment and re-education since simply providing the information does not insure that the child has learned it. In fact, other authors have noted that a patient's lack of recall for their physicians' recommendations (Page, Verstraete, Robb, & Etzwiler, 1981) and an inability to understand either the oral instructions or the reading materials given by the physician (Johnson, 1988) may be barriers to self-management adherence. Children may appear knowledgeable even when they are not. Adherence may be improved if the diabetes care team uses simple language and clarifies information to a greater extent (Johnson & Rosenbloom, 1982).

Family Knowledge

At least one study has found family knowledge of diabetes to be associated with diabetes regimen adherence (Hanson et al., 1987b). Families of children with diabetes must learn considerable new information and many new skills in order to assist the child in adequately managing the disease (Delamater et al., 1990; Prazar & Felice, 1975). They must know information about the nature of the disease, the theory of management, and the recognition and treatment of complications (Christensen, 1983; Guthrie & Jackson, 1975; Hanson et al., 1987b; Johnson, Pollak et al., 1982). Just as with the child, family knowledge about diabetes is a necessary prerequisite, but is not alone sufficient for optimal disease management.

Patient/Provider Relationship

An often overlooked aspect of regimen adherence is the influence of the health care provider. Although most of the research is focused on physicians, increasing emphasis on the diabetes team, including a number of disciplines, underscores the need to focus on relationships with all health care providers. Some studies have found no relationship between adherence and the patient/physician relationship (Bobrow et al., 1985), whereas others maintain the relationship is an important influence (Cox & Gonder-Frederick, 1992; Jacobson, Adler, Derby, Anderson, & Wolfsdorf, 1991). At least two studies have found higher levels of adherence to be associated with youths' positive perceptions of the physicians' personal qualities, such as caring and empathy (Hanson et al., 1988; Reid & Appleton, 1991).

Adolescents who view the physician as an authority figure may be reluctant to discuss their nonadherence, especially with a stern, judgmental physician (Orr, 1986). Thus, adolescence may be a particularly important time to facilitate patient/provider rapport. Furthermore, health care professionals may fail to identify nonadherence, especially if they do not have a confidential relationship with the patient (DiMatteo & DiNicola, 1985).

Cooperation and collaboration between the provider and the family is important, because most of the management of diabetes is carried out at home (Marteau, Johnston, Baum, & Bloch, 1987). Lack of agreement between parents and providers on management goals may pose an adherence problem. For example, in a study conducted by Marteau and colleagues (1987), parents preferred children to show higher glycemic levels than did doctors. In this study, parents were more concerned with avoidance of the short-term threat of diabetes (hypoglycemia), whereas doctors were guided more by the long-term threat (complications from hyperglycemia). In sum, the nature of the relationships between the members of the diabetes care team and the child and family may play an important role in influencing diabetes self-management. Therefore, more research is needed to examine this topic, especially since the results of the DCCT highlight the importance of the involvement of a multidisciplinary team in the management of diabetes.

IMPACT OF INTERVENTIONS

Several approaches have been employed with the goal of facilitating diabetes self-management adherence in children. Much earlier work in this area involved family systems approaches. Family systems theory has provided a widely used framework for treating children with psychiatric and psychosomatic symptoms, including diabetes (Ackerman, 1958; Minuchin, Rossman, & Baker, 1978; Wynne & Singer, 1963). Indeed, many therapists have based their view of the role of the family in chronic illness on Minuchin, Rosman, and Baker's (1978) theory of the "psychosomatic family." Interventions guided by this theory have generally focused on helping families deal with hidden conflicts. Reviews of the literature (Surwit, Feinglos & Scovern, 1983; Coyne & Anderson, 1989) have suggested that this widely accepted theory of the link between family functioning and problems in the management of diabetes has not been verified and should be reconsidered. It has been suggested that focus on the "psychosomatic family" might lead a family therapist to miss important opportunities to assist families in changing behaviors related to diabetes and its management. Given the important role of the family in diabetes management in children, empirical studies of family-based interventions are greatly needed.

A variety of other interventions have been examined for their impact on diabetes adherence behaviors in children. Behavioral strategies that have been examined and found to be helpful in improving regimen adherence include use of a contingency management system (Carney, Schechter, & Davis, 1983; Epstein et al., 1981), goal setting and behavioral contracts (Schafer et al., 1982), feedback training on accuracy in determining blood glucose concentrations (Epstein, Figueroa, Farkas, & Beck, 1981), and peer-modeling of children learning self-injection (Gilbert et al., 1982).

Family-based self-management training utilizing behavioral principles has also been shown to improve adherence (Delamater et al., 1990; Gross, Magalnick, & Richardson, 1985). Such training generally emphasizes proper blood glucose self-monitoring techniques, reinforcement by the parents for accurate monitoring and recording, and the use of blood glucose data to understand and make appropri-ate behavioral changes depending on blood glucose fluctuations. Another study that examined stress management training found that it did not have an effect on regimen adherence (Boardway, Delamater, Tomakowsky, & Gutai, 1993), even though children showed a significant reduction in diabetes-specific stress.

Educational programs have also been evaluated for their effectiveness in improving adherence. For example, children who attended a therapeutic summer camp oriented toward educating them about their diabetes demonstrated improved adherence to self-injection and blood-glucose monitoring (Holden et al., 1991). In another study (Marrero, Fremion, & Golden, 1988), children were taught a structured at-home aerobics fitness program, including the objectives of aerobic exercise and how to adjust insulin and diet to compensate for it. The result was an increase in the fitness level of sedentary adolescents with diabetes, implying that they were more adherent to their exercise regimen. Children who participated in a diabetes-specific educational program showed improved confidence in handling obstacles to dietary adherence (Pichert, Flannery, Kline, Hodge, Meek, & Kinzer, 1994).

Outpatient group therapy also may have potential for improving adherence to the regimen (Anderson, Wolf, Burkhart, Cornell, & Bacon, 1989; Francis, Grogan, Hardy, Jensen, Xenakis, & Kearney; Satin, LaGreca, Zigo, & Skyler, 1989). Such groups have focused on problem-solving, negotiating levels of responsibility, and enhancing communication and cooperation. Additionally, adolescents who participated in a social learning group showed improvement in regimen adherence (Kaplan, Chadwick, & Schimmel, 1985). In that program, adolescents were taught coping skills to help them deal effectively with social situations related to regimen nonadherence.

Given that intervening with self-management adherence is one of the key roles that health psychologists play in working with individuals with diabetes, more research needs to be focused on developing feasible and effective intervention approaches. As underscored in a recent review of psychosocial interventions for children with chronic health conditions (Bauman, Drotar, Leventhal, Perrin, & Pless, 1997), the field would be best served by maintaining a focus on conducting theory-based methodologically sound outcome evaluation.

SUMMARY AND FUTURE DIRECTIONS

The findings of the DCCT, that intensive management helps better control blood glucose in the short term and reduce complications in the long term, makes this both an exciting and challenging time for health psychology. Applying the message of the DCCT as the "modus operandi for type 1 diabetes care" as recommended by Brink and Moltz (1997) will place increased behavioral demands and psychosocial challenges on young people with diabetes. Health psychologists, in collaboration with a multidisciplinary diabetes care team, as well as the child and family, play a key role in facilitating adherence with the self-management tasks needed for intensive management of diabetes. Therefore, the focus will be on this discipline to provide the clinical and research expertise to facilitate adherence to the complex self-management behaviors required to best control glucose levels in youth.

This chapter presented a biopsychosocial perspective on self-management adherence in children with diabetes. This perspective acknowledges the complexity of the interrelationships of key influencing factors and offers a useful framework to guide the examination of factors that have an impact on self-management. In particular, this approach encourages examination of biological, psychosocial, environmental, and provider/treatment factors, all of which may be interrelated and are likely to affect self-management adherence.

The chapter also reviewed the findings of studies that examined the impact of these factors on self-management adherence in children with diabetes. Although much research has been conducted to date, few firm conclusions may be drawn. Throughout the chapter, it has been noted that more research is needed to clarify the biopsychosocial variables that are most related to regimen adherence, as well as to identify the specific nature of these relationships.

Given increased attention to the role of behavior in diabetes management, researchers must take care to be as scientifically rigorous as possible. In particular, it is important to develop standard operational definitions of self-management adherence and use measures which have demonstrated reliability and validity. This will enhance confidence in interpretation of study results and comparison across studies.

In addition, more focus on methodologically rigorous theory-driven research, especially regarding intervention (Bauman, Drotar, Leventhal, Perrin, & Pless, 1997), is needed to advance the knowledge base in this area. There have been several models proposed to explain adherence behaviors with adults with diabetes. For example, several studies have examined the Health Belief Model in people with diabetes (Schlenk & Hart, 1984). Additionally, Glasgow (1991) has proposed the Personal Models approach to understanding and enhancing diabetes self-management. Researchers have also begun to study the application of the Transtheoretical model to diabetes self-management (Ruggiero & Prochaska, 1993). It is noteworthy that in a review of studies on psychosocial interventions for children with chronic health conditions conducted over a 15-year period (1979–1993) (Bauman et al., 1997), only 16 of 266 studies met minimal content and methodological eligibility criteria and none of these were in the area of diabetes. Thus, increased focus needs to be placed on development and controlled evaluation of theory-based interventions designed to improve diabetes self-management in children.

In summary, the chief DCCT finding—that is, intensive diabetes management has a positive impact on long-term complications—and its behavioral implications underscore the important contributions that health psychologists have to offer to the area of diabetes management. There is an increasing role for health psychology in this field and it is an important time for health psychologists to rise to this challenge.

REFERENCES

Ackerman, N. W. (1958). *The psychodynamics of family life: Diagnosis and treatment of family relationships.* New York: Basic Books.

Albisser, A. M. (1991). Insulin infusion devices: Open-loop and closed-loop. In J. K. Davidson (Ed.), *Clinical diabetes mellitus* (pp. 323–329). New York: Thieme Medical Publishers.

Allen, D. A., Tennen, H., McGrade, B. J., Affleck, G., & Ratzan, S. (1983). Parent and child perceptions of the management of juvenile diabetes. *Journal of Pediatric Psychology, 8,* 129–141.

American Diabetes Association (1995). Self-monitoring of blood glucose. *Diabetes Care, 18,* 47–52.

American Diabetes Association (1996). *Diabetes 1996 Vital Statistics.* Alexandria, VA: Author.

Amiel, S. A., Sherwin, R. S., Somonson, D. C., Lauritano, A. A., & Tamborlane, W. V. (1986). Impaired insulin action in puberty: A contributing factor to poor glycemic control in adolescents with diabetes. *New England Journal of Medicine, 315,* 215–219.

Anderson, B. J., & Auslander, W. F. (1980). Research on diabetes management and the family: A critique. *Diabetes Care, 6,* 696–702.

Anderson, B. J., Auslander, W. F., Jung, K. C., Miller, J. P., & Santiago, J. V. (1990). Assessing family sharing of diabetes responsibilities. *Journal of Pediatric Psychology, 15,* 477–492.

Anderson, B. J., Ho, J., Brackett, J., Finkelstein, D., & Laffel, L. (1997) Parental involvement in diabetes management tasks: Relationships to blood glucose monitoring adherence and metabolic control in young adolescents with insulin-dependent diabetes mellitus. *Journal of Pediatrics, 130* (2), 257–265.

Anderson, B. J., & Laffel, L. B. (1997). Behavioral and psychosocial research with school-aged children with type 1 diabetes. *Diabetes Spectrum, 10,* 277–281.

Anderson, B. J., Wolf, R. M., Burkhart, M. T., Cornell, R. G., & Bacon, G. E. (1989). Effects of peer-group intervention on metabolic control of adolescents with IDDM: Randomized outpatient study. *Diabetes Care, 12,* 179–183.

Anderson, B. J., & Rubin, R. R. (1996). *Practical psychology for diabetes clinician: How to deal with the key behavior issues faced by patients & health care teams.* Virginia: American Diabetes Association.

Anderson, L. A. (1990). Health-care communication and selected psychosocial correlates of adherence in diabetes management. *Diabetes Care, 13,* 66–76.

Auslander, W. F., Anderson, B. J., Bubb, J., Jung, K., & Santiago, J. V. (1990). Risk factors to health in diabetic children: A prospective study from diagnosis. *Health and Social Work, 15,* 133–142.

Barkley, R. A. (1981). *Hyperactive children.* New York: Guilford.

Bauman, L. J., Drotar, D., Leventhal, J. M., Perrin, E. C., & Pless, I. B. (1997). A review of psychosocial interventions for children with chronic health conditions. *Pediatrics, 100,* 244–251.

Betschart, J. E. (1997). Diabetes control: Guidelines for parents. *Diabetes Spectrum, 10,* 299–300.

Blackard, W. G. (1991). Insulin deficiency. In J. K. Davidson (Ed.), *Clinical diabetes mellitus* (pp. 68–77). New York: Thieme Medical Publishers.

Blechman, E. A., & Delamater, A. M. (1993). Family communication and Type 1 diabetes: A window on the social environment of chronically ill children. In R. E. Cole & D. Reiss (Eds.), *How do families cope with chronic illness?* (pp. 1–24). Hillsdale, NJ: Lawrence Erlbaum.

Boardway, R. H., Delamater, A. M., Tomakowsky, J., & Gutai, J. (1993). Stress management training for adolescents with diabetes. *Journal of Pediatric Psychology, 18,* 29–45.

Bobrow, E. S., AvRuskin, T. W., & Siller, J. (1985). Mother-daughter interaction and adherence to diabetes regimens. *Diabetes Care, 8,* 146–151.

Bojsen, J., Deckert, T., Kolendorf, K., & Lorup, B. (1979). Patient-controlled portable insulin infusion pump in diabetes. *Diabetes, 28,* 974–979.

Bond, G. G., Aiken, L. S., & Somerville, S. C. (1992). The Health Belief Model and adolescents with insulin-dependent diabetes mellitus. *Health Psychology, 11,* 190–198.

Brink, S. J., & Moltz, K. (1997) The message of the DCCT for children and adolescents. *Diabetes Spectrum 10* (4), 259–267.

Cahill, G. F. (1982). Disorders of carbohydrate metabolism: Diabetes mellitus. In J. B. Wyngaarden & L. H. Smith (Eds.), *Cecil textbook of medicine* (pp. 1053–1072). Philadelphia: W. B. Saunders.

Cahill, G. F., Etzwiler, D. D., & Freinkel, N. (1976). Control and diabetes. *New England Journal of Medicine, 294,* 1004.

Carney, R. M., Schechter, K., & Davis, T. (1983). Improving adherence to blood glucose testing in insulin-dependent diabetic children. *Behavior Therapy, 14,* 247–254.

Charron-Prochownik, D., Becker, M. H., Brown, M. B., Liang, W. M., & Bennett, S. (1993). Understanding young children's health beliefs and diabetes regimen adherence. *The Diabetes Educator, 19,* 409–418.

Christensen, K. S. (1983). Self-management in diabetic children. *Diabetes Care, 6,* 552–555.

Christensen, N. K., Terry, R. D., Wyatt, S., Pichert, J. W., & Lorenz, R. A. (1983). Quantitative assessment of dietary adherence in patients with insulin-dependent diabetes mellitus. *Diabetes Care, 6,* 245–250.

Cox, D. J., & Gonder-Frederick, L. (1992). Major developments in behavioral diabetes research. *Journal of Consulting and Clinical Psychology, 60,* 628–638.

Cox, D. J., Irvine, A., Gonder-Frederick, L., Nowacek, G., & Butterfield, J. (1987). Fear of hypoglycemia: Quantification, validation, and utilization. *Diabetes Care, 10,* 617–621.

Cox, D. J., Taylor, A. G., Nowacek, G., Holley-Wilcox, P., Pohl, S. L., & Guthrow, E. (1984). The relationship between psychological stress and insulin-dependent diabetic blood glucose control: Preliminary investigations. *Health Psychology, 3,* 63–75.

Coyne, J. C., & Anderson, B. J. (1989). The "psychosomatic family" reconsidered II: Recalling a defective model and looking ahead. *Journal of Marital and Family Therapy, 15,* 139–148.

Davidson, J. K., Galloway, J. A., & Chance, R. E. (1991). Insulin therapy. In J. K. Davidson (Ed.), *Clinical diabetes mellitus* (pp. 266–322). New York: Thieme Medical Publishers.

Delamater, A. M., Bubb, J., Davis, S. G., Smith, J. A., Schmidt, L., White, N. H., & Santiago, J. V. (1990). Randomized prospective study of self-management training with newly diagnosed diabetic children. *Diabetes Care, 13,* 492–498.

Delamater, A. M., Kurtz, S. M., Bubb, J., White, N. H., & Santiago, J. V. (1987). Stress and coping in relation to metabolic control of adolescents with Type 1 diabetes. *Developmental and Behavioral Pediatrics, 8,* 136–140.

Diabetes Control and Complications Trial Group (DCCT). (1993). The effect of intensive treatment of diabetes on the development and progression of long-term complications in insulin-dependent diabetes mellitus. *New England Journal of Medicine, 14,* 977–985.

DiMatteo, R., & DiNicola, D. (1985). *Achieving patient compliance: The psychology of the medical practitioner's role.* New York: Pergamon General Psychology Series.

Drash, A. L. (1981). The child with diabetes mellitus. In H. Rifkin & P. Raskin (Eds.), *Diabetes mellitus* (Vol. 5). Bowie, MD: Robert J. Brady Company, Prentice-Hall.

Drash, A. L. (1993). The child, the adolescent, and the diabetes control and complications trial. *Diabetes Care, 16,* 1515–1516.

Drash, A. L., & Becker, D. (1978). Diabetes mellitus in the child: Course, special problems, and related disorders. In H. M. Katzen & R. J. Mahler (Eds.), *Diabetes, obesity, and vascular disease: Advances in modern nutrition* (Vol. 2, pp. 615–643). Washington, DC: Hemisphere.

Eaton, W. W., Mengel, M., Mengel, L., Larson, D., Campbell, R., & Montague, R. B. (1992). Psychosocial and psychopathologic influences on management and control of insulin-dependent diabetes. *International Journal of Psychiatry in Medicine, 22,* 105–117.

Epstein, L. H., Beck, S., Figueroa, J., Farkas, G., Kazdin, A. E., Daneman, D., & Becker, D. (1981). The effects of targeting improvements in urine glucose on metabolic control in children with insulin dependent diabetes. *Journal of Applied Behavior Analysis, 14,* 365–375.

Epstein, L. H., Figueroa, J., Farkas, G. M., & Beck, S. (1981). The short-term effects of feedback on accuracy of urine glucose determinations in insulin dependent diabetic children. *Behavior Therapy, 12,* 560–564.

Erickson, E. (1963). *Childhood and society.* New York: W. W. Norton.

Etzwiler, D. B., & Sines, L. K. (1962). Juvenile diabetes and its management: Family, social and academic implications. *Journal of the American Medical Association, 181,* 304–308.

Ferrari, M. (1986). Perceptions of social support by parents of chronically ill versus healthy children. *Children's Health Care, 15,* 26–31.

Francis, G. L., Grogan, D., Hardy, L., Jensen, P. S., Xenakis, S. N., & Kearney, H. (1990). Group psychotherapy in the treatment of adolescent and preadolescent military dependents with recurrent diabetic ketoacidosis. *Military Medicine, 155,* 351–354.

Frenzel, M. P., McCaul, K. D., Glasgow, R. E., & Schafer, L. C. (1988). The relationship of stress and coping to regimen adherence and glycemic control of diabetes. *Journal of Social and Clinical Psychology, 6,* 77–87.

Garner, A. M., & Thompson, C. W. (1975). Psychological factors in the management of juvenile diabetes. *Journal of Clinical Child Psychology, 4,* 43–45.

Garrison, W. T., Biggs, D., & Williams, K. (1990). Temperament characteristics and clinical outcomes in young children with diabetes mellitus. *Journal of Child Psychology and Psychiatry, 31,* 1079–1088.

Gilbert, B. O., Johnson, S. B., Spillar, R., McCallum, M., Silverstein, J. H., & Rosenbloom, A. (1982). The effects of a peer-modeling film on children learning to self-inject insulin. *Behavior Therapy, 13,* 186–193.

Glasgow, R. E. (1991). Compliance to diabetes regimens: Conceptualization, complexity, and determinants. In J. A. Cramer & B. Spilker (Eds.), *Patient compliance in medical practice and clinical trials* (pp. 209–224). New York: Raven Press.

Glasgow, R. E., McCaul, K. D., & Schafer, L. C. (1987). Self-care behaviors and glycemic control in Type I diabetes. *Journal of Chronic Disease, 40,* 399–412.

Glasgow, A. M., Tynan, D., Schwartz, R., Hicks, J. M., Turek, J., Driscol, C., O'Donnell, R. M., & Getson, P. R. (1991). Alcohol and drug use in teenagers with diabetes mellitus. *Journal of Adolescent Health, 12,* 11–14.

Grey, M., Cameron, M. E., Lipman, T. H., & Thurber, F. W. (1995). Psychosocial status of children with diabetes in the first 2 years after diagnosis. *Diabetes Care, 18,* 1330–1336.

Gross, A. M., Magalnick, L. J., & Richardson, P. (1985). Self-management training with families of insulin-dependent diabetic children: A controlled long-term investigation. *Child and Family Behavior Therapy, 7,* 35–50.

Guthrie, R. A., & Jackson, R. L. (1975). Control of diabetes in children: Recent concepts concerning vascular complications and growth retardation. *Pediatric Annals, 4,* 342–350.

Hanson, C. L., DeGuire, M. J., Schinkel, A. M., Henggeler, S. W., & Burghen, G. A. (1992). Comparing social learning and family systems correlates of adaptation in youths with IDDM. *Journal of Pediatric Psychology, 17,* 555–572.

Hanson, C. L., Harris, M. A., Relyea, G., Cigrang, J. A., Carle, D. L., & Burghen, G. A. (1989). Coping styles in youths with insulin-dependent diabetes mellitus. *Jour-*

nal of Consulting and Clinical Psychology, 57, 644–651.

Hanson, C. L., & Henggeler, W. (1984). Metabolic control in adolescents with diabetes: An examination of systemic variables. *Family Systems Medicine, 2,* 5–16.

Hanson, C. L., Henggeler, S. W., & Burghen, G. A. (1987a). Social competence and parental support as mediators of the link between stress and metabolic control in adolescents with insulin-dependent diabetes mellitus. *Journal of Consulting and Clinical Psychology, 55,* 529–533.

Hanson, C. L., Henggeler, S. W., & Burghen, G. A. (1987b). Model of associations between psychosocial variables and health-outcome measures of adolescents with IDDM. *Diabetes Care, 10,* 752–758.

Hanson, C. L., Henggeler, S. W., Rodrigue, J. R., Burghen, G. A., & Murphy, W. D. (1988). Father-absent adolescents with insulin-dependent diabetes mellitus: A population at risk? *Journal of Applied Developmental Psychology, 9,* 243–252.

Harkavy, J., Johnson, S. B., Silverstein, J., Spillar, R., McCallum, M., & Rosenbloom, A. (1983). Who learns what at diabetes summer camp. *Journal of Pediatric Psychology, 8,* 143–153.

Hauser, S. T., Jacobson, A. M., Lavori, P., Wolfsdorf, J. I., Herskowitz, R. D., Milley, J. E., Bliss, R., Gelfand, E., Wertbieb, D., Stein, J. (1990). Adherence among children and adolescents with insulin-dependent diabetes mellitus over four-year longitudinal follow-up. II. Immediate and long-term linkages with the family milieu. *Journal of Pediatric Psychology, 15,* 527–542.

Hauser, S. T., Jacobson, A. M., Wertlieb, D., Weiss-Perry, B., Follansbee, D., Wolfsdorf, J. I., Herskowitz, R. D., Houlihan, J., & Rajapark, D. C. (1986). Children with recently diagnosed diabetes: Interactions within their families. *Health Psychology, 5,* 275–296.

Hauser, S. T., & Solomon, M. L. (1985). Coping with diabetes: Views from the family. In P. Ahmed & M. Ahmed (Eds.), *Coping with diabetes* (pp. 234–266). Springfield, IL: Thomas.

Haynes, R. B. (1979). Determinants of compliance: The disease and the mechanics of treatment. In R. B. Haynes, D. W. Taylor, & D. L. Sackett (Eds.), *Compliance in health care* (pp. 49–62). Baltimore: Johns Hopkins University Press.

Hoffman, R. G., Speelman, D. J., Hinnen, D. A., Conley, K. L., Guthrie, R. A., & Knapp, R. K. (1989). Changes in cortical functioning with acute hypoglycemia and hyperglycemia in Type I diabetes. *Diabetes Care, 12,* 193–197.

Holden, E. W., Friend, M., Gault, C., Kager, V., Foltz, L., & White, L. (1991). Family functioning and parental coping with chronic childhood illness: Relationships with self-competence, illness adjustment, and regimen adherence behaviors in children attending diabetes summer camp. In J. H. Johnson & S. B. Johnson (Eds.), *Advances in child health psychology* (pp. 265–276). Gainesville, FL: University of Florida Press.

Holmes, C. S., Hayford, J. T., Gonzalez, J. L., & Weydert, J. A. (1983). A survey of cognitive functioning at different glucose levels in diabetic persons. *Diabetes Care, 6,* 180–185.

Horan, P. F., Gwynn, C., & Renzi, D. (1986). Insulin-dependent diabetes mellitus and child abuse: Is there a relationship? *Diabetes Care, 9,* 302–307.

Ingersoll, G., Orr, D., Herrold, A., & Golden, M. (1986). Cognitive maturity and self-management among adolescents with insulin-dependent diabetes mellitus. *Journal of Pediatrics, 108,* 620–623.

Jacobson, A. M., Adler, A. G., Derby, L., Anderson, B. J., & Wolfsdorf, J. I. (1991). Clinic attendance and glycemic control: Study of contrasting groups of patients with IDDM. *Diabetes Care, 14,* 599–601.

Jacobson, A. M., Hauser, S. T., Lavori, P., Wolfsdorf, J. I., Herskowith, R. D., Milley, J. E., Bliss, R., Gelfand, E., Wertlieb, D., & Stein, J. (1990). Adherence among children and adolescents with insulin-dependent diabetes mellitus over four-year longitudinal follow-up. I. The influence of patient coping and adjustment. *Journal of Pediatric Psychology, 15,* 511–526.

Jacobson, A. M., Hauser, S. T., Wolfsdorf, J. I., Houlihan, J., Milley, J. E., Herskowitz, R. A., Wertlieb, D., & Watt, E. (1987). Psychologic predictors of compliance in children with recent onset of diabetes mellitus. *Journal of Pediatrics, 110,* 805–811.

Janis, I. L. (1983). The role of social support in adherence to stressful decisions. *American Psychologist, 38,* 143–160.

Johnson, S. B. (1982). Behavioral management of childhood diabetes. In J. Kuldau (Ed.), *New directions for mental health services: Treatment for psychosomatic problems* (Vol. 15, pp. 5–18). San Francisco: Jossey-Bass.

Johnson, S. B. (1984). Knowledge, attitudes, and behavior: Correlates of health in childhood diabetes. *Clinical Psychology Review, 4,* 503–524.

Johnson, S. B. (1988a). Diabetes mellitus in childhood. In D. K. Routh (Ed.), *Handbook of pediatric psychology* (pp. 9–31). New York: The Guilford Press.

Johnson, S. B. (1988b). Psychological aspects of childhood diabetes. *Journal of Child Psychology and Psychiatry, 29,* 729–738.

Johnson, S. B., Freund, A., Silverstein, J., Hansen, C. A., & Malone, J. (1990). Adherence-health status relationships in childhood diabetes. *Health Psychology, 9,* 606–631.

Johnson, S. B., Kelly, M., Henretta, J. C., Cunningham, W. R., Tomer, A., & Silverstein, J. H. (1992). A longitudinal analysis of adherence and health status in childhood diabetes. *Journal of Pediatric Psychology, 17,* 537–553.

Johnson, S. B., Pollak, T., Silverstein, J. H., Rosenbloom, A. L., Spillar, R., McCallum, M., & Harkavy, J. (1982). Cognitive and behavioral knowledge about insulin-dependent diabetes among children and parents. *Pediatrics, 69,* 708–713.

Johnson, S. B., & Rosenbloom, A. L. (1982). Behavioral aspects of diabetes mellitus in childhood and adolescence. *Psychiatric Clinics of North America, 5,* 357–369.

Johnson, S. B., Silverstein, J, Rosenbloom, A., Carter, R., & Cunningham, W. (1986). Assessing daily management in childhood diabetes. *Health Psychology, 5,* 545–564.

Johnson, S. B., Tomer, A., Cunningham, W. R., & Henretta, J. C. (1990). Adherence in childhood diabetes: Results of a confirmatory factor analysis. *Health Psychology, 9,* 493–501.

Jones, P. M. (1990). Use of a course on self-control behavior techniques to increase adherence to prescribed frequency for self-monitoring blood glucose. *Diabetes Educator, 16,* 296–303.

Kaplan, R. M., Chadwick, M. W., & Schimmel, L. E. (1985). Social learning intervention to promote metabolic control in type 1 diabetes mellitus: Pilot experiment results. *Diabetes Care, 8,* 152–155.

Kovacs, M., Finkelstein, R., Feinberg, T. L., Crouse-Novak, M., Paulauskas, S., & Pollock, M. (1985). Initial psychologic responses of parents to the diagnosis of insulin-dependent diabetes mellitus in their children. *Diabetes Care, 8,* 568–575.

Kovacs, M., Goldston, D., Obrosky, D. S., & Bonar, L. K. (1997a). Psychiatric disorders in youths with IDDM: Rates and risk factors. *Diabetes Care, 20,* 36–44.

Kovacs, M., Goldston, D., Obrosky, S., & Iyengar, S. (1992). Prevalence and predictors of pervasive noncompliance with medical treatment among youths with insulin-dependent diabetes mellitus. *Journal of the American Academy of Child and Adolescent Psychiatry, 31,* 1112–1119.

Kovacs, M., Iyengar, S., Goldston, D., Obrosky, D. S., Stewart, J., & Marsh, J. (1990). Psychological functioning among mothers of children with insulin-dependent diabetes mellitus: A longitudinal study. *Journal of Consulting and Clinical Psychology, 58,* 189–195.

Kovacs, M., Kass, R. E., Schnell, T. M., Goldston, D., & Marsh, J. (1989) Family functioning and metabolic control of school-aged children with IDDM. *Diabetes Care, 12* (6) 409–414.

Kovacs, M., Obrosky, D. S., Goldston, D., & Drash, A. (1997b). Major depressive disorder in youths with IDDM. *Diabetes Care, 20,* 45–51.

Kravitz, A. R., Isenberg, P. L., Shore, M. F., & Barnett, D. M. (1971). Emotional factors in diabetes mellitus. In A. Marble, R. Bradley, & L. Krall (Eds.), *Joslin's diabetes mellitus* (11th ed.) (pp. 767–782). Philadelphia: Lea & Febinger.

Kurtz, S. M., & Delamater, A. M. (1984). Family interactions, adherence, and metabolic control in IDDM. *Diabetes, 33* (Suppl. 1), 78A.

Kuttner, M. J., Delamater, A. M., & Santiago, J. V. (1990). Learned helplessness in diabetic youths. *Journal of Pediatric Psychology, 15,* 581–594.

LaGreca, A. M. (1982). Behavioral aspects of diabetes management in children and adolescents. *Diabetes, 32* (Suppl. 2), 47.

LaGreca, A. M. (1988). Children with diabetes and their families: Coping and disease management. In T. Field, P. McCabe, & N. Schneiderman (Eds.), *Stress and coping across development* (pp. 139–159). Hillsdale, NJ: Erlbaum.

LaGreca, A. M. (1990). Social consequences of pediatric conditions: Fertile area for future investigation and intervention? *Journal of Pediatric Psychology, 15,* 285–308.

LaGreca, A. M., Follansbee, D., & Skyler, J. S. (1990). Developmental and behavioral aspects of diabetes management in youngsters. *Children's Health Care, 19,* 132–139.

LaGreca, A. M., & Hanna, N. C. (1983a). *The health beliefs of children with diabetes and their mothers: Implications for treatment.* Paper presented at the Annual Meeting of the American Diabetes Association, San Antonio, TX. Abstract in: *Diabetes, 32* (Suppl. 1), 66.

LaGreca, A. M., & Hanna, N. C. (1983b). Poster presented at the Annual Meeting of the American Diabetes Association, New Orleans, LA. Abstract in: *Diabetes, 43* (Suppl. 1), 8A.

LaGreca, A. M., Schwarz, L. T., & Satin, W. (1987). Eating patterns in young women with IDDM: Another look. *Diabetes Care, 10,* 659–660.

Lernmark, A. (1991). Insulin-dependent diabetes mellitus. In J. K. Davidson (Ed.), *Clinical diabetes mellitus* (pp. 35–49). New York: Thieme Medical Publishers.

Littlefield, C. H., Craven, J. L., Rodin, G. M., Daneman, D., Murray, M. A., & Rydall, A. C. (1992). Relationship of self-efficacy and bingeing to adherence to diabetes regimen among adolescents. *Diabetes Care, 15,* 90–94.

Marrero, D. G., Fremion, A. S., & Golden, M. P. (1988). Improving compliance with exercise in adolescents with insulin-dependent diabetes mellitus: Results of a self-motivated home exercise program. *Pediatrics, 81,* 519–525.

Marrero, D. G., Lau, N., Golden, M. P., Kershnar, A., & Myers, G. C. (1982). Family dynamics in adolescent diabetes mellitus: Parental behavior and metabolic control. In Z. Laron & A. Galatzer (Eds.), *Psychological aspects of diabetes in children and adolescents* (Vol. 10, pp. 77–82). Basel, Switzerland: Karger.

McCaul, K. D., Glasgow, R. E., & Schafer, L. D. (1987). Diabetes regimen behavior: Predicting adherence. *Medical Care, 25,* 868–881.

McKelvey, J., & Borgersen, M. (1990). Family development and the use of diabetes groups: Experience with a model approach. *Patient Education and Counseling, 16,* 61–67.

Minuchin, S., Rosman, B. L., & Baker, L. (1978). *Psychosomatic families: Anorexia nervosa in context.* Cambridge, MA: Harvard University Press.

Nagasawa, M., Smith, M. C., Barnes, J. H., & Fincham, J. E. (1990). Meta-analysis of correlates of diabetes patients' compliance with prescribed medications. *Diabetes Educator, 16,* 192–200.

Newbrough, J. R., Simpkins, C. G., Maurer, H. (1985). A family development approach to studying factors in the management and control of childhood diabetes. *Diabetes Care, 8,* 83–92.

Olefsky, J. M. (1992) Diabetes mellitus. In J. B. Wyngaarden, L. H. Smith & J. C. Bennett Jr. (Eds.), *Cecil textbook of medicine* (pp. 1291–1310). Philadelphia: W. B. Saunders.

Orme, C. M., & Binik, Y. M. (1989). Consistency of adherence across regimen demands. *Health Psychology, 8,* 27–43.

Orr, D. P. (1986). Psychosocial problems of diabetic teenagers. *Medical Aspects of Human Sexuality, 20,* 88–100.

Page, P., Verstraete, D. G., Robb, J. R., & Etzwiler, D. D. (1981). Patient recall of self-care recommendations in diabetes. *Diabetes Care, 4,* 96–98.

Partridge, J. W., Garner, A. M., Thompson, C. W., & Cherry, T. (1972). Attitudes of adolescents toward their diabetes. *American Journal of Diseases of Children, 124,* 226–229.

Peveler, R. C., Fairburn, C. G., Boller, I., & Dunger, D. (1992). Eating disorders in adolescents with IDDM. *Diabetes Care, 15,* 1356–1359.

Peyrot, M., & McMurray, J. F. (1985). Psychosocial factors in diabetes control: Adjustment of insulin-treated adults. *Psychosomatic Medicine, 47,* 542–557.

Pichert, J., Flannery, M. E., Kline, S., Hodge, M., Meek, J., & Kinzer, C. (1994). Improving teens' confidence about handling situational obstacles to dietary adherence (SODA).

Pinhas-Hamiel, O., Dolan, Daniels, L. M., Standiford, D., Khoury, P. R., & Zeitler, P. (1996). Increased incidence of non-insulin dependent diabetes mellitus among adolescents. *Journal of Pediatrics, 128,* 608–615.

Pinhas-Hamiel, O., & Zeitler, P. (1997). A weighty problem—diagnosis and treatment of type 2 diabetes in adolescents. *Diabetes Spectrum, 10,* 292–296.

Polivy, J., & Herman, C. P. (1985). Dieting and bingeing: A causal analysis. *American Psychologist, 40,* 193–201.

Prazar, G., & Felice, M. (1975). The psychologic and social effects of juvenile diabetes. *Pediatric Annals, 4,* 351–358.

Rabin, C., Amir, S., Nardi, R., & Ovadia, B. (1986). Compliance and control: Issues in group training for diabetics. *Health and Social Work, 11,* 141–151.

Reid, P., & Appleton, P. (1991). Insulin dependent diabetes mellitus: Regimen adherence in children and young people. *The Irish Journal of Psychology, 12,* 17–32.

Reid, P., Ellis, N., Owens, G., & Jones, H. (1992). Diabetic management skills in a paediatric population: Accuracy, responsibility and satisfaction. *The Irish Journal of Psychology, 13,* 295–306.

Riley, W. J., Silverstein, J. H., Rosenbloom, A., L., Spillar, R., & McCallum, M. (1980). Ambulatory diabetes management with pulsed subcutaneous insulin using a portable pump. *Clinical Pediatrics, 19,* 609–614.

Rodin, G., Craven, J., Littlefield, C., Murray, M., & Daneman, D. (1991). Eating disorders and intentional insulin undertreatment in adolescent females with diabetes. *Psychosomatics, 32,* 171–176.

Rodin, G. M., Johnson, L. E., Garfinkel, P. E., Daneman, D., & Kenshole, A. B. (1986). Eating disorders in female adolescents with insulin dependent diabetes mellitus. *International Journal of Psychiatry in Medicine, 16,* 49–57.

Rosenstock, J., Strowig, S., & Raskin, P. (1985). Insulin pump therapy: A realistic appraisal. *Clinical Diabetes, 3,* 25–31.

Rovet, J., Ehrlich, R. M., & Hoppe, M. (1988). Specific intellectual deficits in children with early onset diabetes mellitus. *Child Development, 59,* 226–234.

Rubin, R., Young-Hyman, D., & Peyrot, M. (1989). Parent-child responsibility and conflict in diabetes care (abstract). *Diabetes, 38* (Suppl. 2), 28.

Ruggiero, L., & Prochaska, J. O. (1993). Application of the transtheoretical model to diabetes. *Diabetes Spectrum, 6,* 22–59.

Ryan, C., Vega, A., Longstreet, C., & Drash, A. (1985). Cognitive deficits in adolescents who developed diabetes early in life. *Pediatrics, 75,* 921–927.

Satin, W., LaGreca, A. M., Zigo, M. A., & Skyler, J. S. (1989). Diabetes in adolescence: Effects of multifamily group intervention and parent simulation of diabetes. *Journal of Pediatric Psychology, 14,* 259–275.

Savinetti-Rose, B. (1994). Developmental issues in managing children with diabetes. *Pediatric Nursing, 20,* 11–15.

Schafer, L. C., Glasgow, R. E., & McCaul, K. D. (1982). Increasing the adherence of diabetic adolescents. *Journal of Behavioral Medicine, 5,* 353–362.

Schafer, L., Glasgow, R., McCaul, K., & Dreher, M. (1983). Adherence to IDDM regimens: Relationship to psychosocial variables and metabolic control. *Diabetes Care, 6,* 493–498.

Schlenk, E., & Hart, L. (1984). Relationship between health locus of control, health value, and social support and compliance of persons with diabetes mellitus. *Diabetes Care, 7,* 566–74.

Shouval, R., Ber, R., & Galatzer, A. (1982). Family social climate and the health status and social adaptation of diabetic youth. In Z. Laron & A. Galatzer (Eds.), *Psychological aspects of diabetes in children and adoles-*

cents: Pediatric and adolescent endocrinology (Vol. 10, pp. 89–93). Basel, Switzerland: Karger.

Simonds, J. F. (1979). Emotions and compliance in diabetic children. *Psychosomatics, 20,* 544–551.

Steel, J. M., Young, R. J., Lloyd, G. G., & Macintyre, C. (1989). Abnormal eating attitudes in young insulin-dependent diabetics. *British Journal of Psychiatry, 155,* 515–21.

Stevens, A. B., McKane, W. R., Bell, P. M., Bell, P., King, D. J., & Hayes, J. R. (1989). Psychomotor performance and counterregulatory response during mild hypoglycemia in healthy volunteers. *Diabetes Care, 12,* 12–17.

Striegel-Moore, R. H., Nicholson, T. J., & Tamborlane, W. V. (1992). Prevalence of eating disorder symptoms in preadolescent and adolescent girls with IDDM. *Diabetes Care, 15,* 1361–1368.

Surwit, R. S., Feinglos, M. N., & Scovern, A. W. (1983). Diabetes and behavior: A paradigm for health psychology. *American Psychologist, 38,* 255–262.

Surwit, R. S., & Schneider, M. S. (1993). Role of stress in the etiology and treatment of diabetes mellitus. *Psychosomatic Medicine, 55,* 380–393.

Tarnow, J. D., & Silverman, S. W. (1981–1982). The psychophysiologic aspects of stress in juvenile diabetes mellitus. *International Journal of Psychiatry in Medicine, 11,* 25–44.

Tarnow, J. D., & Tomlinson, N. (1978). Juvenile diabetes: Impact on the child and family. *Psychosomatics, 19,* 487–491.

Tattersall, R. B., & Lowe, J. (1981). Diabetes in adolescence. *Diabetologia, 20,* 517–523.

Travis, L. (1987). Stress, hyperglycemia, and ketosis. In L. Travis, B. H. Brouhard, & B. D. Schreiner (Eds.), *Diabetes mellitus in children and adolescents* (pp. 137–146). Philadelphia: Saunders.

Viederman, M., & Hymowitz, P. (1988). A developmental-psychodynamic model for diabetic control. *General Hospital Psychiatry, 10,* 34–40.

Waller, D., Chipman, J. J., Hardy, Hightower, M. S., North, A. J., Williams, S. B., & Babick, A. J. (1986). Measur-

ing diabetes-specific family support and its relation to metabolic control: A preliminary report. *Journal of the American Academy of Child Psychology, 25,* 415–418.

Watkins, J. D., Williams, T. F., Martin, D. A., Hogan, M. D., & Anderson, E. (1967). A study of diabetic patients at home. *American Journal of Public Health, 57,* 452–459.

Weiner, M. F., & Skipper, F. P. (1979). Euglycemia: A psychological study. *International Journal of Psychiatry in Medicine, 9,* 281–288.

Wilson, D., & Endres, R. (1986). Compliance with blood glucose monitoring in children with type 1 diabetes mellitus. *Journal of Pediatrics, 108,* 1022–1024.

Wing, R. R., Nowalk, M. A., Marcus, M. D., Koeske, R., & Finegold, D. (1986). Subclinical eating disorders and glycemic control in adolescents with type 1 diabetes. *Diabetes Care, 9,* 162–167.

Wishner, W. J., & O'Brien, M. D. (1978). Diabetes and the family. *Medical Clinics of North America, 62,* 849–856.

Wolfsdorf, J. I., Anderson, B. J., & Pasquarello, C. (1994). Treatment of the child with diabetes. In C. R. Kahn & G. C. Weir (Eds.), *Joslin's diabetes mellitus* (13th ed.) (pp. 530–551). Philadelphia: Lea & Febiger.

Wynne, L. C., & Singer, M. (1963). Thought disorder and family relations of schizophrenics, I and II. *Archives of General Psychiatry, 9,* 191–206.

Wysocki, T., Hough, B. S., Ward, K. M., & Green, L. B. (1992). Diabetes mellitus in the transition to adulthood: Adjustment, self-care, and health status. *Developmental and Behavioral Pediatrics, 13,* 194–201.

Wysocki, T., Taylor, A., Hough, B. S., Linscheid, T., Yeates, K. O., Naglieri, J. A. (1996). Deviation from developmentally appropriate self-care autonomy. *Diabetes Care, 19* (2), 119–125.

Younger, D., Brink, S. J., Barnett D. M., Wentworth, S. M., Leibovich, J., & Madden, P. B. (1985). In A. Marble, L. P. Krall, R. F. Bradley, A. R. Christlieb, & J. S. Soeldner (Eds.), *Joslin's diabetes mellitus* (12th ed.). Philadelphia: Lea & Febiger.

CHAPTER 5

ANOREXIA AND BULIMIA NERVOSA

Susan E. Barker, MEDICAL UNIVERSITY OF SOUTH CAROLINA
Patrick Mahlen O'Neil, MEDICAL UNIVERSITY OF SOUTH CAROLINA

The most common eating disorders in adolescents and young adults are anorexia nervosa and bulimia nervosa. This chapter provides an overview of relevant findings pertaining to diagnosis of anorexia and bulimia nervosa, epidemiology, health risks, etiological theories, risk factors, comorbidity with other psychiatric disorders, assessment, and treatment planning and outcome.

Since anorexia and bulimia nervosa have been thought to be largely disorders of adolescents and adults, research conducted with prepubertal children is rare and consists mainly of case reports of anorexia nervosa. It is likely that occurrence both of anorexia and of bulimia nervosa among children is low. However, eating-related attitudes and behaviors that are developed during childhood may place the child at risk for subsequent development of an eating disorder. For example, picky eating and digestive problems during early childhood are predictive of later symptoms of anorexia nervosa, whereas childhood pica (eating nonnutritive substances such as clay) has been found to predict subsequent bulimia nervosa (Marchi & Cohen, 1990).

Since most research has examined postpubertal eating disorders, information presented in this chapter focuses primarily on anorexia nervosa and bulimia nervosa during adolescence and young adulthood.

DIAGNOSIS AND CLINICAL DESCRIPTION

Anorexia Nervosa

Anorexia nervosa was first recognized as a psychiatric syndrome in 1868 when it was described by Sir William Gull. Although the term *anorexia* literally means "loss of appetite," the central feature of the disorder is not lack of appetite but an intense fear of fatness, which motivates the anorexic toward extreme methods for weight loss despite being very thin. Most anorexics use extreme dieting and excessive exercise to achieve and maintain an abnormally low body weight. Anorexics may or may not binge eat; it has been estimated that 40 percent of anorexics develop problems with bingeing within two years of the onset of anorexia nervosa (Hsu, 1990). Approximately half of patients diagnosed with anorexia also use purgative methods (self-induced vomiting or misuse of laxatives, diuretics, or enemas) as a means of controlling weight (Halmi & Falk, 1982).

In the fourth edition of the *Diagnostic and Statistical Manual for Mental Disorders (DSM-IV;* American Psychiatric Association, 1994), *anorexia nervosa* is defined as a disorder characterized by a refusal to maintain a minimum normal body weight (less than 85 percent of expected weight for age and height). In addition, anorexics exhibit an intense fear of gaining weight, a disturbance in body image, and amenorrhea (in postmenarcheal females). *DSM-IV* diagnostic criteria for anorexia nervosa are summarized in Figure 5. 1.

These criteria represent a distinct change from the earlier *DSM-III-R* (APA, 1987) description for anorexia nervosa. In *DSM-III-R* nomenclature, an individual was diagnosed with both anorexia nervosa and bulimia nervosa if she or he met criteria for both disorders. In the *DSM-IV* system, the anorexic can be subclassified into either a binge eating/purging subtype (in which she or he regularly engages in binge eating and purgative behaviors) or a nonbulimic or restricting subtype. DaCosta and Halmi (1992) reviewed studies comparing these subtypes and concluded that the distinction between bulimic and nonbulimic types of anorexia appears to be warranted. Bulimic-anorexics were consistently found to demonstrate more impulsive behaviors, including stealing, drug abuse, suicide attempts, and self-mutilation as compared to anorexic-restrictors. In addition, bulimic-anorexics were found to have a longer duration of illness and a higher prevalence of premorbid and familial obesity and familial psychopathol-

Figure 5.1 Summary of *DSM-IV* Diagnostic Criteria for Anorexia Nervosa

---

1. One refuses to attain or maintain a minimum normal body weight (is 15 percent or more below expected weight for age and height).
2. One has a strong fear of "fatness" and weight gain, even though underweight.
3. One is disturbed in the way one's body weight and shape is experienced, excessive influence of body shape and weight on self-evaluation, or denial of the seriousness of low body weight.
4. There is an absence of three or more consecutive menstrual cycles (amenorrhea) in postmenarcheal females.

Binge Eating/Purging Type: The person currently engages in regular binge eating or purgative behavior (self-induced vomiting or misuse of laxatives, enemas, or diuretics).

Restricting Type: The person does not currently binge eat or engage in purgative behavior.

Source: Adapted from *Diagnostic and Statistical Manual of Mental Disorders,* 4th ed. Washington, DC: America Psychiatric Association.

ogy. There was no consistent difference between the two groups in amount of depression or general psychological distress.

In *DSM-III-R,* the construct of body image disturbance in anorexia nervosa focused on body size overestimation, indicated by the anorexic claiming to "feel fat" when emaciated, or to believe one area of the body to be too fat, even when obviously underweight (APA, p. 67). Indeed, many studies have found greater body size overestimation in both anorexics and bulimics as compared to controls (for a review, see Slade, 1985). However, as reviewed by Hsu and Sobkiewicz (1991), other studies have provided conflicting evidence. Of the research reviewed for both anorexics and bulimics, 14 studies found that clinical subjects overestimated their body size to a greater degree than normal controls, and 12 studies found no differences between the two groups. Hsu and Sobkiewicz concluded that size overestimation should not be considered characteristic of all or even most persons with an eating disorder.

Accordingly, diagnostic criteria for anorexia nervosa in *DSM-IV* do not require overestimation of body size, but define body image disturbance as "denial of the seriousness of current low body weight, or undue influence of body shape and weight on self-evaluation" (APA, p. 545). Garfinkel (1992) reviewed the salient literature and reported that patients with anorexia consistently demonstrate higher levels of concern about weight and shape than do noneating-disordered controls.

Bulimia Nervosa

Bulimia nervosa is an eating disorder characterized by frequent episodes of uncontrolled binge eating, followed by use of compensatory behaviors to control weight. These behaviors include both "purgative" techniques (self-induced vomiting or misuse of laxatives, diuretics, or enemas) and "nonpurgative" compensatory behaviors (excessive exercise and strict dieting or fasting). Like anorexics, bulimic individuals are thought to engage in these behaviors because of body image disturbances and an intense fear of weight gain. Unlike anorexics, bulimic patients are usually within the normal weight range, since they are not as successful in restricting their caloric intake.

The *DSM-IV* diagnostic criteria for bulimia nervosa (which are summarized in Figure 5.2) are also somewhat different from the *DSM-III-R* system of diagnosing bulimia nervosa. First, the *DSM-IV* system allows for subclassification of bulimics into "purging" or "nonpurging" types, depending on their use of purgative or nonpurgative compensatory behaviors to control weight. *DSM-III-R* did not differentiate purgative and nonpurgative compensatory techniques. In addition, specification in *DSM-III-R* that bingeing involves rapid eating has been eliminated from the *DSM-IV* criteria, since there is little evidence that rapidity of eating is a defining characteristic of a binge (Wilson, 1992).

There has been much debate about how a *binge* should be defined. Laboratory studies of binge eating have shown that average binges by bulimics consist of 3,500 kcals to 4,477 kcals (Kaye, Gwirtsman, George, Weiss, & Jimerson, 1986; Kissileff, Walsh, Kral, & Cassidy, 1986). However, other studies have shown that self-reported binges may consist of fewer than 1,000 kcals (Rossiter, Agras, & Losch, 1988). *DSM-IV* diagnostic criteria attempt to operationally define a *binge* as uncontrollably "eating, in a discrete period of time . . . an amount of food that is definitely larger than most people would eat during a similar period of time and under similar circumstances" (p. 549). The *DSM-III-R* requirement of binge frequency (i.e., two or more times per week) was retained in *DSM-IV*, although there is conflicting evidence as to whether bulimics who binge more frequently have more concurrent psychopathology or whether binge frequency affects treatment outcome (Wilson, 1992).

Bulimic individuals display weight and shape concerns similar to those experienced by anorexics (Garfinkel, 1992). Garfinkel and associates (1992), using a structured interview procedure, found that only 3 of 104 bulimic patients did *not* exhibit overconcern for shape or weight. More than 80 percent of these patients classified their weight and shape as "moderately" to "supremely" important. In the *DSM-IV* diagnostic criteria, body image disturbance is indicated when the bulimic's self-evaluation is "unduly influenced" by body shape and weight (APA, p. 550).

Figure 5.2 Summary of *DSM-IV* Diagnostic Criteria for Bulimia Nervosa

1. One experiences episodes of binge eating, characterized by *both*:
   a. Eating, within any two-hour period, an amount of food that is larger than most people would eat under similar circumstances and during a similar period of time.
   b. A feeling of lack of control over what or how much is eaten during the binge episode.
2. One uses compensatory behaviors to prevent weight gain (self-induced vomiting; use of laxatives, diuretics, or enemas; excessive exercise; or fasting).
3. Binge-eating episodes and compensatory behaviors occur a minimum average of two times a week for three months.
4. Self-evaluation is excessively influenced by body shape and weight.
5. Bulimic behaviors do not occur exclusively during episodes of anorexia nervosa.

Purging Type: The person regularly engages in self-induced vomiting or in use of laxatives, diuretics, or enemas to prevent weight gain.

Nonpurging Type: The person does not regularly engage in self-induced vomiting or use of laxatives, diuretics, or enemas to prevent weight gain, but does use other compensatory behaviors (fasting or excessive exercise).

Source: Adapted from *Diagnostic and Statistical Manual of Mental Disorders,* 4th ed. Washington, DC: American Psychiatric Association.

PREVALENCE OF ANOREXIA AND BULIMIA NERVOSA

Prevalence estimates of eating disorders have varied widely, and prevalence studies are limited by several methodological problems. First, subjects sampled have consisted mostly of college students, instead of individuals from the general population. In addition, many studies have relied exclusively on self-report questionnaires to detect cases of eating disorders. Prevalence rates based on these investigations are consistently higher than those derived from interview-based studies (Fairburn, Hay, & Welch, 1993). Diagnostic criteria for the eating disorders have changed through the years and continue to be revised, producing different estimates of prevalence. Finally, Fairburn and Beglin (1990) have suggested that prevalence figures from even the best interview-based studies may be underestimates of true rates, since eating-disordered individuals may choose not to participate in these studies.

Studies consistently have shown that the prevalence of eating disorders is increasing (Lucas, Beard,

O'Fallon, & Kurlan, 1991) and that they are more common in females than in males (Eller, 1993). Eating disorders are especially common in girls and women whose occupations or avocations emphasize slimness and competitiveness, such as ballet dancers (Garner, Garfinkel, Rockert, & Olmsted, 1987) and athletes (Rosen & Hough, 1988). Bulimia is more common than anorexia. In interview-based studies using *DSM-III-R* or equivalent definitions, prevalence rates for anorexia nervosa have generally been between 0.7 percent and 2.1 percent, whereas those for bulimia nervosa are between 1 percent and 4.5 percent of adolescent girls and women in the general population (Fairburn & Beglin, 1990; Hsu, 1990; Brewerton, Dansky, O'Neil, & Kilpatrick, 1993). There currently are no available estimates of the prevalence of anorexia or bulimia nervosa in prepubertal children. Eating disorders are more common in Caucasians than in other racial and ethnic groups (Fairburn & Beglin, 1990) and are rare in people from developing countries (Mumford, Whitehouse, & Choudry, 1992).

Both anorexia nervosa and bulimia nervosa typically emerge during late adolescence (Hsu, 1990), and younger women are more at risk for eating disorders than older women (Bushnell, Wells, Hornblow, Oakley-Browne, & Joyce, 1990). Halmi, Casper, Eckert, Goldberg, and Davis (1979) found a bimodal distribution in age of onset of anorexia, with peaks at 14 and 18 years. These researchers hypothesized that emergence of eating-disorder symptoms occurs during developmental periods that are challenging to the adolescent (i.e., entering and leaving high school). Some researchers have also suggested that physical changes associated with puberty play an important role in the development of eating disorders (Levine & Smolak, 1992).

Whereas eating disturbances severe enough to meet diagnostic criteria occur at a relatively low rate, the occurrence of pathological eating behaviors is more common, especially among adolescent and young adult females. For example, Rosen, Tacy, and Howell (1990) found that 68 percent of adolescent girls were attempting to lose weight, although few of them were actually overweight. Occasional binge eating, self-induced vomiting, and diet pill use have also been found to occur frequently in adolescents and children (Fairburn & Beglin, 1990; Childress, Brew-

erton, Hodges, & Jarrell, 1993). Maloney, McGuire, Daniels, and Specker (1989) found that 45 percent of elementary school children wanted to be thinner, and 37 percent had already dieted.

HEALTH RISKS ASSOCIATED WITH ANOREXIA AND BULIMIA

The anorexic's visible emaciation is a stark symbol of the grave health risks associated with the disorder. Other common physical signs of anorexia include dry skin and thinning hair, yellowish discoloration of the skin, edema, and growth of fine hair (lanugo) on the face, trunk, and extremities. Stunted growth and arrested sexual maturation may occur in prepubertal anorexics, and prolonged amenorrhea is often associated with irreversible bone mineral density loss and a correspondingly higher risk of fractures (Ehrenkranz, 1993). Anorexics commonly suffer from dehydration, gastrointestinal problems, and metabolic and nutritional deficiencies; prolonged starvation may cause infertility. The most acute and life-threatening complication of anorexia nervosa is cardiac arrhythmia associated with electrolyte disturbances and the pathologic effects of starvation on the heart (Ehrenkranz, 1993). The long-term mortality from untreated anorexia nervosa is over 10 percent; the most common causes of death are suicide and starvation (APA, 1993).

Physical signs of bulimia nervosa include swelling of the salivary (particularly the parotid) glands due to bingeing and vomiting, dental erosion and resulting dental caries, and callouses on the fingers if they are used to induce a gag reflex for vomiting (Mitchell, 1986). Evidence of small hemorrhages may be seen on the cornea and face if the bulimic is examined soon after vomiting (Hsu, 1990). Physical complications of vomiting and of laxative and diuretic abuse include electrolyte imbalances (particularly hypokalemia) leading to cardiac disturbances, fluid imbalances and edema, irritation and potential tearing of the esophagus, gastrointestinal problems, and bowel abnormalities. Resting bradycardia and hypotension are observed in some bulimic patients. Use of syrup of ipecac to induce vomiting causes muscle damage, including cardiomyopathy (Ehrenkranz, 1993).

COMORBIDITY WITH OTHER PSYCHIATRIC DISORDERS

Depression

An association between depression and eating disorders is well established (Marx, 1993). Studies show significant prevalence rates of both depressive disorders and symptoms of depression in eating-disordered patients. For example, Halmi and colleagues (1991) found a lifetime prevalence of 68 percent for major depression in patients with anorexia nervosa. Other estimates have ranged from 44 percent (Laessle, Kittl, Fitcher, Wittchen, & Pirke, 1987) to 77 percent in patients with bulimia nervosa (Lee, Rush, & Mitchell, 1985).

Most studies examining families of eating-disordered patients have also shown greater prevalence of mood disorders than in families of control subjects (e.g., Kassett et al., 1989). There is conflicting evidence as to whether there are differences in depressive symptoms among the types of eating disorders and whether the depression or the eating disorder develops first. One possibility that has been raised is that malnutrition caused by starvation itself may produce detrimental effects on mood (Strober & Katz, 1988).

Personality Disorders

Estimates of the comorbidity of personality disorders and eating disorders have varied widely. Skodol and colleagues (1993) recently conducted a thorough investigation of personality disorders in 42 eating disordered patients, using a conservative method for diagnosis (i.e., consensus between two clinician-administered personality disorder interviews). The rate of one or more personality disorders in eating-disordered inpatients was 74 percent and among outpatients, 54 percent. These rates were significantly greater than those among 158 noneating-disordered psychiatric controls. Skodol and colleagues found a strong relationship between borderline personality disorder and bulimia nervosa, even when binge eating was not counted as impulsivity for diagnosing borderline personality disorder. Anorexia nervosa was found to be most strongly related to avoidant personality disorder. Finally, eating disorders with concurrent personality disorders were found to be characterized by greater chronicity and lower overall functioning. Personality disorders have also been implicated in negative treatment outcome (Johnson, Tobin, & Dennis, 1990).

Obsessive-Compulsive Disorder

Eating disorders appear to share many topographic features with obsessive-compulsive disorder (OCD). In fact, anorexia can be conceptualized as an obsessive-compulsive disorder in which one experiences obsessional thoughts about weight, and compulsively avoids eating to reduce these thoughts. The disorders have been found to coexist at a substantial rate: Hudson, Pope, Yurgelun-Todd, Jonas, and Frankenburg (1987) found that 33 percent of their bulimic sample met criteria for a diagnosis of OCD. Halmi and associates (1991) found that OCD was the fourth most common comorbid disorder in anorexic subjects in a 10-year follow-up study. Conversely, several studies have found an increased prevalence of eating disorders among OCD patients (e.g., Kasvikis, Tsakiris, Marks, Basoglu, & Noshirvani, 1986).

Some researchers have hypothesized that eating disorders may be etiologically related to OCD, citing evidence that pharmacological treatments that are effective for OCD are also effective for anorexia and bulimia (e.g., Fluoxetine Bulimia Nervosa Collaborative Study Group, 1992). Hsu, Kaye, and Weltzin (1993) reviewed evidence supporting this idea and concluded that although the available evidence is intriguing, it is premature at this time to conclude that eating disorders are a variant of OCD.

Substance Abuse Disorders

Lifetime prevalence rates for alcoholism have been estimated to be 6.7 percent in anorexia nervosa subjects (Eckert, Goldberg, Halmi, Casper, & Davis, 1979), as compared to the prevalence rate of 4.6 percent in U.S. women (Robins, Helzer, Pryzbeck, & Regier, 1988). Estimates of the prevalence of alcohol abuse and/or dependence in bulimia nervosa patients range from 2.9 percent to 48.6 percent, with a median of 22.9 percent (for a review, see Holderness, Brooks-Gunn, & Warren, 1994).

Helzer and Pryzbeck (1988) caution that these high rates may be an artifact of "an increased tendency for persons with multiple diagnoses to seek and receive treatment and thus fall into study populations drawn from treatment sources" (p. 219). Using data from an epidemiological catchment area survey, Helzer and Pryzbeck found no association between anorexia nervosa and alcoholism. In another population-based study, however, Kendler and colleagues (1991) found that 15.5 percent of bulimic subjects had a lifetime diagnosis of alcoholism.

RISK FACTORS ASSOCIATED WITH EATING DISORDERS

Most researchers agree that the etiology of eating disorders is complex and multifactorial. It is generally thought that eating disorders occur in the context of a society in which standards for feminine beauty rely predominantly on unrealistic thinness (Thompson, 1990). Current sociocultural emphasis on extreme thinness in women is thought to play a primary role in producing desire to lose weight and a strong belief that one must be thin (Brownell, 1991; Levine & Smolak, 1992). Striegel-Moore, Silberstein, and Rodin (1986) wrote, "The more a woman believes that 'what is fat is bad, what is thin is beautiful, and what is beautiful is good,' the more she will work toward thinness and be distressed about fatness" (p. 247).

However, although most girls and women in developed countries are exposed to societal pressure to be thin, only a minority develops severe eating disturbance. Identification of more specific risk factors for eating disorders is therefore important. Eating disorders are seen more frequently in girls who experience parental pressure to be thin (Pike & Rodin, 1991) and who have high needs for achievement (Steiner-Adair, 1986). Other variables implicated as risk factors for eating disturbance include depression (Gross & Rosen, 1988), low self-esteem (Rosen et al., 1990), and a history of being teased about weight (Brown, Cash, & Lewis, 1989).

Studies investigating a possible relationship between eating disorders and sexual abuse have reported highly discrepant results. Overall, around 30 percent of eating-disordered patients were found to have histories of sexual abuse (Pope & Hudson, 1992; Connors & Morse, 1993; Dansky, Kilpatrick, Brewerton, & O'Neil, 1993), a figure that is comparable to rates found in normal populations (Finkelhor, Hotaling, Lewis, & Smith, 1990). Gleaves and Eberenz

(1994), however, report higher rates of abuse in treatment-resistant bulimia nervosa patients (about 71 percent) as compared to a rate of 15 percent in patients with successful treatment outcome.

Finally, family dysfunction has been implicated in the development of eating disorders (Humphrey, 1988). However, similar patterns of dysfunction exist in families of children with other psychological problems, and it is not clear whether family problems may be the cause or the result of eating-disordered behaviors.

THEORIES OF ETIOLOGY

Cognitive-Behavioral Theories

Cognitive and behavioral researchers (Rosen & Leitenberg, 1982; Williamson, 1990) have proposed etiological models for anorexia and bulimia nervosa that emphasize the proximal cognitions and behaviors that cause and maintain the disorders. The hypothesized starting point of both anorexia and bulimia nervosa is dietary restriction as an attempt to control weight and to avoid anxiety caused by fear of fatness and overconcern with body shape and size. Anorexic behavior is maintained by the positive consequences of dieting, including thinness, feelings of self-control, and initial approval from others. Binge eating is thought to develop in some individuals after dietary restraint is broken due to caloric deprivation, food cravings, and hunger. A cycle develops in which breaking of dietary restraint is precipitated by emotional distress or the consumption of "forbidden" foods (Polivy & Herman, 1985). Bingeing causes anxiety to increase, and purging serves the function of reducing such anxiety; purgative behaviors are therefore negatively reinforced. Binge eating is maintained by the normal pleasurable effects of eating as well as the reduction of negative mood (Heatherton & Baumeister, 1991).

Biological Theories

First- and second-degree relatives of eating-disordered patients are four to five times more likely than the general population to develop an eating disorder themselves (Strober, Morrell, Burroughs, Salkin, & Jacobs, 1985). Hsu (1990) reviewed twin studies and found concordance rates for anorexia nervosa of about 50 percent in monozygotic female twins, as compared to 7 percent in dizygotic twins. In bulimia nervosa, concordance rates of 22.9 percent have been found in monozygotic twins, as compared to 8.7 percent in dizygotic twins (Kendler et al., 1991).

Biological theories of the eating disorders have focused on the potential dysfunction of serotonergic and endogenous opioid systems in the brain. Serotonergic theories are based on evidence that anorexics and bulimics have decreased activity of this neurotransmitter (Fava, Copeland, Schweiger, & Herzog, 1989) and on studies showing that medications that increase serotonin activity are effective for the treatment of bulimia nervosa (Fluoxetine Bulimia Nervosa Collaborative Study Group, 1992). Brewerton and colleagues have suggested that postsynaptic serotonin receptor sensitivity may be altered in bulimia nervosa, and that anorexia nervosa may be associated with pre- or postsynaptic disturbances in serotonin function (Brewerton et al., 1992; Brewerton, 1993; Brewerton & Jimerson, 1993).

Insatiety during a binge episode may reflect deficient activity of serotonergic systems. Evidence in support of this theory has found that bulimic subjects exhibit a slower turnover rate of serotonin than do anorexic patients (Kaye, Ebert, & Gwirtsman, 1984). A recent study by Jimerson, Lesom, Kaye, and Brewerton (1992) found that in comparison with normal controls, bulimic subjects had significantly lower levels of serotonin and dopamine metabolites in cerebrospinal fluid. Levels of both metabolites were negatively correlated with binge frequency. However, these findings are contradicted by results of a study by Kaye and associates (1990), which found comparable levels of serotonin activity in bulimics and control subjects.

There is evidence that the gastrointestinal hormone cholecystokinin (CCK) induces satiety and reduces food intake in both animals (Weller, Smith, & Gibbs, 1990) and humans (Kisseleff, Pi-Sunyer, Thornton, & Smith, 1981). Geracioti and Liddle (1988) found that 14 bulimic subjects had significantly lower plasma CCK levels after eating, as compared to 10 age- and sex-matched normal controls. A recent study by Lydiard and colleagues (1993) found significantly lower levels of cholecystokinin in the cerebrospinal fluid of 11 bulimic patients than in 16 normal controls. The authors of both these studies hypothesized that impaired cholecystokinin activity in the central nervous system and the periphery (whether primary or secondary to the disorder) may contribute to the impaired satiety and binge eating of patients with bulimia nervosa.

Cholecystokinin levels have been studied in anorexic patients with mixed results. Tamai and associates (1993) found abnormally high levels in plasma of untreated anorexic subjects (thus, possibly promoting premature satiety), both after fasting and after an oral glucose tolerance test and further found that these levels normalized after psychological therapy and restoration of body weight. However, Geracioti, Liddle, Altemus, Demitrack, and Gold (1992) found that six patients with anorexia nervosa (both before and after weight normalization) and six healthy control subjects had comparable fasting and postprandial plasma cholecystokinin concentrations.

Some researchers (e.g., Reid, 1990) have theorized that eating disorders and alcoholism might be explained by a common opioidergic mechanism, citing evidence that naltrexone, an opiate antagonist which reduces craving in alcoholics, has been shown in uncontrolled studies to decrease binge eating in bulimia nervosa (Jonas, 1990). However, double-blind, placebo-controlled studies of naltrexone in bulimia have shown only modest effects (Mitchell, Laine, Morley, & Levine, 1986) or no effects at all (Mitchell et al., 1989).

Body Image Theories

Rosen (1992) and Thompson (1992) have recently suggested that eating abnormalities and extreme attempts to control weight are secondary to overconcern with body shape and weight. Individuals who are dissatisfied with their body shape may attempt to control the negative feelings associated with body image through strict dieting behaviors, thus predisposing them to development of an eating disorder.

Body dissatisfaction has been shown to be the best predictor of bulimic eating behaviors and concerns in teenage girls (Brown et al., 1989; Gross & Rosen, 1988). Striegel-Moore, Silberstein, Frensch, and Rodin (1989) found that measures of body dissatisfaction and perceived attractiveness were the best predictors of dieting and eating disturbance in college freshmen. Similarly, Attie and Brooks-Gunn (1989) found that dissatisfaction with body size was a significant predictor of eating problems in adolescent girls after a two-year interval.

ASSESSMENT OF ANOREXIA AND BULIMIA NERVOSA

Individuals suspected of having eating disorder symptoms should receive complete examinations by a physician and a registered dietitian. At entry to treatment, nearly all anorexics and many bulimics are malnourished and biologically starved (Pirke, Pahl, Schweiger, & Warnhoff, 1985).

The psychological consequences of malnutrition and excess weight loss have been shown among eating-disordered patients (Casper & Davis, 1977) and among formerly normal-weight men undergoing severe food restriction as prisoners of war (Polivy, Zeitlin, Herman, & Beal, 1994) or volunteers (Keys, Brozek, Henschel, Michelson, & Taylor, 1950). The initial psychological presentation of eating-disordered patients may reflect the effects of starvation more than any characteristic psychological functioning. Therefore, initial psychological assessment should be directed to obtaining a differential diagnosis, description of the eating disorder, and identification of factors maintaining the eating disorder. Comorbid psychopathological characteristics are best diagnosed after normalization of weight and eating behaviors have been established.

The remainder of this section will review methods for conducting the initial assessment of an eating disorder, including clinical interviews, self-report inventories, body image assessment, and behavioral assessment techniques, such as self-monitoring and test meals.

Structured Interviews

Advantages of using structured interviews for the assessment of eating disorders are the breadth and depth of information they provide for treatment planning. However, all structured interviews rely on patient self-report, which may not be accurate or reliable. Williamson (1990) has recommended that parents and significant others also be interviewed to gather more accurate information.

Three structured interviews have shown promise for the assessment of anorexia and bulimia nervosa. The Eating Disorder Examination (Cooper & Fairburn, 1987; Cooper, Cooper, & Fairburn, 1989) assesses current bulimic and anorexic symptomatology (over the past four weeks) and was originally designed as a treatment outcome measure. The Clinical Eating Disorder Rating Instrument (Palmer, Christie, Cordle, Davies, & Kendrick, 1987) measures eating-disorder symptoms as well as depression, anxiety, obsessions, and psychosis. The Interview for Diagnosis of Eating Disorders (Williamson, 1990) elicits detailed diagnostic and historical information. All of these interviews have been shown to have good interrater reliability and internal consistency.

Self-Report Inventories

Numerous self-report inventories assess the symptoms of eating disorders. Advantages of using these inventories include ease of administration, efficiency, and the ability to assess large groups of subjects. In addition, self-report instruments can be administered repeatedly to assess change. However, these measures do not typically provide sufficient information for diagnosis, and they are subject to the same limitations of self-reported information as are structured interviews.

The 40-item Eating Attitudes Test (EAT; Garner & Garfinkel, 1979) is best used as a general index of anorexic characteristics. Research has shown that it can discriminate both anorexic and bulimic subjects from normals, and anorexic subjects from normals; however, no study has shown that it differentiates anorexics from bulimics (Williamson, 1990).

The Bulimia Test-Revised (BULIT-R; Thelen, Farmer, Wonderlich, & Smith, 1991) is a 28-item test designed to measure *DSM-III-R* symptoms of bulimia nervosa. Its questions concern binge eating, purgative behavior, negative affect related to eating, and weight fluctuations. This measure has been shown to differentiate bulimics from normal controls (Thelen et al., 1991).

The Eating Disorder Inventory-2nd edition (EDI-2; Garner, 1991) is a multiscale instrument designed to assess the psychopathological features of anorexia and bulimia nervosa. It contains 11 subscales that measure different eating-disorder symptoms, including drive for thinness and body dissatisfaction. Satisfactory internal consistency and criterion-related validity have been reported for the entire scale and for the subscales (Garner & Olmsted, 1984). The EDI-2 has been shown to differentiate patients with diagnosed eating disorders from normal controls (Garner, 1991).

Two self-report inventories have been developed to assess pathological eating behaviors in children. The 14-item Kids Eating Disorder Survey (KEDS; Childress, Jarrell, & Brewerton, 1993) measures weight dissatisfaction and purging/dieting behaviors in boys and girls (grades 5–8). For younger children (grades 3–6), the Children's Eating Attitudes Test (ChEAT; Maloney, McGuire, & Daniels, 1988) consists of 26 items that assess dieting behaviors, food preoccupation, bulimic behaviors, and concerns about being overweight. Both of these inventories have adequate internal consistency and test-retest reliability; however, their efficacy in diagnosing childhood eating disorders has not been tested.

Body Image Assessment

Body image assessment procedures include perceptual (body size estimation) methods that require the subject to make a judgment about the size of his or her body and reproduce that image; questionnaires that assess subjective aspects of body image; and silhouette methods that can measure both perceptual and subjective components. Questionnaires have been developed recently that assess behavioral avoidance (Rosen, Srebnik, Saltzberg, & Wendt, 1991) and situational (Cash, 1994) components of body image disturbance. For thorough reviews of body image assessment instruments, the reader is directed to Thompson (1990, 1992).

The Body Image Assessment procedure (Williamson, Davis, Bennett, Goreczny, & Gleaves, 1989) is a useful index of both size estimation and body dissatisfaction. This procedure utilizes nine silhouettes of female body shapes, ranging from very thin to very large. Subjects are asked to select the silhouettes that most accurately depict their current and ideal body sizes. The Body Image Assessment procedure differentiates bulimia nervosa subjects from normal controls (Williamson, Kelley, Davis, Ruggiero, & Blouin, 1985) and from nonpurging binge eaters

(Davis, Williamson, Goreczny, & Bennett, 1989). A discrepancy score, which can be derived from the Body Image Assessment procedure (current body size minus ideal body size), has been found to be a valid measure of body size dissatisfaction (Williamson, Gleaves, Watkins, & Schlundt, 1993).

Behavioral Assessment

Behavioral assessment techniques can be used to obtain more direct information about eating-disorder behaviors. The use of test meals can be particularly useful for evaluating patients who minimize problems associated with eating in order to avoid treatment (Williamson, 1990). Parameters that can be measured include amount and caloric density of the food consumed, avoidance tactics used, speed of eating, and subjective or objective indices of anxiety before, during, and after eating. Standardized test meals can also be used to assess progress over the course of treatment. In an attempt to establish the validity of this type of assessment, Rosen, Leitenberg, Fondacaro, Gross, and Willmuth (1985) found that bulimic eaters, when prevented from vomiting, ate less than normal eaters in both laboratory and at-home standardized test-meal situations.

Self-monitoring is one of the most widely used procedures in the behavioral assessment of the eating disorders. Ideally, self-monitoring records should include time of day, location, type and amount of food consumed, and the social, emotional, and environmental context in which the food was eaten. Also, the patient should identify whether eating episodes are identified as binges, and whether she or he felt in control while eating. Data derived from self-monitoring records can be used for diagnosis, for developing a functional analysis for treatment planning, and for evaluation of treatment outcome.

TREATMENT PLANNING AND TREATMENT OUTCOME

The first goals of treatment for the eating disorders are nutritional rehabilitation and the restoration of normal eating patterns. Hospitalization may be required to accomplish these goals in patients with anorexia nervosa. Bulimic patients can often be treated successfully on an outpatient basis.

Weight restoration and normalization of eating should be initial treatment goals for seriously underweight anorexics, who may present for treatment in medical crisis. Nasogastric tube feeding or total parenteral nutrition may be required if the anorexic is unwilling or unable to eat; however, the physical dangers of rapid refeeding (severe fluid retention and cardiac failure) must be considered.

Several therapeutic approaches for anorexia and bulimia nervosa have been developed. Most controlled treatment outcome studies have been conducted with bulimic patients, since the health risks associated with anorexia nervosa preclude the use of waiting list or placebo control conditions. Most outcome studies of the treatment of bulimia nervosa have focused on pharmacological treatments, psychotherapeutic approaches, and combinations of pharmacotherapy and psychotherapy. These studies have generally used percent reduction in binge eating and purging, along with rates of remission, as primary outcome variables.

Pharmacological Treatments

No medication has proved to be useful for maintaining long-term weight gain, changing attitudes about weight and shape, or preventing relapse in anorexia nervosa. Several psychotropic medications—including neuroleptics (Vandereycken, 1984), tricyclic antidepressants (Halmi, Eckert, LaDau, & Cohen, 1986), and lithium carbonate (Gross et al., 1981)—have been shown to have marginal effects at best. Cyproheptadine, an appetite stimulant, was somewhat effective in inducing weight gain in restrictive (but not bulimic) anorexics (Halmi et al., 1986). A small, uncontrolled study suggested that low doses of fluoxetine may help some anorexic patients with weight restoration and weight maintenance (Gwirtsman, Guze, Yager, & Gainsley, 1990).

Medications, particularly antidepressants, have been shown to be more effective in the treatment of bulimia nervosa. Double-blind placebo controlled studies have demonstrated the efficacy of imipramine (Agras, Dorian, Kirkley, Arnow, & Bachman, 1987), desipramine (Barlow, Blouin, Blouin, & Perez, 1988), monoamine oxidase inhibitors (Walsh et al., 1988), and fluoxetine (Fluoxetine Bulimia Nervosa Collaborative Study Group, 1992). To date, fluoxe-

tine is the only medication to receive FDA approval for the treatment of bulimia nervosa.

Several studies have shown improvements in eating disorder symptoms in nondepressed subjects, implying that these drugs do not work primarily by relieving mood disturbance. However, high attrition rates have been noted in patients treated with antidepressants (Wilson & Fairburn, 1993), and long-term treatment may be required because bulimic subjects have been found to relapse after discontinuation of the medication (Pyle et al., 1990; Walsh, Hadigan, Devlin, Gladis, & Roose, 1991).

Psychotherapeutic Treatments

Treatment outcome studies using psychological treatments have similarly focused on bulimia nervosa; much less is known about the treatment of anorexia nervosa. There is evidence that medical management plus psychotherapy, particularly behavior therapy utilizing positive and negative reinforcers, is more effective in the treatment of anorexia than medical management alone (APA, 1993). Positive reinforcers may consist of praise and social attention, the ability to engage in pleasurable activities, or the opportunity to engage in light physical exercise. Effective negative reinforcers might include removal of various restrictions and, ultimately, the opportunity to leave the hospital. Family therapy is considered to play an important role in the treatment of anorexia nervosa, particularly for patients with early adolescent onset of the disorder (Russell, Szmukler, Dare, & Eisler, 1987).

There are several controlled treatment outcome studies of cognitive behavior therapy (CBT) in bulimia nervosa, and it has been recommended as the psychological treatment of choice (APA, 1993). Cognitive behavior therapy for eating disorders generally comprises three components (Fairburn, 1985): (1) education about eating disorders and behavioral techniques such as self-monitoring, exposure with response prevention, and stimulus control; (2) an emphasis on learning to identify and alter dysfunctional thoughts and attitudes about shape, weight, and eating; and (3) a focus on the use of relapse prevention strategies. CBT has been shown to be more effective than waiting list controls in six studies (Wilson & Fairburn, 1993) and has also been shown to be more effective than other types of psychotherapy. For example, Garner and associates (1993) compared CBT to psychodynamic psychotherapy and found that CBT was more effective in decreasing purging and psychological distress and in changing attitudes toward weight. The two treatments were equally effective in reducing rates of bingeing.

Fairburn and colleagues (Fairburn et al., 1991; Fairburn, Jones, Peveler, Hope, & O'Connor, 1993) compared CBT to (1) behavior therapy techniques, including education about healthy eating, self-monitoring, and stimulus control measures to regain control over eating; and (2) a modification of interpersonal therapy (Klerman, Weissman, Rounsaville, & Chevron, 1984), which focused on major interpersonal problems associated with the onset of the eating disorder, with no attention paid to eating habits or attitudes about shape and weight.

CBT was superior to behavior therapy at both posttreatment and at one-year follow-up. About half of the patients in the behavior therapy condition dropped out of or were withdrawn from treatment. At posttreatment, CBT and interpersonal therapy were equally effective in reducing binge eating, but CBT was superior to interpersonal therapy in decreasing purging frequency and in changing attitudes about weight. However, these differences were absent at four-month and one-year follow-ups as a result of the continued improvement of the subjects treated with interpersonal therapy. Fairburn and colleagues (1993) hypothesized that since the effects of interpersonal therapy followed a different temporal course than those of CBT, the two treatments must have operated through different, though equally effective, psychological mechanisms.

Studies examining combinations of CBT and pharmacological therapies (including desipramine and imipramine) have not found that either treatment enhances the other (Mitchell et al., 1990; Agras et al., 1992).

Little is known about the long-term outcome of patients receiving treatment for anorexia and bulimia nervosa. The overall short-term success rate (i.e., as long as one year) for treated bulimia nervosa patients is about 34 percent with full remission of bingeing and purging (Mitchell, Raymond, & Specker, 1993); about 70 percent of patients report substantial reduction of symptoms (APA, 1993). Reviews of follow-up studies conducted on hospitalized anorexics at least four years after onset of the disorder indicate that about 44 percent of patients had an overall good outcome (weight restoration to within normal limits), 24 percent had a poor outcome (less than 85 percent of recommended weight), 28 percent had an intermediate outcome (between poor and good), and about 4 percent had died (APA, 1993).

SUMMARY

Anorexia and bulimia nervosa are complex, chronic psychiatric disorders with severe physical sequelae. These disorders have been the focus of extensive research since the early 1980s, and significant progress has been made in understanding descriptions, epidemiology, and risk factors for their development. Researchers have recently begun to explore risk factors for eating disorder symptoms in pre-pubertal children. It is hoped that identification of these precipitating factors at younger ages may lead to development of useful preventive approaches.

Treatment outcome research in the eating disorders has led to development of effective therapeutic techniques for anorexia and bulimia nervosa. Future research efforts should be directed to ensuring long-term maintenance of improvements made during treatment, as well as tailoring specific treatment components to individuals with varying presentations.

REFERENCES

Agras, W. S., Dorian, B., Kirkley, B. G., Arnow, B., & Bachman, J. (1987). Imipramine in the treatment of bulimia: A double-blind controlled study. *International Journal of Eating Disorders, 6,* 29–38.

Agras, W. S., Rossiter, E. M., Arnow, B., Schneider, J. A., Telch, C. F., Raeburn, S. D., Bruce, B., Perl, M., & Koran, L. M. (1992). Pharmacologic and cognitive-behavioral treatment for bulimia nervosa: A controlled comparison. *American Journal of Psychiatry, 149,* 82–87.

American Psychiatric Association. (1987). *Diagnostic and statistical manual of mental disorders* (3rd ed., rev.). Washington, DC: Author.

American Psychiatric Association. (1993). Practice guidelines for eating disorders. *American Journal of Psychiatry, 150,* 212–228.

American Psychiatric Association. (1994). *Diagnostic and statistical manual of mental disorders* (4th ed.). Washington, DC: Author.

Attie, I., & Brooks-Gunn, J. (1989). Development of eating problems in adolescent girls: A longitudinal study. *Developmental Psychology, 25,* 70–79.

Barlow, J., Blouin, J., Blouin, A., & Perez, E. (1988). Treatment of bulimia with desipramine: A double-blind crossover study. *Canadian Journal of Psychiatry, 33,* 129–133.

Brewerton, T. D. (1993). Studies of 5HT function in the eating disorders. *Advances in the Biosciences, 90,* 49–57.

Brewerton, T. D., Dansky, B. S., O'Neil, P. M., & Kilpatrick, D. G. (1993). The prevalence of bulimia nervosa and binge eating disorder in a national sample of women. Manuscript submitted for publication.

Brewerton, T. D., & Jimerson, D. C. (1993, September). *Studies of serotonin function in anorexia nervosa.* Paper presented for the proceedings of the WHO Collaborating Center for Research and Training in the Neurosciences —Study Group on Anorexia Nervosa. Geneva, Switzerland.

Brewerton, T. D., Mueller, E. A., Lesom, M. D., Brandt, H. A., Quearry, B., George, D. T., Murphy, D. L., & Jimerson, D. C. (1992). Neuroendocrine responses to m-chlorphenylpiperazine and L-tryptophan in bulimia. *Archives of General Psychiatry, 49,* 852–861.

Brown, T. A., Cash, T. F., & Lewis, R. J. (1989). Body image disturbances in adolescent female binge-purgers: A brief report of the results of a national survey in the USA. *Journal of Child Psychology and Psychiatry, 30,* 605–615.

Brownell, K. D. (1991). Dieting and the search for the perfect body: Where culture and physiology collide. *Behavior Therapy, 22,* 1–12.

Bushnell, J. A., Wells, J. E., Hornblow, A. R., Oakley-Browne, M. A., & Joyce, P. (1990). Prevalence of three bulimia syndromes in the general population. *Psychological Medicine, 20,* 671–680.

Cash, T. F. (1994). The Situational Inventory of body-image dysphoria: Contextual assessment of a negative body image. *The Behavior Therapist, 17,* 133–134.

Casper, R. C., & Davis, J. M. (1977). On the course of anorexia nervosa. *American Journal of Psychiatry, 134,* 974–978.

Childress, A. C., Brewerton, T. D., Hodges, E. L., & Jarrell, M. P. (1993). The Kids Eating Disorder Survey (KEDS): A study of middle school students. *Journal of the American Academy of Child and Adolescent Psychiatry, 32,* 843–850.

Childress, A. C., Jarrell, M. P., & Brewerton, T. D. (1993). The Kids Eating Disorder Survey (KEDS): Internal consistency, component analysis, and reliability. *Eating Disorders, 1,* 123–133.

Connors, M. E., & Morse, W. (1993). Sexual abuse and the eating disorders: A review. *International Journal of Eating Disorders, 13,* 1–11.

Cooper, Z., Cooper, P. J., & Fairburn, C. G. (1989). The validity of the Eating Disorder Examination and its subscales. *British Journal of Psychiatry, 154,* 807–812.

Cooper, Z., & Fairburn, C. G. (1987). The Eating Disorder Examination: A semi-structured interview of the assessment of the specific psychopathology of eating disorders. *International Journal of Eating Disorders, 6,* 1–8.

DaCosta, M., & Halmi, K. A. (1992). Classifications of anorexia nervosa: Question of subtypes. *International Journal of Eating Disorders, 11,* 305–313.

Dansky, B. S., Kilpatrick, D. G., Brewerton, T. D., & O'Neil, P. M. (1993, March). *The relationship between bulimia and victimization in a national representative sample of women.* Proceedings of the Society of Behavioral Medicine's 14th Annual Scientific Sessions, San Francisco, CA.

Davis, C. J., Williamson, D. A., Goreczny, A. J., & Bennett, S. M. (1989). Body image disturbances and bulimia nervosa: An empirical analysis of recent revisions of the DSM-III. *Journal of Psychopathology and Behavioral Assessment, 11,* 61–69.

Eckert, E. D., Goldberg, S. C., Halmi, K. A., Casper, R. C., & Davis, J. M. (1979). Alcoholism in anorexia nervosa. In R. W. Pickens & L. L. Heston (Eds.), *Psychiatric factors in drug abuse* (pp. 267–283). New York: Grune & Stratton.

Ehrenkranz, J. R. L. (1993). The medical care of the patient with an eating disorder. In A. J. Giannini & A. E. Slaby (Eds.), *The eating disorders* (pp. 147–157). New York: Springer-Verlag.

Eller, B. (1993). Males with eating disorders. In A. J. Giannini & A. E. Slaby (Eds.), *The eating disorders* (pp. 133–146). New York: Springer-Verlag.

Fairburn, C. G. (1985). Cognitive-behavioral treatment for bulimia. In D. M. Garner & P. E. Garfinkel (Eds.), *Handbook of psychotherapy for anorexia and bulimia nervosa.* New York: Guilford.

Fairburn, C. G., & Beglin, S. J. (1990). Studies of the epidemiology of bulimia nervosa. *American Journal of Psychiatry, 147,* 401–408.

Fairburn, C. G., Hay, P. J., & Welch, S. L. (1993). Binge eating and bulimia nervosa: Distribution and determinants. In C. G. Fairburn & G. T. Wilson (Eds.), *Binge eating: Nature, assessment, and treatment.* New York: Guilford.

Fairburn, C. G., Jones, R., Peveler, R. C., Carr, S. J., Solomon, R. A., O'Connor, M. E., Burton, J., & Hope, R. A. (1991). Three psychological treatments for bulimia nervosa. *Archives of General Psychiatry, 48,* 463–469.

Fairburn, C. G., Jones, R., Peveler, R. C., Hope, R. A., & O'Connor, M. E. (1993). Psychotherapy and bulimia nervosa: Longer-term effects of interpersonal therapy, behavior therapy, and cognitive behavior therapy. *Archives of General Psychiatry, 50,* 419–428.

Fava, M., Copeland, P. M., Schweiger, U., & Herzog, D. B. (1989). Neurochemical abnormalities of anorexia and bulimia nervosa. *American Journal of Psychiatry, 146,* 963–971.

Finkelhor, D., Hotaling, G., Lewis, I. A., & Smith, C.

(1990). Sexual abuse in a national survey of adult men and women: Prevalence, characteristics, and risk factors. *Child Abuse and Neglect, 14,* 19–28.

Fluoxetine Bulimia Nervosa Collaborative Study Group. (1992). Fluoxetine in the treatment of bulimia nervosa. *Archives of General Psychiatry, 49,* 139–147.

Garfinkel, P. E. (1992). Evidence in support of attitudes to shape and weight as a diagnostic criterion of bulimia nervosa. *International Journal of Eating Disorders, 11,* 321–325.

Garfinkel, P. E., Goldbloom, D., Davis, R., Olmsted, M., Garner, D. M., & Halmi, K. A. (1992). Body dissatisfaction in bulimia nervosa: Relationship to weight and shape concerns and psychological functioning. *International Journal of Eating Disorders, 11,* 151–161.

Garner, D. M. (1991). *Eating Disorders Inventory-2.* Odessa, FL: Psychological Assessment Resources.

Garner, D. M., & Garfinkel, P. E. (1979). The Eating Attitudes Test: An index of the symptoms of anorexia nervosa. *Psychological Medicine, 9,* 273–279.

Garner, D. M., Garfinkel, P. E., Rockert, W., & Olmsted, M. P. (1987). A prospective study of eating disturbances in the ballet. *Psychotherapy and Psychosomatics, 48,* 170–175.

Garner, D. M., & Olmsted, M. P. (1984). *Manual for the Eating Disorders Inventory-EDI.* Odessa, FL: Psychological Assessment Resources.

Garner, D. M., Rockert, W., Davis, R., Garner, M. V., Olmsted, M. P., & Eagle, M. (1993). Comparison of cognitive-behavioral and supportive-expressive therapy for bulimia nervosa. *American Journal of Psychiatry, 150,* 37–46.

Geracioti, T. D., & Liddle, R. A. (1988). Impaired cholecystokinin secretion in bulimia nervosa. *New England Journal of Medicine, 319,* 683–688.

Geracioti, T. D., Liddle, R. A., Altemus, M., Demitrack, M. A., & Gold, P. W. (1992). Regulation of appetite and cholecystokinin secretion in anorexia nervosa. *American Journal of Psychiatry, 149,* 958–961.

Gleaves, D. H., & Eberenz, K. P. (1994). Sexual abuse histories among treatment-resistant bulimia nervosa patients. *International Journal of Eating Disorders, 15,* 227–231.

Gross, H. A., Ebert, M. H., Faden, V. B., Goldberg, S. C., Lee, L. E., & Kaye, W. H. (1981). A double-blind controlled trial of lithium carbonate in primary anorexia nervosa. *Journal of Clinical Psychopharmacology, 1,* 376–381.

Gross, J., & Rosen, J. C. (1988). Bulimia in adolescents: Prevalence and psychosocial correlates. *International Journal of Eating Disorders, 7,* 51–61.

Gwirtsman, H. E., Guze, B. H., Yager, J., & Gainsley, B. (1990). Fluoxetine treatment of anorexia nervosa: An open clinical trial. *Journal of Clinical Psychiatry, 51,* 378–382.

Halmi, K. A., Casper, R., Eckert, E., Goldberg, S. C., & Davis, J. M. (1979). Unique features associated with

age of onset of anorexia nervosa. *Psychiatry Research, 1,* 209–215.

Halmi, K. A., Eckert, E., LaDau, T. J., & Cohen, J. (1986). Anorexia nervosa: Treatment efficacy of cyproheptadine and amitriptyline. *Archives of General Psychiatry, 43,* 177–181.

Halmi, K. A., Eckert, E., Marchi, P., Sampugnaro, V., Apple, R., & Cohen, J. (1991). Comorbidity of psychiatric diagnoses in anorexia nervosa. *Archives of General Psychiatry, 48,* 712–718.

Halmi, K. A., & Falk, J. R. (1982). Anorexia nervosa: A study of outcome discriminators in exclusive dieters and bulimics. *Journal of the American Academy of Child Psychiatry, 21,* 369–375.

Heatherton, T. F., & Baumeister, R. F. (1991). Binge eating as escape from self-awareness. *Psychological Bulletin, 110,* 86–108.

Helzer, J. E., & Pryzbeck, T. R. (1988). The co-occurrence of alcoholism with other psychiatric disorders in the general population and its impact on treatment. *Journal of Studies on Alcohol, 49,* 219–224.

Holderness, C. C., Brooks-Gunn, J., & Warren, M. P. (1994). Co-morbidity of eating disorders and substance abuse: A review of the literature. *International Journal of Eating Disorders, 16,* 1–34.

Hsu, L. K. G. (1990). *Eating disorders.* New York: Guilford.

Hsu, L. K. G., Kaye, W., & Weltzin, T. (1993). Are the eating disorders related to obsessive-compulsive disorder? *International Journal of Eating Disorders, 14,* 305–318.

Hsu, L. K. G., & Sobkiewicz, T. A. (1991). Body image disturbance: Time to abandon the concept for eating disorders? *International Journal of Eating Disorders, 10,* 15–30.

Hudson, J. I., Pope, H. G., Yurgelun-Todd, D., Jonas, J. M., & Frankenburg, F. R. (1987). A controlled study of lifetime prevalence of affective and other psychiatric disorders in bulimic outpatients. *American Journal of Psychiatry, 144,* 1283–1287.

Humphrey, L. L. (1988). Relationships within subtypes of anorexic, bulimic, and normal families. *Journal of the American Academy of Child and Adolescent Psychiatry, 27,* 544–551.

Jimerson, D. C., Lesom, M. D., Kaye, W. H., & Brewerton, T. D. (1992). Low serotonin and dopamine metabolite concentrations in cerebrospinal fluid from bulimic patients with frequent binge episodes. *Archives of General Psychiatry, 49,* 132–138.

Johnson, C., Tobin, D. L., & Dennis, A. (1990). Differences in treatment outcome between borderline and nonborderline bulimics at one-year follow-up. *International Journal of Eating Disorders, 9,* 617–627.

Jonas, J. M. (1990). Do substance abuse, including alcoholism, and bulimia covary? In L. D. Reid (Ed.), *Opioids, bulimia, and alcohol abuse and alcoholism* (pp. 247–258). New York: Springer-Verlag.

Kassett, J. A., Gershon, E. S., Maxwell, M. E., Guroff, J. J., Kazuba, D. M., Smith, A. L., Brandt, H. A., & Jimerson, D. C. (1989). Psychiatric disorders in the first-degree relatives of probands with bulimia nervosa. *American Journal of Psychiatry, 146,* 1468–1471.

Kasvikis, Y. G., Tsakiris, F., Marks, L. M., Basoglu, M., & Noshirvani, H. F. (1986). Past history of anorexia nervosa in women with obsessive-compulsive disorder. *International Journal of Eating Disorders, 5,* 1069–1075.

Kaye, W. H., Ballenger, J. C., Lydiard, B., Stuart, G. W., Laraia, M. T., O'Neil, P. M., Fossey, M. D., Stevens, V., Lesser, S., & Hsu, G. (1990). CSF monoamine levels in normal-weight bulimia: Evidence for abnormal noradrenergic activity. *American Journal of Psychiatry, 147,* 225–229.

Kaye, W. H., Ebert, M. H., & Gwirtsman, H. E. (1984). Differences in brain serotonergic metabolism between nonbulimic and bulimic patients with anorexia nervosa. *American Journal of Psychiatry, 141,* 1598–1601.

Kaye, W. H., Gwirtsman, H. E., George, D. T., Weiss, S. R., & Jimerson, D. C. (1986). Relationship of mood alterations to bingeing behavior in bulimia. *British Journal of Psychiatry, 149,* 470–485.

Kendler, K. S., MacLean, C., Neale, M., Kessler, R., Heath, A., & Eaves, L. (1991). The genetic epidemiology of bulimia nervosa. *American Journal of Psychiatry, 148,* 1627–1637.

Keyes, A., Brozek, J., Henschel, A., Michelson, O., & Taylor, H. L. (1950). *The biology of human starvation.* Minneapolis, MN: University of Minnesota Press.

Kisseleff, H. R., Pi-Sunyer, F. X., Thornton, J., & Smith, G. P. (1981). C-terminal octapeptide of cholecystokinin decreases food intake in man. *American Journal of Clinical Nutrition, 34,* 154–160.

Kisseleff, H. R., Walsh, B. T., Kral, J. G., & Cassidy, S. M. (1986). Laboratory studies of eating behavior in women with bulimia. *Physiology and Behavior, 38,* 563–570.

Klerman, G. L., Weissman, M. M., Rounsaville, B. J., & Chevron, E. S. (1984). *Interpersonal therapy of depression.* New York: Basic Books.

Laessle, R. G., Kittl, S., Fichter, M. M., Wittchen, H., & Pirke, K. (1987). Major affective disorder in anorexia nervosa and bulimia. *British Journal of Psychiatry, 151,* 785–789.

Lee, N. F., Rush, A. J., & Mitchell, J. E. (1985). Bulimia and depression. *Journal of Affective Disorders, 9,* 231–238.

Levine, M. P., & Smolak, L. (1992). Toward a model of the developmental psychopathology of eating disorders: The example of early adolescence. In J. Crowther, D. Tennenbaum, S. Hobfoll, & M. A. P. Stephens (Eds.), *The etiology of bulimia nervosa: The individual and family context.* Washington, DC: Hemisphere Publishers.

Lucas, A. R., Beard, C. M., O'Fallon, W. M., & Kurlan, L. T. (1991). 50-year trends in the incidence of anorexia nervosa in Rochester, MN: A population-based study. *American Journal of Psychiatry, 148,* 917–922.

Lydiard, R. B., Brewerton, T. D., Fossey, M. D., Laraia, M. T., Stuart, G., Beinfeld, M. C., & Ballenger, J. C. (1993). CSF cholecystokinin octapeptide in patients with bulimia nervosa and in normal comparison subjects. *American Journal of Psychiatry, 150,* 1099–1101.

Maloney, M. J., McGuire, J. B., & Daniels, S. R. (1988). Reliability testing of a children's version of the Eating Attitudes Test. *Journal of the American Academy of Child and Adolescent Psychiatry, 27,* 541–543.

Maloney, M. J., McGuire, J., Daniels, S. R., & Specker, B. (1989). Dieting behavior and eating attitudes in children. *Pediatrics, 84,* 482–489.

Marchi, M., & Cohen, P. (1990). Early childhood eating behaviors and adolescent eating disorders. *Journal of the American Academy of Child and Adolescent Psychiatry, 29,* 112–117.

Marx, R. D. (1993). Depression and eating disorders. In A. J. Giannini & A. E. Slaby (Eds.), *The eating disorders* (pp. 110–127). New York: Springer-Verlag.

Mitchell, J. E. (1986). Bulimia: Medical and physiological aspects. In K. D. Brownell & J. P. Foreyt (Eds.), *Handbook of eating disorders.* New York: Basic Books.

Mitchell, J. E., Christenson, G., Jennings, J., Huber, M., Thomas, B., Pomeroy, C., & Morley, J. (1989). A placebo-controlled double-blind crossover study of naloxone hydrochloride in outpatients with normal weight bulimia. *Journal of Clinical Psychopharmacology, 9,* 94–97.

Mitchell, J. E., Laine, D., Morley, J. E., & Levine, A. S. (1986). Naloxone but not CCK-8 may attenuate binge-eating behavior in patients with the bulimia syndrome. *Biological Psychiatry, 21,* 1399–1406.

Mitchell, J. E., Pyle, R. L., Eckert, E. D., Hatsukami, D., Pomeroy, C., & Zimmerman, R. (1990). A comparison study of antidepressants and structured intensive group psychotherapy in the treatment of bulimia nervosa. *Archives of General Psychiatry, 47,* 149–157.

Mitchell, J. E., Raymond, N., & Specker, S. (1993). A review of the controlled trials of pharmacotherapy and psychotherapy in the treatment of bulimia nervosa. *International Journal of Eating Disorders, 14,* 229–247.

Mumford, D. B., Whitehouse, A. M., & Choudry, I. Y. (1992). Survey of eating disorders in English-medium schools in Lahore, Pakistan. *International Journal of Eating Disorders, 11,* 173–184.

Palmer, R., Christie, M., Cordle, C., Davies, D., & Kendrick, J. (1987). The Clinical Eating Disorder Rating Instrument (CEDRI): A preliminary description. *International Journal of Eating Disorders, 6,* 9–16.

Pike, K. M., & Rodin, J. (1991). Mothers, daughters, and disordered eating. *Journal of Abnormal Psychology, 100,* 198–204.

Pirke, K. M., Pahl, J., Schweiger, U., & Warnhoff, M. (1985). Metabolic and endocrine indices of starvation in bulimia: A comparison with anorexia nervosa. *Psychiatry Research, 15,* 33–39.

Polivy, J., & Herman, C. P. (1985). Dieting and bingeing: A causal analysis. *American Psychologist, 40,* 193–201.

Polivy, J., Zeitlin, S. B., Herman, C. P., & Beal, A. L. (1994). Food restriction and binge eating: A study of former prisoners of war. *Journal of Abnormal Psychology, 103,* 409–411.

Pope, H. G., & Hudson, J. I. (1992). Is childhood sexual abuse a risk factor for bulimia nervosa? *American Journal of Psychiatry, 149,* 455–563.

Pyle, R. L., Mitchell, J. E., Eckert, E. D., Hatsukami, D. K., Pomeroy, C., & Zimmerman, R. (1990). Maintenance treatment and six-month outcome for bulimic patients who respond to initial treatment. *American Journal of Psychiatry, 147,* 871–875.

Reid, L. D. (1990). *Opioids, bulimia, and alcohol abuse and alcoholism.* New York: Springer-Verlag.

Robins, L. N., Helzer, J. E., Pryzbeck, T. R., & Regier, D. A. (1988). Alcohol disorders in the community: A report from the Epidemiologic Catchment Area. In R. M. Rose & J. Barrett (Eds.), *Alcoholism: Origins and outcome* (pp. 15–29). New York: Raven Press.

Rosen, J. C. (1992). Body image disorder: Definition, development, and contribution to eating disorders. In J. H. Crowther, D. L. Tennenbaum, S. E. Hobfoll, & M. A. P. Stephens (Eds.), *The etiology of bulimia: The individual and family context.* Washington, DC: Hemisphere Publishers.

Rosen, J. C., & Leitenberg, H. (1982). Bulimia nervosa: Treatment with exposure and response prevention. *Behavior Therapy, 13,* 117–124.

Rosen, J. C., Leitenberg, H., Fondacaro, K. M., Gross, J., & Willmuth, M. E. (1985). Standardized test meals in assessment of eating behavior in bulimia nervosa: Consumption of feared foods when vomiting is prevented. *International Journal of Eating Disorders,* 4, 59–70.

Rosen, J. C., Srebnik, D., Saltzberg, E., & Wendt, S. (1991). Development of a Body Image Avoidance Questionnaire. *Psychological Assessment, 3,* 32–37.

Rosen, J. C., Tacy, B., & Howell, D. (1990). Life stress, psychological symptoms, and weight-reducing behavior in adolescent girls: A prospective analysis. *International Journal of Eating Disorders, 9,* 17–26.

Rosen, L. W., & Hough, D. O. (1988). Pathogenic weight-control behaviors of female college gymnasts. *Physician and Sports Medicine, 16,* 141–146.

Rossiter, E. M., Agras, W. S., & Losch, M. (1988). Changes in self-reported food intake in bulimics as a consequence of antidepressant treatment. *International Journal of Eating Disorders, 7,* 779–783.

Russell, G. F., Szmukler, G. I., Dare, C., & Eisler, I. (1987). An evaluation of family therapy in anorexia nervosa and bulimia nervosa. *Archives of General Psychiatry, 44,* 1047–1056.

Skodol, A. E., Oldham, J. M., Hyler, S. E., Kellman, H. D., Doidge, N., & Davies, M. (1993). Comorbidity of DSM-III-R eating disorders and personality disorders. *International Journal of Eating Disorders, 14,* 403–416.

Slade, P. (1985). A review of body image studies in anorexia and bulimia nervosa. *Journal of Psychiatric Research, 19,* 255–265.

Steiner-Adair, K. (1986). The body politic: Normal female adolescent development and the development of eating disorders. *Journal of the American Academy of Psychoanalysis, 14,* 95–114.

Striegel-Moore, R. H., Silberstein, L., Frensch, P., & Rodin, J. (1989). A prospective study of disordered eating among college students. *International Journal of Eating Disorders, 8,* 499–509.

Striegel-Moore, R. H., Silberstein, L., & Rodin, J. (1986). Toward an understanding of risk factors for bulimia. *American Psychologist, 41,* 246–263.

Strober, M., & Katz, J. (1988). Depression in the eating disorders: A review and analysis of descriptive, family, and biological findings. In D. Garner & P. E. Garfinkel (Eds.), *Diagnostic issues in anorexia nervosa and bulimia nervosa.* New York: Brunner/Mazel.

Strober, M., Morrell, W., Burroughs, J., Salkin, B., & Jacobs, C. (1985). A controlled family study of anorexia nervosa. *Journal of Psychiatric Research, 19,* 239–246.

Tamai, H., Takemura, J., Kobayashi, N., Matsubayashi, S., Matsukura, S., & Nakagawa, T. (1993). Changes in plasma cholecystokinin concentrations after oral glucose tolerance test in anorexia nervosa before and after therapy. *Metabolism, 42,* 581–584.

Thelen, M. H., Farmer, J., Wonderlich, J., & Smith, M. C. (1991). A revision of the Bulimia Test: BULIT-R. *Psychological Assessment, 3,* 119–124.

Thompson, J. K. (1990). *Body image disturbance: Assessment and treatment.* New York: Pergamon.

Thompson, J. K. (1992). Body image: Extent of disturbance, associated features, theoretical models, assessment methodologies, intervention strategies, and a proposal for a new DSM-IV diagnostic category—Body image disorder. In M. Hersen, R. M. Eisler & P. M. Miller (Eds.), *Progress in behavior modification.* Sycamore, IL: Sycamore Publishing.

Vandereycken, W. (1984). Neuroleptics in the short term treatment of anorexia nervosa—A double blind placebo-controlled study with sulpiride. *British Journal of Psychiatry, 144,* 288–290.

Walsh, B. T., Gladis, M., Roose, S. P., Stewart, J. W., Stetner, F., & Glassman, A. H. (1988). Phenelzine vs. placebo in 50 patients with bulimia. *Archives of General Psychiatry, 45,* 471–475.

Walsh, B. T., Hadigan, C. M., Devlin, M. J., Gladis, M., & Roose, S. P. (1991). Long-term outcome of antidepressant treatment for bulimia nervosa. *American Journal of Psychiatry, 148,* 1206–1212.

Weller, A., Smith, G. P., & Gibbs, J. (1990). Endogenous cholecystokinin reduces feeding in young rats. *Science, 247,* 1589–1591.

Williamson, D. A. (1990). *Assessment of eating disorders: Obesity, anorexia, and bulimia nervosa.* New York: Pergamon Press.

Williamson, D. A., Davis, C. J., Bennett, S. M., Goreczny, A. J., & Gleaves, D. H. (1989). Development of a simple procedure for body image assessment. *Behavioral Assessment, 11,* 433–446.

Williamson, D. A., Gleaves, D. H., Watkins, P. C., & Schlundt, D. G. (1993). Validation of self-ideal body size discrepancy as a measure of body size dissatisfaction. *Journal of Psychopathology and Behavioral Assessment, 15,* 57–68.

Williamson, D. A., Kelley, M. L., Davis, C. J., Ruggiero, L., & Blouin, D. C. (1985). Psychopathology of eating disorders: A controlled comparison of bulimic, obese, and normal subjects. *Journal of Consulting and Clinical Psychology, 53,* 161–166.

Wilson, G. T. (1992). Diagnostic criteria for bulimia nervosa. *International Journal of Eating Disorders, 11,* 315–319.

Wilson, G. T., & Fairburn, C. G. (1993). Cognitive treatments for eating disorders. *Journal of Consulting and Clinical Psychology, 61,* 261–269.

CHAPTER 6

HEADACHE

Kenneth R. Lofland, PAIN AND REHABILITATION CLINIC OF CHICAGO
James M. Sturges, UNIVERSITY OF MISSISSIPPI MEDICAL CENTER
Thomas J. Payne, UNIVERSITY OF MISSISSIPPI MEDICAL CENTER
AND DEPARTMENT OF VETERANS AFFAIRS MEDICAL CENTER

Historically, pain-related disorders have received little scientific attention relative to other health care issues. Some authors have noted that, relative to pain disorders, less pervasive and disabling conditions have received much more scrutiny (Saper, Silberstein, Gordon, & Hamel, 1993). This is certainly true with regard to pain syndromes experienced by children. In particular, childhood headache has been one of the least studied pain syndromes, as a likely result of the view that it is relatively unimportant (Kuttner, 1993). However, a growing awareness of the disability caused by headaches has stimulated an increase in interest and research activity in this area.

Estimates of the disabling sequelae of headache derive from several epidemiological and longitudinal studies. There are approximately 60 million headache sufferers in the United States (Ford & Ford, 1994). The prevalence of headaches increases during childhood and adolescence (especially for females as they approach puberty), and headache pain is responsible for one million days of missed school per year (Linet, Stewart, Celentano, Ziegler, & Sprecker, 1989). In addition, although there is considerable individual variation in the frequency and severity of headache episodes, chronic and severe symptoms challenge a child's coping ability, thus increasing the likelihood of depressive symptoms, behavioral problems, and other somatic complaints (Andrasik, Burke, Attanasio, & Rosenblum, 1985; Prensky & Sommer, 1979).

Migraines comprise the most common form of headache afflicting children (Barlow, 1984), with estimates approaching 1 out of 10 school-aged children (Winner, 1994). Several longitudinal studies have documented the course of childhood migraine. Bille (1981) reassessed 73 migraineurs studied 23 years earlier as children (Bille, 1962) and found the 60 percent were still suffering from migraines. Hockaday (1978) found that 73 percent of a sample of children and adolescents reported that they continued to experience migraine headaches into adulthood. Similarly, Sillanpaa (1983) found that 78 percent of children with migraines at age seven continued to have headaches at age 14, with 37 percent having improved somewhat but the other 41 percent experiencing symptoms that remained unchanged or became worse. All three of these studies reported that migraine symptoms were more debilitating in childhood than in adulthood, and although some children outgrow the disorder, most must learn to cope with it for a substantial portion of their lives.

The purpose of this chapter is to provide a broad overview of the current understanding about headaches in children and adolescents. First, background information and current controversies about the pathogenesis and diagnostic criteria for the major headache types are presented. A description of medical and psychological approaches to the assessment of headache follows. Last, a description of primary treatment options, including pharmacological and nonpharmacological interventions is presented, along with a review of the available treatment outcome literature.

CLASSIFICATION AND PATHOGENESIS

There has been documentation regarding the experience of headache since ancient times, with the first written reference dating back 5,000 years (see Bille, 1962). However, it was only recently that health care professionals developed the first diagnostic nosology of headache (Ad Hoc Committee on Classification of Headache, 1962). This classification scheme identified and differentiated many of the major headache disorders. Despite its utility, it was evident that a classification system for headache required greater delineation and more objective diagnostic criteria than the original classification scheme provided. The International Headache Society (IHS) accepted the challenge of revising the headache nomenclature, ultimately producing the currently used diagnostic nosology (Headache Classification Committee of the International Headache Society, 1988). Because migraine and tension-type headaches are the most prevalent forms of headache and, by far, have received the most scientific attention, they are the primary focus of consideration throughout this chapter.

Migraine Headache

Diagnostic Criteria

Migraine derives from the Greek, *hemicrania*, meaning half of the head. A headache meets current diagnostic criteria for *Migraine without aura* (previously *Common migraine*) if it lasts between 4 and 72 hours with two or more of the following: (1) unilateral location, (2) pulsating quality, (3) moderate or severe intensity, and (4) aggravation of headache during routine physical activity. Additionally, there must be at least five occurrences of this type of pain with at least

one of the following present: (1) nausea and/or vomiting or (2) sensitivity to light (photophobia) and sound (phonophobia). Last, the headache must not be due to an organic disorder, and if it occurs in children below the age of 15 years, attacks may last between 2 and 48 hours. *Migraine with aura* (previously *Classic migraine*) is a less common form of migraine and must include at least two attacks of aura symptoms lasting less than 60 minutes and followed by a migraine within 60 minutes. Aura symptoms may include visual disturbances, unilateral paresthesias and/or numbness, unilateral weakness, and aphasia or a similar language difficulty (Headache Classification Committee of the International Headache Society, 1988). There is some evidence that migraines have a significant genetic component (Williamson, Baker, & Cubic, 1993).

Current IHS criteria for migraine in children and adults are the same, except for the allowance of a shorter duration in childhood migraine. However, the assumption that these two disorders closely relate to one another has become a matter of debate. Many specialists in the field have suggested that childhood migraine differs from its adult counterpart based on discriminable symptom patterns. Winner (1994) stated that children's migraines differ from those of adults in that they are often bilateral rather than unilateral. In addition, the duration of attacks is much shorter for children, lasting only 30 minutes to one or two hours, versus the longer adult counterpart. Many other researchers are in agreement that the criteria for migraine requires modification for the pediatric population (e.g., Gladstein, Holden, Peralta, & Raven, 1993). One study compared the current IHS criteria to a proposed IHS revision for pediatric migraine and found that the diagnostic sensitivity was 53 percent and 80 percent, respectively, using clinical diagnosis by a pediatric neurologist as the criterion (Winner, Martinez, Mate, & Bello, 1994). A second edition of the IHS criteria, originally planned for publication in 1993, but not yet begun at the time of publication of this text, will likely include criteria for migraine in children that are separate from those used to diagnose migraine in adults.

Pathophysiology

Although the exact mechanisms producing the benign, recurrent pain of migraine remain unknown, researchers have developed various models in an attempt to understand this phenomenon. Williamson and associates (1993) summarized the traditional theory for the pathogenesis of migraine as occurring in three phases. The *preheadache phase* is identified by the prodromal symptoms of an aura, as described previously. Theoretically, these symptoms result from vasoconstriction of both the innervated cerebral vascular system and the extracranial arteries. A series of events follow, including decreased oxygenation of cerebral tissue, increased serotonin output, increased platelet aggregation, and a state of cerebral lactic acidosis, all thought to play a role in the production of aura symptoms.

The *headache phase* follows, characterized by the vasodilatory response of the noninnervated cerebral vascular system and the extracranial arteries, which represents an attempt to meet the needs of the deoxygenated brain tissue. In addition, the body releases several biochemical substances, including histamine and polypeptides, that produce edema and a reduction in pain threshold. These changes result in distended arteries and inflammation of the nerves innervating these vessels, causing pain with each pulse of blood. The *postheadache phase* coincides with the return of vascular and biochemical functioning to homeostasis, although swelling and tenderness may remain for days after the headache has remitted.

Recent studies on the pathogenesis of migraine have identified inconsistencies with this theory. Not all migraines exhibit the initial constriction of blood vessels. In addition, recent research supports a neurogenic theory that posits the cause of migraine to be a primary disturbance of brain function, with vascular changes being secondary to this disturbance (Gillies & Lance, 1993). Premonitory symptoms (aura) are suggestive of a hypothalamic origin, and the interaction between activities of the hypothalamus and serotonin levels is receiving considerable attention. The hypothalamus, centrally located, interacts with the limbic system (important in the control of emotions), the brain stem (relevant to pain mediation), and the pituitary (involved in regulation of hormonal changes and body cycles, such as menstruation).

In ways that are not yet fully understood, these structures communicate with the assistance of the neurotransmitter serotonin (5-HT), which possesses powerful vasoactive properties. Support for the role of serotonin comes from observations that introducing reserpine, a serotonin-depleting agent, will trigger a migraine, which will subsequently abate with the introduction of serotonin and serotonin agonists (Saper et al., 1993). Recent pharmacotherapeutic efforts have focused on drugs that affect serotonin directly or indirectly. A $5-HT_1$ agonist, sumatriptan, has proven to be effective in terminating acute migraine headaches, whereas $5-HT_2$ antagonists are effective in their prevention (Gillies & Lance, 1993). Although much still remains undetermined regarding the pathogenesis of migraine, elucidation of the roles of serotonin and the hypothalamus represents an exciting and fruitful direction for future research.

Tension-Type Headache

Diagnostic Criteria

A diagnosis of *episodic tension-type headache* (previously *Muscle-contraction*) requires that headaches have occurred at least 10 times, with fewer than 15 days of headache pain within a single month and fewer than 180 days of headache pain within a year. The headache must last between 30 minutes and seven days, and at least two of the following pain characteristics must exist: (1) pressing/tightening (nonpulsating) quality, (2) mild or moderate intensity, (3) bilateral location, and (4) no aggravation by routine physical activity. In addition, both of the following must be true: (1) no nausea or vomiting and (2) the presence of no more than one of the following: photophobia or phonophobia. Last, the headache must not be due to an organic disorder. *Chronic tension-type headache* is diagnosed if the headache is essentially the same as just stated but with a frequency of 15 or more days per month (180 or more days per year) for six or more months (Headache Classification Committee of the International Headache Society, 1988).

Pathophysiology

Like migraine, the pathogenesis of tension-type headache is a matter of debate. The traditional theory posits that muscular contraction in the pericranial and nearby muscle groups (e.g., cervical paraspinals, trapezius) leads to increased pressure on the cranium and the constriction of blood vessels (Saper et al., 1993). Theoretically, the muscle tension is a direct source of pain, whereas the constricted of blood vessels decrease the supply of blood to the brain, thus inhibiting the necessary activities of providing nutrients and eliminating waste products. Contrary to this formulation, researchers have not reliably detected significant differences in muscle tension, as measured by surface electromyography (EMG), among tension-type headache sufferers versus others (Jensen, Tuxen, & Olesen, 1988). Additional research evaluating muscle tension in areas other than the frontalis region may add clarity to this literature.

Migraine and Tension-Type Headaches: Additional Issues

Literature on the pharmacological treatment of migraine and tension-type headache diagnoses identifies areas of significant overlap. Current guidelines recommend only some medications for the treatment of migraine headache, but not for tension-type headache (e.g., corticosteroids, phenothiazines/neuroleptics, sumatriptan, antihistamines, lithium carbonate, ergotamine derivatives, pizotofen). In contrast, the literature supports many medications for the treatment of both migraine and tension-type headache (e.g., most analgesics, nonsteroidal anti-inflammatory drugs [NSAIDs], isometheptene, beta and calcium-channel blockers, antidepressants, monamine oxidase inhibitors [MAOIs], and anticonvulsants; see Saper et al., 1993).

This lack of specificity regarding treatment for migraine and tension-type headaches has fueled the debate about whether these are distinct disorders or variations of the same disorder (Silberstein, 1990). The severity model posits that headaches fall on a continuum, with episodic tension-type at one end and migraine with aura at the other end. Other headaches with equivocal diagnoses fall between the extremes of this continuum of severity, rather than being artificially forced into one or another distinct category (Gladstein et al., 1993).

Empirical literature regarding this debate remains mixed. For example, physiological comparisons have identified consistencies between migraine and tension-type headache (Jensen et al., 1988; Langemark & Olesen, 1987). In addition, similar biochemical changes—such as the depletion of beta endorphin in cerebral spinal fluid, alterations in serotonin and platelet physiology, and sympathetic

hypofunction—exist during both types of headache (Anderson & Frank, 1981; Arena, Blanchard, Andrasik, Appelbaum, & Myers, 1985). These findings coincide with the lack of specificity of drug treatment studies and support the concept that these two headache types may indeed be variants of a single headache disorder.

On the other hand, investigations examining symptom clusters in headache patients tend to support the notion that migraine and tension-type headaches are distinct. Merikangas and Frances (1993) suggested that use of statistical techniques, such as cluster analysis, is necessary to provide information regarding the validity of current IHS criteria. A recent study utilizing this approach in a sample of 408 headache sufferers found that symptoms reported by these patients formed two distinct clusters that were clearly identifiable as migraine-like and tension-like, thereby supporting current IHS criteria (Bruehl, Lofland, Penzien, Rains, & Semenchuk, 1994). It is important to acknowledge that different symptom clusters do not necessarily indicate the presence of distinct disorders, although this certainly appears to be a reasonable hypothesis warranting further investigation.

Cluster Headache and Chronic Paroxysmal Hemicrania

Cluster headaches are extremely rare in children, as the average age of onset is 27 to 30 years. Cluster headaches are rare even in the adult population, affecting only 0.09 to 0.40 percent of adult males, with the prevalence for males being five to six times higher than for females (Linet & Stewart, 1984; Maytal, Lipton, Solomon, & Shinnar, 1992). Due to the low prevalence in children and adolescents, this section will provide only a clinical description of this disorder. When cluster headaches do occur in children, they share the same characteristics as cluster headaches in adults. The symptom pattern includes severe, unilateral head pain (especially around the eye and temple), with ipsilateral lacrimation (eye tearing), ptosis (drooping eyelid), miosis (pupillary constriction), conjunctival injection (red eye), rhinorrhea (running nose), forehead and facial sweating, eyelid edema, and nasal congestion. Cluster headaches typically last from 15 minutes to several hours and can occur up to eight times a day (Headache

Classification Committee of the International Headache Society, 1988).

Chronic paroxysmal hemicrania (CPH), closely related to cluster headache, shares some of the symptoms of cluster headache, including unilateral pain with severe intensity in the same location and accompanying autonomic phenomena, temporal pattern of attacks, and typical onset in adulthood. However, CPH a is different from cluster headache in that CPH attacks are more frequent, of shorter duration, occur most frequently in females, and there is absolute effectiveness of treatment with indomethacin (Headache Classification Committee of the International Headache Society, 1988).

Other Headache Types

The vast majority of scientific work on child and adolescent headaches has emphasized migraine and tension-type headaches. Therefore, this chapter will focus on these two headaches, with the remaining IHS headache types being listed for reference purposes only. Interested readers should examine the IHS criteria for these other headaches in order to become familiar with their symptom presentations. The remaining headache types include the following:

1. Miscellaneous headaches not associated with structural lesion
2. Headache associated with head trauma
3. Headache associated with vascular disorders
4. Headache associated with nonvascular intracranial disorder
5. Headache associated with substances or their withdrawal
6. Headache associated with noncephalic infection
7. Headache associated with metabolic disorder
8. Headache or facial pain associated with disorder of cranium, neck, eyes, ears, nose, sinuses, teeth, mouth or other facial or cranial structures
9. Cranial neuralgias, nerve trunk pain, and deafferentation pain
10. Headache not classifiable (Headache Classification Committee of the International Headache Society, 1988)

It is important to note that the diagnostic system for headache is still in its infancy. Considerable research is underway and new findings are continually refining the classification nosology. This is an important process because identification of reliable, meaningful subgroups of headache patients is a necessary prerequisite to the development of maximally effective treatments.

ASSESSMENT

A detailed, comprehensive interview is the most important component of an effective headache evaluation (Rothner, 1993; Saper et al., 1993). Collection of information about headache history, frequency, severity, temporal characteristics, concomitant activities, and other vital information typically provides headache specialists with the necessary information to make an accurate diagnosis. The exception to this scenario is the relatively rare case in which a patient's presentation and historical data lead one to suspect an organic lesion, requiring further diagnostic testing. The authors cannot overemphasize the importance of a comprehensive assessment conducted by a trained clinician, especially given its relevance to the development and evaluation of an appropriate treatment plan.

Medical Assessment

Most headaches are benign in nature, although serious etiologies (e.g., trauma, infectious disease, neoplasm) occasionally produce headache symptoms. Clinicians must first address these concerns and rule out such serious organic pathology prior to initiation of any headache treatment. Any patient experiencing a headache with concomitant neurological signs (e.g., visual disturbance, limb weakness) must first receive a complete neurological evaluation with appropriate tests (Williamson et al., 1993).

Although history and physical examination for neurological signs will generally rule out headaches due to underlying conditions, such as a brain tumor (Masek & Hoag, 1990), reliance on sophisticated testing equipment is necessary in some cases. An electroencephalogram (EEG) is effective in detecting subtle abnormalities, but given these abnormalities often occur in children without headache, the utility of this test appears limited (Rothner, 1993).

Magnetic resonance imaging (MRI) and computerized tomography (CT) results are useful in ruling out tumors or other structural or inflammatory pathology (McAbee, Siegel, Kadakia, & Cantos, 1993; Rothner, 1993). However, a recent investigation found that CT scans detected important pathology in less than one-half of one percent of cases in a group of chronic headache patients with normal neurological examinations (Akpek et al., 1994). This study concluded that CT is an expensive and unrewarding technique for the evaluation of headache patients unless significant neurological signs are present. Similarly, the Quality Standards Subcommittee of the American Academy of Neurology (1994) reviewed the literature on the use of neuroimaging (CT and MRI) in patients with headache, and concluded with the following practice guideline:

> In adult patients with recurrent headaches that have been defined as migraine, including those with visual aura, with no recent change in pattern, no history of seizures, and no other focal neurologic signs or symptoms, the routine use of neuroimaging techniques is not warranted. In patients with atypical headache patterns, a history of seizures, or focal neurologic signs or symptoms, CT or MRI may be indicated.

Although there are many other medical tests available that vary in their utility, invasiveness, and expense, it is beyond the scope of this chapter to provide a thorough review of these technologies. In general, the guidelines for deciding whether to use such tests include the specificity and sensitivity of the test, the likelihood that the additional test data will facilitate determination of an accurate diagnosis, and the knowledge that this information will impact the course of treatment.

Psychological/Behavioral Assessment

Interview

Interviews are necessary to collect initial information, establish a therapeutic relationship, and evaluate potential associations between environmental events and headache episodes. This is a necessary first step in the formulation of an individualized treatment plan targeting relevant situations and responses. For exam-

ple, interviewers must carefully explore social and school-related factors (and preferably include information from the child's parents and teachers) in order to identify any associations related to the exacerbation of pain behavior.

Separate interviews with the parents and child/adolescent must explore the history of pain experiences in the family. Clinicians also need to raise questions regarding other physical sensations experienced by the patient, typical situations in which headaches occur, responses of others to the headaches, and responses by the patient that ameliorate and exacerbate pain (see Masek & Hoag, 1990).

Questions about family history of headaches may suggest inherited conditions as well as potentially relevant observational learning. Identifying existing coping strengths and resources that the patient and family have used to successfully handle prior difficulties of any kind can greatly facilitate treatment efforts. The reader may refer to Rothner (1993) and colleagues (1993) for further discussion.

Self-Report Measures

Recommended self-report measures include two headache questionnaires developed for use with children: The Childhood Headache Questionnaire (CHQ: modification by Labbe, Williamson, & Southard, 1985, of the Headache Questionnaire; Blanchard, Theobald, Williamson, Silver, & Brown, 1978) and the Headache Symptom Questionnaire-Revised (Mindell & Andrasik, 1987). The CHQ has children rate 35 questions on a Likert-based frequency scale. Questions address temporal factors related to headache occurrence and duration as well as the presence of specific symptoms. Because the CHQ is an adaptation of an adult measure, some questions appear inappropriate for young children, such as whether headaches occur after drinking coffee or alcohol.

The Headache Symptom Questionnaire-Revised consists of 20 questions of a nature similar to the CHQ, and one study reported this questionnaire accurately classified 66.2 percent of headache sufferers, using a diagnostic interview based on the Ad Hoc Committee criteria as the criterion (Mindell & Andrasik, 1987). Preliminary research indicates scores from these two measures correlate well with parent report and suggest they may provide useful information in determining diagnosis.

Headache Diaries

Unfortunately, retrospective self-report of headache activity (e.g., frequency, severity, duration) often does not yield accurate estimates (Andrasik et al., 1985). However, use of child and parent daily headache diaries is a useful alternative. There is an overall tendency for diary data to reveal lower and presumably more accurate estimates of headache parameters relative to child and parent retrospective monthly reports. Comparison of parent and child diaries suggest lower frequency ratings by parents but equivalent intensity ratings (Andrasik et al., 1985). Obtaining diaries recorded on a daily basis from both child and parent appears to maximize reliability and provide the most useful data for clinical decision making.

Provision of booklets and instructions, as well as enlisting patients' assistance in developing the recording system, can facilitate adherence to daily monitoring instructions. Common instructions include having the patient rate headache information (e.g., presence, intensity, duration, medication usage) at regular intervals, such as meals and bedtime. This record keeping provides reliable headache data that clinicians can use later to evaluate treatment efficacy and reinforce patients' efforts (Labbe et al., 1985).

In a similar manner, patients and others can observe, describe, and rate a child's activities and environmental circumstances. Understanding situational and temporal antecedents, as well as consequences of children's pain behavior, may shed light on a variety of relevant learning factors. These may include classically conditioned stimuli that serve to elicit headache episodes as well as sources of secondary gain that serve to maintain pain behaviors and complaints via operant mechanisms (see McGrath, 1987).

Headache diary ratings of pain intensity using a visual analog scale, such as a 10 cm. line with the ends representing no pain and severe pain, can be an effective tool, even with very young children (Feuerstein & Dobkin, 1990). Choices among a series of cartoon drawings of varying facial expressions have also been useful in representing levels of physical and emotional pain or anchoring the ends of the scales (Ross et al., 1993).

Issues to consider when using diaries and other self-report measures with young children include concerns about their reliability and validity as a function of differing levels of cognitive and affective development (Marcon & Labbe, 1990). The following strategies may help clinicians obtain consistent, accurate data: (1) using visual analog scales in lieu of verbal descriptions of pain severity, (2) using pictures instead of verbally requesting information about headache locations, (3) discussing durations of headache episodes in terms of familiar activities of a similar duration, and (4) selecting an appropriate level of wording and concepts when using verbal discussion (Marcon & Labbe, 1990).

Psychological/Emotional Assessment

It is important to assess psychological adjustment in chronic headache sufferers. This appears to be especially true for adolescent males who, as a group, seem more likely than other groups to have clinically significant adjustment problems, as measured by the Personality Inventory for Children (Andrasik et al., 1988; Wirt, Loeber, Klinedinst, & Seat, 1977). Measures such as the Child Behavior Checklist (Achenbach, 1991), Fear Survey Schedule for Children-Revised (Ollendick, 1983), Children's Manifest Anxiety Scale (Reynolds & Richmond, 1978), the State-Trait Anxiety Inventory for Children (Spielberger, 1973), and the Children's Depression Inventory (Kovacs, 1992) can also be useful in exploring potential problem areas.

Sequelae to chronic headaches can include developmentally inappropriate behaviors, fears, anxieties, sadness, and social difficulties. To the extent that these problems are clinically significant, a primary treatment emphasis on these issues may be necessary. For many children, affective and behavioral problems may develop as a result of headaches and subsequently show positive change with headache improvement (Andrasik et al., 1988; Kowal & Pritchard, 1990). For other children, clinicians may need to address affective and behavioral problems specifically, regardless of their course of development, to reduce their interference with adherence to treatment recommendations. For children with somatic preoccupations or long histories of somatic complaints, depression may be an important mediating factor related to poor treatment outcome (Osterhaus et al., 1993). Special considerations are thus necessary when developing cognitive-behavioral interventions for these children.

An early study of psychological characteristics of headache sufferers concluded that children with headaches are more anxious than other children (Bille, 1962). However, reliability and validity of the measures used in this study were unknown. More recently, Andrasik and associates (1988) concluded that younger children with headaches do not demonstrate elevated anxiety relative to controls but that adolescents with headaches do demonstrate significantly increased anxiety. They hypothesized that the anxiety and inappropriate externalizing behaviors they observed among the male adolescents resulted from their frustration with the headache chronicity.

Once a clinician becomes satisfied that a child's headache condition is not a result of known trauma, disease, or other serious pathology and that other factors suggesting poor prognosis are not present, then it is appropriate to develop and implement the first stage of a treatment plan. If difficulties arise during the course of treatment—such as adherence problems, failure of symptoms to remit, or continuation/ development of psychosocial difficulties—then further assessment may be necessary.

TREATMENT

Recent advances suggest a growing arsenal of effective interventions for children and adolescents who suffer from headaches. Although pharmacological options comprise an important and growing area of headache treatment, many medications pose considerably greater risks for children, relative to adults. Due to such concerns, clinicians must remain aware of pharmacological interventions but consider initiating a conservative course of nonpharmacological treatment when possible. This section will review the primary medication and nondrug approaches and then summarize the treatment outcome literature.

Overview of Treatment Options

Pharmacological Interventions

As discussed earlier, headache, particularly migraine, is a qualitatively different experience for children than adults (Winner, 1994). Due to difficulties inherent in conducting pharmacological treatment outcome studies with minors, there is a paucity of published information on the efficacy or safety of many drugs used to treat children (Wilkinson, 1993). Use of medications is often a double-edged sword with adults, and there are additional concerns when using drugs with children. Clinicians must always evaluate medications using a cost-benefit analysis, paying particular attention to negative side-effects. This must occur for all types of medications because even analgesics cause negative side-effects, including the perpetuation and worsening of headaches (Rapoport & Sheftell, 1993).

There are several medications that can assist in the abortive (symptomatic) treatment of headache. These medications include various prescription and nonprescription analgesics (aspirin, acetaminophen, butalbital, propoxyphene napsylate), ergotamine compounds, NSAIDs (ibuprofen, naproxen, indomethacin), isometheptene, corticosteroids (prednisone, methylprednisone), phenothiazines/ neuroleptics (chlorpromazine, promethazine hydrochloride), and sumatriptan (Saper et al., 1993). Adequate treatment outcome data for the use of many of these agents with children is not available. Therefore, the primary concern for most of these medications is that although there are known negative side-effects when used with adults, practitioners are not fully aware of the degree to which they negatively affect children.

One commonly reported caution is that children below the age of 15 years must not take aspirin, especially during the course of an acute viral syndrome, due to the potential risk of developing Reye's syndrome (Rapoport & Sheftell, 1990). Therefore, the analgesic treatment of choice for children is acetaminophen because of its similar efficacy to aspirin without the antiinflammatory activity. However, one must take caution against exceeding the recommended daily dosage of acetaminophen due to the potential for hepatic damage, which may not become apparent for several days (Wilkinson, 1993). There are additional concerns for children, including kidney and gastrointestinal complications in response to NSAIDs and cardiac sensitivities when using some of the prophylactic medications described below.

Prophylactic (preventive) pharmacologic treatment for children is appropriate only in cases when the headaches are frequent and severe enough to be disabling. It is important to remember that migraine is a benign, recurring disability, with no insidious underlying structural pathology. Therefore, it is essential that treatment providers take precautions to ensure that the treatment of headache is less unpleasant or damaging than the disorder itself. Medications used in the prophylactic treatment of migraine include beta-blockers (propranolol), calcium-channel blockers (verapamil hydrochloride, nifedipine), antidepressants (amitriptyline, doxepin hydrochloride), antihistamines (cyproheptadine hydrochloride), tranquilizers (diazepam, alprazolam), NSAIDs (naproxen sodium, ibuprofen), serotonergic drugs (pizotofen), and anticonvulsants (phenytoin sodium, carbamazapine).

Nonpharmacological Interventions

In contrast with pharmacological interventions for headache, nondrug treatments typically produce no negative side-effects and often result in positive side-effects (e.g., improved mood, improved sleep, increased energy, physical fitness, increased ability to manage diverse stressors; Rapoport & Sheftell, 1990). The primary drawback associated with nonpharmacological approaches is the lengthier interval between treatment onset and evidence of effect; this is due to the training requirements. However, evidence for long-term maintenance of treatment gains is quite good (Andrasik, Blanchard, Edlund, & Attanasio, 1983; Grazzi, Leone, Frediani, & Bussone, 1990; Labbe & Ward, 1990).

Nonpharmacological treatments may include a variety of cognitive-behavioral interventions, such as relaxation therapy; biofeedback; stress management; education; communication training; time management; regulating sleep patterns; minimizing intake of caffeine, nicotine, and other chemicals; and other lifestyle changes. Given the importance of factors that may affect treatment adherence and outcome—such as the nature of family relationships, evidence of pain behavior, and potential for secondary gain—appropriate administration of therapy requires expert professionals well versed in headache disorders (Saper et al., 1993).

Relaxation and Biofeedback Training. Relaxation therapy achieved increased popularity in the Western hemisphere in the 1970s when researchers determined that transcendental meditation could reliably evoke a "relaxation response" of lowered physiological arousal in those who regularly practice it (Wallace

& Benson, 1972; Wallace, Benson, & Wilson, 1971). Researchers subsequently hypothesized that this reduction in arousal may have many physical and psychological benefits, and this belief led to its wide popularity. Current beliefs are that the level of relaxation attained by individuals relates to a variety of factors beyond a specific technique's capacity to lower physiological arousal (e.g., individual differences in acceptability of different techniques, differential efficacy of techniques due to the nature of the disorder, other factors related to the "match" between patient and technique) and that therapists must account for significant individual variation when conducting relaxation therapy with patients (Smith, 1990).

Biofeedback is a highly effective treatment approach whereby patients learn to control a physiological response with the assistance of an auditory or visual signal that provides feedback/information about the ongoing status of that physiological system. For example, many headache patients may not be aware of the level of muscle tension in their head, neck, and shoulder muscles as it varies throughout the day. EMG biofeedback techniques help increase an individual's awareness of muscle tension and then provide immediate feedback and reinforcement regarding efforts to reduce the level of muscle tension. This is important because the control of some headaches may depend on early detection of tension to prevent it from rising to increasingly higher levels; high levels of muscle tension over prolonged periods can cause muscle fatigue, increase the likelihood of muscle strain, restrict local blood flow, and exacerbate pain (Cram, 1990; Price, Clare, & Ewerhardt, 1948).

The biofeedback apparatus allows patients to experiment with different strategies (e.g., various relaxation techniques, correcting poor posture) to control the targeted physiological response. Different types of biofeedback facilitate control over various specific physiological responses, such as heart rate, blood pressure, muscle tension, blood flow (either directly, as in cephalic vasomotor feedback, or indirectly, as in skin temperature), and others.

Biofeedback and relaxation have several advantages that render them first-line treatment approaches for headache disorders. First, once patients acquire the requisite skills, they can produce the desired effect without further assistance from a clinician or any external apparatus. Second, there are no negative side-effects from these treatments, and for many patients, there is the additional positive side-effect of increased control over diverse stressors in their lives (Ford & Ford, 1994). Third, this therapy is a time-limited and cost-effective intervention (Burke & Andrasik; 1989), typically requiring a total of 7 to 10 sessions, including primary treatment, as well as follow-up sessions to promote maintenance and generalization. The one caveat of these approaches is the necessity of sufficient practice to attain proficiency. Patients usually respond well to the rationale for nonpharmacological interventions, but in cases of limited treatment success, clinicians must reevaluate patient motivation and place an emphasis on closely monitoring daily practice.

Treatment Outcome

Placebo Effects

Prior to summarizing the treatment outcome literature for drug and nondrug treatments for headache pain, a brief discussion of the placebo effect is appropriate. The *placebo effect* refers to the well-documented improvements (in various medical and psychological conditions) that patients obtain when they receive a theoretically nonactive intervention (e.g., sugar pill, "fake" biofeedback), but believe that they are obtaining a therapeutic intervention. For example, when empirically testing headache pain medications against placebos that have no pain relieving qualities at all, up to 40 percent of the placebo group report as much relief as those taking the active medication (Rapoport & Sheftell, 1990).

Similarly, providing biofeedback signals that indicate a patient is producing appropriate physiological changes, despite the actual lack of any such changes, can have positive effects on headache activity, suggesting the role of cognitive or other factors in pain perception (cf. Holroyd et al., 1984). This underscores the necessity of including placebo groups in controlled experimental designs to adequately assess the efficacy of an intervention.

Pharmacological Interventions

The most striking observation regarding the status of the pharmacological treatment outcome literature for headache in children and adolescents concerns the overall paucity of controlled studies. Whereas the adult literature is developing to a point where researchers can now reach reasonable conclusions regarding treatment efficacy, this is simply not the case in the pediatric literature. The few studies conducted on pharmacological interventions have almost exclusively focused on migraines. Recent reviews of this literature indicate that many medications remain widely used in clinical practice, despite their lack of empirical support (Igarashi, May, & Golden, 1992).

Abortive Medications. The use of abortive agents in the pharmacological treatment of pediatric migraine is often problematic because many children have difficulty recognizing early headache stages, thus resulting in frequent failure (Igarashi et al., 1992). Ergotamine, used effectively and well studied in adults, has limited empirical support for use with children. The only study that has investigated ergotamine in children was unsuccessful due to a high dropout rate (Congdon & Forsythe, 1979). Parenteral (i.e., by injection) administration of dihydroergotamine for severe migraine attacks has been beneficial for adults and adolescents (Callahan & Raskin, 1986). Aspirin, acetaminophen, and ibuprofen may be effective, especially if the attack is mild. Ibuprofen, investigated in a randomized, double-blind crossover trial in adults, resulted in a significant reduction in headache compared with placebo (Havanka-Kanniainen, 1989). No study has yet replicated these results with children or adolescents.

One study compared isometheptene to placebo in adults, with partial or complete relief occurring in 42 percent of the isometheptene group and 29 percent of the placebo group (Diamond & Medina, 1979). Unfortunately, there are no reported treatment outcome results of isometheptene with children or adolescents. Two calcium-channel blockers, flunarizine (not yet approved for use in the United States) and verapamil, have undergone evaluation in double-blind studies with adults. Flunarizine has had mixed results, but verapamil obtained a positive response in 74 percent of patients compared to 28 percent of the placebo group (Pfaffenrath, Wolfgang, & Wolfgang, 1990; Soyka, Taneri, Oestereich, & Schmidt, 1989). Data on calcium-channel blockers used as abortive agents with children are not currently available. Last, sumatriptan appears promising in its efficacy with adults (Subcutaneous Sumatriptan International

Study Group, 1991), but studies with children have not yet appeared in the published literature. Thus, the available research on abortives suggests that some of these agents may be efficacious; unfortunately, this literature base is too limited to offer much guidance regarding the use of many specific medications, or allow for a meaningful comparative analysis across medications.

Prophylactic Medications. Treatment outcome studies for prophylactic pharmacological agents are similarly lacking. Anticonvulsants (phenobarbital) have been useful for migraine prophylaxis, with similar reported efficacy to propranolol (Barlow, 1984), but neither drug has undergone adequate evaluation, especially in the child or adolescent population (Igarashi et al., 1992). In addition, phenobarbital has several negative side-effects, including attention/concentration deficits and agitated behavior. Antidepressant medications (amitriptyline, imipramine, phenelzine) have proven useful in the prevention of migraines and in the treatment of concomitant emotional disorders, with amitriptyline being the most commonly used psychotropic medication for migraine prophylaxis in all age groups (Saeed, Pumariega, & Cinciripini, 1992).

Some studies have compared amitriptyline to propranolol and placebo in adults, with both active medications producing similar effects that are significantly superior to placebo (Couch & Hassanein, 1979; Ziegler et al., 1987). Phenelzine, a monoamine oxidase inhibitor (MAOI), is one of the preferred agents for resistant adult headaches, but it has not received adequate study in children. Similarly, clinicians have used imipramine for headache prophylaxis in children despite the lack of controlled investigations for children or adults (Igarashi et al., 1992). One recent study compared fluvoxamine, a new serotonin reuptake inhibitor, to amitriptyline for adult migraine prophylaxis, with both drugs significantly reducing headache frequency, but amitriptyline produced greater negative side-effects (severe drowsiness) than fluvoxamine (Bank, 1994). This study suggests that fluvoxamine may be a useful alternative for amitriptyline, but its efficacy needs to be evaluated in children.

Clinicians have used antiserotonergic drugs (methysergide and cyproheptadine) with children and adults despite very little empirical evidence regarding their efficacy. Methysergide is not appropriate for children due to a potentially serious side-effect (retroperitoneal fibrosis). Cyproheptadine has not undergone evaluation in any controlled outcome study, but an uncontrolled pilot study found positive effects for 17 of 19 children, aged 6 to 16 years, with weight gain and drowsiness reported as the primary side-effects (Bille, Ludvigsson, & Sanner, 1977). Several studies have revealed that prostaglandin inhibitors (NSAIDs, such as naproxen) reduce the frequency of migraine attacks, vomiting and nausea, and other medication usage in adults (Bellavance & Meloche, 1990; Welch, Ellis, & Keenan, 1985), but indomethacin was not an effective prophylactic agent in a controlled study with adults (Anthony & Lance, 1968), and neither naproxen nor indomethacin have received adequate study in children (Igarashi et al., 1992).

Clinical researchers have used several beta-blockers for migraine prophylaxis. Andersson and Vinge (1990) reviewed the double-blind treatment outcome studies using beta-blockers with adults and found that propranolol, metoprolol, timolol, nadolol, and atenolol reduced the frequency of classic and common migraine attacks, but their effects on the duration and intensity of attacks were not clear. Other beta-blockers—including pindolol, atenolol, oxprenolol, and acebutolol—were not effective for migraine prophylaxis. Only one of the reviewed studies reported differential effectiveness for the beta-blockers, finding nadolol more effective than propranolol in adults (Sudtlovsky et al., 1987). There have been three studies investigating propranolol in pediatric migraine, with one study finding reduced frequency of migraine attacks and nausea and no notable side-effects (Ludvigsson, 1974). However, the other two studies showed no significant differences between propranolol and placebo with regard to frequency, severity, or duration of headache episodes (Forsythe, Gilles, & Sills, 1987; Olness, MacDonald, & Uden, 1987). Also, timolol produced no significant difference from placebo in pediatric migraineurs (Frenken & Nuijten, 1984).

Andersson and Vinge (1990) reviewed the double-blind studies on calcium-channel blockers and concluded that flunarizine effectively reduced the frequency of classic and common migraine, with less clear effects on severity and duration. Of three controlled studies of flunarizine conducted with children, two showed significant reductions in headache frequency and duration (Sorge & Marano, 1985; Sorge et al., 1988), but the third study noted flunarizine's significant impact on headache frequency was equivalent to that of aspirin (Pothmann, 1987). Other calcium-channel blockers—including verapamil, nifedipine, nimodipine, and dilitiazem—appeared promising, but the authors were not able to draw any definitive conclusions. Of the remaining prophylactic medications reviewed, papaverine showed positive effects (Sillanpaa & Kaponen, 1978), whereas clonidine produced negative effects (Sillanpaa, 1977; Sills, Cogdon, & Forsythe, 1982) and is not appropriate for the prophylactic treatment of childhood migraine (Igarashi et al., 1992).

As is the case with abortives, the literature on prophylactic medications is still too preliminary to allow definitive conclusions regarding their use with children and adolescents. However, sufficient data presently exist to suggest reasonable therapeutic options and potentially fruitful research directions. Wilkinson (1993) stated that of the drugs available in the United States, the current prophylactic drugs of choice for children are cyproheptadine or propranolol; ergot derivatives, such as methysergide maleate, are not recommended alternatives. Saeed and associates (1992) were in partial agreement, stating however that clinicians must first consider amitriptyline and propranolol because of their potential efficacy and better side-effect profiles (Fenichel, 1985; Woody & Kearns, 1986).

Nonpharmacological Interventions

The literature on the use of nonpharmacological treatments for headache is quite positive. Numerous studies have compared different cognitive-behavioral techniques with biofeedback (thermal, EMG), relaxation procedures (breathing, imagery), pharmacological interventions (amitriptyline, propranolol), and placebos across different headache types (migraine, tension). In general, nonpharmacological interventions performed significantly better than placebo, typically resulting in 50 to 70 percent of patients obtaining significant reductions in frequency, severity, and/or duration of headache pain (Hoelscher & Lichstein, 1984; Rapoport & Sheftell, 1990).

Studies of tension-type headache sufferers have found that EMG biofeedback is highly effective at reducing headache symptoms (i.e., greater than 50 percent reduction in headache frequency, severity, and/or duration) in children and that the results persist for long periods of time after discontinuation of treatment (Andrasik et al., 1983; Labbe & Ward, 1990). One treatment outcome study reported clinical improvement in 9 out of 10 patients at the end of treatment and 10 out of 10 patients at one-year follow-up (Grazzi et al., 1990). Across the studies reviewed, follow-up assessments varied from none to two years, with long-term clinical improvements maintained. These results are very encouraging and indicate the need for larger-scale treatment outcome studies to replicate these findings.

The treatment outcome literature on migraine headache in children is also encouraging. All but one out of several treatment outcome studies found various psychological interventions (e.g., cognitive-behavioral therapy, thermal and EMG biofeedback, imagery, breathing relaxation, and progressive muscle relaxation [PMR]) significantly more effective than placebo and control conditions (see Williamson et al., 1993). One study found relaxation to be more effective than propranolol (Olness et al., 1987). Another controlled study tested the efficacy of a cognitive coping intervention versus relaxation versus placebo (Richter et al., 1986). The cognitive coping intervention was as effective as relaxation therapy, and both were more effective than the attention-placebo intervention. Two other studies found no significant difference in treatment effects between a home-based treatment approach using nonpharmacological techniques and a traditional clinic-based approach (Burke & Andrasik, 1989; Guarnieri & Blanchard, 1990), further suggesting the efficacy and potential cost effectiveness of nonpharmacological approaches.

A recent meta-analysis provides an excellent summary of the treatment outcome studies conducted on migraine in children to date, comparing the efficacy of nonpharmacological interventions to prophylactic pharmacological interventions (Hermann, Kim, & Blanchard, 1995). Results indicated that both pharmacological and nonpharmacological approaches performed significantly better than placebos. Further, two nonpharmacological techniques were significantly more effective than two drug interventions.

Specifically, thermal biofeedback was significantly more effective in reducing headache than serotonergic drugs, and PMR in combination with biofeedback was significantly more effective than calcium-channel blockers. Thus, current data suggest the overall efficacy of treatments for migraine and the superior efficacy for particular nonpharmacological approaches over the prophylactic medications studied. Additional reviews comparing other treatment options as further research accumulates will be very helpful.

Combined Pharmacological/ Nonpharmacological Treatments

To date, the utility of combined interventions for children and adolescents with headache remains untested. Indeed, the literature evaluating such options for adults is also virtually nonexistence. However, this represents a potentially important direction for future research. Holroyd, Holm, and Penzien (1988) observed this and provided guidelines for research in this area that warrant repeating. The first and most obvious potential application is that these treatment modalities may complement each other, thereby improving overall treatment efficacy. Although this possibility seems plausible and deserves attention, the authors wisely caution that certain combinations may not be beneficial (e.g., some drugs may interfere with the acquisition of self-regulation skills during biofeedback training).

A second direction for research involves the training of self-management skills to facilitate the proper administration of medications and adherence to regimens (e.g., education as to the manner in which medications work and misconceptions about side-effects, proper timing for administration, particularly for abortives). Finally, psychological assessment may be helpful in identifying patients who are good versus poor candidates for particular treatment modalities. It is the authors' belief that all these areas are potentially applicable to children as well.

Multidisciplinary Headache Clinics

Comprehensive headache management from a multi-disciplinary approach is cost effective for quality and breadth of care. A multidisciplinary team generally includes a physical therapist, physician, and psychologist, and may include other disciplines as well. This approach is particularly beneficial for difficult cases of severe or persistent headache. Treatment outcome studies in multidisciplinary clinics have shown significant and sustained reductions in headache and related symptoms, such as depression, symptomatic drug use, emergency-room utilization, and level of disability (Lake, Saper, Madden, & Kreeger, 1990; Silberstein, 1992).

Generally, recommended criteria for referral to a comprehensive center for headache management include (1) history of recurring acute care needs or progressive, debilitating headache; (2) multiple diagnostic and therapeutic interventions by qualified health care professionals without success; (3) excessive utilization of health care services (e.g., outpatient services, diagnostic procedures, hospital admissions, medications); (4) inconclusive diagnosis; and (5) when pain appears to have a multifactorial make-up requiring comprehensive, multidisciplinary interventions (Saper et al., 1993). This comprehensive approach is typically available only for adults and, to a lesser degree, adolescents; little is known about its utility for children. However, the impact of removing a child from his or her home for an inpatient hospitalization must be considered in the cost-benefit decision-making process.

SUMMARY

Although the treatment outcome literature for headache in children and adolescents is still in its infancy, preliminary evidence suggests that several efficacious interventions are now available. As always, the development of a treatment protocol must occur on an individual basis, keeping in mind empirically supported treatment outcome findings, knowledge of treatment history, and psychological, social, or familial factors likely to have an impact on the effective implementation of any intervention.

Of particular importance with this population, however, is that health care providers give primary consideration to conservative interventions that are likely to produce positive outcomes. Specifically, there are many pharmacological treatment options available, although most medications have negative side-effects that are of particular concern in their use with children. Nonpharmacological interventions discussed must be a first-line intervention whenever possible, because they generally produce similar, or in some cases, better treatment effects when compared with pharmacological interventions without the associated risks. Clinicians must discuss expectations for treatment outcome with patients so that the patients will understand that although elimination of headaches is possible, the most frequent outcome is a significant reduction in the frequency, severity, and/or duration of headache pain.

CONCLUSIONS

The status of the literature on childhood headache is at a point where one can draw preliminary conclusions and pursue new directions. It is important to acknowledge, however, that current controversies regarding headache nomenclature have broad implications for the accurate assessment and treatment of headaches. As research addressing the pathophysiology and symptom patterns of headaches advances, resultant improvements in the diagnostic system will facilitate the efforts to develop individualized treatment packages that are maximally effective.

Treatment outcome studies indicate that although most headache sufferers do not receive complete remission from current treatments, most show a significant reduction in headache frequency, severity, and/or duration (Rapoport & Sheftell, 1990). This is promising in that there is much to offer patients in the way of ameliorating the physical and psychological disability associated with headaches. Also, although clinicians have not yet attained the ultimate goal of matching treatments to headache diagnosis, it appears that they can significantly improve most headaches via a variety of headache treatments.

Perhaps the issue of greatest concern regarding the treatment of headache is that approximately two out of every three headache sufferers do not seek care (Lipton & Stewart, 1994; Stewart & Lipton, 1993). Dissemination of information describing treatment options such that a larger proportion of the headache population obtains therapy that is available remains an important priority.

NOTE

The authors would like to thank Jeffrey E. Cassisi, Ph.D., of Jackson State University, and David A. Fitzgerald, M. D., of the Pain and Rehabilitation Clinic of Chicago, for their contributions.

REFERENCES

Achenbach, T. M. (1991). *Manual for the Child Behavior Checklist / 4–18 and 1991 profile*. Burlington, VT: University of Vermont Department of Psychiatry.

Ad Hoc Committee on Classification of Headache, National Institute of Neurological Diseases and Blindness. (1962). Classification of headache. *Journal of the American Medical Association, 179,* 717–718.

Akpek, S., Arac, M., Atilla, S., Onal, B., Yucel, C., & Isik, S. (1994). Cost effectivity of computed tomography in the evaluation of patients with headache. *Headache, 34,* 301–302.

Anderson, C. D., & Frank, R. D. (1981). Migraine and tension headache: Is there a difference? *Headache, 21,* 63–71.

Andersson, K. E., & Vinge, E. (1990). Beta-adrenoceptor blockers and calcium agonists in the prophylaxis and treatment of migraine. *Drugs, 39,* 355–373.

Andrasik, F., Blanchard, E. B., Edlund, S. R., & Attanasio, V. (1983). EMG biofeedback in the treatment of a child with muscle contraction headache. *American Journal of Clinical Biofeedback, 6,* 96–102.

Andrasik, F., Burke, E. J., Attanasio, V., & Rosenblum, E. L. (1985). Child, parent, and physician reports of a child's headache pain: Relationship prior to and follow-up treatment. *Headache, 25,* 421–425.

Andrasik, F., Kabela, E., Quinn, S., Attanasio, V., Blanchard, E. B., & Rosenblum, E. L. (1988). Psychological functioning of children who have recurrent migraine. *Pain, 34,* 43–52.

Anthony, M., & Lance, J. W. (1968). Indomethacin in migraine. *Medical Journal of Australia, 1,* 56–57.

Arena, J. G., Blanchard, E. B., Andrasik, F., Appelbaum, K., & Myers, P. E. (1985). Psychophysiological comparisons of three kinds of headache subjects during and between headache states: Analysis of post-stress adaptation periods. *Journal of Psychosomatic Research, 29,* 427–441.

Bank, J. (1994). A comparative study of amitriptyline and fluvoxamine in migraine prophylaxis. *Headache, 34,* 476–478.

Barlow, C. F. (1984). *Headaches and migraine in childhood*. London: Spastics International Medical Publications.

Bellavance, A. J., & Meloche, J. P. (1990). A comparison study of naproxen sodium, pizotyline and placebo in migraine prophylaxis. *Headache, 30,* 710–715.

Bille, B. S. (1962). Migraine in school children. *Acta Paediatrica Scandanavia, 51 (Suppl 136),* 1–151.

Bille, B. S. (1981). Migraine in childhood and its prognosis. *Cephalalgia, 1,* 71–75.

Bille, B. S., Ludvigsson, J., & Sanner, G. (1977). Prophylaxis of migraine in children. *Headache, 17,* 61–63.

Blanchard, E. B., Theobald, E. E., Williamson, D. A., Silver, B. V., & Brown, D. (1978). Temperature biofeedback in the treatment of migraine headaches. *Archives of General Psychiatry, 35,* 581–588.

Bruehl, S., Lofland, K. R., Penzien, D. P., Rains, J. C., & Semenchuk, E. M. (1994). Cluster analysis of headache symptoms: Support for the IHS diagnostic criteria for migraine and tension-type headache. *Headache, 34,* 303.

Burke, E. J., & Andrasik, F. (1989). Home vs. clinical based biofeedback treatment for pediatric migraine: Results of treatment through one-year follow-up. *Headache, 29,* 434–440.

Callahan, M., & Raskin, N. H. (1986). A controlled study of dihydroergotamine in the treatment of acute migraine headache. *Headache, 26,* 168–171.

Congdon, P. J., & Forsythe, W. I. (1979). Migraine in childhood: A study of 300 children. *Developmental Medical Child Neurology, 21,* 209–216.

Couch, J. R., & Hassanein, R. S. (1979). Amitriptyline in migraine prophylaxis. *Archives of Neurology, 36,* 695–699.

Cram, J. R. (1990). *Clinical EMG for surface recording, volume 2.* Nevada City, CA: Clinical Resources.

Diamond, S., & Medina, J. L. (1979). Isometheptene: A nonergot drug in the treatment of migraine. *Headache, 15,* 211–213.

Fenichel, G. M. (1985). Migraine in children. *Neurological Clinics of North America, 3,* 77–94.

Feuerstein, M., & Dobkin, P. L. (1990). Recurrent abdominal pain in children. In A. M. Gross & R. S. Drabman (Eds.), *Handbook of clinical behavioral pediatrics* (pp. 291–309). New York: Plenum.

Ford, R. G., & Ford, K. T. (1994). *Conquer your headaches: How to get rid of your headaches and on with your life* (p. 93). International Headache Management, Inc.

Forsythe, W. I., Gilles, D., & Sills, M. A. (1987). Propranolol ("Inderal") in the treatment of childhood migraine. *Developmental Medicine & Child Neurology, 26,* 737–741.

Frenken, C. W. G. M., & Nuijten, S. T. M. (1984). Flunarizine, a new preventive approach to migraine: A double-blind comparison with placebo. *Clinical Neurology & Neurosurgery, 86,* 17–20.

Gillies, J. D., & Lance, J. W. (1993). Pathophysiology of migraine. In C. D. Tollison & R. S. Kunkel (Eds.), *Headache: Diagnosis and treatment* (pp. 77–84). Baltimore: Williams & Wilkins.

Gladstein, J., Holden, E. W., Peralta, L., & Raven, M. (1993). Diagnoses and symptom patterns in children presenting to a pediatric headache clinic. *Headache, 33,* 497–500.

Grazzi, L., Leone, M., Frediani, F., & Bussone, G. (1990). A therapeutic alternative for tension headache in children: Treatment and 1-year follow-up results. *Biofeedback and Self-Regulation, 15,* 1–6.

Guarnieri, P., & Blanchard, E. B. (1990). Evaluation of home-based thermal biofeedback treatment of pediatric migraine headache. *Biofeedback and Self-Regulation, 15,* 179–184.

Havanka-Kanniainen, H. (1989). Treatment of acute migraine attack: Ibuprofen and placebo compared. *Headache, 29,* 507–509.

Headache Classification Committee of the International Headache Society. (1988). Classification and diagnostic criteria for headache disorders, cranial neuralgias and facial pain. *Cephalalgia, 8(Suppl 7),* 9–96.

Hermann, C., Kim, M., & Blanchard, E. B. (1995). Behavioral and prophylactic pharmacological intervention studies of pediatric migraine: An exploratory meta-analysis. *Pain, 60,* 239–255.

Hockaday, J. M. (1978). Late outcome of childhood onset migraine and factors affecting outcome, with particular reference to early and late EEG findings. In R. Green (Ed.), *Current concepts in migraine research* (pp. 41–48). New York: Raven.

Hoelscher, J. M., & Lichstein, K. L. (1984). Behavioral assessment and treatment of child migraine: Implications for clinical research and practice. *Headache, 24,* 94–103.

Holroyd, K. A., Holm, J. E., & Penzien, D. B. (1988). Clinical issues in the behavioral treatment of recurrent headache. In P. A. Keller & S. R. Heyman (Eds.), *Innovations in clinical practice: A source book, volume 7* (pp. 433–437). Sarsota, FL: Professional Resource Exchange.

Holroyd, K. A., Penzien, D. B., Hursey, K. G., Tobin, D. L., Rogers, L., Holm, J. E., Marcille, P. J., Hall, J. R., & Chila, A. G. (1984). Change mechanisms in EMG biofeedback training: Cognitive changes underlying improvements in tension headache. *Journal of Consulting and Clinical Psychology, 62,* 1039–1053.

Igarashi, M., May, W. N., & Golden, G. S. (1992). Pharmacologic treatment of childhood migraine. *The Journal of Pediatrics, 120,* 653–657.

Jensen, K., Tuxen, C., & Olesen, J. (1988). Pericranial muscle tenderness and pressure-pain threshold in the temporal region during common migraine. *Pain, 35,* 65–70.

Kovacs, M. (1992). *Children's Depression Inventory Manual.* North Tonawanda, NY: Multi-Health Systems.

Kowal, A., & Pritchard, D. (1990). Psychological characteristics of children who suffer from headache: A research note. *Journal of Child Psychology and Psychiatry, 31,* 637–649.

Kuttner, L. (1993). Managing pain in children. *Canadian Family Physician, 39,* 563–568.

Labbe, E. E., & Ward, C. H. (1990). Electromyographic biofeedback with mental imagery and home practice in the treatment of children with muscle-contraction headaches. *Developmental and Behavioral Pediatrics, 11*, 65–68.

Labbe, E.E., Williamson, D. A., & Southard, D. R. (1985). Reliability and validity of children's reports of migraine headache symptoms. *Journal of Psychopathology and Behavioral Assessment, 7*, 375–383.

Lake, A. E., Saper, J. R., Madden, S., & Kreeger, C. (1990). Inpatient treatment for chronic daily headache: A prospective long-term outcome study. *Headache, 30*, 299.

Langemark, M., & Olesen, J. (1987). Pericranial tenderness in tension headache—A blind controlled study. *Cephalalgia, 7*, 249–255.

Linet, M. S., & Stewart, W. F. (1984). Migraine headache: Epidemiologic perspectives. In N. Nathanson, L. Gordis, M. Gregg, & M. Szklo (Eds.), *Epidemiological review* (pp.107–129). Baltimore, MD: The Johns Hopkins University Press.

Linet, M. S., Stewart, W. F., Celentano, D. D., Ziegler, D., & Sprecker, M. (1989). An epidemiological study of headache among adolescents and young adults. *Journal of the American Medical Association, 261*, 2211–2216.

Lipton, R. B., & Stewart, W. F. (1994). Medical consultation for migraine: Results from the American Migraine Study [abstract]. *Headache, 34*, 294.

Ludvigsson, J. (1974). Propranolol used in prophylaxis of migraine in children. *Acta Neurologica Scandinavia, 50*, 109–115.

Marcon, R. A., & Labbe, E. E. (1990). Assessment and treatment of children's headaches from a developmental perspective. *Headache, 30*, 586–592.

Masek, B. J., & Hoag, N. L. (1990). Headache. In A. M. Gross & R. S. Drabman (Eds.), *Handbook of clinical behavioral pediatrics* (pp. 99–109). New York: Plenum.

Maytal, J., Lipton, R. B., Solomon, S., & Shinnar, S. (1992). Childhood onset cluster headaches. *Headache, 32*, 275–279.

McAbee, G. N., Siegel, S. E., Kadakia, S., & Cantos, E. (1993). Value of MRI in pediatric migraine. *Headache, 33*, 143–144.

McGrath, P. A. (1987). The multidimensional assessment and management of recurrent pain syndromes in children. *Behaviour Research and Therapy, 25*, 251–262.

Merikangas, K. R., & Frances, A. (1993). Development of diagnostic criteria for headache syndromes: Lessons from psychiatry. *Cephalalgia, 13*, 34–38.

Mindell, J. A., & Andrasik, F. (1987). Headache classification and factor analysis with a pediatric population. *Headache, 27*, 96–101.

Ollendick, T. H. (1983). Reliability and validity of the revised Fear Survey Schedule for Children (FSSC-R). *Behavior Research and Therapy, 21*, 685–692.

Olness, K., MacDonald, J. T., & Uden, D. L. (1987). Comparison of self-hypnosis and propranolol in the treatment of juvenile classic migraine. *Pediatrics, 79*, 593–597.

Osterhaus, S. O. L., Passchier, J., Helm-Hylkema, H., Jong, K.T., Orlebeke, J. F., Grauw, A. J. C., & Dekker, P. H. (1993). Effects of behavioral psychophysiological treatment on schoolchildren with migraine in a nonclinical setting: Predictors and process variables. *Journal of Pediatric Psychology, 18*, 697–715.

Pfaffenrath, V., Wolfgang, O., & Wolfgang, H. (1990). Flunarizine (10 and 20mg) I. V. versus placebo in the treatment of acute migraine attacks: A multicenter double-blind study. *Cephalagia, 10*, 77–81.

Pothmann, R. (1987). Calcium-antagonist flunarizine vs. low-dose acetylsalicylic acid in childhood migraine: A double-blind study. *Cephalalgia, 7(Suppl 6)*, 385–386.

Prensky, A. L., & Sommer, D. (1979). Diagnosis and treatment of migraine in children. *Neurology, 29*, 506–510.

Price, J. P., Clare, M. H., & Ewerhardt, R. H. (1948). Studies in low backache with persistent muscle spasm. *Archives of Physical Medicine and Rehabilitation, 29*, 703–709.

Quality Standards Subcommittee of the American Academy of Neurology. (1994). Practice parameter: The utility of neuroimaging in the evaluation of headache in patients with normal neurological examinations. *Neurology, 44*, 1353–1354.

Rapoport, A. M., & Sheftell, F. D. (1990). *Headache relief.* New York: Simon & Schuster.

Rapoport, A. M., & Sheftell, F. D. (1993). Headache associated with medication and substance withdrawal. In C. D. Tollison & R. S. Kunkel (Eds.), *Headache: Diagnosis and treatment* (pp. 227–231). Baltimore: Williams & Wilkins.

Reynolds, C. R., & Richmond, B. O. (1978). What I think and feel: A revised measure of children's manifest anxiety. *Journal of Abnormal Child Psychology, 6*, 271–280.

Richter, I. L., McGrath, P. J., Humphreys, P. J., Goodman, J. T., Firestone, P., & Keene, D. (1986). Cognitive and relaxation treatment of pediatric migraine. *Pain, 25*, 195–203.

Ross, C. K., Lavigne, J. V., Hayford, J. R., Berry, S. L., Sinacore, J. M., & Pachman, L. M. (1993). Psychological factors affecting reported pain in juvenile rheumatoid arthritis. *Journal of Pediatric Psychology, 18*, 561–573.

Rothner, A. D. (1993). Management of headaches in children and adolescents. *Journal of Pain and Symptom Management, 8*, 81–86.

Saeed, M. A., Pumariega, A. J., & Cinciripini, P. M. (1992). Psychopharmacological management of migraine in children and adolescents. *Journal of Child and Adolescent Psychopharmacology, 2*, 199–211.

Saper, J. R., Silberstein, A., Gordon, C. D., & Hamel, R. L. (1993). *Handbook of headache management: A practical guide to diagnosis and treatment of head, neck, and facial pain.* Baltimore: Williams & Wilkins.

Silberstein, S. D. (1990). Twenty questions about headaches in children and adolescents. *Headache, 30,* 716–724.

Silberstein, S. D. (1992). Intractable headache: Inpatient and outpatient treatment strategies. *Neurology, 42 (Suppl 2),* 6–10.

Sillanpaa, M. (1977). Clonidine prophylaxis of childhood migraine and other vascular headache. *Headache, 17,* 28–31.

Sillanpaa, M. (1983). Changes in the prevalence of migraine and other headaches during the first seven school years. *Headache, 23,* 15–19.

Sillanpaa, M., & Kaponen, M. (1978). Papaverine in the prophylaxis of migraine and other vascular headache in children. *Acta Paediatrica Scandanavia, 67,* 209–212.

Sills, M., Cogdon, P., & Forsythe, I. (1982). Clonidine and childhood migraine: A pilot and double-blind study. *Developmental Medicine & Child Neurology, 24,* 837–841.

Smith, J. C. (1990). *Cognitive-behavioral relaxation training: A new system of strategies for treatment and assessment.* New York: Springer.

Sorge, F., DeSimone, R., Marano, E., Nolano, M., Orefice, G., & Carrieri, P. (1988). Flunarizine in prophylaxis of childhood migraine: A double-blind, placebo-controlled, crossover study. *Cephalalgia, 8,* 1–6.

Sorge, F., & Marano, E. (1985). Flunarizine vs. placebo in childhood migraine: A double-blind study. *Cephalalgia, 5(Suppl 2),* 145–148.

Soyka, D., Taneri, Z., Oestereich, W., & Schmidt, R. (1989). Flunarizine I.V. in the acute treatment of common or classical migraine attack: A placebo-controlled double-blind trial. *Headache, 29,* 21–27.

Spielberger, C. D. (1973). *Manual for the State-Trait Anxiety Inventory for Children.* Palo Alto, CA: Consulting Psychologists Press.

Stewart, W. F., & Lipton, R. B. (1993). Migraine headache: Epidemiology and health care utilization. *Cephalalgia, 13 (Suppl 12),* 41–46.

Subcutaneous Sumatriptan International Study Group. (1991). Treatment of migraine attacks with sumatriptan. *New England Journal of Medicine, 325,* 316–321.

Sudtlovsky, A., Elkind, A. H., Ryan, R. E., Saper, J. R., Stern, M. A., & Meyer, J. H. (1987). Comparative efficacy of nadolol and propranolol in the management of migraine. *Headache, 27,* 421–426.

Wallace, R. K., & Benson, H. (1972). The physiology of meditation. *Scientific American, 226,* 84–90.

Wallace, R. K., Benson, H., & Wilson, K. (1971). A wakeful hypometabolic physiologic state. *American Journal of Physiology, 221,* 795–799.

Welch, K. M. A., Ellis, D. J., & Keenan, P. A. (1985). Successful migraine prophylaxis with naproxen sodium. *Neurology, 35,* 1304–1319.

Wilkinson, M. (1993). Headaches in children. In A. M. Rapoport & F. D. Sheftell (Eds.), *Headache: A clinician's guide to diagnosis, pathophysiology, and treatment strategies* (pp. 185–205). Los Alamitos, CA: PMA.

Williamson, D. A., Baker, J. D., & Cubic, B. A. (1993). Advances in pediatric headache research. In T. H. Ollendick & R. J. Prinz (Eds.), *Advances in clinical child psychology* (pp. 275–304). New York: Plenum Press.

Winner, P. (1994). Migraine in children. *American Council for Headache Education, 5,* 1–3.

Winner, P., Martinez, W. C., Mate, L. J., & Bello, L. E. (1994). Classification of pediatric migraine: Proposed revisions to the IHS criteria. [Summary]. *Headache, 34,* 299.

Wirt, R. D., Loeber, D., Klinedinst, J. K., & Seat, P. (1977). *Personality Inventory for Children.* Los Angeles: Western Psychological Services.

Woody, R. C., & Kearns, G. L. (1986). Amitriptyline and nortriptyline plasma concentrations in the treatment of childhood migraine. *Annals of Neurology, 20,* 432.

Ziegler, D. K., Hurwitz, A., Hassanein, R. S., Kodanaz, H. A., Preskorn, S. H., & Mason, J. (1987). Migraine prophylaxis: A comparison of propranolol and amitriptyline. *Archives of Neurology, 44,* 486–489.

CHAPTER 7

PSYCHOSOCIAL CONSEQUENCES OF EPILEPSY

Albert P. Aldenkamp, "MEER & BOSCH" EPILEPSY CENTRE, THE NETHERLANDS
Olaf G. Mulder, "MEER & BOSCH" EPILEPSY CENTRE, THE NETHERLANDS

> Epilepsy represents one of the most exquisite experiments of nature and its study may provide insight into fundamental functions of the brain. (Jasper, 1969)

This quotation from Jasper illustrates that epilepsy is often considered to be a unique opportunity to study brain-behavior relationships. The majority of the studies in this field are, however, clinical observations that do not allow such inferences. Moreover, research is complicated by methodological pitfalls, such as sample selection bias, absence of adequate control groups, controversies as to measures of psychopathology (such as using validated tests), the possible influence of various confounding variables such as the use of antiepileptic medication, and the effects of economic and social stress associated with chronic disorders in general (Hermann & Whitman, 1984). Nonetheless, the enormous body of research that has been carried out over a period of more than a century (the studies by Reynolds in 1861 and Gowers in 1885 are generally considered an important starting point) contains ample evidence to illustrate that children and adolescents with epilepsy, as a group, have more emotional and social problems than several control populations of healthy subjects. In some individuals, such problems may be more debilitating than the seizures themselves.

The topics reviewed here represent problem areas on which considerable debate has centered and will be discussed from two approaches, starting with *indirect effects of epilepsy*. Having epilepsy itself (or, in fact, any other chronic condition, such as arthritis or asthma) may have consequences that often seem severe enough to explain anything from mild depression to paranoid delusions as an understandable psychological reaction to the stress induced by living with the disorder. It would be surprising if factors such as the unpredictable and traumatic nature of the seizures, ignorance, and stigma still associated with epilepsy, or limitations of activities and aspirations resulting from having a chronic disease, did not have a considerable influence on a child's psychological status.

There are, however, also effects that are *directly* related to the epilepsy. These emotional and personality correlates of epilepsy represent more than simply an understandable psychological reaction to the emotional trauma of physical, social, or cognitive disability. That is, neurophysiological-neurochemical mechanisms, particularly those reflecting limbic system dysfunction, may be involved as well. Because the temporal lobe, and the limbic structures contained within it, are known to be important in the mediation of emotional, sexual, and social behavior, one might expect that epilepsies originating in the temporal lobe are at special risk for developing emotional and social difficulties, psychiatric disorders, and personality problems. Indeed, a high incidence of emotional disorders in persons with temporal lobe epilepsy, suggesting that psychological factors are less important determinants of these disorders than the location of the epileptogenic focus within temporal structures, has been reported since the 1950s (Gibbs & Stamps, 1953). A very large body of literature now exists concerning the etiological importance of temporal lobe dysfunction in the psychological and social difficulties of people with epilepsy.

Both types of relationships between psychosocial problems and epilepsy (direct and indirect) will be considered here. A related distinction that is often used in literature does not focus on the condition (i.e., epilepsy) itself, but on the major symptoms: the seizures. This distinction is between *ictal/peri-ictal effects* (effects observed as direct aftermaths of the ictus or seizures) and *inter-ictal consequences* (effects observed independent of the seizures). When using such classification, clinicians should keep in mind that both factors are not independent. Limbic system dysfunction may indeed be an important factor predisposing children with epilepsy to emotional and behavioral disorders, but in individual cases, the form and severity of such disorders presumably depends on an interaction with other factors, including an individual's past experience and his or her current psychological and social status (Hermann et al., 1982).

EPILEPSY

By definition, *epilepsy* is a chronic disorder, characterized by recurrent seizures. Therefore, those patients who have seizures elicited by drugs such as neuroleptics and antidepressants, or in connection with transient changes in cerebral function due to various forms of organic psychosyndromes (e.g. withdrawal from sedatives or alcohol), are not classed as epileptic patients (Dreifuss & Henriksen, 1992). Seizures are classified mainly according to the presumed site of pathology in the brain in generalized or partial (focal) seizures.

Generalized seizures are those in which the first clinical changes indicate initial involvement of both hemispheres of the brain. The ictal electroencephalographic patterns initially are bilateral and presumably reflect neuronal discharge that is widespread in both hemispheres and may be generated by structures in the brain stem. There are a number of different types of generalized seizures, but the most important are tonic-clonic seizures and absence seizures. *Tonic-clonic seizures* (formerly known as "grand mal") are characterized by a sudden loss of consciousness (in a minority, preceded by a vague warning), a sudden contraction of the muscles, a tonic state (in which cyanosis may occur), followed by clonic convulsive movements. Postictal drowsiness may occur. This seizure is the most impressive seizure type and often epilepsy is erroneously associated only with tonic-clonic seizures.

The hallmark of the *absence seizure* (formerly known as "petit mal") is a sudden onset, interruption of ongoing activities, a blank stare, and possibly a brief upward rotation of the eyes. The child may continue with his or her activities during this seizure (e.g., if the child is speaking, he or she may continue, but with slowed speech). The child cannot, however, respond to questions.

Partial (focal) seizures are those in which the first clinical and electroencephalographic changes indicate excessive activation of a limited part of one cerebral hemisphere (the epileptic focus). In general, two types of partial seizures are distinguished based on whether consciousness is impaired (Dreifuss & Henriksen, 1992). When consciousness is impaired, the seizure is classified as a *complex partial seizure*; in *simple partial seizures,* consciousness is not impaired. A form of epilepsy with complex partial seizures is *temporal lobe epilepsy*, where the seizures originate from a focus in the temporal lobe. In this type of epilepsy, the limbic system is often involved. This is related to a considerable increase of risk for emotional and social impairment.

A phenomenon in partial seizures that requires separate description is the aura. The *aura* is described as a warning signal before the seizure occurs. Recent research has demonstrated that the aura is, in fact, the part of the seizure experienced before loss of consciousness occurs.

Epidemiological studies show that epilepsy is the most common neurological problem in childhood and adolescence, usually with serious consequences for this most critical period of development. The lifetime prevalence of epilepsy (the percentage of people that suffer from or have suffered from epilepsy during some period in their lives) is 3.2 percent (Hauser et al., 1983). The yearly incidence rate varies roughly around 100 per 100,000 per year, and point prevalence rates (the percentage of people who actually suffer from the disease) is estimated to be approximately 0.75 percent of the population. This illustrates that epilepsy is a condition with a high prevalence that is, for example, 10 times higher than multiple sclerosis.

The difference between the 0.75 percent point prevalence and the 3.2 percent lifetime prevalence illustrates that, although epilepsy is a chronic disease, a large number of patients "outgrow" or are cured of their condition. In fact, the existing epidemiological data show that two subgroups exist. In the largest group, seizure remission is achieved soon after seizure onset. If the patients are evaluated 15 years after seizure onset, approximately 80 percent have been seizure-free during the preceding two years. In 42 to 47 percent, seizure remission is in fact already achieved within one year after seizure onset (Goodridge & Shorvon, 1983). In the second group (probably 10 percent of all patients with epilepsy), epilepsy is therapy-resistant and becomes a chronic refractory condition (with an average duration of 20 to 30 years). In this latter group, the possibility of social and emotional consequences is greater, and so this chapter will therefore focus on this subgroup. Incidence of epilepsy is increased considerably during childhood. In fact, the majority of the epilepsies have their onset during childhood.

DEVELOPMENTAL PROBLEMS

Although some of the epilepsy syndromes may also cause developmental problems (e.g., the West Syndrome and the Lennox-Gastaut Syndrome) (Arzimanoglou & Aicardi, 1992), there is no evidence for a *direct* relationship between seizures and social-emotional development.

Nonetheless, epilepsy with onset in early childhood may have a large *indirect* effect on development through adverse impact on parental and peer-group attitudes and the learning of social skills. Restrictions on a child's activities and life-style due to epilepsy may interfere with personality maturation and contribute to psychosocial difficulties later in life (Fenton, 1981). Parents may worry about the seizures, about the side effects of antiepileptic medication, or about possible future social handicaps (West, 1979; Ward & Bower, 1978; Suurmeijer, 1978). Parents also tend to have differential expectations of their children with epilepsy relative to their healthy children, such as more emotional problems, poorer concentration, lower academic achievement, and fewer employment opportunities (Long & Moore, 1979; Suurmeijer, 1978).

Because of such special concerns and expectations, parents may behave differently toward their children with epilepsy. However, there is considerable variation among parents and other members of the family in their reactions to a child with epilepsy, which may range from overprotection to rejection and scapegoating. Various developmental problems may occur due to such extreme reactions. Examples are low self-esteem, lack of social skills (Fenton, 1981), feelings of guilt, or the adoption of a sick role (Lechtenberg, 1984), which may have significant effects in adult life. The importance of parental expectations is emphasized in studies on so-called outgrown epilepsies. In these studies, children are studied after they are considered to be cured of their epilepsy. Most of the studies report that, although the children tend to adapt to new situations, their parents still remain worried, and new behavior patterns of the children are not immediately evaluated positively by the parents (Aldenkamp et al., 1994).

LEARNING AND EDUCATIONAL PROBLEMS

There is only one peri-ictal phenomenon showing a *direct* relation between ictal discharge and learning impairment: the *transitory cognitive impairment*. This concept followed from early observations (Gibbs et al., 1936) that, although epileptic discharge (as recorded with an electroencephalogram) will mostly result in overt clinical symptoms such as automatisms, movements, or impaired consciousness (the seizures), epileptic EEG-discharge was also found to occur without observable clinical symptoms, even in persons who are not known to suffer from epilepsy: the *subclinical* (or *masked* or *larval*) epilepsy. Some years later, Schwab (1939) disclosed the possibility of EEG-discharge, not accompanied by seizures but by transitory changes in higher cortical functions. In fact, transitory cognitive impairment was found to be a seizure with impairment of cognitive function and learning as its only symptom. It is often considered a subclinical form of the absence seizure.

Transitory cognitive impairment was studied extensively during a large time period (cf. Prechtl et al., 1965; Aarts et al., 1984). The concept has proven its value for explaining impairment of complex behavior patterns (e.g., episodic learning difficulties [Siebelink et al., 1988] and fluctuations during intelligence testing [Aldenkamp et al., 1992a]). In fact, based on the large impact of transitory cognitive impairment, some authors (Stores, 1987; Binnie, 1987) recommend the combination of EEG recording with psychological testing in any child who shows inconsistent behavior.

As with developmental processes, the *indirect* effects of epilepsy may have a far greater impact on learning. Children with epilepsy, as a group, also run a greater risk for developing learning problems. However, *learning problems* has been used as a rather ill-defined category and there is no uniformity in assessment methods. Consequently, prevalence estimates of learning problems in children with epilepsy vary widely, percentages mentioned in the literature ranging from 5 to 50 percent (Thompson, 1987). Approximately one-third receive some form of special educational support (Aldenkamp, 1983; Thompson, 1987; Aldenkamp et al., 1990).

Academic underachievement in children with epilepsy relative to their own abilities has been noted by several authors (Aldenkamp et al., 1990; Seidenberg et al., 1986). Parental attitudes and behavior may be expected to influence the child's learning behavior (Suurmeijer et al., 1978). However, specific cognitive deficits may be responsible for learning problems and underachievement, as well. Slowing on speeded tasks involving complex information processing, quick decision making, and attention and concentration difficulties are all well-established phenomena in epilepsy

(Aldenkamp et al., 1992b; Alpherts & Aldenkamp, 1990). Factors such as the localization of the epileptogenic focus, the seizure activity, and the central side effects of antiepileptic medication may underlie such cognitive deficits and thus interfere with learning processes (Vermeulen et al., 1994). Disappointing school achievement, regardless of its origin, may have a considerable impact on self-perception of the child with epilepsy, and may lead to reduced employment choices and earning potential as an adult, as will be discussed later in this chapter.

AFFECTIVE DISORDERS

Four types of affective disorders will be presented here: aggression, sexual behavior, mania, and depression. Although most of the findings that are reported come from studies on adults with epilepsy, they are also valid for childhood epilepsy and epilepsy in adolescents.

Aggression

Despite anecdotal reports in the medico-legal literature suggesting that violent events might occur as a peri-ictal phenomenon, the weight of the evidence does not support such allegations (Treiman, 1986; Treiman & Delgado-Escueta, 1983). It is extremely unusual for patients with epilepsy to behave aggressively during a seizure. Also, limbic stimulation rarely evokes anger or aggression. Aggressive behavior sometimes occurs as a post-ictal phenomenon (as a direct aftermath of a seizure) because the patient is restrained in an attempt to protect him or her. Aggressive behavior during seizures, if it occurs at all, is typically simple, stereotyped, unsustained, unplanned, and never supported by a consecutive series of purposeful acts. It is not premeditated and does not occur in response to pre-ictal provocation (Strauss, 1989). It therefore is not likely that a coordinated act of violence or aggression against others could occur as part of a seizure.

Inter-ictal aggression that has been studied in surveys of hospital-based clinics fail to reveal increased aggression in people with epilepsy (or extreme behavioral disturbances in children) in general, and temporal lobe epilepsy in particular. Surveys of penal institutions (where more violence-prone individuals might be found) in the United States and England have revealed an increased prevalence of epilepsy relative to the general population. However, prisoners with epilepsy did not commit more serious crimes or more crimes of violence compared to their nonepileptic counterparts. Prisoners with temporal lobe epilepsy did not commit more violent crimes than those having other seizure types (Hermann & Whitman, 1984).

Sexual Behavior

Peri-ictal sexual behavior may consist of somatosensory sensations in the genitalia occurring during seizures, probably due to discharges from the post central gyrus, that may be unpleasant or emotionally neutral. Sexual automatisms (i.e., mannerisms such as exhibitionism and other sexual activities that may be related to frontal seizure origin, and erotic feelings that typically indicate the involvement of temporal-limbic structures) may also occur both in adults and in children (Strauss, 1989).

Few methodologically sound studies have been carried out on inter-ictal sexual function in people with epilepsy. However, the existing data suggest that sexual dysfunction is not uncommon in epilepsy. Hyposexuality, usually in the form of a global loss of performance as well as interest in sex, is the most prominent abnormality, and appears to be specifically associated with temporal lobe epilepsy. However, presence of temporal lobe epilepsy is presumably only one of the several factors that may contribute to sexual dysfunction in epilepsy. The individual's overall mental health is an important consideration. Indeed, depressed or anxious subjects may have little interest in sex. The chronic use of antiepileptic drugs may produce alterations in sex hormone levels and thus affect sexual functioning. Adolescents with epilepsy may have limited opportunities for social interactions and subsequently sexual contacts because of their isolated position in peer groups (Hermann & Whitman, 1984; Strauss, 1989). Thus, a large number of indirect relationships exist between epilepsy and the reported problems of sexual behavior.

Euphoria, Mania, and Hypomania

Pleasurable emotions, such as feelings of euphoria or gladness, can also occur as part of a peri-ictal event,

but are extremely rare (Strauss, 1989). Periods of peri-ictal laughing are also observed. This is called *gelastic epilepsy* or *ictal laughter* (Daly & Mulder, 1957). The laughing is mostly inappropriate and is not triggered by environmental cues. The epileptic focus is predominantly found in the left temporal lobe. Ictal crying seems to be a rare phenomenon and is only described in a handful of case reports.

Also, inter-ictal reports on elation are not common (Robertson, 1992). In fact, an extensive literature search (Robertson, 1992) revealed a total of 42 cases with some form of euphoria, mania, or hypomania. In most of these cases, a bipolar illness (with manic-depressive presentation) was described. As one inspects correlations with epileptic conditions, contribution of right-sided temporal lobe epilepsy is apparent in patients who become hypomanic. Often, the mood delusions of these patients have a predominantly religious theme.

Depression and Anxiety

Peri-ictal depression—manifested in feelings of sadness, futility, and the like, and unmotivated by the context—may occur as an aura during the seizure or as a sequel to the seizure. Peri-ictal depression is fairly uncommon, occurring in about 1 percent of the patients with epilepsy, and it is associated with temporal-limbic discharges (Robertson, 1987). The duration of the depression may be brief, lasting for minutes, but unlike other ictal emotions, the mood may persist for days after the seizure. Naturally, the sequelae of such effects may lead to serious emotional complications, especially in adolescents (Robertson, 1992).

Fear is much more common as part of a seizure and is experienced as a peri-ictal phenomenon in about 3 percent of patients with epilepsy. It may also be produced by experimental electrical stimulation of limbic structures, especially the amygdala. Peri-ictal fear typically occurs with temporal lobe seizures. About 20 percent of subjects with such seizures report episodes of peri-ictal fear, which differs from the normal state in that it arises suddenly out of context and is undirected. Its duration varies from seconds to minutes, and its intensity ranges from mild anxiety to overwhelming terror.

The major inter-ictal affective disorders in epilepsy are depression and anxiety, though their exact prevalence is not known—especially in children. Relevant studies are too few to establish a specific association with specific factors (e.g., temporal lobe epilepsy) (Hermann & Whitman, 1984). Psychosocially oriented explanations have emphasized the various psychological and social stress factors associated with having seizures. Seizures are essentially unpredictable traumatic events over which the individual has little or no control. The nature of epilepsy thus may be conducive to "learned helplessness" (Seligman, 1975), and it has been suggested that this may be one way of understanding some of the inter-ictal behavioral concomitants of epilepsy, particularly the apparent high rates of anxiety and depression (Hermann, 1979).

Medical misinformation, fear of seizures, and fear of death from seizures is widespread among patients—especially in adolescents—and this may affect behavior in adverse ways. Patients have many concerns about what they think are the potentially destructive effects of epilepsy (i.e., progressive brain damage, mental deterioration, mental illness, loss of intelligence). A common approach to dealing with such fears and concerns is social and emotional withdrawal. Depression and anxiety in epilepsy may, in part, be due to such mechanisms.

PSYCHIATRIC IMPAIRMENT

A wide variety of simple and complex sensory and perceptual experiences as well as alterations in cognitive and emotional states can be elicited by temporal lobe seizures. Many of the phenomena experienced during partial seizures can also occur in psychiatric illness (e.g., hallucinations and illusions, feelings of depersonalization, or forced thinking). When occurring as peri-ictal events, they have a sudden onset and rapid resolution, and the attacks have a stereotyped quality.

There is little doubt that overall rates of inter-ictal psychopathology of any type are elevated in epilepsy relative to healthy controls. This increased tendency toward psychopathology appears to be due to presence of a chronic disorder rather than the epilepsy in itself, thus emphasizing the importance of indirect relationships between epilepsy and psychosocial problems. Comparisons with patients with other chronic disorders generally fail to reveal increased overall psychopathology rates in epilepsy. A good example is the issue of a typical "epileptic personality" that is reported frequently. Traits that have traditionally been associated with this term include excessive religiosity, mental slowness, viscosity, hyposexuality, circumstantiality, irritability, impulsivity, and mood fluctuations. However, these symptoms have never been demonstrated relative to other subjects with chronic brain-related disorders (Hermann & Whitman, 1984; Strauss, 1989).

Psychopathology, when present in epilepsy, is more likely to manifest itself as psychosis, particularly schizophrenia-like and paranoid states, than in chronically ill controls (Whitman et al., 1984). This finding might account for the observed overrepresentation of patients with epilepsy in psychiatric hospitals and the increased rates of previous psychiatric hospitalizations in epilepsy, as patients with psychotic disorders are more likely to receive treatment in inpatient psychiatric settings (Hermann & Whitman, 1984). However, as yet there are no population-based studies on the prevalence of psychosis in epilepsy that might resolve the question as to whether the combination of epilepsy and psychosis is coincidental.

Despite such uncertainties, various explanations for a causal link between epilepsy and psychosis have been advanced (see Toone, 1981). It is theorized that the repeated intrusions into consciousness of bizarre and alien seizure-related experiences and affects could have deleterious effects on a patient's mental health, and could prepare the ground for a later psychotic development (Pond, 1957). There are some data supporting this hypothesis. For example, patients with complex auras manifest more psychopathology than those with simple auras (Standage & Fenton, 1975). Patients with auras consisting of illusions, hallucinations, and complex automatisms are at increased risk for psychosis relative to other types of auras (Jensen & Larsen 1979).

PSEUDO-SEIZURES

A common psychosocial problem in epilepsy is the combination of pseudo-seizures and epileptic seizures (Aldenkamp & Mulder, 1990). Pseudo-seizures are frequently found—for example 7 to 10 percent of the patients referred to a specialized epilepsy center in the Netherlands suffer from pseudo-epileptic seizures (Aldenkamp & Mulder, 1990).

In theory, the distinction between epileptic and pseudo-epileptic seizures is evident. Epileptic seizures are the manifestation of a sudden abnormal change in brain function, accompanied by excessive electrical discharge of brain cells. Pseudo-epileptic seizures are not accompanied by abnormal paroxysmal discharges, but are symptoms of emotional disturbances (Williams et al., 1978). However, EEG-recording of the actual seizure is not always possible. In the case of the coexistence of pseudo-epileptic and epileptic seizures in the same patient, this may lead to serious diagnostic problems, as interictal EEG-registration does not rule out the possibility of pseudo-epileptic seizures in a patient with epilepsy. Consequently, these patients may be diagnosed as suffering from intractable epilepsies and might be overtreated (Ramani et al., 1980).

The definition of *pseudo-epileptic seizures* is hindered by the diversity in often conflicting terminology, such as *hysterical seizures, psychogenic seizures,* and *functional seizures.* Different models have been proposed to explain pseudo-epileptic seizures. In some studies, pseudo-seizures are seen as a symptom of internalized emotional conflicts or coping ego mechanisms to avoid unconscious conflicts. In other studies, these seizures are seen as learned behavior, mostly applied in situations that overrun the individual's stress capacity. In some cognitive-behavioristic theories, pseudo-epileptic seizures are evaluated as a form of dissociation. This may explain the observation that people with epilepsy are highly hypnotizable (Gross, 1979), as hypnosis is also as a state of dissociation.

Using *DSM-III* criteria, Stewart and associates (1982) were able to uncover several forms of psychopathology behind the pseudo-epileptic symptomatology. There was a clear tendency in their study for the combination of borderline and antisocial personality disorders for patients with pseudo-epileptic seizures. Hysteria was not a common diagnosis for the patients in this study. One must conclude that pseudo-seizures are probably a symptom of various affective and psychiatric factors that may seriously complicate the evaluation of relationships between epileptic conditions and psychosocial reactions.

SOCIOECONOMIC STATUS

Although somewhat beyond the scope of the target group (i.e., children and adolescents), the authors consider briefly the "endpoint" of several critical influences and focus on the socioeconomic status of the adolescent and young adult with epilepsy. Being able to obtain and maintain a satisfactory job and income is obviously relevant to an individual's psychosocial functioning, if only because unemployment introduces economic pressure and may reduce the opportunities for social interaction and leisure activities. Unfortunately, unemployment and underemployment of people with epilepsy are much more frequent than in the general population. According to So and Penry (1981), the unemployment rate for people with epilepsy is two times the national average in the United States. Many young adults with epilepsy experience problems finding work (Fraser, 1980, gives an estimate of 50 percent), and it is by no means uncommon that people lose their job because of seizures. Not surprisingly, people with epilepsy generally have lower than average income.

The relationship between epilepsy and lower socioeconomic status is, however, complex. Characteristics of the seizures may be such that they limit an individual's employment opportunities. Bothersome personality or behavioral characteristics may contribute to difficulties with employment. Cognitive functioning may be a significant factor in determining successful or unsuccessful employment status. Neuropsychological investigations of epilepsy have found, for example, that measures of higher cortical function predict vocational status and adequacy of psychosocial functioning (Dikmen & Morgan, 1980; Dodrill, 1980). Also, epilepsy continues to be associated with considerable stigma and ignorance, manifesting itself in various forms of social discrimination, (e.g., difficulties in obtaining a driver's license, discrimination in obtaining employment [Fraser, 1980], and difficulty in obtaining all types of insurance).

The National Commission for the Control of Epilepsy and Its Consequences (1978) has outlined the societal sanctions in greater detail. Such sanctions are conducive to social exclusion and ostracism, which may result in limited opportunities for extended social contact. Public attitudes toward epilepsy and misconceptions about this condition may go a long way in accounting for the difficulties experienced in getting employment.

SUMMARY

A very heterogeneous group of psychosocial problems is associated with epilepsy. These include, among others, personality and behavior difficulties, learning and educational problems, changed affect, and psychiatric problems. Readers must realize that this review focused on the group where such factors coincide. Fortunately, there is evidence that this group has a limited size (i.e., 10 percent of the children with epilepsy) and larger groups may not be at risk for the majority of the problems described here.

Among the factors that may increase the risk of serious emotional and social problems are the type of epilepsy, temporal lobe epilepsy being the most critical risk factor (possibly because of limbic system involvement). Also social factors that in fact are similar in other chronic conditions must be included, such as the popular misconceptions and prejudices still surrounding epilepsy.

When one examines the outcome of a development with psychosocial complications, one may find a dissatisfying socioeconomic position of the adolescent and young adult with epilepsy. Because the problems in socioeconomic position seem rather common in people with epilepsy (e.g., the average income is lower for the total group), some studies suggest that the psychosocial consequences of epilepsy may not be limited to specific groups. Several epidemiological studies have been initiated (e.g., the ERG population-based study in the Netherlands) that may produce data on this topic in the near future.

REFERENCES

Aarts, J. H. P., Binnie C. D., Smit, A. M., & Wilkins, A. J. (1984). Selective cognitive impairment during focal and generalised epileptiform EEG activity. *Brain, 107,* 293–308.

Aldenkamp, A. P. (1983). Epilepsy and learning behavior. In M. Parsonage, R. H. E. Grant, A. G. Graig, & A. A. Ward (Eds.), *Advances in epileptology* (pp. 221–229). New York: Raven Press.

Aldenkamp, A. P., Alpherts, W. C. J., Blennow, G., Elmqvist, D., Heijbel, J., Nilsson, H., Sandstedt, P., Tonnby, B., Wahlander, L., & Wosse, E. (1994). Computerized assessment of cognitive function and quality of life. In W. E. Dodson & M. R. Trimble (Eds.), *Quality of life in epilepsy*. New York: Raven Press.

Aldenkamp, A. P., Alpherts, W. C. J., Dekker, M. C. A., & Overweg, J. (1990). Neuropsychological aspects of learning disabilities in epilepsy. *Epilepsia, 31,* 9–20.

Aldenkamp, A. P., Gutter, T., & Beun, A. M. (1992). The effect of seizure activity and paroxysmal electroencephalographic discharge on cognition. *Acta Neurologica Scandinavica, 86,* 111–122.

Aldenkamp, A. P., & Mulder, O. G. (1990). Some considerations on diagnosis and treatment of pseudo-epileptic seizures in adolescents. *International Journal of Adolescent Medicine and Health, 4,* 81–91.

Aldenkamp, A. P., Vermeulen, J., Alpherts, W. C. J., Overweg, J., Van Parijs, J. A. P., & Verhoeff, N. P. L. G. (1992). Validity of computerized testing: Patient dysfunction and complaints versus measured changes. In W. E. Dodson & M. Kinsbourne (Eds.), *Assessment of cognitive function* (pp. 51–68). New York: Demos.

Alpherts, W. C. J., & Aldenkamp, A. P. (1990). Computerized neuropsychological assessment of cognitive functioning in children with epilepsy. *Epilepsia, 31,* 35–40.

Arzimanoglou, A., & Aicardi, J. (1992). The epilepsy of Sturge-Weber syndrome. *Acta Neurologica Scandinavica, 86,* 18–23.

Bear, D. M. (1979). Temporal lobe epilepsy: A syndrome of sensory-limbic hyperconnection. *Cortex, 15,* 357–384.

Binnie, C. D. (1987). Seizures, EEG discharges and cognition. In M. R. Trimble & E. H. Reynolds (Eds.), *Epilepsy, behaviour and cognitive function* (pp. 45–51). New York: John Wiley & Sons.

Daly, D., & Mulder, D. (1957). Gelastic epilepsy. *Neurology, 7,* 189–192.

Dikmen, S., & Morgan, S. F. (1980). Neuropsychological factors related to employability and occupational status in persons with epilepsy. *Journal of Nervous and Mental Disease, 168,* 236–240.

Dodrill, C. B. (1980). Interrelationships between neuropsychological data and social problems in epilepsy. In R. Canger, F. Angeleri, & J. K. Penry (Eds.), *Advances in epileptology: XIth Epilepsy International Symposium* (pp. 191–197). New York: Raven Press.

Dreifuss F. E., & Henriksen, O. (1992). Classification of epileptic seizures and the epilepsies. *Acta Neurologica Scandinavica, 86,* 8–18.

Fenton, G. W. (1981). Personality and behavioral disorders in adults with epilepsy. In E. H. Reynolds & M. R. Trimble (Eds.), *Epilepsy and psychiatry* (pp. 77–91). Edinburgh: Churchill Livingstone.

Fraser, R. T. (1980). Vocational aspects of epilepsy. In B. P. Hermann (Ed.), *A multidisciplinary handbook of epilepsy* (pp. 74–105). Springfield, IL: Charles C. Thomas.

Gibbs, F. A., & Stamps, F. W. (1953). *Epilepsy handbook*. Springfield, IL: Charles C. Thomas.

Gibbs, F. A., Lennox, W. G., & Gibbs, E. L. (1936). The electroencephalogram in diagnosis and in localization of epileptic seizures. *Archives of Neurology and Psychiatry, 36,* 1225–1235.

Goodridge, D. M. G., & Shorvon, S. D. (1983). Epileptic seizures in a population of 6000: II. Treatment and prognosis. *British Medical Journal, 287,* 645–647.

Gross, M. (1979). Hypnosis a diagnostic tool in epilepsy. In G. D. Burrows, D. R. Collison, & L. Dennerstein (Eds.), *Hypnosis.* Biomedical Press.

Hauser, W. A., Annegers, J. F., & Anderson, V. E. (1983). Epidemiology and genetics of epilepsy. In A. A. Ward, J. K. Penry, & D. Purpura (Eds.), *Epilepsy* (pp. 274–285). New York: Raven Press.

Hermann, B. F. (1979). Psychopathology in epilepsy and learned helplessness. *Medical Hypotheses, 5,* 723–729.

Hermann, B. P., Dikmen, S., Schwarz, M. S., & Karnes, W. E. (1982). Psychopathology in TLE patients with ictal fear: A quantitative investigation. *Neurology, 32,* 7–11.

Hermann, B. P., & Whitman, S. (1984). Behavioral and personality correlates of epilepsy: A review, methodological critique, and conceptual model. *Psychological Bulletin, 95,* 451–497.

Jasper, H. (1969). Neurophysiological basis of generalized epilepsies. In H. Gastaut, H. Jasper, J. Bancaud, & A. Weltregny (Eds.), *The physiopathogenesis of the epilepsies* (pp. 201–208). Springfield, IL: Charles C. Thomas.

Jensen, I., & Larsen, J. K. (1979). Psychoses in drug resistant temporal lobe epilepsy. *Journal of Neurology Neurosurgery and Psychiatry, 42,* 948–954.

Lechtenberg, R. (1984). *Epilepsy and the family.* Cambridge, MA: Harvard University Press.

Long, C. G., & Moore, J. L. (1979). Parental expectations for their epileptic children. *Journal of Child Psychology and Psychiatry, 20,* 299–312.

Pond, D. A. (1975). Psychiatric aspects of epilepsy. *Journal of the Indian Medical Profession, 3,* 1441–1451.

Prechtl, H. F. R., Boeke, P. E., & Schut, T. (1965). The electroencephalogram and performance in epileptic patients. *Neurology, 11,* 296–302.

Ramani, S. V., Quesney, L. F., Olson, D., & Gumnit, R. J. (1980). Diagnosis of hysterical seizures in Epileptic patients. *American Journal of Psychiatry, 137,* 705–709.

Robertson, M. M. (1987). Epilepsy and mood. In M. R. Trimble & E. H. Reynolds (Eds.), *Epilepsy, behaviour and cognitive function* (pp. 145–157). New York: John Wiley & Sons.

Robertson, M. M. (1992). Affect and mood in epilepsy: An overview with a focus on depression. *Acta Neurologica Scandinavica, 86,* 127–133.

Schwab, R. S. (1939). A method of measuring consciousness in petit mal epilepsy. *Journal of Nervous and Mental Disease, 89,* 690–691.

Seidenberg, M., Beck, N., Geisser, M., Giordani, B., Sackellaris, J. C., Berent, S., Dreifuss, F. E., & Boll, T. J. (1986). Academic achievement of children with epilepsy. *Epilepsia, 29,* 753–759.

Seligman, M. E. P. (1975). *Helplessness.* San Francisco: Freeman.

Siebelink, B. M., Bakker, D. J., & Binnie, C. D. (1988). Psychological effects of sub-clinical EEG discharges in children: General intelligence tests. *Epilepsy Research, 2,* 117–121.

So, E. L., & Penry, J. K. (1981). Epilepsy in adults. *Annals of Neurology, 9,* 3–16.

Standage, K. F., & Fenton, G. W. (1975). Psychiatric symptom profiles of patients with epilepsy: A controlled investigation. *Psychological Medicine, 5,* 152–160.

Stewart, R. S., Lovitt, R., & Stewart, R. M. (1982). Are hysterical seizures more than hysteria? A research diagnostic criteria, DSM-III, and psychometric analysis. *American Journal of Psychiatry, 139,* 926–929.

Stores, G. (1987). Effects on learning of "subclinical" seizure discharge. In A. P. Aldenkamp, W. C. J. Alpherts, H. Meinardi, & G. Stores (Eds), *Education and epilepsy* (pp. 14–21). Lisse/Berwyn: Swets & Zeitlinger.

Strauss, E. (1989). Ictal and interictal manifestations of emotions in epilepsy. In F. Boller & J. Grafman (Eds.), *Handbook of neuropsychology* (Vol. 3, pp. 315–344). Amsterdam: Elsevier.

Suurmeijer, T. P. B. M., Dam, A. van, & Blijham, M. (1978). Socialization of the child with epilepsy and school achievement. In H. Meinardi & J. Rowan (Eds.), *Advances in epileptology—1977.* Lisse: Swets & Zeitlinger.

Thompson, P. J. (1987). Educational attainment in children and young people with epilepsy. In J. Oxley & G. Stores (Eds.), *Epilepsy and education* (pp. 15–24). London: The Medical Tribune Group.

Toone, B. K. (1981). Psychoses of epilepsy. In E. H. Reynolds & M. R. Trimble (Eds.), *Epilepsy and psychiatry* (pp. 113–137). Edinburgh: Churchill Livingstone.

Treimann, D. M. (1986). Epilepsy and violence: Medical and legal issues. *Epilepsia, 27,* 77–104.

Treimann, D. M., & Delgado-Escueta, A. V. (1983). Violence and epilepsy: A critical review. In T. A. Pedley & B. S. Meldrum (Eds.), *Recent advances in epilepsy* (Vol. 1, pp. 179–209). London: Churchill Livingstone.

Vermeulen, J., Kortstee, S. W. A. T., Alpherts, W. C. J., & Aldenkamp, A. P. (1994). Cognitive performance in learning disabled children with and without epilepsy. *Seizure, 3,* 13–21.

Ward, F., & Bower, B. D. (1978). A study of certain social aspects of epilepsy in childhood. *Developmental Medicine and Child Neurology, 39,* 1–50.

Waxman, S. G., & Geschwind, N. (1975). The interictal behavior syndrome of temporal lobe epilepsy. *Archives of General Psychiatry, 32,* 1580–1588.

West, P. (1979). An investigation into the social construction and consequences of the label epilepsy. *Sociological Review, 27,* 719–741.

Whitman, S., Hermann, B. P., & Gordon, A. (1984). Psychopathology in epilepsy: How great is the risk? *Biological Psychiatry, 19,* 213–236.

Williams, D. T., Spiegel, H., & Mostofsky, D. I. (1978). Neurogenic and hysterical seizures in children and adolescents: Differential diagnostic and therapeutic considerations. *American Journal of Psychiatry, 135,* 82–86.

CHAPTER 8

BURN INJURIES

Kenneth J. Tarnowski, FLORIDA GULF COAST UNIVERSITY
Ronald T. Brown, EMORY UNIVERSITY SCHOOL OF MEDICINE

This chapter provides an overview of pediatric burn epidemiology, medical management, acute psychosocial problems and treatment considerations, long-term sequelae, and prevention strategies. The purpose of the chapter is to acquaint readers with medical and surgical aspects of pediatric burns and to highlight typical points of psychological interface with this population from the time of injury through extended follow-up. The following presentation is based, in part, on Tarnowski (1994a, 1994b,) and Tarnowski and Brown (in press a).

EPIDEMIOLOGY

In the United States, approximately two million people sustain burn injuries each year (American Burn Association, 1984; Silverstein & Lack, 1987). Injuries result in hospitalization for approximately 70,000 individuals (American Burn Association, 1984; Frank, Berry, Wachtel, & Johnson, 1987), about 50 percent of whom are children and adolescents. Of hospitalized burn patients, 38 percent are less than 15 years of age (Barrow & Herndon, 1990).

The fatality rate for thermal injuries is 3.9 per 100,000 (National Safety Council, 1979), and 1,400 of these deaths involve children. Two-thirds of burn fatality victims are less than 15 years old, with a 2:1 male to female ratio (U.S. Fire Administration, 1978).

Fire and burn injuries are the third leading cause of death for youth to age 19 and second to motor vehicle accidents for young children (ages 1 to 4 years) (Guyer & Gallagher, 1985). House fires are responsible for the majority (84 percent) of burn-related pediatric mortality. However, mortality is largely attributable to smoke inhalation and is not a direct result of burn insult.

Victims frequently survive massive burns (e.g., more than 80 percent total body surface area [TBSA]). Advances in medical and surgical care, however, have enhanced the survival rate for burn victims (Fratianne & Brandt, 1994). Approximately 50 percent of patients with more than 70 percent TBSA currently survive such injuries (Burn Injury Reporting System, 1986). Concurrent with the impressive advances in medical care has been a marked increase in the number of specialized burn care facilities, including those subspecializing in pediatric care (1,800 beds in the burn units of 146 U.S. hospitals).

Burn injuries are among the most serious of all human injuries (McLoughlin & McGuire, 1990) and account for more hospitalization days than any other type of injury. McLoughlin and McGuire (1990) estimated that in 1985 alone, pediatric burn mortality and morbidity resulted in the loss of 101,000 life years, with a societal cost exceeding 3.5 billion dollars.

Developmental Aspects

In general, the manner in which children sustain burn injuries varies as a function of their developmental levels, (McLoughlin & Crawford, 1985). Most children (80 percent) who suffer a burn injury usually incur the injury as a result of their own behavior (Carvajal, 1990), and the majority of pediatric victims (more than 50 percent) are less than five years of age.

Infants often sustain injury (75 to 80 percent of cases) due to scalding from excessively hot bath water temperature or pullover liquid spills (El-Muhtaseb, Qaryoute, & Ragheb, 1984; Libber & Stayton, 1984). Expectedly, more than 90 percent of the burn injuries that children sustain from birth to age 2 occur indoors. Toddlers are at increased risk for liquid and food spills and hot tap water scalds. As development progresses, children are more likely to incur injuries during play and experimentation with matches, lighters, stoves, and microwaves than from spills and scalds. A common misperception is that the majority of severe pediatric burns are due to flame injuries. Although flame burns frequently prove to be lethal, they are, in fact, relatively infrequent. Such injuries account for approximately 20 percent of pediatric hospitalizations but 80 percent of the mortality (Breslin, 1975). On the other hand, scalds account for about 50 percent of the cases and 20 percent of the fatalities.

During adolescence, a shift occurs whereby 60 percent of burn injuries occur outdoors and the minority (20 percent) of burns are scalds (Green, 1984). Older children and adolescents often sustain injury by experimenting with dangerous flammables (gasoline) or high-voltage electrical sources (McLoughlin Joseph, & Crawford, 1976). Consistent with findings for other forms of pediatric injury (Rosen & Peterson, 1990), data indicate a gender discrepancy that increases as a function of age: Older adolescents present with an approximate male to female ratio of 4:1 (Clark & Lerner, 1978). Burns from fireworks (McCauley et al., 1991) and those associated with the use of common household devices, including hair dryers (Prescott, 1990) and microwaves (Hibbard & Blevins, 1988), also comprise a subset of serious burns. Although estimates vary widely, abuse-related burns account for 4 to 2 percent of all admissions to pediatric burn unit admissions (Deitch & Staats, 1982; Stone, Rinaldo, Humphrey, & Brown, 1970).

OVERVIEW OF BURN INJURIES

Burn injuries are described in terms of percentage of TBSA affected and burn type (degree). Percentage TBSA is calculated using standard body diagrams that display dorsal and ventral body aspects fractionated into discrete areas of known percentage body surface area (Lund & Browder, 1944). Burns are categorized as thermal, radiation, chemical, or electrical.

Heat intensity and duration of skin contact determine the extent and depth of skin damage. *First-degree* burns are those in which injury involves only the epidermis (comprised of several layers of epidermal cells). *Second-degree* or partial-thickness burns involve damage to the dermis (a vascular plexus consisting of arterioles, venules, and capillaries). Epidermal appendages (sweat glands, sebaceous glands, and hair follicles) are present in the dermis, as are nerve endings and connecting tissue. The subcutaneous fascia, muscle, and bone lie below this structural foundation. *Third-degree* burns, also known as full-thickness burns, are massive injuries that involve several layers of skin and typically compromise subcutaneous tissue and peripheral nerve tracts. According to American Burn Association classification criteria (American Burn Association, 1984), burns can be minor, moderate, or severe.

Treatment

Treatment of burn patients consists of three overlapping phases: emergency period, acute phase, and rehabilitation phase (Miller, Elliott, Funk, & Pruitt, 1988; Wernick, 1983). Articles by Dyer and Roberts (1990) and Fratianne and Brandt (1994) provide the basis for the following discussion.

At the scene of a burn injury, emergency treatment entails removing the source of heat, ensuring a clear airway, and assessing respiratory, circulatory, and shock status. Cardiopulmonary resuscitation can be required. Upon arrival to the hospital, clinicians obtain an account of the injury and institute efforts to stabilize respiration. A bronchoscopic evaluation may be necessary to assess inflammation. Cases involving severe inhalation injuries require placement of endotracheal tubes. Burns cause diffusion of intravascular fluid into extravascular fluid (Demling, 1987). Several fluid resuscitation formulas are available that correct homeostatic imbalances, including those involving electrolyte imbalance and decreased blood volume. Emergency personnel infuse fluids via a central line placed in a major vein and evaluate bladder output with a Foley catheter.

During the first two days following injury, a "fluid shift," associated with marked diuresis and increased cardiac output occurs. Possible complications at this time include pulmonary edema (infiltration of the lung with fluid) and congestive heart failure (Rubin, Mani, & Hiebert, 1986). Continuous monitoring of vital signs, cardiac functions, temperature, and intravenous (IV) fluid titration is necessary. Gastrointestinal (GI) complications may result as blood moves away from the GI tract. Patients who are unconscious and those with TBSAs over 20 percent may need low-suction nasogastric tubes to decrease GI distention.

Once a patient has stabilized, treatment shifts to the burn wound itself. The acute phase of treatment is often the most painful and traumatic because patients must repeatedly endure a variety of highly aversive procedures (e.g., dressing changes, wound cleansing, grafting). A central concern during this phase of treatment is the possibility of serious infection due to accelerated bacterial invasion. Within a few days of injury, untreated burn wounds contain gram-positive and gram-negative organisms. Burn sepsis (infection) looms as a major threat to patient survival. Clinical signs include changes in mental status, hypo- or hyperthermia, GI disturbances, degradation of grafted burn sites, and conversion of partial-thickness to full-thickness wounds. Treatment involves aggressive parenteral administration of antibiotics, autografting (transplanting healthy skin from undamaged areas to the site of injury), and comprehensive nutritional support. If such interventions fail, sepsis is most often fatal.

Eschar (burned tissue) combines with edema to produce circulatory compromise. For this reason, it is important that clinicians surgically remove eschar as soon as feasible. Escharotomy is often necessary to treat circumferential burns (injuries that affect an entire limb) of the hands, arms, fingers, neck, trunk, and feet. Patients undergo debridement procedures one to two times a day. This procedure involves vigorous removal of necrotic (devitalized) tissue and typically occurs in a hydrotherapy tub that contains hypochlorite solution. Patients undergo minor debridement upon admission, and clinical staff take great care to maintain the protective surface covering of the blisters. Topical antimicrobials, applied to the wounds, inhibit infection. Daily debridement and application of topical dressings are typically the most painful procedures. Serious patient management problems often occur as patients repeatedly endure these procedures over extended periods of time.

Partial-thickness wounds heal in about two to four weeks, and full-thickness injuries heal in three to five weeks. Physiological dressings comprised of transplanted skin from cadavers (heterografts), animals (zenografts) or artificial preparations are often useful during this phase of treatment. The body will ultimately reject these dressings, but they temporarily serve as a barrier to decrease heat and fluid loss. Autografting procedures are necessary for severe injuries, and this most frequently occurs in phases. Pressure dressings and garments maintain physiological integrity of autografts.

During the rehabilitation phase, physical therapy, nutritional, medical, surgical, and self-care procedures continue (e.g., wearing pressure garments, movement exercises). Plastic and reconstructive surgeries often entail repeated hospitalizations.

PSYCHOLOGICAL ASPECTS

Burns share several characteristics of chronic disease (e.g., compromised functioning, protracted course of treatment) (Hobbs & Perrin, 1985) and often result in long-term physical and psychosocial morbidity (Patterson et al., 1993; Tarnowski, 1994a; Tarnowski, Rasnake, Gavaghan-Jones, & Smith, 1991). Early reports regarding psychological functioning of pediatric burn victims consisted of uncontrolled case reports (Long & Cope, 1961; Watson & Johnson, 1958; Woodward, 1959), with conclusions about patient adjustment based largely on anecdotal data. To a large extent, the psychological aspects of pediatric burns has been a neglected topic. Unfortunately, with few exceptions, the relative dearth of basic and applied interest in this population has continued to the present. For example, a 1987 review of the pediatric burn behavioral assessment and treatment literature revealed only 14 investigations (Tarnowski, Rasnake, & Drabman, 1987). The appearance of a specialty journal,

Journal of Burn Care and Rehabilitation, has focused increased attention on the plight of burn survivors. To date, researchers have focused primarily on adult patients. However, a comprehensive text on behavioral aspects of pediatric burns recently appeared (Tarnowski, 1994a) and hopefully will serve to increase clinical and research efforts in the area.

In several ways, burns are unique in the challenges they pose to children and families and offer novel opportunities to study coping and adaptation. As noted by Tarnowski (1994b), burn injuries and their causes often share characteristics of acute disorders as well as those of chronic illness, simultaneously affect multiple family members, and can result in losses not usually associated with other forms of injury (e.g., parents, siblings, home, possessions, pets). Burn injuries, often associated with premorbid parent/child psychopathology, can also result in characteristic forms of physical disfigurement and psychiatric sequelae that are disproportionate to the extent of injury. Burns also result in extended periods of severe pain that may be recalcitrant to pharmacologic intervention and present challenges that often exceed the coping capabilities of children, families, and staff (Tarnowski, 1994a,1994b).

Psychological variables are integral to treatment planning and provision of comprehensive care to pediatric burn survivors and their families. To acquaint readers with the range of these issues, we provide a brief overview of psychological considerations involved in consultation, rehabilitation, and prevention.

Onset

Behavioral factors often contribute to injury occurrence. A subset of injuries are due to child abuse. Often, such injuries consist of immersion burns, which occur as part of attempts to "quiet" or "punish" infants and toddlers (Caniano, Beaver, & Boles, 1986; Purdue, Hunt, & Prescott, 1988).

Neglect is also an important consideration. The topography of neglect can vary widely (e.g., lapse in parental supervision, failure to make matches and lighters inaccessible to children, compromised caregiver judgment). However, an entry of "parental neglect" in patients' charts does little to enhance one's understanding of environmental variables, setting events, and psychological processes involved in injury occurrence. For example, children may sustain injury during a lapse in caregiver supervision. However, a detailed analysis may reveal that child developmental variables (e.g., curiosity) combined with underestimation of a child's developmental competencies (e.g., motor skills) interact with environmental variables (e.g., availability of potentially dangerous items), setting factors (e.g., variables associated with economically disadvantaged living conditions), and psychological states (e.g., negative affect) to increase risk for accidental injury. In sum, identification of neglect is a subjective process, and there appears to be marked bias in the labeling of injuries that occur under similar circumstances as *neglect* in one instance and *accidental* in another.

When considering the circumstances under which children receive injuries, the interaction between specific environmental factors and family variables becomes a central concern (Tarnowski & Brown, in press b). For example, the probability of sustaining a burn injury increases as one descends in socioeconomic status (SES) (Center for Disease Control, 1987). Economically disadvantaged families may not be able to secure adequate housing. Substandard living quarters may pose specific risks of injury (e.g., crowding, faulty electrical systems). In other instances, a lack of basic resources may induce caregivers to use hazardous means to meet basic needs (e.g., heating homes with makeshift stoves).

Low SES populations also appear to be at heightened risk for specific psychological disorders (e.g., depression) (Belle, 1990). The symptoms of such disorders may contribute to risk of injury. For example, depressive symptoms result in a decreased ability to maintain the vigilance needed to prevent child injuries (Davidson, Hughes, & O'Connor, 1988). Other setting events (e.g., recent geographic move, children with acute injuries) may also function to increase injury risk (Knudson-Cooper & Leuchtag, 1982; Wilson, Buckland, & Sully, 1988).

Behavioral variables may also contribute to injury occurrence in other ways. For example, a significant subset of children with severe burn injuries present with marked premorbid psychopathology (Tarnowski et al., 1991). Children with certain symptoms (e.g., attention problems, impulsivity) present unique supervision challenges and may be more likely to respond in ways (high risk taking) that increase risk of injury. Although infrequent, a subset of youth also receive injuries or die by self-immolation (Hammond, Ward, & Pereira, 1988).

A subset of burns (e.g., nonintentional immersion burns) relate to parental nonadherence. Although frequently advised to reduce hot water tank temperatures, to safeguard electrical outlets and flammables, to purchase fire-retardant sleepwear, many parents fail to engage in such preventive measures (Cole, Herndon, Desai, & Abston, 1986; MacKay & Rothman, 1982; McLoughlin & McGuire, 1990).

Acute Phase

Developmental Factors

Children's capacity to cope with any chronic illness or severe injury is, in large part, a function of their cognitive and emotional development. An understanding of such factors is critical to providing effective psychological consultation to staff and families. Knowledge of and sensitivity to developmental variables are central in shaping intervention strategies. Expectedly, the stressors associated with illness may cause children to regress cognitively and emotionally, and clinicians must consider such variables during all phases of treatment.

Bibace and Walsh (1980) invoked Piaget's theory of cognitive development in their conceptualization of children's understanding of illness. During the sensorimotor stage, infants understand their environment largely through manipulation and activity. During this period, injured children react adversely to the highly restrictive hospital environment, and frequent contact with caregivers is critical to their well-being. The prelogical thinking of children 2 to 7 years old involves phenomenism (attribution of the illness/injury to a remote cause) and contagion (attribution of an illness/injury to a proximate object). Preschool children may attribute distress to events such as separation from family rather than to their actual injuries. Concrete, logical explanations of illness (7 to 11 years) center on contamination (i.e., person, object, or bad behavior) and internalization (looking for the source of the illness inside the body). Youth in this phase may see discomfort as resulting from caregivers or their own negative behavior. Logical thinking that develops after 12 years of age, entails physiological cause and effect relationships (Bibace & Walsh,

1980). Adolescents, relative to younger children, have a more realistic understanding of the nature of burn injuries, scar development, need for grafting, and specific rehabilitation goals.

Premorbid Psychopathology

There appears to be several premorbid risk factors associated with children who sustain burn injury. Included are demographic and environmental variables as well as the general psychological stability of children and their families (Miller et al., 1988). Evidence supports the existence of marked premorbid emotional and behavioral disturbances, including aggression, overactivity, history of prior accidents, and general behavioral and emotional handicaps (Borland, 1967; Libber & Stayton, 1984; Long & Cope, 1961; Tarnowski, Rasnake, Linscheid, & Mulick, 1989a). Other reports suggest high rates of family dysfunction and marital discord (Kaslow, Koon-Scott, & Dingle, 1994) as well as environmental stressors (Knudson-Cooper & Leuchtag, 1982; Libber & Stayton, 1984) among the families of pediatric burn victims.

Assessment of child and family premorbid psychopathology has proven to be very challenging (Tarnowski et al., 1991). Although there exist several methodologic problems associated with identification of premorbid competence, such an assessment is key to the differentiating acute reactions and long-term psychological sequelae that are unique to the injury versus those responses associated with preexisting conditions. Such data may also contribute to development of prevention strategies.

Mental Status

Burn injuries frequently produce central nervous system (CNS) effects, and for this reason continued evaluation of mental status during the acute phase of the injury is important. CNS effects include carbon monoxide inhalation, other hypoxic or anoxic conditions, electrical injury and related cardiac dysrhythmias, generalized burn encephalopathies, burn psychosis, and intensive care unit (ICU) syndrome (Brown, Dingle, & Koon-Scott, 1994; Tarnowski, Rasnake, Linscheid, & Mulick, 1989b). Furthermore, alterations in mental status may result from infections and metabolic complications (Brown et al., 1994).

Burn psychosis may also occur during the initial phase of hospitalization but typically dissipates within several days. Symptoms of burn psychosis include delirium, disorientation, impairments in memory and judgment, and hallucinations or delusions. Burn psychosis likely results from CNS effects and sleep and sensory deprivation. Consequently, management of burn psychosis includes correcting electrolyte imbalances and continued orientation of children by the use of calendars, clocks, windows with outside views, and familiar staff.

Pain

Routh and Sanfilippo (1991) suggested that burns are one of the most painful pediatric injuries. Thermal sources can differentially stimulate unmyelinated C-nerve fibers and open the pain "gate," thereby increasing pain sensitivity of the skin. In addition to the pain of the original injury, pain and stress often accompany some of the treatment procedures (e.g., hydrotherapy and dressing changes).

Pain behavior in children varies as a function of the child's developmental level. Infants and toddlers are not able to distinguish pain with negative affective states, but older children are able to describe the location, intensity, duration, and sensation of pain (Tarnowski & Brown, in press c). Personnel who are familiar with developmental issues will be of significant importance to burn unit staff in the assessment and treatment of pain. Successful management of pain requires a team effort and early agreement regarding appropriate strategies and goals for children and adolescents. Recent research has indicated that involvement of a child's family in the treatment program increases adherence to the pain management program (Kazak & Nachman, 1991; Sharpe, Brown, Thompson, & Eckman, in press).

Behavioral, cognitive, and pharmacologic approaches have been the modalities of choice on pediatric burn units (Bush & Maron, 1994). Certain widely-researched techniques have demonstrated efficacy for the management of pain during stressful procedures. These techniques include relaxation, imagery, modeling, contingency management, distraction, and hypnotherapy (Tarnowski & Brown, in press c). According to the stress inoculation model (Wernick, 1983), these techniques are employed concurrently, although few research studies are available that assess their efficacy (Elliott & Olson, 1983). The

scant studies that are available are lacking in methodologic rigor, which includes absence of control groups and failure to employ physiologic measurements (Tarnowski & Brown, in press b).

Pharmacotherapy is typically the treatment of choice in the management of pain during the acute phase (McGrath, 1991; Tarnowski & Brown, in press b). Pain management initially involves use of narcotics, at times accompanied by psychotropic medications, including benzodiazepines, neuroleptics, and tricyclic antidepressants for synergy (McGrath, 1991). After acute pain has come under control, antipyretics, which have demonstrated efficacy regarding the maintenance of pain management, may be of assistance (McGrath, 1991). Children are frequently reluctant to request pain medications, fearing intramuscular injections. For this reason, initial pain control is typically intravenous, followed by oral administration once healing has begun.

Patient-controlled analgesia (PCA) is an effective alternative to as needed (prn) and intramuscular injections (Bush & Maron, 1994). Gaukroger, Chapman, and Davey (1991) found that PCA resulted in superior analgesia and that the children in their study benefited from an increased sense of control over pain. Nursing personnel strongly favored PCA because it reduced their workload and resulted in less interruption of the children's sleep. Moreover, excess sedation is not a likely result of PCA (Gaukroger et al., 1991). Although preliminary research has suggested the efficacy of PCA, further research efforts are necessary to validate their clinical utility.

Despite availability of appropriate pain medication, pediatric burn patients frequently obtain inadequate amounts of medication (McGrath, 1991). By way of explanation, Eland and Anderson (1977) noted that this may result from the misconceptions that children do not experience the same pain intensity as adults, that they are at greater risk for addiction and respiratory depression, and that they are unable to convey their pain. A consensus of the clinical and research literature is that adequate management of pain in children must include both pharmacotherapy and nonsomatic forms of therapy (Bush & Maron, 1994). For this reason, medical personnel must receive adequate information regarding the limitations of psychologically based interventions for managing pain.

Sleep Disturbances and Nutritional Intake

Because burns frequently occur under life-threatening circumstances, recent evidence suggests that children may exhibit symptoms associated with post-traumatic stress disorder (PTSD), particularly during the acute phase of treatment (Tarnowski et al., 1991). Symptoms may include dysthymia, anxiety, guilt, sleep disturbances, and nightmares (Noyes, Andreasen, & Hartford, 1971). Unfortunately, there is a dearth of documented intervention studies in this area. Roberts and Gordon (1979) instituted a response-prevention procedure with a 5-year-old girl who evidenced 10 to 20 nightmares a night after discharge. Her mother received instructions on the use of a hierarchy of pictorially presented, fire-related stimuli. Although fearful responses to fire-related stimuli ceased, criticisms of the study include the change of criteria used to define target behaviors and lack of reliability data (Tarnowski et al., 1987). Although behavioral techniques show some promise for the treatment of PTSD, endorsement of these therapies for clinical use awaits further empirical support.

A crucial component of treatment during the acute phase involves maintenance of high fluid and caloric intake. Tube feedings are often necessary due to children's frequent refusals of food and inadequate dietary intake. Use of contingency management and behavioral contracting are effective for enhancing food intake (Miller et al., 1988; Simons et al., 1978; Zide & Pardoe, 1976). Children also need to learn that if they do not consume their required total daily calories orally, tube feeding will be necessary. Miller and colleagues (1988) recommended that children receive as many food options as possible, with small meals offered throughout the day. Furthermore, because many burn injuries involve the arms, face, and hands, children may find their capacities to eat seriously compromised (Miller et al., 1988). Occupational therapy may be useful for assisting children with adaptive devices for self-feeding.

Compliance

During the acute and rehabilitative phases of burn injuries, children typically receive occupational and physical therapies to prevent scar contractures and loss of range of motion. Such therapies frequently include lengthening exercises and the use of Jobst garments, which apply light pressure to a newly healed area. Consistent with other pediatric chronic illnesses, lack of compliance with treatment demands is frequent and may impede optimal recovery. Operant techniques and token economy systems are effective at encouraging children to wear pressure garments, use splints, and perform therapeutic exercises (Tarnowski et al., 1987). Because parents frequently get involved in the treatment regimens of their children, problems with compliance must target parents as well as children.

Body Image

Earlier studies regarding adaptation and disfigurement have suggested significant problems with social adjustment and peer relationships (Molinaro, 1978; Woodward, 1959). Furthermore, for youths with burned injures, problems with peer relationships intensify during adolescence due to increased concern with body image and peer conformity at this developmental stage (Sawyer, Minde, & Zuker, 1982). Some earlier studies have suggested reduced maladjustment as a function of time since burn injury (Goldberg, 1974; Martin, 1970; Woodward, 1959). However, Sawyer and associates (1982) provided support for ongoing psychological evaluation of youth throughout all phases of rehabilitation. Such ongoing consultation addresses the possibility of adjustment difficulties that may not surface for months or even years following injury.

Unfortunately the aforementioned studies have methodological concerns, including small sample sizes, failure to consider children and adults separately, and inclusion of inappropriate statistical analyses (Tarnowski & Brown, in press b). Finally, Pruzinsky and Doctor (1994) conceded that prediction of a child's image and sense of competence may have limited usefulness because children differ in terms of the emphasis they place on appearance.

Sensitive preparation of and truthful discussion with children and adolescents who have disfigurements is imperative. It is necessary for a member from health care teams to assist with appropriate coping strategies and accompany children when they first encounter social situations (Brown et al., 1994). Parents are instrumental in children's body image development, and they, along with other family members, will influence a child's adaptation to the burn injury (Pruzinsky & Doctor, 1994). Use of cognitive-behavioral therapies may also assist in adjustment, with the goal of replacing maladaptive cognitions with more adaptive ones, thereby changing behavioral patterns (Pruzinsky & Doctor, 1994).

Self-Excoriation

One problem frequently encountered on burn units is intense itching, which typically begins when burn surfaces begin to heal. Younger children are at particular risk for impeding the healing process by self-abrading tissue. Use of medication and wrappings applied to the hands and legs have shown limited success for a toddler (St. Lawrence & Drabman, 1983). However, in one study with a toddler burn victim, a response-interruption device, which fits over the waist, eliminated the self-inflicted abrasions yet permitted the toddler to engage in other developmentally appropriate movements (St. Lawrence & Drabman, 1983).

Behavioral Problems

When children begin to adjust to the environment of the burn unit and learn hospital rules, the staff frequently report disruptive behavioral problems (Tarnowski et al., 1987). These externalizing behaviors may correspond to the learned helplessness phenomenon observed in studies of laboratory animals (Routh & Sanfilippo, 1991). In short, behavioral problems increase in response to procedures, such as debridement and hydrotherapy, that are aversive and that children perceive to be random. Such behaviors are a manifestation of a child's attempt to regain control of an environment characterized by dependency on medical personnel (Kavanaugh, 1983; Simons et al., 1978).

Due to the hypothesized origins of these behavioral problems, Tarnowski and colleagues (1987) recommended that hospital environments be predictable and conducive to clear expectations as to what will occur and when. In one study, children were placed in an environment with a great deal of predictability and maximum control was accorded depending on the developmental level of the child. In this situation, children reported less depression, anxiety, hostility, and stress analgesia than controls who did not participate in the program (Kavanaugh, 1983).

Family Coping

Children who evidence the most positive adjustment to their burn injuries tend to come from families who have strong social support networks and realistic appraisals of their child's medical condition and the rehabilitative process (Kaslow et al., 1994). This finding is consistent with the literature of other pediatric chronic illness groups. Furthermore, adjusted families tend to be cohesive, able to communicate effectively, and support age-appropriate independence.

In contrast, children who evidence maladaptive patterns of adjustment and coping frequently come from more dysfunctional families. These families, characterized by enmeshment and overprotectiveness, tend to support passive or dependent stances in their children. Other important predictors of a child's and family's positive adjustment include absence of premorbid psychopathology (Kaslow et al., 1994), increased time since injury (Tarnowski et al., 1991), and burn severity (Byrne et al., 1986; Tarnowski et al., 1991).

Given the many stressors associated with procedures during hospitalization, parents and other family members may be significant sources of support to children. For this reason, family involvement is important in both the decisions that medical personnel and families must make regarding treatment as well as protocols they must follow (Gwyther & Smith, 1980). A recent study demonstrated an association between children's coping with pain and their parents' coping (Sharpe et al., in press). Thus, family involvement in pain management and other stressful procedures during hospitalization will likely attenuate difficulties regarding transition from a hospital to a home, where family members must assume the major responsibility for care (Brown et al., 1994).

Rehabilitation Phase

The rehabilitative phase often poses challenging compliance demands and may represent the critical point at which children and their families must face the reality that recovery is not yet complete. It is during this time that children must wear customized elastic pressure garments, receive physical therapy, and endure repeated hospitalizations for reconstructive surgeries and release of contractures. Body image, coping, and adherence with treatment procedures are critical matters as children make the transition from hospital to school environment.

The clinical literature cites several adjustment problems, including difficulties with self-esteem, dysfunctional peer relationships, coping with disfigurement, and increased family stressors (Brown et al., 1994; Tarnowski & Brown, in press b, in press c). However, Tarnowski and Brown (in press b) advised caution regarding acceptance of these clinical observations and suggested that a complex of multitudinous factors, including child and family resource variables and severity of injury, likely mediate adjustment. Empirical findings indicate that the majority of children do not exhibit severe psychopathology at follow-up. Thus, research that will likely prove fruitful must address resistance and risk factors to predict children's adaptations to burn injuries (Tarnowski & Brown, 1994c; Wallander & Varni, 1992).

Finally, a formidable task during the rehabilitation of pediatric burn victims is their return to school. There is a dearth of research in the area of school reentry after a chronic illness, particular for pediatric burn survivors. Sexson and Madan-Swain (1993) provided recommendations for a reentry plan for teachers and offered recommendations for preparation of a child's class. Moreover, they advised that a member of the health-care team consult with school personnel during the rehabilitative phase and beyond until the injured child has evidenced good adjustment.

Finally, Blakeney (1994) suggested that health care teams tailor plans for each child in accordance with individual developmental level, extent of physical impairment, visibility of scars, and premorbid functioning. The quality of life of these youngsters will depend greatly on intervention programs that target school reintegration with follow-up evaluations. Such interventions will not just benefit burn-injured youth but will help children with other chronic illnesses as well.

PREVENTION

Recently, there has been increased interest in burn prevention research. The impetus for such research has been that burn injuries are a leading cause of death for children, notwithstanding the resultant emotional hardships such injuries pose for families as well as the economic burden placed on the health care system (McLoughlin & McGuire, 1990). Successful intervention efforts have focused on prevention of scald burns via use of antiscald devices, education, and home visits to monitor water temperature (Webne, Kaplan, & Shaw, 1989); prevention of hair dryer burns by cautioning pediatricians and parents regarding use of dryers to prevent diaper rash (Deans, Slater, & Goldfarb, 1990); careful supervision of toddlers during busy mealtimes (Schubert, Arenholz, & Solem, 1990); and development of special wall cover designs to prevent child access to electrical sockets (Baker & Chiavello, 1989).

Although education of parents remains an essential component of prevention activities, some promising prevention efforts have focused on children. Recently, some investigators have developed a series of programs to teach children fire-emergency skills that include safe escape and assistance seeking (Jones & Zaharopoulos, 1994; Varas, Carbone, & Hammond, 1988; Wade, Purdue, Hunt, & Childers, 1990). Such programs show particular promise in both the prevention of fires and burns, although additional data are necessary concerning efficacy and cost effectiveness.

Finally, several premorbid factors that designate children at risk for burn injuries include demographics, with lower SES children being at particular risk; physiologic factors; and psychosocial parameters (Tarnowski & Brown, in press b; Tarnowski et al., 1987, Tarnowski et al., 1991). A greater understanding of behavioral competencies as well as premorbid adjustment difficulties to define at risk-children and their families remains an important research goal in the prevention of burn injuries. No doubt, identification of at-risk children and their families who will benefit from specific types of prevention programs constitutes a crucial research component of future prevention activities.

CONCLUSIONS

Burns often cause severe life-threatening injuries that frequently result in serious acute and long-term psychosocial sequelae in addition to permanent physical disfigurement and disability. Thermal injuries share characteristics of acute injuries as well as those found in a variety of chronic illnesses. Recent medical and surgical advances have dramatically increased the survival rate for pediatric burn victims. Unfortunately, development of the psychological database has not paralleled progress in the medical/surgery areas. Research is necessary to address a variety of unanswered questions concerning child and family coping and adjustment from the time of injury through rehabilitation, with increased attention to prevention issues.

Data indicate that burn injuries place severe demands on the coping resources of patients, families, and staff. During the acute phase, children and families often present with multiple problems that require sophisticated and comprehensive intervention strategies. In general, consultants will need to have expertise in evaluation and treatment of acute CNS dysfunction, pain, eating disorders, family coping, abuse, body image problems, procedural adherence, disruptive behavior, affective disturbance, and school and community reentry consultation issues. A detailed knowledge of developmental psychopathology will be necessary to estimate child and family levels of premorbid psychological competence. Finally, given that data suggest that most pediatric burn injuries are avoidable, prevention research is a priority for future work.

REFERENCES

American Burn Association. (1984). Guidelines for service standards and severity classifications in the treatment of burn injuries. *Bulletin of the American College of Surgeons, 69,* 24–28.

Baker, M. D., & Chiaviello, C. (1989). Household electrical injuries in children: Epidemiology and identification of avoidable hazards. *American Journal of Diseases of Children, 143,* 59–62.

Barrow, R. E., & Herndon, D. N. (1990). Incidence of mortality in boys and girls after severe thermal burns. *Surgery, Gynecology, and Obstetrics, 170,* 295–298.

Belle, D. (1990). Poverty and women's mental health. *American Psychologist, 45,* 385–389.

Bibace, R., & Walsh, M. E. (1980). Development of children's concepts of illness. *Pediatrics, 66,* 912–917.

Blakeney, P. (1994). School reintegration. In K. J. Tarnowski (Ed.), *Behavioral aspects of pediatric burns* (pp. 217–241). New York: Plenum.

Borland, B. L. (1967). Prevention of childhood burns: Conclusions drawn from an epidemiologic study. *Clinical Pediatrics, 6,* 693–695.

Breslin, P. W. (1975). The psychological reactions of children to burn traumata: A review. *Illinois Medical Journal, 148,* 514–519, 595–597, 602.

Brown, R. T., Dingle, A., & Koon-Scott, K. (1994). Inpatient consultation and liaison. In K. J. Tarnowski (Ed.), *Behavioral aspects of pediatric burns* (pp. 119–146). New York: Plenum.

Burn Injury Reporting System. (1986). *Report from the secretary of state.* Albany, NY: New York State Department of State Office of Fire Prevention and Control.

Bush, J. P., & Maron, M. T. (1994). Pain management. In K. J. Tarnowski (Ed.), *Behavioral aspects of pediatric burns* (pp. 147–168). New York: Plenum.

Byrne, C., Love, B., Browne, G., Brown, B., Roberts, J., & Streiner, D. (1986). The social competence of children following burn injury: A study of resilience. *Journal of Burn Care, 7,* 247–252.

Caniano, D. A., Beaver, B. L., & Boles, E. T. (1986). Child abuse: An update on surgical management of 256 cases. *Annals of Surgery, 203,* 219–224.

Carvajal, H. F. (1990). Burns in children and adolescents: Initial management as the first steps in successful rehabilitation. *Pediatrician, 17,* 237–243.

Center for Disease Control Division of Epidemiology and Control. (1987). Regional distribution of deaths from residential fires—United States, 1978–1984. *Journal of the American Medical Association, 258,* 2355–2356.

Clark, W. R., & Lerner, D. (1978). Regional burn survey: Two years of hospitalized burned patients in New York. *Journal of Trauma, 18,* 524–532.

Cole, M., Herndon, D. N., Desai, M. H., & Abston, S. (1986). Gasoline explosions, gasoline sniffing: An epidemic in young adolescents. *Journal of Burn Care and Rehabilitation, 7,* 532–534.

Davidson, L. L., Hughes, S. J., & O'Connor, P. A. (1988). Preschool behavior problems and subsequent risk of injury. *Pediatrics, 82,* 644–651.

Deans, L., Slater, H., & Goldfarb, I. W. (1990). Bad advice; Bad burn: A new problem in burn prevention. *Journal of Burn Care and Rehabilitation, 11,* 563–564.

Deitch, E. A., & Staats, M. (1982). Child abuse through burning. *Journal of Burn Care and Rehabilitation, 3,* 89–94.

Demling, R. H. (1987). Fluid replacement in burned patients. *Surgical Clinics of North America, 67,* 15–70.

Dyer, C., & Roberts, D. (1990). Thermal trauma. *Nursing Clinics of North America, 25,* 85–117.

Eland, J. M., & Anderson, J. E. (1977). The experience of pain in children. In A. K. Jacox (Ed.), *Pain: A source book for nurses and other health professionals* (pp. 453–471). Boston: Little, Brown.

Elliott, C. H., & Olson, R. A. (1983). The management of children's distress in response to painful medical treatment for burn injuries. *Behaviour Research and Therapy, 21,* 675–683.

El-Muhtaseb, H., Qaryoute, S., & Ragheb, S. A. (1984). Burn injuries in Jordan: A study of 338 cases. *Burns, 10,* 116–120.

Frank, H. A., Berry, C., Wachtel, T. L., & Johnson, R. W.

(1987). The impact of thermal injury. *Journal of Burn Care and Rehabilitation, 8,* 260–262.

Fratianne, R. B., & Brandt, C. P. (1994). Medical management. In K. J. Tarnowski (Ed.), *Behavioral aspects of pediatric burns* (pp. 23–53). New York: Plenum.

Gaukroger, P. B., Chapman, M. J., & Davey, R. B. (1991). Pain control in pediatric burns: The use of patient-controlled analgesia. *Burns, 17,* 396–399.

Goldberg, R. T. (1974). Adjustment of children with invisible and visible handicaps: Congenital heart disease and facial burns. *Journal of Counseling Psychology, 21,* 428–432.

Green, A. (1984). Epidemiology of burns in childhood. *Burns Including Thermal Injuries, 10,* 368–371.

Guyer, B., & Gallagher, S. S. (1985). An approach to the epidemiology of childhood injuries. *Pediatric Clinics of North America, 32,* 5–15.

Gwyther, O. A., & Smith, J. (1980). Social work with burn patients. *Physiotherapy, 66,* 188–191.

Hammond, J. S., Ward, C. G., & Pereira, E. (1988). Self-inflicted burns. *Journal of Burn Care and Rehabilitation, 9,* 178–179.

Hibbard, R. A., & Blevins, R. (1988). Palatal burn due to bottle warming in a microwave oven. *Pediatrics, 82,* 382–383.

Hobbs, N., & Perrin, J. M. (Eds.). (1985). *Issues in the care of children with chronic illnesses.* San Francisco: Jossey-Bass.

Jones, R. T., & Zaharopoulos, V. (1994). Prevention. In K. J. Tarnowski (Ed.), *Behavioral aspects of pediatric burns* (pp. 243–264). New York: Plenum.

Kaslow, N. J., Koon-Scott, K., & Dingle, A. (1994). Family considerations and interventions. In K. J. Tarnowski (Ed.), *Behavioral aspects of pediatric burns* (pp. 193–215). New York: Plenum.

Kavanaugh, C. (1983). Psychological intervention with the severely burned child: Report of an experimental comparison of two approaches and their effects on psychological sequelae. *Journal of the American Academy of Child and Adolescent Psychiatry, 22,* 145–156.

Kazak, A. E., & Nachman, G. S. (1991). Family research on childhood chronic illness: Pediatric oncology as an example. *Journal of Family Psychology, 4,* 462–483.

Knudson-Cooper, M. S., & Leuchtag, A. K. (1982). The stress of a family move as a precipitating factor in children's burn accidents. *Journal of Human Stress, 8,* 32–38.

Libber, S. M., & Stayton, D. J. (1984). Childhood burns reconsidered: The child, the family and the burn injury. *Journal of Trauma, 24,* 245–252.

Long, R. T., & Cope, O. (1961). Emotional problems of burned children. *New England Journal of Medicine, 264,* 1121–1127.

Lund, C. C., & Browder, J. R. (1944). An estimation of areas of burns. *Surgery, Gynecology, and Obstetrics, 79,* 224–252.

MacKay, A. M., & Rothman, K. J. (1982). The incidence and severity of burn injuries following Project Burn Prevention. *American Journal of Public Health, 72,* 248–252.

Martin, H. L. (1970). Parents' and children's reactions to burns and scalds in children. *British Journal of Medical Psychology, 43,* 183–191.

McCauley, R. L., Stenberg, B. A., Rutan, R. L., Robson, M. C., Heggers, J. P., & Herndon, D. N. (1991). Class C firework injuries in a pediatric population. *Journal of Trauma, 31,* 389–391.

McGrath, P. J. (1991). Intervention and management. In J. P. Bush & S. W. Harkins (Eds.), *Children in pain: Clinical and research issues from a developmental perspective* (pp. 83–115). New York: Springer Verlag.

McLoughlin, E., & Crawford, J. D. (1985). Types of burn injuries. *Pediatric Clinics of North America, 32,* 61–75.

McLoughlin, E., Joseph, M. P., & Crawford, J. D. (1976). Epidemiology of high tension injuries in children. *Journal of Pediatrics, 89,* 62–65.

McLoughlin, E., & McGuire, A. (1990). The causes, cost, and prevention of childhood burn injuries. *American Journal of Diseases of Children, 144,* 677–683.

Miller, M. D., Elliott, C. H., Funk, M., & Pruitt, S. D. (1988). Implications of children's burn injuries. In D. K. Routh (Ed.), *Handbook of pediatric psychology* (pp. 426–447). New York: Guilford.

Molinaro, J. R. (1978). The social fate of children disfigured by burns. *American Journal of Psychiatry, 135,* 979–980.

National Safety Council. (1979). *Accident safety facts.* Chicago: Author.

Noyes, R., Andreasen, N. O., & Hartford, C. (1971). The psychological reaction to severe burns. *Psychosomatics, 12,* 416–422.

Patterson, D. R., Everett, J. J., Bombardier, C. H., Questad, K. A., Lee, V. K., & Marvin, J. A. (1993). Psychological effects of severe burn injuries. *Psychological Bulletin, 113,* 362–378.

Prescott, P. R. (1990). Hair dryer burns in children. *Pediatrics, 86,* 692–697.

Pruzinsky, T., & Doctor, M. (1994). Body images and pediatric burn injury. In K. J. Tarnowski (Ed.), *Behavioral aspects of pediatric burns* (pp. 169–191). New York: Plenum.

Purdue, G. F., Hunt, J. L., & Prescott, P. R. (1988). Child burning by abuse—An index of suspicion. *Journal of Trauma, 28,* 221–224.

Roberts, R. N., & Gordon, S. B. (1979). Reducing childhood nightmares subsequent to a burn trauma. *Child Behavior Therapy, 1,* 373–381.

Rosen, B. N., & Peterson, L. (1990). Gender differences in children's outdoor play injuries: A review and integration. *Clinical Psychology Review, 10,* 187–205.

Routh, D. K., & Sanfilippo, M. D. (1991). Helping children cope with painful medical procedures. In J. P. Bush & S. W. Harkins (Eds.), *Children in pain: Clinical and* research issues from a developmental perspective (pp. 397–424). New York: Springer-Verlag.

Rubin, W. D., Mani, M. M., & Hiebert, J. M. (1986). Fluid resuscitation of the thermally injured patient. *Clinics in Plastic Surgery, 13,* 9–20.

Sawyer, M. G., Minde, K., & Zuker, R. (1982). The burned child: Scarred for life? *Burns, 9,* 201–213.

Sexson, S. B., & Madan-Swain, A. (1993). School reentry for the child with chronic illness. *Journal of Learning Disabilities, 26,* 115–125.

Sharpe, J. N., Brown, R. T., Thompson, N. J., & Eckman, J. (in press). Predictors of coping with pain in mothers and their children with sickle cell syndrome. *Journal of the American Academy of Child and Adolescent Psychiatry.*

Schubert, W., Arenholz, D. H., & Solem, L. D. (1990). Burns from hot oil and grease: A public health hazard. *Journal of Burn Care and Rehabilitation, 11,* 558–562.

Silverstein, P., & Lack, B. O. (1987). Epidemiology and prevention. In J. A. Boswick (Ed.), *The art and science of burn care* (pp. 11–17). Rockville, MD.

Simons, R. D., McFadd, A., Frank, H. A., Green, L. C., Malin, R. M., & Morris, J. L. (1978). Behavioral contracting in a burn care facility: A strategy of patient participation. *Journal of Trauma, 18,* 257–260.

St. Lawrence, J. S., & Drabman, R. S. (1983). Interruption of self- excoriation in a pediatric burn victim. *Journal of Pediatric Psychology, 8,* 155–159.

Stone, N. H., Rinaldo, L., Humphrey, C. R., & Brown, R. H. (1970). Child abuse by burning. *Surgical Clinics of North America, 50,* 1419–1424.

Tarnowski, K. J. (Ed.). (1994a). *Behavioral aspects of pediatric burns.* New York: Plenum.

Tarnowski, K. J. (1994b). Overview. In K. J. Tarnowski (Ed.), *Behavioral aspects of pediatric burns* (pp. 1–22). New York: Plenum.

Tarnowski, K. J., & Brown, R. T. (in press a). Pediatric burns. In M. C. Roberts (Ed.), *Handbook of pediatric psychology* (2nd ed.). New York: Guilford.

Tarnowski, K. J., & Brown, R. T. (in press b). Psychological aspects of pediatric disorders. In M. Hersen & R. T. Ammerman (Eds.), *Advanced abnormal child psychology.* New York: Lawrence Erlbaum.

Tarnowski, K. J., & Brown, R. T. (in press c). Pediatric pain. In R. T. Ammerman & M. Hersen (Eds.), *Handbook of child behavior therapy in the psychiatric setting.* New York: Wiley.

Tarnowski, K. J., & Brown, R. T. (1994). Future directions. In K. J. Tarnowski (Ed.), *Behavioral aspects of pediatric burns* (pp. 265–276). New York: Plenum.

Tarnowski, K. J., Rasnake, L. K., & Drabman, R. S. (1987). Behavioral assessment and treatment of pediatric burns: A review. *Behavior Therapy, 18,* 417–441.

Tarnowski, K. J., Rasnake, L. K., Gavaghan-Jones, M. P., & Smith, L. (1991). Psychosocial sequelae of pediatric burn injuries: A review. *Clinical Psychology Review, 11,* 371–398.

Tarnowski, K. J., Rasnake, L. K., Linscheid, T. R., & Mulick, J. A. (1989a). Behavioral adjustment of pediatric burn victims. *Journal of Pediatric Psychology, 14,* 607–615.

Tarnowski, K. J., Rasnake, L. K., Linscheid, T. R., & Mulick, J. A. (1989b). Ecobehavioral characteristics of a pediatric burn injury unit. *Journal of Applied Behavioral Analysis, 22,* 101–109.

U.S. Fire Administration. (1978). *First in the United States.* Washington, DC: U.S. Department of Commerce, National Fire Data Center.

Varas, R., Carbone, R., & Hammond, J. S. (1988). A one-hour burn prevention program for grade school children: Its approach and success. *Journal of Burn Care and Rehabilitation, 9,* 69–71.

Wade, J., Purdue, G. F., Hunt, J. L., & Childers, L. (1990). Crawl on your belly like GI Joe. *Journal of Burn Care and Rehabilitation, 11,* 261–263.

Wallander, J. L., & Varni, J. W. (1992). Adjustment in children with chronic physical disorders: Programmatic research on a disability-stress-coping model. In A. M. LaGreca, L. J. Siegel, J. L. Wallander, & C. E. Walker (Eds.), *Stress and coping in child health* (pp. 279–298). New York: Guilford.

Watson, E. J., & Johnson, A. M. (1958). The emotional significance of acquired physical disfigurement in children. *American Journal of Orthopsychiatry, 28,* 85–97.

Webne, S., Kaplan, B. J., & Shaw, M. (1989). Pediatric burn prevention: An evaluation of the efficacy of a strategy to reduce tap water temperature in a population at risk for scald burns. *Developmental and Behavioral Pediatrics, 10,* 187–191.

Wernick, R. L. (1983). Stress inoculation in the management of clinical pain: Application to burn pain. In D. Meichenbaum & M. E. Jaremko (Eds.), *Stress reduction and prevention* (pp. 191–217). New York: Plenum.

Wilson, G. R., Buckland, R., & Sully, L. (1988). Childhood illness as an aetiological factor in burns. *Burns, 14,* 237–238.

Woodward, J. (1959). Emotional disturbances of burned children. *British Medical Journal, 1,* 1009–1113.

Zide, B., & Pardoe, R. (1976). The use of behavior modification therapy in a recalcitrant burned child. *Plastic and Reconstructive Surgery, 57,* 378–382.

CHAPTER 9

CYSTIC FIBROSIS

Deborah L. Miller, DUPONT HOSPITAL FOR CHILDREN/JEFFERSON MEDICAL COLLEGE
Elissa Jelalian, RHODE ISLAND HOSPITAL/BROWN UNIVERSITY SCHOOL OF MEDICINE
Lori J. Stark, RHODE ISLAND HOSPITAL/BROWN UNIVERSITY SCHOOL OF MEDICINE

As the most common autosomal recessive disease in Caucasians, cystic fibrosis (CF) affected approximately 30,000 individuals in 1990 in the United States, in addition to 7 million symptom-free carriers of the CF gene (FitzSimmons, 1993). CF is a lethal disorder of the exocrine system that affects the gastrointestinal, pancreatic, hepatic, respiratory, and reproductive systems, and sweat glands (Matthews & Drotar, 1984). In CF, a thick, viscous mucus accumulates in the affected organs, resulting in the progressive scarring and destruction of excretory ducts (Oppenheimer & Esterley, 1975). The disease is typically characterized by pancreatic insufficiency, chronic lung disease with acute and chronic bacterial infections, as well as liver disease and diabetes mellitus in some patients (Scanlin, 1988). The median projected life expectancy for individuals with CF has increased from 4 years in 1950 (CF Foundation, 1980) to 28 years in 1990 (FitzSimmons, 1993).

Cystic fibrosis, then, is a chronic illness that affects multiple organ systems and ultimately results in premature death. Currently, there is no cure for CF, so medical treatment must target the symptoms of the disease in an effort to increase longevity. The prescribed treatment regimen is complex, time consuming, and expensive, affecting not only the individual with CF but also immediate and extended family members. Additionally, as with any chronic illness, different challenges arise as the individual with CF progresses developmentally. Finally, as median life expectancy increases, individuals with CF are facing new challenges associated with adulthood. The role of health psychologists in the care of patients with CF is rich and varied and includes assessment and treatment of patients and families, consultation to inpatient and outpatient health care providers, and research.

MEDICAL ASPECTS

Identification of the CF gene, the cystic fibrosis transmembrane regulator, and its corresponding defective protein (Kerem et al., 1989; Riordan et al., 1989), has expanded the possibilities that a cure for CF will be discovered via gene therapy. However, there is currently no cure for CF, and medical treatment targets the associated symptoms of the disease in an effort to reduce morbidity and mortality.

Lung disease is the most serious complication of CF, with approximately 78 percent of deaths caused by cardiorespiratory factors (FitzSimmons, 1993). A progression of lung disease, caused by impedance of the normal cleaning mechanism, results in mucous plugging of the bronchi and bronchioles and leads to a chronic cycle of obstruction and infection. Although lung transplantation is a recent development for patients with CF, it is reserved for those with end-stage disease.

Aggressive treatment of the pulmonary complications associated with CF is necessary to prolong survival and includes antibiotic therapy, chest physiotherapy, and inhalation therapy. Chest physiotherapy (CPT) is believed to reduce the rate of lung function deterioration by assisting in clearing the lungs of excessive mucus (Bauer, McDougal, & Schoumacher, 1994). CPT is prescribed one to four times daily and involves clapping on the chest of the patient while he or she assumes up to 11 positions to promote movement of mucus out of the lungs. CPT may be preceded by inhalation therapy, which serves to wet and thin the mucous, or followed by inhalation therapy to deliver antibiotics. CPT is a common treatment prescription, but the long-term effects have not been demonstrated and the optimal treatment regimen has not been determined (Eigen, Clark, & Wolle, 1987).

Exercise training programs have also been advocated as an alternative to CPT in clearing the lungs, improving pulmonary functioning, and increasing exercise tolerance (Edlund et al., 1986; Orenstein et al., 1981). These programs may offset the restriction of physical activity observed in many individuals with CF, which results from a vicious cycle of deteriorating pulmonary functioning and inactivity (Sherrill, 1976). In the short term, exercise has been found to lead to improved exercise tolerance and cardiorespiratory fitness but has rarely been shown to affect clinical status (Edlund et al., 1986) or pulmonary function. Orenstein and colleagues (1981) suggest investigation of long-term conditioning programs to determine whether pulmonary function could be positively affected.

Pancreatic involvement results from accumulation of mucus in the pancreatic ducts, preventing secretion of sufficient digestive enzymes, thus producing pancreatic insufficiency (PI) (Kopelman, 1991). As many as 93 percent of CF patients may be affected by PI (FitzSimmons, 1993). Patients with PI cannot digest fat, fat-soluble vitamins, or protein, thus necessitating a regimen of vitamin-mineral supplementation and pancreatic replacement enzymes that must be taken with all meals and snacks. Despite this regimen,

malabsorption continues to be a problem for many CF patients.

The nutritional status of patients with CF is frequently problematic and is strongly associated with health status and long-term survival (Corey, McLaughlin, Williams, & Levison, 1988) as the immune system and the course of respiratory disease may be adversely affected by malnutrition (Pencharz, Hill, Archibald, Levy, & Newth, 1984). Malnutrition in CF appears to be multidetermined by fat and micronutrient malabsorption, loss of bile salts and bile acids, reduced appetite and consumption secondary to potential recurrent vomiting, gastroesophageal reflux, psychosocial stress (Ramsey, Farrell, Pencharz, & the Consensus Committee, 1992), and increased energy expenditure secondary to chronic pulmonary infection, medication side effects, and a possible metabolic defect. Thus, CF patients often exhibit growth failure, with approximately 50 percent of patients falling below the tenth percentile for weight or height (FitzSimmons, 1993).

Nutritional status has been linked to disease severity in CF, wherein those exhibiting mild clinical manifestations of CF do not differ from healthy controls on most growth and body composition variables. However, changes in body composition, such as depletion of percent body fat, may be a risk factor for disease progression and may signal the onset of clinical deterioration (Tomezsko, Scanlin, & Stallings, 1994).

Given the close association between malnutrition and clinical status, early identification and treatment of malnutrition are important (Steinkamp & von der Hardt, 1994). Nutritional management includes consumption of 125 to 150 percent of the recommended daily allowance (RDA) of calories for healthy individuals (Ramsey et al., 1992), with a normal to high fat intake (MacDonald, Holden, & Harris, 1991), pancreatic-enzyme replacement and vitamin-mineral supplementation for patients with PI, and, in the case of nutritional failure (i.e., less than 85 percent of ideal weight-for-height ratio), enteral feeds via nasogastric tubes, gastrostomy, or jejunostomy (Ramsey et al., 1992).

From 1969 to 1990, the population of individuals with CF increased in age fourfold, thus indicating new challenges in terms of medical and psychosocial problems to be encountered by a new generation of older patients (FitzSimmons, 1993). As CF patients age, medical complications such as insulin-dependent diabetes mellitus, liver disease, gallbladder disease, and pancreatitis become more common. Although the majority of males with CF are sterile (Webb, 1991), adult women with CF can carry pregnancy to term and deliver without additional morbidity and mortality (FitzSimmons, 1993)

ADHERENCE

The review of CF symptoms and treatment reveal that it is a progressive disease for which there is no cure and that necessitates a time- and labor-intensive regimen. Also, many aspects of the CF medical regimen may be prescribed prophylactically, often do not provide obvious benefit in terms of symptomatic relief or improved health status, and thus are not inherently reinforcing (Bartholomew, Parcel, Swank, & Czyzewski, 1993). Unfortunately, research investigating adherence to the CF medical regimen has been limited in scope and has been largely conducted outside a theoretical framework (Stark, Jelalian, & Miller, in press).

Generally, adherence to the CF regimen is considered to be good (Gudas, Koocher, & Wypij, 1991; Geiss, Hobbs, Hammersley-Maercklein, Kramer, & Henley, 1992; Passero, Remor, & Solomon, 1981; Schultz & Moser, 1992). Almost uniformly across studies, high adherence rates have been observed for medication (Gudas et al., 1991; Passero et al., 1981). However, adherence to CPT, diet, and exercise prescriptions are often cited as problematic (Gudas et al., 1991; Hobbs, Geiss, Hammersley, Kramer, & Henley, 1985; Schultz & Moser, 1992). In any regimen consisting of multiple health care tasks, adherence is often lowest for those treatment components that interfere most with life-style, as may be the case for CPT, diet, and exercise prescriptions (Hobbs et al., 1985; LaGreca, 1990).

In an effort to provide a conceptual formulation for understanding medical nonadherence in CF, Koocher, McGrath, and Gudas (1990) proposed a typology based on a critical incident survey of 223 patients and their families. The three categories include inadequate knowledge, psychosocial resistance, and educated nonadherence. Inadequate knowledge represents those patients whose nonadherence is secondary to an inadequate understanding of available disease-related information.

Empirical support for this category was provided by Henley and Hill (1990), who demonstrated several misconceptions on the part of both patients and parents regarding the CF regimen. For example, 22 percent of patients and 14 percent of parents in their sample believed that CPT is unnecessary when the patient is well. Half of parents and 90 percent of patients reported that fat should be excluded from the CF diet, and 30 percent of parents and 17 percent of patients did not know that enzyme-replacement dosages should be varied with percent of fat intake. Other researchers have reported similar information deficits regarding dietary, CPT (Gudas et al., 1991), and exercise prescriptions (Hobbs et al., 1985). Unfortunately, adherence was assessed in only one study, which indicated that increased knowledge was associated with better adherence to medication and CPT (Gudas et al., 1991).

Resistance is conceptualized as stemming from psychosocial and demographic factors. Psychosocial factors examined thus far include optimism and family functioning. In general, high optimism is positively associated with better adherence, particularly in older children (Gudas et al., 1991). Another investigation reported that high levels of family expressiveness and the coping styles of cooperation and optimism were positively associated with adherence (Patterson, 1985).

Several sociodemographic factors are also related to adherence. Illness severity is associated with adherence, in that more severe disease is typically associated with lower adherence ratings. Adherence also tends to decrease as children grow older although this may simply reflect deteriorating health status (Gudas et al., 1991; Hobbs et al., 1985; Patterson, 1985). Other factors found to be negatively associated with adherence include number of children in the family and maternal employment (Patterson, 1985).

Educated, or adaptive, nonadherence applies to patients who have made quality-of-life decisions regarding their treatment regimens. These patients have decided that the costs of adhering to the CF regimen outweigh the benefits and thus adhere less than might be medically optimal (Koocher et al., 1990). Results of two studies support the existence of this type of nonadherence. For example, mothers exhibiting low levels of marital satisfaction and adult social contact (Geiss et al., 1992) and mothers not employed outside the home (Patterson, 1985) have children with higher-rated levels of adherence. Perhaps the time needed to ensure good child adherence interferes with maternal social relationships and recreational activities or, conversely, mothers experiencing low levels of marital satisfaction and social contact may have more time to ensure child adherence.

The literature to date on adherence in children and adolescents with CF is limited although promising. Researchers have begun to explore the psychosocial and medical concomitants of adherence and nonadherence; Koocher and colleagues (1990) have outlined a conceptual framework of adherence in the CF population. Such conceptual models have the capacity to guide clinical care and research and thus further the understanding of treatment adherence (LaGreca, 1990).

Assessment of adherence to the CF regimen, however, remains problematic in that a reliable and objective measure has not yet been developed. For example, many researchers rely on self-reports, which may produce overestimates of compliance (Passero et al., 1981). Development of direct measures of adherence is worthwhile, in that they might produce less biased ratings and identify specific behaviors to be targeted for intervention. That is, global ratings of adherence do not provide the depth of information needed to design interventions and do not capture problematic parent/child interactions that may ensue in the process of obtaining child adherence. Optimally, assessment of adherence would be objective, be multidimensional, include multiple raters, and be conducted within longitudinal and prospective research designs so as to best identify relevant variables and the way in which they affect and are affected by the CF treatment regimen (LaGreca, 1990).

PSYCHOLOGICAL ADAPTATION

Individual Adaptation

Given the chronic, progressive, and ultimately fatal nature of the disease, it would certainly seem that cys-

tic fibrosis poses a considerable challenge to affected children and adolescents. Research on the psychosocial adjustment of children with CF, as with other chronic illnesses, has progressed from a descriptive to an empirical, theoretically driven approach (Bennett, 1994; Thompson, Gustafson, George, & Spock, 1994). Consequent to the use of theoretically derived models of adjustment, empirical assessment techniques, and multiple informants, recent research has found much lower rates of adjustment difficulties in children with CF in comparison to earlier studies (Thompson, Merritt, Keith, Murphy, & Johndrow, 1993). Indeed, although children and adolescents with CF are at increased risk for adjustment problems, many can anticipate good adjustment (Thompson et al., 1994).

Infancy and Preschool Age

Goldberg and colleagues have longitudinally examined infant and toddler adaptation in terms of infant/mother attachment and medical status. Results indicated that infants with CF exhibit a similar pattern of attachment as healthy peers and a normative sample (Goldberg, Washington, Morris, Fischer-Fay, & Simmons, 1990). Longitudinal assessment, however, revealed that infants exhibiting insecure attachment at age 1 year evidenced significant decline in weight for height percentile through age 3, in contrast to securely attached infants whose status on this variable increased over the first year of life and remained above 100 percent to age 4 (Goldberg, Washington, Simmons, & MacClusky, 1992; Simmons, Goldberg, Washington, & MacClusky, 1991). Interestingly, medical severity was not related to nutritional status, suggesting that early mother/infant relationships may significantly affect the infant's vulnerability to failure to thrive (Goldberg et al., 1992).

In a cross-sectional investigation of preschool children, Cowen and associates (1985) found that parents of healthy children reported significantly more child-related problems than parents of children with CF, although the latter group described their children as significantly more hostile-aggressive than did a normative sample. Together, these studies suggest that infants and toddlers with CF may be vulnerable to certain adjustment difficulties, which may in turn be related to some aspects of medical status (i.e., nutritional status). The degree of vulnerability and the relationships between these variables are unclear and merit further investigation.

School-Age and Adolescence

Very few studies have focused exclusively on school-age children (Simmons et al., 1987; Thompson, Gustafson, Hamlett, & Spock, 1992a) or adolescents (Cappelli et al., 1989; Quittner, DiGirolamo, & Regolio, 1993; Simmons et al., 1985), thus making it difficult to delineate areas of good or poor adjustment specific to any developmental phase. The literature pertaining to adaptation of children and adolescents will be presented together, although findings relevant to any one age group will be indicated.

Internalizing Problems

Evidence suggesting that children with CF are at particular risk for developing internalizing problems is accumulating (Kashani, Barbero, Wilfley, Morris, & Shepperd, 1988; Thompson, 1985; Thompson, Hodges, & Hamlett, 1990). When compared to psychiatrically referred and nonreferred children, Thompson and associates (1990) reported that children with CF generally exhibited equivalent levels of psychological disturbance to the nonreferred group. However, children with CF were similar to the referred sample in terms of worries, self-image, and separation anxiety, with 37 percent of the CF sample meeting *DSM-III* criteria for an anxiety disorder. Indeed, anxiety disorders seem to be more common than depressive disorders in children with CF. Thompson and colleagues (1992a) also reported a high rate of anxiety diagnoses (44 percent) and a comparably lower rate of depression (9 percent) in a sample of 7- to 12-year-old children with CF.

Additionally, results of a meta-analysis indicated that children with CF are at reduced risk for depressive symptomatology in comparison to children with other chronic illnesses (e.g., asthma, sickle cell anemia) (Bennett, 1994). Age may be a critical factor in determining whether a child with CF experiences anxiety or depression, in that younger children may be at greater risk for anxiety disorders (Thompson et al., 1990) whereas adolescents and adults tend to exhibit increased depressive symptoms (Pearson, Pumariega, & Seilheimer, 1991; Simmons et al., 1985; Thompson et al. 1990). Perhaps younger children are buffered by the degree of active family involvement required by

their treatment regimen (Bennett, 1994), whereas adolescents, who may be striving for increased independence, may experience depressive symptomatology secondary to their deteriorating health status and the realization that premature death is probable (Thompson et al., 1990). Finally, several studies reported that children with CF exhibit more somatic complaints than non-chronically ill children (Kashani et al., 1988; Simmons et al., 1987; Thompson et al., 1990), although the clinical significance of these findings is unclear (Stark et al., in press).

Externalizing Problems

Although less prevalent than internalizing behavior problems, externalizing problems have been observed in children with CF, though not to a greater degree than in the general population (Kashani et al., 1988; Simmons et al., 1987; Thompson et al., 1990). Within the spectrum of externalizing disorders, children with CF may be at particular risk for oppositional disorders, as typified by disobedience, stubbornness, and provocativeness—a pattern observed in 23 to 24 percent of children assessed (Thompson et al., 1990, 1992a). Examination of the relationship between oppositional symptoms and other behavioral disturbances in CF, such as nonadherence, would be worthwhile (Thompson et al., 1990).

Although children are often described as exhibiting either internalizing or externalizing behavior problems, a mixed profile of internalizing and externalizing behavior problems was most common in a sample of 7- to 12-year-old children with CF (Thompson et al., 1992a; Thompson et al., 1994). In these studies, a transactional stress and coping model, which examines maternal and child adaptational processes in the context of illness and demographic parameters, was applied to the psychological adjustment of children with CF. Interestingly, both internalizing and externalizing behavior problems may be mediated by the same processes. Results indicated that maternal anxiety and child self-worth accounted for a significant amount of variance in child- and mother-reported child adjustment, above and beyond that accounted for by demographic and illness parameters and prior levels of child adjustment.

Generally, research focusing specifically on adolescents with CF suggests that their psychological adjustment is equivalent to that of nonchronically ill peers (Cappelli et al., 1989; Simmons et al., 1985). Two studies, however, investigated adolescent adjustment via more innovative assessment methodologies (e.g., phone diaries, interviews) than the behavior checklists most typically used (Cappelli et al., 1989; Quittner et al., 1993). Adolescents identified problems relating to extended family, parents, health, and clinic/hospital as most difficult. Illness severity had an impact on the domain of eating and gaining weight, with more severely ill adolescents rating this domain as more problematic than less ill adolescents. Thus, adolescents with CF experience typical, developmentally appropriate concerns (i.e., school, family relationships) as well as concerns specific to their disease (i.e., medications and treatment, clinic, hospitalizations).

When considering the literature on the psychological adjustment of children and adolescents with CF, caution should be exercised. First, despite statistical elevations on measures of adjustment above those obtained for comparison groups, scores may not be clinically meaningful. For example, although children with CF were reported to exhibit significantly more behavior problems than a healthy control sample, Kashani and colleagues (1988) acknowledged that scores on the CBCL were within one-half of a standard deviation of the mean.

Another concern is the potential interaction between maternal adjustment and child behavior problems. One study revealed that statistically significant levels of child behavior problems were no longer significant when maternal depression was statistically controlled. Therefore, prior reports of child behavior problems in chronically ill children may have overestimated the incidence of such problems by not controlling for maternal depression (Walker, Ortiz-Valdez, & Newbrough, 1989).

Intellectual and Academic Functioning

Thompson and associates (1992) examined the intellectual and academic functioning of a representative sample of children and adolescents using standardized assessment measures. Results indicated that the intelligence and achievement of children and adolescents with CF is normally distributed and not affected by disease severity. Age, however, was negatively as-

sociated with intellectual functioning. That is, children exhibited significantly higher levels of intellectual functioning than adolescents, perhaps indicating the impact of the chronic strain associated with CF and its treatment.

Parental Adaptation

Several investigators have examined relations between parental adaptation to CF and other psychological variables. For example, coping styles have been implicated in parents' adjustment. Generally, parents utilizing emotion-focused strategies—such as avoidance, self-blame, and wishful thinking—exhibit greater degrees of distress than parents who utilize active, problem-focused strategies such as seeking social support, cognitive restructuring, and seeking information (Mullins et al., 1991; Thompson, Gustafson, Hamlett, & Spock, 1992b).

Two studies examined parent adjustment during the diagnostic phase, which is typically considered a difficult time for families. Using a global measure of parenting stress, Goldberg, Morris, Simmons, Fowler, and Levison (1990) found that parents of infants with CF reported equivalent levels of parenting stress to a normative sample. Alternatively, Quittner and colleagues (Quittner, DiGirolamo, Jacobsen, & Eigen, 1991; Quittner, DiGirolamo, Michel, & Eigen, 1992) proposed a contextual approach to assess parental adaptation to the diagnostic phase. They argued that a fine-grained analysis would provide richer and more detailed information unique to specific medical conditions, illness phases, developmental stages, and family processes. Results indicated that mothers experienced higher levels of role strain than fathers. Specifically, mothers perceived that they carried an unequal share of child care responsibilities. Similarly, Nagy and Ungerer (1990) reported that mothers receiving more support from their husbands exhibited better adjustment, particularly if their husbands placed a high value on child-rearing activities (Nagy & Ungerer, 1990).

Together, these studies provide support for the stress-buffering effect of social support on maternal adjustment. Additionally, in the Quittner, DiGirolamo, and associates (1992) study, mothers and fathers reported elevated levels of depressive symptomatology, though mothers reported significantly greater symptomatology than fathers. Results further indicated that maternal perceptions of increased role strain contributed significantly to maternal depression, as did lower levels of marital adjustment. Results supported the contextual approach, which allowed identification of specific conditions that might predispose parents to adjustment difficulties and which might indicate effective interventions (Quittner, DiGirolamo, et al., 1992).

Reports on the impact of having a preschooler with CF have been inconsistent. In one study that compared a group of healthy preschool children to a group with CF, the latter exhibited equivalent adjustment for family functioning (Cowen et al., 1985). Walker and colleagues (1991; Walker, Ford, & Donald, 1987), however, found that parents of preschool children with CF experience greater levels of depressive symptomatology than do mothers of medically healthy children in the same age group. In another study, Quittner, Opipari, Regolio, Jacobsen, and Eigen (1992) included both behavioral and perceptual measures in their comparison of daily activities of mothers of preschoolers with CF and matched controls. Mothers of children with CF were observed to spend significantly more time engaged in medical care throughout the week and more time in chores and child care on weekends. Also, mothers of children with CF spent significantly less time engaged in play and recreation.

One variable that may buffer mothers from stress and depression is employment. Walker and associates (1989) examined a conceptual model of the relationship among maternal employment, maternal depression, and child behavior problems in mothers whose children were mentally retarded, had CF or diabetes, or were healthy. Regardless of child health status, mothers employed outside the home exhibited less depressive symptomatology than those not so employed. Quittner, DiGirolamo, and colleagues (1992) also reported lower levels of maternal role strain and depression in mothers employed outside the home, although these results were based on post hoc analyses. The buffering effect of maternal employment may derive from increased opportunities for stimulation and accomplishment, relief from caregiving responsibilities, and access to additional

social support (Quittner, DiGirolamo, et al., 1992; Walker et al., 1989).

Sibling Adaptation

Minimal attention has been directed toward the psychosocial functioning of siblings of children with CF. As with research on the adaptation of the child with CF, early reports of sibling adaptation revealed significant problems in adjustment, whereas more recent work relying on objective measures has failed to reveal such problems (Cowen et al., 1986; Phillips, Bohannon, Gayton, & Friedman, 1985). However, a subsample of parents reported some difficulties, including expression of jealous feelings and complaints about lack of parent attention by the healthy sibling (Phillips et al., 1985). Indeed, Quittner and Opipari (1994) reported that mothers spent proportionately more time with younger affected children than with their older healthy children, a finding not evident in a healthy control group. Also, older siblings of children with CF experienced more negative interactions with their mothers than healthy sibling pairs and younger siblings with CF.

Thus, children with CF generally exhibit similar patterns of adjustment to healthy peers but appear to be vulnerable to specific psychosocial adjustment problems. During infancy, the distribution of attachment patterns is equivalent to that of healthy infants, although those infants with CF that exhibit attachment difficulties may be predisposed to malnutrition. Screening for infant attachment difficulties might be a productive way of identifying children at nutritional risk who might benefit from early intervention targeting dietary intake. School-age children with CF, in turn, are at risk for developing internalizing disorders, particularly anxiety disorders, and oppositional disorders as well. Adolescents seem to be particularly at risk for depression, rather than anxiety, and frequently report disease-specific concerns in addition to concerns typically expressed by adolescents.

Further, having a child with CF can adversely affect the entire family constellation. For example, although siblings do not generally exhibit adaptational problems, there is some evidence suggesting that they experience interactional difficulties with their parents. In terms of mothers versus fathers, mothers appear to be at particular risk for depression, social isolation, and role strain, particularly if they are not employed outside the home. Also, the interaction of maternal and child adjustment is vital to the understanding of either.

Clinical Implications and Intervention

The findings on psychological adaptation and adherence have implications for clinical practice and demonstrate the need for psychological interface with medicine in the management of this disease. Much of the research addressing clinical interventions focuses on adherence to the CF treatment regimen (i.e., chest physiotherapy, diet, and exercise). The following is a review of interventions that have been used to target adherence to the CF regimen as well as interventions that address adaptational difficulties associated with CF.

Chest physiotherapy (CPT) is especially problematic because it is administered prophylactically, and patients will not likely feel any improvement as a result of a single treatment. Indeed, CPT may produce negative side effects (i.e., coughing, choking, and vomiting), thus further reducing the likelihood of future adherence (Gudas et al., 1991). CPT is administered one to four times daily and may take up to an hour to perform a single treatment. In the only intervention study reported to date, Stark, Miller, Plienes, and Drabman (1987) described the use of behavioral contracting to mitigate parent/child conflict and increase CPT in an 11-year-old girl with CF. Privileges and activities, previously available noncontingently, were provided contingently upon meeting prespecified goals that delineated the number and timing of CPT each day. The procedure effectively increased the child's performance of CPT to the prescribed level and decreased mother/child conflict. On follow-up, treatment effects had been maintained and the child exhibited improved health status as reflected by increased weight percentile for age and improved pulmonary function (Stark et al., 1987).

Diet is often problematic because parents and patients do not understand that it is a formal treatment recommendation (Gudas et al., 1991) and, once they do, there is often a control struggle in attempts to meet caloric recommendations (Bowen & Stark, 1991). Stark and colleagues have designed an intervention package intended to improve parent/child interactions during meals and increase caloric consumption of children with CF to the recommended levels.

The intervention is implemented by a multidisciplinary team and includes nutritional education and behavioral parent training. This treatment has been conducted on both a group (Stark, Bowen, Tyc, Evans, & Passero, 1990; Stark et al., 1993) and individual basis (Stark, Powers, Jelalian, Rape, & Miller, 1994). Parents and children are seen in simultaneous but separate groups where nutritional education can be presented at a developmentally appropriate level. In their group, children practice appropriate eating skills and try new foods during meals that are managed by group leaders who implement the behavioral skills of differential attention and contingency management being taught to parents.

Results have consistently indicated marked increases in calorie consumption, to or above the recommended levels, and increases in weight (Stark, Bowen, et al., 1990; Stark et al., 1993, 1994) with maintenance at 9 (1990) and 24 months posttreatment (1993). In addition, treatment has been found to positively affect parent/child interactions (Stark et al., 1994). Singer, Nofer, Benson-Szekely, and Brooks (1991) implemented a similar treatment program in four young children with CF and reported increased caloric intake with marked catch-up growth at follow-up.

Exercise

Minimal attention has been directed to the evaluation of programmatic exercise for children with CF. Hobbs, Stratton, Geiss, Kramer, and Ozturk (1987) reported preliminary results of a study in which children were assigned to either a clinic- or home-based exercise program. Both 10-week programs involved four 30- to 45-minute sessions per week, which children spent swimming, bicycling, playing basketball, running, and/or walking. The home-based program included participation of a partner and behavioral contracting. Contracts between parents and children specified rewards that children could earn contingent upon completing exercise sessions.

Preliminary results suggested that children in the home-based program completed more exercise sessions over 10 weeks than those in the clinic condition. All participants exhibited significant improvements in pulmonary function (i.e., FEV_1, FVC, PEF) and ventilation equivalent posttreatment. Additionally, child-reported depressive symptomatology was significantly reduced, and there was a trend toward lower levels of mother-reported child somatic concerns and maternal depression.

Biofeedback

One promising application of behavior therapy in CF is biofeedback-assisted breathing retraining (Delk, Gevirtz, Hicks, Carden, & Rucker, 1994). Using an age- and disease severity-matched control group with random assignment to experimental versus placebo conditions, Delk and associates (1994) examined the effects of respiratory muscle feedback and breathing retraining on lung function in adults and children with CF. Treatment resulted in statistically and clinically significant improvements in FEV_1 and $FEF_{25\%-75\%}$, and a clinically significant improvement in FVC for individuals in the experimental condition, whereas control subjects remained stable on all measures. Thus, biofeedback-assisted breathing retraining can be used to improve respiratory function in patients with CF, and future research should examine its long-term effects on clinical status.

Self-Management

Given the complex, long-term nature of the medical regimen for CF and increasing life expectancy, interventions seeking to enhance self-management are certainly warranted. In a summer camp program for adolescents with CF, McCracken and Budd (1992) provided intensive education in CF, home and health maintenance skills, and group psychotherapy. In comparison to an age-, sex-, and disease severity-matched control group, adolescents who participated in the self-care program exhibited significant improvements on measures of functional status (i.e., weight for height & FEV_1) and knowledge about self-care. Their program also had a positive impact on psychosocial adaptation. Following the intervention, group participants exhibited significant improvements on measures of adjustment (i.e., behavior and anxiety) and family functioning over adolescents in a matched control group. Further details on the intervention were not provided, which is unfortunate, as the intervention might be appropriate in other settings. Additionally, the multimodal nature of the in-

tervention, coupled with the research design utilized, precludes the determination of the efficacy of any one treatment component.

Bartholomew and colleagues (1991) have also developed a comprehensive self-management program that includes the development of coping and medical management skills via the techniques of modeling, goal setting, self-monitoring, skill training, and positive reinforcement. Additionally, the program includes age-appropriate modules spanning several developmental stages. Although promising, this program has yet to be empirically examined.

Stark, Spirito, and Hobbs (1990) describe use of cognitive and behavioral self-management strategies to encourage more adaptive and autonomous behaviors in adolescents and young adults with CF, particularly during end-stage disease. Self-instruction to reinterpret bodily cues and replacing anxious responses with more adaptive behaviors, such as deep breathing, is one application of cognitive-behavior therapy the authors describe. They also recommend use of relaxation, via imagery, autogenics, and deep muscle relaxation, to aid with anxiety and pain reduction and sleep difficulties.

One study investigated use of relaxation and self-instructional training in a group of adolescents and young adults with CF. Four to six months posttreatment, participants reported that the intervention had been useful and had produced an increased sense of control (Spirito, Russo, & Masek, 1984). Stark, Spirito, and associates caution, however, that due to the complexity of the CF disease process, relaxation strategies must be individually tailored in terms of medical conditions (e.g., coughing, use of an oxygen mask).

Another consideration is the application of relaxation strategies with younger children. Koeppen (1974) devised a relaxation script for use with young children that was implemented by Stark and colleagues (1993) to help children cope with feelings of fullness at meals. Use of this procedure for other target problems (e.g., anxiety) in young children is worth investigating, as is the use of biofeedback to enhance relaxation.

In terms of designing and investigating new interventions, Bennett (1994) recommended utilizing an approach that combines components specific to a certain disease with those typically implemented with healthy children. For example, interventions targeting oppositional behaviors in children with CF could certainly be drawn from the existing clinical literature. The parent training program described by Forehand and McMahon (1981) was specifically designed to help parents learn to modify child oppositional behaviors. This program could be implemented to target oppositional behaviors, in general, and disease-related oppositional behaviors as well. A good illustration of this approach was conducted by Stark and colleagues (1990, 1993, 1994) who utilized the Forehand and McMahon program as a framework around which to design an intervention targeting dietary adherence. Their results, as reported earlier in this chapter, are promising, and application of similar interventions to other oppositional behavior problems would be beneficial.

The impact of parent-focused interventions on both parent and child adaptation merits consideration. Coping skills, depression, social isolation, and marital discord would certainly be suitable targets for intervention. Also, interventions for parents of children with CF might focus on improving support-related interactions between spouses and helping couples achieve a satisfactory division of child care and household responsibilities. Potentially, such interventions might yield concurrent, positive effects on parent child interactions, child adaptation, and maternal perceptions of child distress.

SUMMARY

Cystic fibrosis remains a challenging arena for psychologists, given the chronicity and life-threatening nature of the disease; a medical regimen that is complex, time consuming, and often has uncertain benefits; and the impact of the disease and its treatment on affected individuals and their families. Certainly, for psychologists to be able to positively affect adherence and psychosocial adaptation in children and adolescents with CF, direct and objective assessment techniques must be developed. Additionally, use of multiple raters and incorporation of a context-specific assessment approach into longitudinal research designs is desirable. Finally, efforts should be made to isolate age and developmental status as variables for future study. In order to accomplish the latter goal, cross-center collaborative research may be necessary to ensure adequate sample sizes and reduce site-specific biases (Lavigne & Faier-Routman, 1992). In these ways, psychologists will be able to better understand the specific vulnerabilities that confront individuals with CF across the life span, and they therefore will be able to identify specific, operationalized behaviors for which appropriate interventions can be designed.

Much remains to be accomplished in terms of psychosocial interventions for children with CF and their families. One promising approach is the implementation of treatment by multidisciplinary teams that yield comprehensive care for the patient with CF (e.g., Bartholomew et al., 1991; Stark et al., 1990, 1993, 1994). Inclusion of psychologists and other mental health professionals on these teams would help ensure that the medical regimen is understood and that families are given guidance as to how best to implement the regimen. An important aspect of future research would thus include methodologies that permit the examination of individual treatment components within multimodal interventions. Finally, long-term follow-up assessment will help determine the extent to which positive outcomes produced by psychosocial interventions persist.

Although psychological research on CF has become more theoretically driven, as evidenced by the construction and empirical investigation of models of adjustment and adherence (e.g., Thompson et al. 1992a, 1994; Quittner, Digirolamo et al., 1992), several authors have provided suggestions as to how to further advance the development of these models. First, future research should integrate conceptually similar models, as no one model has accounted for all of the variance in maternal or child adjustment (Thompson et al., 1994). For example, the risk and resistance model (Wallander, Varni, Babani, Banis, & Wilcox, 1989; Wallander, Varni, Babani, DeHaan, et al., 1989) might be appropriate, as it is not specific to any particular chronic illness, includes adaptational processes that are not included in the transactional stress and coping model, and thus may account for an additional proportion of the variance (Thompson et al., 1994). Bennett (1994), on the other hand, recommends a normative approach whereby factors implicated in healthy children are examined along with factors both common across disorders and unique to specific chronic illnesses. Any of these proposed models will require empirical validation via path analysis.

Again, psychosocial research in CF has been progressing, although psychologists must continue to advance the methodologies used and build the current knowledge base in order to keep pace with rapidly advancing medical technology and increasing life expectancy for patients with CF. Indeed, with the impact of new therapies (i.e., gene therapy) and continued aggressive treatment of the pulmonary and gastrointestinal complications, there is increasing optimism as to the prognosis for patients with CF (FitzSimmons, 1993).

REFERENCES

Bartholomew, L. K., Parcel, G. S., Seilheimer, D. K., Czyzewski, D. I., Spinelli, S. H., & Congdon, B. (1991). Development of a health education program to promote the self-management of cystic fibrosis. *Health Education Quarterly, 18,* 429–443.

Bartholomew, L. K., Parcel, G. S., Swank, P. R., & Czyzewski, D. I. (1993). Measuring self-efficacy expectations for the self-management of cystic fibrosis. *Chest, 103,* 1524–1530.

Bauer, M. L., McDougal, J., & Schoumacher, R. A. (1994). Comparison of manual and mechanical chest percussion in hospitalized patients with cystic fibrosis. *Journal of Pediatrics, 124,* 250–254.

Bennett, D. S. (1994). Depression among children with chronic medical problems: A meta-analysis. *Journal of Pediatric Psychology, 19,* 149–169.

Bowen, A. M., & Stark, L. J. (1991). Malnutrition in cystic fibrosis: A behavioral conceptualization of cause and treatment. *Clinical Psychology Review, 11,* 315–331.

Cappelli, M., McGrath, P. J., Heick, C. E., MacDonald, N. E., Feldman, W., & Rowe, P. (1989). Chronic disease and its impact: The adolescent's perspective. *Journal of Adolescent Health Care, 10,* 283–288.

Corey, M., McLaughlin, F. J., Williams, M., & Levison, H. (1988). A comparison of survival, growth, and pulmonary function in patients with cystic fibrosis in Boston and Toronto. *Journal of Clinical Epidemiology, 41,* 483–491.

Cowen, L., Corey, M., Keenan, N., Simmons, R., Arndt, E., & Levison, H. (1985). Family adaptation and psychosocial adjustment to cystic fibrosis in the preschool child. *Social Science Medicine, 20,* 553–560.

Cowen, L., Mok, J., Corey, M., McMillan, H., Simmons, R., & Levison, H. (1986). Psychologic adjustment of the family member who has cystic fibrosis. *Pediatrics, 77,* 745–753.

Cystic Fibrosis Foundation. (1980). *Report of the 1978 patient registry.* Rockville, MD: Author.

Delk, K. K., Gevirtz, R., Hicks, D. A., Carden, F., & Rucker, R. (1994). The effects of biofeedback assisted breathing retraining on lung functions in patients with cystic fibrosis. *Chest, 105,* 23–28.

Edlund, L. D., French, R. W., Herbst, J. J., Ruttenberg, H. D., Ruhling, R. O., & Adams, T. D. (1986). Effects of a swimming program on children with cystic fibrosis. *American Journal of Diseases of Children, 140,* 80–83.

Eigen, H., Clark, N. M., & Wolle, J. M. (1987). Clinical-behavioral aspects of cystic fibrosis: Directions for future research. *American Review of Respiratory Disease, 136,* 1509–1513.

FitzSimmons, S. C. (1993). The changing epidemiology of cystic fibrosis. *Journal of Pediatrics, 122,* 1–9.

Forehand, R. L., & McMahon, R. J. (1981). *Helping the noncompliant child: A clinician's guide to parent training.* New York: Guilford Press.

Geiss, S. K., Hobbs, S. A., Hammersley-Maercklein, G., Kramer, J. C., & Henley, M. (1992). Psychosocial factors related to perceived compliance with cystic fibrosis. *Journal of Clinical Psychology, 48,* 99–103.

Goldberg, S., Morris, P., Simmons, J., Fowler, R. S., & Levison, H. (1990). Chronic illness in infancy and parenting stress: A comparison of three groups of parents. *Journal of Pediatric Psychology, 15,* 347–358.

Goldberg, S., Washington, J., Morris, P., Fischer-Fay, A., & Simmons, R. J. (1990). Early diagnosed chronic illness in mother-child relationships in the first two years. *Canadian Journal of Psychiatry, 35,* 726–733.

Goldberg, S., Washington, J., Simmons, R. J., & MacClusky, I. (1992). Nutrition is more than calories: Infant-mother relationship and nutritional status in the first four years. *Pediatric Pulmonology, 11* (Suppl. 8), 321.

Gudas, L. J., Koocher, G. P., & Wypij, D. (1991). Perceptions of medical compliance in children and adolescents with cystic fibrosis. *Developmental and Behavioral Pediatrics, 12,* 236–242.

Henley, L. D., & Hill, I. D. (1990). Errors, gaps, and misconceptions in the disease-related knowledge of cystic fibrosis patients and their families. *Pediatrics, 85,* 1008–1014.

Hobbs, S. A., Geiss, S. K., Hammersley, G., Kramer, J. C., & Henley, M. (1985, March). *Compliance with cystic fibrosis treatment: Patient, parent, and physician reports.* Paper presented at the meeting of the Society of Behavioral Medicine, New Orleans, LA.

Hobbs, S. A., Stratton, R., Geiss, S. K., Kramer, J. C., & Ozturk, A. (1987, March). *Effects of programmed exercise on children with cystic fibrosis.* Paper presented at the meeting of the Society of Behavioral Medicine, Washington, DC.

Kashani, J. H., Barbero, G. J., Wilfley, D. E., Morris, D. A., & Shepperd, J. A. (1988). Psychological concomitants of CF in children and adolescents. *Adolescence, 23,* 873–880.

Kerem, B. S., Rommens, J. M., Buchanan, J. A., Mark-iewicz, D., Cox, T. K., Chakravarti, A., Buchwald, M., & Tsui, L. C. (1989). Identification of the cystic fibrosis gene: Genetic analysis. *Science, 245,* 1073–1080.

Koeppen, A. S. (1974). Relaxation training for children. *Elementary School Guidance Counseling, 9,* 14–21.

Koocher, G. P., McGrath, M. L., & Gudas, L. J. (1990). Typologies of nonadherence in cystic fibrosis. *Developmental and Behavioral Pediatrics, 11,* 353–358.

Kopelman, H. (1991). Gastrointestinal and nutritional aspects. *Thorax, 46,* 261–267.

LaGreca, A. M. (1990). Issues in adherence with pediatric regimens. *Journal of Pediatric Psychology, 15,* 423–436.

Lavigne, J. V., & Faier-Routman, J. (1992). Psychological adjustment to pediatric physical disorders: A meta-analytic review. *Journal of Pediatric Psychology, 17,* 133–157.

MacDonald, A., Holden, C., & Harris, G. (1991). Nutritional strategies in cystic fibrosis: Current issues. *Journal of the Royal Society of Medicine, 84* (Suppl. 18), 28–35.

Matthews, L. W., & Drotar, D. (1984). Cystic fibrosis: A challenging long-term chronic disease. *Pediatric Clinics of North America, 31,* 133–152.

McCracken, M. J., & Budd, J. (1992). A study of a self care intervention for adolescents with cystic fibrosis. *Pediatric Pulmonology, 11* (Suppl. 8), 322.

Mullins, L. L., Olsen, R. A., Reyes, S., Bernardy, N., Huszti, H. C., & Volk, R. J. (1991). Risk and resistance factors in the adaptation of mothers of children with cystic fibrosis. *Journal of Pediatric Psychology, 16,* 701–715.

Nagy, S., & Ungerer, J. A. (1990). The adaptation of mothers and fathers to children with cystic fibrosis: A comparison. *Children's Health Care, 19,* 147–154.

Oppenheimer, E. H., & Esterley, J. R. (1975). Pathology of cystic fibrosis: Review of the literature and comparison of 146 autopsied cases. *Perspectives in Pediatric Pathology, 2,* 241–278.

Orenstein, D., Franklin, B., Doershuk, C., Hellerstein, H., German, K., Horowitz, J., & Stern, R. (1981). Exercise conditioning and cardiopulmonary fitness in cystic fibrosis. *Chest, 80,* 392–398.

Passero, M. A., Remor, B., & Solomon, J. (1981). Patient-reported compliance with cystic fibrosis therapy. *Clinical Pediatrics, 20,* 264–268.

Patterson, J. M. (1985). Critical factors affecting family compliance with home treatment for children with cystic fibrosis. *Family Relations, 34,* 79–89.

Pearson, D. A., Pumariega, A. J., & Seilheimer, D. K. (1991). The development of psychiatric symptomatology in patients with cystic fibrosis. *Journal of the American Academy of Child and Adolescent Psychiatry, 30,* 290–297.

Pencharz, P., Hill, R., Archibald, E., Levy, L., & Newth, C. (1984). Energy needs and nutritional rehabilitation in undernourished adolescents and adults with cystic fibrosis. *Journal of Pediatric Gastroenterology and Nutrition, 3* (Suppl. 1), S147–S153.

Phillips, S., Bohannon, W. E., Gayton, W. F., & Friedman, S. B. (1985). Parent interview findings regarding the impact of cystic fibrosis on families. *Developmental and Behavioral Pediatrics, 6,* 122–127.

Quittner, A. L., DiGirolamo, A. M., Jacobsen, J., & Eigen, H. (1991). A contextual model of parenting problems and outcomes for newly diagnosed families. *Pediatric Pulmonology, 10* (Suppl. 6), 310.

Quittner, A. L., DiGirolamo, A. M., Michel, M., & Eigen, H. (1992). Parental response to cystic fibrosis: A contextual analysis of the diagnosis phase. *Journal of Pediatric Psychology, 17,* 683–704.

Quittner, A., DiGirolamo, A. M., & Regolio, M. J. (1993, April). *Developing a measure of problems faced by adolescents with cystic fibrosis: The situational analysis phase.* Paper presented at the meeting of the Florida Conference on Child Health Psychology, Gainesville, FL.

Quittner, A., & Opipari, L. C. (1994). Differential treatment of siblings: Interview and diary analyses comparing two family contexts. *Child Development, 65,* 800–814.

Quittner, A. L., Opipari, L. C., Regolio, M. J., Jacobsen, J., & Eigen, H. (1992). The impact of caregiving and role strain on family life: Comparisons between mothers of children with cystic fibrosis and matched controls. *Rehabilitation Psychology, 37,* 275–289.

Ramsey, B. W., Farrell, P. M., Pencharz, P., & the Consensus Committee. (1992). Nutritional assessment and management in cystic fibrosis: A consensus report. *American Journal of Clinical Nutrition, 55,* 108–116.

Riordan, J. R., Rommens, J. M., Kerem, B. S., Alon, N., Rozmahel, L., Grzelczak, Z., Zielenski, J., Lok, S., Plavsic, N., Chou, J. L., Drumm, M. L., Iannuzzi, M. C., Collins, F. S., & Tsui, L. C. (1989). Identification of the cystic fibrosis gene: Cloning and characterization of complementary DNA. *Science, 245,* 1066–1073.

Scanlin, T. (1988). Cystic fibrosis. In A. Fishman (Ed.), *Pulmonary diseases and disorders* (pp. 1273–1293). New York: McGraw-Hill.

Schultz, J. R., & Moser, A. (1992). Barriers to treatment adherence in cystic fibrosis. *Pediatric Pulmonology, 11* (Suppl. 8), 321.

Sherrill, C. (1976). *Adapted physical education and recreation.* Dubuque, IA: William C. Brown.

Simmons, R. J., Corey, M., Cowen, L., Keenan, N., Robertson, J., & Levison, H. (1985). Emotional adjustment of early adolescents with cystic fibrosis. *Psychosomatic Medicine, 47,* 111–122.

Simmons, R. J., Corey, M., Cowen, L., Keenan, N., Robertson, J., & Levison, H. (1987). Behavioral adjustment of latency-age children with cystic fibrosis. *Psychosomatic Medicine, 49,* 291–301.

Simmons, R., Goldberg, S., Washington, J., & MacClusky, I. (1991). Psychosocial development of children with CF. *Pediatric Pulmonology, 10* (Suppl. 6), 310.

Singer, L. T., Nofer, J. A., Benson-Szekely, L. J., & Brooks, L. J. (1991). Behavioral assessment and management of food refusal in children with cystic fibrosis. *Journal of Developmental and Behavioral Pediatrics, 12,* 115–120.

Spirito, A., Russo, D. C., & Masek, B. (1984). Behavioral interventions and stress management training for hospitalized adolescents and young adults with cystic fibrosis. *General Hospital Psychiatry, 6,* 351–357.

Stark, L. J., Bowen, A. M., Tyc, V. L., Evans, S., & Passero, M. A. (1990). A behavioral approach to increasing calorie consumption in children with cystic fibrosis. *Journal of Pediatric Psychology, 15,* 309–326.

Stark, L. J., Jelalian, E., & Miller, D. L. (in press). Cystic Fibrosis. In M. C. Roberts (Ed.), *Handbook of pediatric psychology* (2nd ed.). New York: Guilford Press.

Stark, L. J., Knapp, L., Bowen, A. M., Powers, S. W., Jelalian, E., Evans, S., Passero, M. A., Mulvihill, M. M., & Hovell, M. (1993). Behavioral treatment of calorie consumption in children with cystic fibrosis: Replication with two year follow-up. *Journal of Applied Behavior Analysis, 26,* 435–450.

Stark, L. J., Miller, S. T., Plienes, A. J., & Drabman, R. S. (1987). Behavioral contracting to increase chest physiotherapy: A study of a young cystic fibrosis patient. *Behavior Modification, 11,* 75–86.

Stark, L. J., Powers, S. W., Jelalian, E., Rape, R. N., & Miller, D. L. (1994). Modifying problematic mealtime interactions of children with cystic fibrosis and their parents via behavioral parent training. *Journal of Pediatric Psychology, 19,* 751–768.

Stark, L. J., Spirito, A., & Hobbs, S. A. (1990). The role of behavior therapy in cystic fibrosis. In A. M. Gross & R. S. Drabman (Eds.), *Handbook of clinical behavioral pediatrics* (pp. 253–265). New York: Plenum.

Steinkamp, G., & von der Hardt, H. (1994). Improvement of nutritional status and lung function after long term nocturnal gastrostomy feedings in cystic fibrosis. *Journal of Pediatrics, 124,* 244–249.

Thompson, R. J., Jr. (1985). Delineation of children's behavior problems: A basis for assessment and intervention. *Journal of Developmental and Behavioral Pediatrics, 6,* 37–50.

Thompson, R. J., Jr., Gustafson, K. E., George, L., & Spock, A. (1994). Change over a 12-month period in the psychological adjustment of children and adolescents with cystic fibrosis. *Journal of Pediatric Psychology, 19,* 189–203.

Thompson, R. J., Jr., Gustafson, K. E., Hamlett, K. W., & Spock, A. (1992a). Psychological adjustment of children with cystic fibrosis: The role of child cognitive processes and maternal adjustment. *Journal of Pediatric Psychology, 17,* 741–755.

Thompson, R. J., Jr., Gustafson, K. E., Hamlett, K. W., & Spock, A. (1992b). Stress, coping, and family functioning in the psychological adjustment of mothers of children and adolescents with cystic fibrosis. *Journal of Pediatric Psychology, 17,* 573–585.

Thompson, R. J., Gustafson, K. E., Meghdadpour, S., Harrell, E. S., Johndrow, D. A., & Spock, A. (1992). The role of biomedical and psychosocial processes in the intellectual and academic functioning of children and adolescents with cystic fibrosis. *Journal of Clinical Psychology, 48,* 3–10.

Thompson, R. J., Hodges, K., & Hamlett, K. W. (1990). A matched comparison of adjustment in children with cystic fibrosis and psychiatrically referred and nonreferred children. *Journal of Pediatric Psychology, 15,* 745–759.

Thompson, R. J., Jr., Merritt, K. A., Keith, B. R., Murphy, L. B., & Johndrow, D. A. (1993). Mother-child agreement on the Child Assessment Schedule with non-referred children: A research note. *Journal of Child Psychology and Psychiatry and Allied Disciplines, 34,* 813–820.

Tomezsko, J. L., Scanlin, T. F., & Stallings, V. A. (1994). Body composition of children with cystic fibrosis with mild clinical manifestations compared with normal children. *American Journal of Clinical Nutrition, 59,* 123–128.

Walker, L. S. (1991). Maternal distress, illness severity, and child adjustment in cystic fibrosis. *Pediatric Pulmonology, 10* (Suppl. 6), 105–106.

Walker, L. S., Ford, M. B., & Donald, W. D. (1987). Cystic fibrosis and family stress: Effects of age and severity of illness. *Pediatrics, 79,* 239–246.

Walker, L. S., Ortiz-Valdes, J. A., & Newbrough, J. R. (1989). The role of maternal employment and depression in the psychological adjustment of chronically ill, mentally retarded, and well children. *Journal of Pediatric Psychology, 14,* 357–370.

Wallander, J. L., Varni, J. W., Babani, L., Banis, H. T., & Wilcox, K. T. (1989). Family resources as resistance factors for psychological maladjustment in chronically ill and handicapped children. *Journal of Pediatric Psychology, 14,* 157–174.

Wallander, J. L., Varni, J. W., Babani, L., DeHaan, C. B., Wilcox, K. T., & Banis, H. T. (1989). The social environment and the adaptation of mothers of physically handicapped children. *Journal of Pediatric Psychology, 14,* 371–387.

Webb, A. K. (1991). Management problems of the adult with cystic fibrosis. *Schweiz Medical Wschr, 121,* 110–114.

CHAPTER 10

ASTHMA

Kathleen L. Lemanek, UNIVERSITY OF KANSAS
Sarah T. Trane, UNIVERSITY OF KANSAS
Ronald E. Weiner, UNIVERSITY OF KANSAS MEDICAL CENTER

Findings from numerous epidemiological investigations show that children and adolescents with a chronic illness and physical disability are at greater risk (threefold increase) of experiencing behavioral and social problems compared to healthy peers; children with only a chronic illness are at somewhat less risk (twofold increase) (Cadman, Boyle, Szatmari, & Offord, 1987; Gortmaker, Walker, Weitzman, & Sobol, 1990; Pless & Roghmann, 1971). However, while at risk, most children do not evidence adjustment problems. Even for those children who do exhibit difficulties in adjustment, the nature and intensity of these problems can be quite variable.

Complicating investigations regarding psychosocial adjustment of children with a chronic illness/disability are difficulties in defining and measuring the construct "adjustment" (Perrin, Ayoub, & Willett, 1993). In a broad sense, adjustment is a complex function of person factors, disease factors, and environmental context, represented by either a decrease in behavioral problems or an increase in competence. In fact, a shift in outcome measurement toward competence or resistance (versus psychopathology) has occurred in the field of pediatric psychology, reflecting

an interest in assessing the heterogeneity of responses to chronic illness/disability (Harper, 1991).

Literature on the psychological aspects of asthma, the most prevalent pediatric chronic condition, exemplifies this variability of adjustment in children, adolescents, and their families. A transactional or biopsychosocial model has helped organize and integrate medical and psychological data about asthma (Creer, Stein, Rappaport, & Lewis, 1992; Miller & Wood, 1991). According to this model, a somatic predisposition in the child may interact with varying psychologic and social variables to govern the clinical nature and morbidity of asthma.

Reflecting this model's multicomponent focus, this chapter surveys literature on specific influences of children, their families, school settings, and physiological aspects of asthma. In the medical domain section, the etiology, clinical symptomatology, and treatment approaches for asthma are discussed. The psychological domain section reviews adaptation in various areas of functioning, including emotional/behavioral functioning, peer and family relationships, academic achievement, and self-management and medical compliance. This chapter concludes with recommendations for future research and practice within both the medical and psychological domains.

MEDICAL DOMAIN

A practical definition of *asthma* is the obstruction, inflammation, and hyperreactivity of airways. Together, these factors lead to breathing difficulties manifested by coughing, wheezing, or shortness of breath. Asthma occurs in approximately 8 to 10 percent of children; is a foremost cause of missed school days, urgent medical visits, and hospitalizations; and frequently leads to restrictions in daily activities if not aggressively treated.

Etiology

Predisposing factors for the development of asthma primarily include heredity and the environment. The risk of inheriting an atopic disease (i.e., asthma, hay fever/allergic rhinitis, eczema/atopic dermatitis) is 50 percent when one parent has such a disease and 60 percent when both parents do. Asthma occurs more frequently in African Americans and less frequently in Native Americans than in the general population. Although more males develop asthma before the age of 10, females outnumber males after this age.

Environmental factors associated with a higher prevalence of asthma include urban locations, certain countries (e.g., 20 percent in New Zealand versus 3 percent in Japan), a large amount of indoor allergens (e.g., dust mite, animal danders), and tobacco smoke exposure in the home (i.e., two to four times increase in prevalence). Smoke exposure also relates to a decreasing probability of having a diminution in the severity and frequency of asthma symptoms as a child progresses through adolescence.

Clinical Symptomatology

Sensitive/hyperreactive airways in patients with asthma react to various triggers that may exacerbate the obstruction (narrowing/blocking) and inflammation (swelling and excess mucus secretion) in the bronchioles. Besides smoke, another nearly universal irritant is cold air, and essentially all patients with asthma will experience an exacerbation of symptoms

with viral respiratory infections (the "common cold"); in individuals with asthma, such exacerbations are often incorrectly diagnosed as bronchitis and inappropriately treated with antibiotics rather than more aggressive asthma therapy. Among most patients with asthma, strenuous exercise will trigger an increase in symptoms, but prevention of this reaction is almost always possible, thereby allowing for full participation in sports and other activities. For the majority of children, inhaling specific allergens—such as pollens, dust mites, airborne molds, or animal danders—will exacerbate their asthma.

Asthma exacerbations lead to airway narrowing by constriction of the smooth muscle surrounding the bronchioles (bronchoconstriction—much like the tightening of rubber bands). Inflammation results in further obstruction as the airway membranes swell and secrete excess mucus. Children may first experience mild symptoms, including coughing with laughing, crying, running, or on exposure to cold air; possibly feel chest tightness; and typically have diminished endurance for strenuous activities. These symptoms may progress to wheezing (i.e., squeaking or whistling noises as air moves through the narrowed airways). However, many patients with asthma rarely, if ever, experience wheezing, which is one reason patients who truly do have asthma frequently receive alternative diagnoses.

Shortness of breath can progress to labored breathing manifested by an increased respiratory rate and use of the accessory muscles to assist in getting more air into the chest. For example, infants' and toddlers' skin will suck in between their ribs/retractions, and older children may utilize the strap muscles in the neck to help expand their chests. In the most severe episodes of asthma, cyanosis (i.e., blue skin color from lack of oxygen) may occur, and further progression can result in respiratory arrest and death.

In 1988, there were 4,580 asthma deaths in the United States, nearly all of which might have been prevented had earlier/more aggressive treatment been received. Of those patients who died, the most common variables related to death included poor communication between children, their parents, and their physicians, as well as feelings of anger and despair about their asthma, subsequently leading to poor compliance with recommended preventive therapy.

Many children with asthma limit themselves by avoiding activities that exacerbate their symptoms or in which they have previously felt discomfort or had their success limited by their asthma. Parents, teachers, and coaches often restrict participation in strenuous activities to avoid triggering the asthma, possibly diminishing the self-esteem of some children with asthma and causing feelings of being fragile and different from one's peers. Aggressive preventive therapy can eliminate nearly all of these restrictions, as proven by the fact that 15 percent of recent Olympic medalists from the United States have asthma.

Treatment Approaches

There are two types of asthma medications in common usage: bronchodilators and antiinflammatory medicines. Bronchodilators (e.g., albuterol, metaproterenol) are adrenaline-like drugs that relax the constriction of smooth muscle surrounding the airways. Antiinflammatory medicines lessen airway hyperreactivity (e.g., cromolyn, nedocromil) and the swelling and mucus secretions of airway membranes (steroids—do not confuse these medications with the testosterone-like anabolic steroids used illegally by some athletes). Recommended delivery of these medications is via an inhaled route whenever possible, allowing use of the lowest dosage with the least potential for side effects. Careful education is necessary for appropriate use of metered-dose inhalers and a spacer device (i.e., a chamber between the mouth and the inhaler) to ensure that optimal amounts of appropriately sized particles reach the airways.

Bronchodilators can be useful prior to exercise and as needed up to every four hours for coughing, wheezing, or shortness of breath. The only common side effects of use of an inhaler in recommended doses include mild, transient tremor and tachycardia (i.e., increased heart rate). Patients must contact their physicians if this medication does not relieve symptoms for at least four hours, because this situation is an indication of the need for urgent evaluation and/or initiation of aggressive antiinflammatory therapy; simply using a bronchodilator more frequently without further intervention could lead to a life-threatening situation. Theophylline is a less efficacious bronchodilator

administered in a pill or syrup. It has much more potential for side effects, including restlessness, nausea, headaches, and, at excessive doses, seizures.

Antiinflammatory medications may serve as daily preventive therapy and have little potential for side effects when inhaled at recommended doses. Use of these medications lessens the frequency of symptoms that would otherwise require more recurrent administration of bronchodilators. Patients can take cromolyn or nedocromil daily and/or prior to exposures likely to trigger their asthma (e.g., exercise, allergen, cold air).

Inhaled steroids (e.g., beclomethasone, triamcinolone), given at daily low doses and increased for periods of time, can lessen airway inflammation. Oral steroids (e.g., prednisone, prednisolone) may be necessary during exacerbations of asthma that do not adequately resolve with inhaled medications (e.g., viral infection/"chest cold" causing increased airway inflammation). Physicians will typically prescribe oral steroids for a 5- to 10-day "burst," with significant side effects potentially occurring only if taken for more than two weeks.

General principles regarding use of asthma medications entails extensive and repeated education about mechanisms of action and potential side effects of each medication, optimal utilization of inhalers, a clear understanding of how to adjust medications at home, and awareness of when to contact one's physician or seek urgent evaluation and treatment. A peak flow meter, which measures airflow, can objectively assess the status of one's asthma and aid in knowing when to adjust medications and/or seek further intervention (i.e., a 20 to 50 percent decrease below typical peak flow). It is important for all prescribed medications to follow a reasonable schedule so as not to interfere with daily activities.

Reasonable avoidance of the triggers for one's asthma, except exercise, can be very helpful and will allow children to manage their asthma with minimal medication. Strict elimination of tobacco smoke from the home and receipt of an annual immunization in the fall to prevent influenza in the winter are standard recommendations for patients with asthma. Having air-conditioning, changing filters frequently, and avoiding the use of attic fans will benefit those patients with positive allergy tests for pollens or molds. Lowering humidity levels will help control dust mite and mold allergies; as such, patients with asthma might consider completely avoiding humidifiers and using a dehumidifier from spring through fall. Eliminating bedroom carpeting helps manage dust mite allergy and, ideally, pets should be removed from homes where residents have allergies to pet dander.

When avoidance precautions and medications are inadequate for strong allergies, immunotherapy, allergy shots, can be very helpful to lessen allergic sensitivity. A text by Kaliner, Barnes, and Persson (1991) and a publication by the National Institute of Health (National Asthma Education Program, 1991) on the diagnosis and management of asthma provide additional information about physiological aspects of asthma and current medical care.

PSYCHOLOGICAL DOMAIN

Past research on psychological adaptation of children and adolescents with asthma has emphasized the psychosomatic nature of the illness, with reference to an emotional predisposition and disease-specific personality characteristics (Creer et al., 1992; Perrin & MacLean, 1988). Recent investigations have moved away from this classification and have focused on tasks and challenges that may interfere with normal growth and development in physical, personal-social, and cognitive domains (Drotar & Bush, 1985; Miller & Wood, 1991; Perrin & MacLean, 1988). Specifically, such issues as physical and emotional sequelae of asthma and its treatment, the impact of asthma on family members, social and academic influences of school settings, and education about asthma and its management have been the focus of attention in these studies. In addition, investigators have indicated the importance of examining reciprocal interactions between these factors in terms of how they either hinder progress or produce a successful balance between emotional, behavioral, and cognitive tasks associated with normal development and asthma-related responsibilities and the abilities to manage these tasks (e.g., Miller & Wood, 1991; Patterson & Geber, 1991).

This section reviews research on psychological adaptation of children and adolescents with asthma regarding individual adjustment, peer and family relationships, school functioning, and medical management.

Psychological Adaptation

Emotional/Behavioral Problems

Studies evaluating the presence of emotional/behavioral problems in children and adolescents with asthma have employed a variety of research strategies. A recent meta-analysis (Bennett, 1994) of 60 studies of children with a chronic illness found an increased risk for depressive symptoms at a rate almost twice that seen among children in the general community. Maternal reports have also consistently indicated internalizing and externalizing problem behaviors at a rate more than twice that of the normative group (Cadman et al., 1987; Hambley, Brazil, Furrow, & Chua, 1989; MacLean, Perrin, Gortmaker, & Pierre, 1992), especially for children and adolescents requiring inpatient treatment for asthma (Furrow, Hambley, & Brazil, 1989).

For example, in the study by Furrow and associates (1989), parents of 16 girls and 32 boys (aged 6 to 16 years) rated the behavior of their children using the Child Behavior Checklist (CBCL; Achenbach & Edelbrock, 1983). Each of the Internalizing, Externalizing, and Total behavior problem T-scores of the children with asthma were significantly higher than the T-scores for the normative group of clinically nonreferred children, with the exception of externalizing behaviors among girls aged 6 to 11. The authors noted, however, that elevations in behavior problems among children with severe asthma does not suggest that all children and adolescents with asthma have behavioral problems; rather, these findings are consistent with previous research demonstrating a higher association between behavior problems and severe asthma requiring hospitalization.

A study by Biederman, Milberger, Faraone, Guite, and Warburton (1994) also indicated the need for greater specificity when identifying behavior problems among children with any chronic illness. In this study, the authors compared rates of asthma among 260 children and adolescents, ages 6 to 17, with and without Attention-Deficit Hyperactivity Disorder (ADHD) and their first-degree biological relatives. The investigators used psychiatric interviews and parent-completed questionnaires to arrive at diagnoses of ADHD and asthma. Results indicated that the rate of asthma among children with ADHD was not significantly different than among children without ADHD. The authors concluded that children and adolescents with ADHD in general were not at higher risk for asthma and that genetically transmitted ADHD and asthma are independent of each other and have separate etiologies.

Anxiety and depression are the two problems most often identified among children and adolescents with asthma who do evidence problems; both problems may trigger asthma symptoms. Depressive symptomatology is most common, with a mean effect size of 0.54 (Bennett, 1994). Biederman and colleagues (1994) found that relatives of children and adolescents with ADHD and asthma were at twice the risk of developing some type of anxiety disorder compared to relatives of children and adolescents with ADHD alone, and that relatives of children with asthma in general were also at twice the risk for multiple anxiety disorders compared to the general population.

Other studies have revealed elevated rates of separation anxiety, overanxious disorder, obsessive compulsive disorder, and depression among children with asthma as compared to their healthy peers (e.g., Bussing & Burket, 1993; Gizynski & Shapiro, 1990; Mascia et al., 1989). In their examination of 155 children with mild to moderate asthma (aged 7 to 12), Butz and Alexander (1993) assessed anxiety levels of children and their parents three to five days following the child's treatment in a pediatric emergency ward for an acute asthma attack. They found that mothers' ratings of both state and trait anxiety were significantly higher than their children's ratings; mothers' ratings also correlated with age of diagnosis of asthma. The authors suggested that the longer course and increased duration of stress experienced by mothers may have accounted for this finding.

Interestingly, the best predictors of children's state anxiety levels were their feelings of being "upset" at the beginning of an attack and their having experienced one or more asthma attacks in the previous 12 months. In contrast, predictors of their trait anxiety levels were feelings of panic, rate of attacks as reported by their mothers, and state anxiety scores. Butz and Alexander (1993) concluded that health care providers need to be aware of both child and maternal levels of anxiety in order to be effective in working with families of children with asthma or other chronic illness groups.

Another area of potential concern involves children's and adolescent's levels of self-esteem and their self-concepts. Published research to date is contradictory. Although some studies have shown lower levels of self-esteem and higher self-reports of depression among adolescents with asthma compared to adolescents without asthma (Hambley et al., 1989; Nelms, 1989; Seigel, Golden, Gough, Lashley, & Sacker, 1990), more evidence exists that there are no differences in self-concept between children and adolescents with asthma and their healthy peers or siblings (Christiaanse, Lavigne, & Lerner, 1989; Kashani, Konig, Sheppard, Wilfley, & Morris, 1988; Townsend et al., 1991; Vazquez, Fontan-Bueso, & Buceta, 1992).

In particular, both Vazquez and colleagues (1992) and Christiaanse and colleagues (1989) found that children with mild to moderate asthma rated their competence the same as healthy peers in most areas assessed by the Self-Perception Profile for Children (Harter, 1985). Only their self-ratings of athletic competence were slightly, but not significantly, lower than their peers.

In summary, there is a significant proportion of children and adolescents with asthma who experience emotional/behavioral difficulties regardless of the severity of their illness. Although some of these difficulties are externalizing in nature (e.g., aggressive, noncompliant), children and adolescents with asthma are more vulnerable to internalizing problems (e.g., depression, anxiety). Bennett (1994) suggested that research on psychosocial adaptation of children with asthma should increase its focus on the role of processes other than specific illness variables, which include life stress and family interactions and their relationships to asthma. On the other hand, it appears that children with asthma are similar to their peers in self-perceptions and self-esteem and do not necessarily feel different or limited because of their illness. Vazquez and associates (1992) proposed that children's self-perceptions are a stable trait, not easily influenced by the effects of asthma.

Peer Relationships

There has been limited research on peer relationships among children with asthma. In general, research on peer relationships and social competence among children with chronic illnesses suggests that the quality of peer relationships is the same for ill and healthy children, with the exception of those diseases that result in changes in physical appearance or restriction of activities (e.g., asthma) (Spirito, DeLawyer, & Stark, 1991). Given that children with asthma experience more psychological difficulties than healthy children (Cadman et al., 1987), one might assume that these children also show increased problems relating to their peers or are at risk for peer rejection. However, there has been little empirical research examining specific similarities and differences among peer relations between children with asthma and their healthy peers.

Eiser, Havermans, Pancer, and Eiser (1992) found that parents of 273 children (mean age = 9.4 years) with various chronic illnesses (i.e., asthma, diabetes, cardiac disease, leukemia, and epilepsy) who perceived their children's activities as restricted due to their illness had poorer adjustment, particularly with peer relationships. Schwam (1987) provided clinical suggestions for working with children with asthma, including the importance of improving social skills and planning time with peers because school absences may affect children's peer relationships. Schwam, however, offered no empirical support for these suggestions. Clearly, this area is in need of further research.

Spirito and associates (1991) outlined common weaknesses in studies on peers and offered several suggestions for future research on peer relations among children with chronic illnesses. Weaknesses in past research have included lack of an appropriate control group, variation in defining asthma severity and other subject characteristics, and use of indirect methods to assess peer relationships (e.g., global constructs of social adjustment rather than those specific to peers). They suggested that future research needs to clarify characteristics of children with asthma by taking a developmental perspective, specifying the impact of the disease on daily functioning rather than severity, and accounting for the course and prognosis of the disease and for family characteristics known to affect children's adjustment.

Family Relationships

Another significant factor in children's adjustment to asthma is their family environments, particularly their relationships with their parents. This relationship is bidirectional: How parents respond to their children's symptoms has effects on how their children in turn will be able to adapt to having the illness. Peri, Molinari, and Taverna (1991) described how an entire family may often get involved with the health of one member and how family members can become the health care provider's largest ally or enemy.

Recently, there has been an increased effort to examine factors that contribute to adjustment within families of children with asthma. Several studies have demonstrated that parental reports of family conflict and increased parenting stress predict heightened difficulties with both externalizing and internalizing child behaviors in children with asthma (Bussing & Burket, 1993; Hamlett, Pellegrini, & Katz, 1992). Parents of children with asthma have also typically reported increased levels of anxiety (Peri et al., 1991) and lower perceived support from friends and neighbors than parents of healthy children (Carson & Schauer, 1992; Peri et al., 1991).

Most of the research to assess family relationships has utilized mothers of children with asthma, with a recurrent theme of mothers' overprotective behaviors and poor communication within the family (Bussing & Burket, 1993; diBlasio, Molinari, Peri, & Taverna, 1990; Morey & Jones, 1993; Schobinger, Florin, Reichbauer, Lindemann, & Zimmer, 1993). For example, Carson and Schauer (1992) found that mothers of 41 children with asthma (aged 8 to 13 years) were more rejecting, overprotective, and overindulgent, as rated by mothers on the Mother-Child Relationship Evaluation (Roth, 1980, as cited in Carson & Schauer). These mothers also reported experiencing more stress from their children than mothers in the normative sample on a measure of parenting stress.

Two interesting prospective studies have examined dyadic adjustment in families with young children at genetic risk for developing asthma (Askildsen, Watten, & Faleide, 1993; Klinnert, Gavin, Wamboldt, & Mirazek, 1992). Klinnert and colleagues (1992) reported that parents experienced linear declines in dyadic adjustment after the birth of their child through the first 18 months, with parents' reports describing increased burden and additive stress. The authors hypothesized that parents' perceptions of increased stress led to disruptions in family cohesiveness and difficulty maintaining communication.

Although Askildsen and associates (1993) did not find any between-group differences of parents with children at risk for asthma versus parents of low-risk children, they noted there were large within-group differences, with parents of children who later developed asthma evidencing very high agreement on dyadic adjustment during their children's infancies. Parents of children with asthma reported that their children caused less disruption in time available for themselves or for the rest of their family members relative to reports given by parents of children without asthma. The authors described these parents of children with asthma as "ambitious" and "invading" because they tended to guide parent/child interactions rather than being receptive to cues provided by their children. The behavior exhibited by the parents of children with asthma are similar to behaviors later seen among parents who are overprotective and overly cautious with their children.

Families are a primary source of social interactions for children. Several studies have begun to outline the influence of family functioning on children's and adolescents' adaptations to asthma, with the majority of studies noting increased levels of generalized anxiety and overprotectiveness among parents and subsequent difficulties in the family members with asthma. Researchers have seldom conducted studies assessing the perspective of perceived support from family members in children with asthma, and there exists only limited research on interactions and adjustment.

Although there has been an increase in research on families of children with asthma and other chronic illnesses, additional in-depth examinations are necessary. Such research might help determine the mediating role of family and other social interactions, including peers and siblings, and to lead to an increase in efficacy of interventions with families and children who are in distress.

School Adaptation

School settings are influential in fostering adequate intellectual and academic development in children and adolescents with asthma (Miller & Wood, 1991). Literature on school adaptation has thus far centered on school absentee rates or the possible effects of theophylline on learning and behavior (Fowler, Dav-

enport, & Garg, 1992). A few studies have, however, examined academic performance and effects of other medications used in the treatment of asthma (e.g., corticosteroids) (e.g., Bender, Lerner, & Kollasch, 1988; Gutstadt et al., 1989). Unfortunately, differences in methodology, such as varying assessment measures and duration of past and current therapy, have resulted in conflicting results (Celano & Geller, 1993; Weinberger, Lindgren, Bender, Lerner, & Szefler, 1987).

This section surveys research on academic performance, school attendance rates, and effects of medications on learning in children and adolescents with asthma.

Academic Performance

Studies directly assessing academic performance of children and adolescents with asthma have been minimal. Hypothesized attributions for deficient academic performance among children with asthma have included increased absenteeism; adverse effects of asthma medications; variability in frequency, duration, and intensity of asthma attacks; and general stress related to a chronic illness (Celano & Geller, 1993). However, available data indicate that children and adolescents with asthma do not evidence deficiencies in academic performance when compared to children in a control group (McLoughlin et al., 1983) or standardized tests of intelligence and academic achievement (Gutstadt et al., 1989; Lindgren et al., 1992).

For example, Gutstadt and associates (1989) studied cognitive functioning and academic achievement in 99 children (9 to 17 years old) with moderately severe to severe asthma referred for evaluation and rehabilitation. Intelligence test scores and standardized achievement scores in reading and mathematics were average to above average in this group. Results of stepwise regression analysis revealed that low socioeconomic status (SES), older age, history of oral steroid use, and greater emotional/behavioral problems were related to low school performance. Severity of asthma and medications used to treat asthma (e.g., theophylline, B-agonists), however, did not relate to performance.

Fowler and colleagues (1992) examined data from the 1988 U.S. National Health Interview Survey on Child Health and subsequently provided national estimates of school outcome (i.e., grade failure, learning disabilities, and suspension/expulsions) and absences in children with various pediatric chronic illnesses. Their data indicated that children with asthma were at moderate risk of academic problems in terms of learning disabilities compared to children without asthma. Low income also significantly related to a higher risk of grade failure. In contrast to Gutstadtand and colleagues (1989), health status interacted with academic performance, with children in fair or poor health evidencing twice the risk of learning disabilities compared to those in good condition. These studies highlight the influence of factors other than a diagnosis of asthma on children's and adolescent's academic performance.

School Attendance Rates

Objective data and reports from families and schools indicate that asthma is responsible for a majority of school days missed in children and adolescents (Fowler et al., 1992; Freudenberg et al., 1980; Parcel, Gilman, Nader, & Bunce, 1979). For instance, in the study by Fowler and associates (1992), the mean number of days absent in the previous 12 months for children with asthma was 7.6 days compared to 2.5 days for well children; children in fair or poor health averaged 17.4 days absent versus 6.7 days for those in good condition. However, the relationship between academic performance, school absenteeism, and illness variables is less clear due to differences in definitions of asthma severity, assessment methodology used to compute absence rates, and sets of predictor variables entered (Celano & Geller, 1993).

Gutstadt and associates (1989) found that school absenteeism did not correlate with other medical and psychological variables, including age of onset, oral steroid dosage/use, SES, emotional/behavioral problems, or performance on standardized tests of achievement. These authors proposed that children with asthma who frequently miss school can succeed if they demonstrate psychological adaptation. On the other hand, Fowler and associates (1992) showed that children with asthma who missed 16 or more days from school were at increased risk for grade failures and suspensions, and those who missed 11 or more days were at risk for learning disabilities.

It seems, therefore, that a threshold exists at which point school absenteeism negatively affects academic performance. As with other chronic illnesses,

school absences of children with asthma is a complex function of physiological, psychological, and social variables that are specific to each child.

Effects of Medications

There have been numerous studies regarding effects of theophylline on the central nervous system and on the behavior of children and adolescents with asthma. Summaries of the results of these studies, as well as their strengths and weaknesses, appear in reviews by Creer and colleagues (e.g., Creer & Gustafson, 1989) and Weinberger and associates (Weinberger et al., 1987). The combination of strengths (e.g., adequate experimental designs, application of standardized assessment measures or recommended neuropsychological tests) and weaknesses (e.g., subjects differed in time on/off theophylline and in severity of asthma, confounds present regarding medication compliance and lack of restrictions on xanthine-containing foods) of these studies led to the conclusion that data on the effects of theophylline on the learning and behavior of children with asthma is preliminary, ambiguous, and contradictory.

To illustrate some of the methodological differences, Rappaport and colleagues (1989) employed a double-blind cross-over design to compare parent and teacher reports of behavior, child reports of anxiety, and performance on a variety of neuropsychological tests in 17 children (aged 6 to 12 years) with mild asthma, who were intermittent theophylline users. No significant worsening was found on measures of performance (assessing attention, memory, and fine-motor skills) or behavior during the induction phase of theophylline compared to the placebo phase. Limitations of this study include assessment of drug effects over only a 3½ day period for each drug and the wide range of compliance to theophylline (i.e., from below therapeutic levels to high levels).

Rachelefsky and associates (1986) found no differences on parent questionnaires or psychological tests in a double-blind, placebo-controlled study with 20 children (aged 6 to 12 years) with mild asthma who had not received oral bronchodilators for at least six months. A four-week theophylline or placebo period, conducted with compliance and therapeutic levels maintained throughout the study, revealed adverse effects in terms of teacher-reported decreased attention and increased activity levels on initiation of treatment. Unfortunately, the authors did not administer any direct measures of academic achievement, and repeated blood drawings (i.e., every three days) only during the theophylline phase of treatment may have negated the double-blind nature of the study (Celano & Geller, 1993; Weinberger et al., 1987).

Schlieper, Alcock, Beaudry, Feldman, and Leikin (1991) used a double-blind, randomized, cross-over design with 31 children (aged 8 to 12 years) with moderate asthma to assess effects of theophylline on behavior, cognitive processing, and mood. The authors of this study instituted restrictions to xanthine-containing foods and beverages and ensured that children maintained therapeutic levels of theophylline. Dependent measures, administered while children were on theophylline/placebo or placebo/theophylline for 10 days with a 2-day wash-out period, identified no significant drug effects on parent-reported attention or activity level, self-reported mood (i.e., depression and anxiety), or cognitive processing (i.e., memory and attention). However, there were individual variations in response to theophylline.

In one of the few studies investigating long-term effects of theophylline, Bender, Lerner, Ikle, Comer, and Szefler (1991) compared performance of children with mild to moderate asthma who were receiving theophylline to those not on the medication and to those without asthma on tests of cognitive processing, behavior, and mood over a six-month period. Families were not blind to treatment condition due to concerns about length of the study. Results revealed that children receiving theophylline evidenced improved scores on laboratory measures of attention but increased behavior problems relative to predrug assessment as reported by parents (i.e., conduct problems and hyperactivity); the authors interpreted these results as indicative of only subtle effects of theophylline.

Based on these studies, there can be no definitive conclusions at this time regarding effects of theophylline on learning or behavior. It appears that individual susceptibility to theophylline may account for some of the inconsistencies in the literature (Celano & Geller, 1993). However, theophylline should still be considered a treatment option when adverse effects are not evident for individual patients (Celano & Geller, 1993; Moffitt & Moffitt, 1989).

Several investigators have examined continuous oral steroid use in relationship to cognitive performance (Suess, Stump, Chai, & Kalisker, 1986), academic performance (e.g., Gutstadt et al., 1989), and mood (e.g., Bender et al., 1988). For example, Suess and associates (1986) compared performance of 120 hospitalized children between the ages of 9 and 18 years old who comprised three groups: those with asthma and receiving theophylline, those with asthma and on both theophylline and steroids, and those without asthma. Findings revealed impaired performance on tests of visual retention and paired associate learning in those children who received both theophylline and steroids when tested 6 to 8 hours postmedication. There were no differences in performance between any of the groups when tested at 22 to 24 hours or 46 to 48 hours postmedication. Although considered a well-controlled study, possible confounds include the wide range in IQ scores achieved by the children (i.e., 84 to 136) and the interaction of theophylline and steroids.

Lindgren and associates (1992) compared academic performance of 25 children with asthma receiving inhaled steroids to their siblings. The researchers found the mean composite achievement scores on the Iowa Testing Program were not significantly different between the two groups. Bender and colleagues (1988) investigated both cognitive and affective processes in 27 inpatients with severe asthma (ages 8 to 16 years old) at high steroid levels (i.e., 61.5 mg/day) and at low steroid levels (i.e., 3.33 mg/day). The authors followed methodological controls to assess attention, impulsivity, hyperactivity, motor control, verbal memory, and mood (i.e., depression and anxiety), as well as lung function and theophylline levels. Results indicated that children on high doses of steroids, compared to those on low doses, evidenced problems with depression, anxiety, and long-term recall of information. There was no association between the psychological variables and asthma severity or theophylline level, suggesting to the authors that steroid use only accounted for previous differences. The authors also proposed that their findings, as well as those of Suess and colleagues (1986), reflect subtle memory deficits that are statistically but not clinically significant. However, Gutstadt and colleagues (1989) suggested that the absence of correlations between academic performance and current dosage and days on and off steroids found in their study implicate cumulative effects of steroids on learning.

As seen from this review, studies have revealed conflicting findings, possibly due to flaws in the studies, such as inadequate sample sizes, influence of attention on memory, and the interaction between different medications (Bender et al., 1988). Overall, subtle effects on memory and mood seem to be evident but dose dependent (Celano & Geller, 1993).

In general, the academic performance of children and adolescents with asthma appears to be similar to that of children and adolescents without asthma. Although factors other than asthma itself may account for any detected academic differences, parents' concerns about school problems, especially in children with a long history of asthma and continuous use of steroids, should not be discounted. Researchers need to continue to conduct studies evaluating relationships between academic performance (using standardized tests) and various illness variables (e.g., severity).

Effects of school absenteeism also seem minimal, with the exceptions being children with a history of psychological difficulties and those from low income families. Influences of theophylline and corticosteroids on the learning and behavior of children and adolescents with asthma are not clear because of methodological differences and flaws in available studies as well as the complex nature of the interaction between physiological and psychological factors. Due to the documented variability in responding to these drugs, there exists a need for investigations into the presence of possible deficits in attention/memory and elevated depression and anxiety symptomatology. Future studies need to involve direct observations of classroom performance and behavior, utilize diagnostic tests that are suited to detecting pharmacologic effects, and focus on determining qualities of children and adolescents who are sensitive to the effects of theophylline or caffeine through, for example, xanthine-challenge tests (Schlieper et al., 1991; Weinberger et al., 1987).

Medical Adaptation

Adaptation to a chronic illness, such as asthma, involves achieving an optimal equilibrium between disease management and quality of life (Miller & Wood,

1991). Successful disease management consists of not only educating children and families about physiological aspects of asthma and its treatment but also complying to a therapeutic regimen.

This section describes features of self-management programs for asthma and studies evaluating their effectiveness, and issues related to compliance and medical management.

Self-Management

Evans and Mellins (1991) delineated obstacles to successful disease management. They cited data indicating that parents and children lack crucial information, skills, and certainty in implementing treatments at home (Clark et al., 1980). For example, some family members reported difficulties recognizing symptoms of asthma or determining whether emergency care is necessary. Families also express problems conversing with physicians and school personnel about asthma (Freudenberg et al., 1980). Specifically, many family members view physicians as too busy or disinclined to discuss difficulties treating asthma at home, and school staff are not fully cooperative in following medication and physical activity guidelines (Clark et al., 1980).

Lewis and Lewis (1990) also described problems similar to those delineated by Clark and associates in terms of the distribution of self-management programs. Their research demonstrated that the fear of loss of control by parents, physicians' reluctance to share power with adult and child patients, and lack of trust in children's decision-making skills are major obstacles in increasing children's self-care skills.

Even in the presence of these obstacles, clinical researchers have developed numerous self-management programs for childhood asthma. Wigal, Creer, Kotses, and Lewis (1990) and Creer, Wigal, Kotses, and Lewis (1990) have reviewed and critiqued 19 educational and self-management programs developed since the 1970s. These programs have emphasized education of children and families regarding various medical and psychological aspects of asthma and its management due to the increasing number of deaths (for unknown reasons) in children and adolescents with asthma during the past 5 to 10 years. The burden of asthma on the family's income (i.e., 33 to 35 percent of annual income) is also emphasized.

Reflecting the diversity of available self-management programs, examples include Asthma Care Training (A.C.T.) for Kids (Lewis, Rachelefsky, & Lewis, 1981) and Open Airways (Feldman & Clark, 1981), suitable for outpatient and hospital clinics; Camp Wheeze, a summer camp program (Blessing-Moore, Landon, Miya, & Berman, 1981); Sunair, a residential treatment program (Richards, Church, Roberts, Newman, & Garon, 1981); Teaching My Parents/Myself about Asthma, a school-based education program (Parcel, Nader, & Tiernan, 1980); and Asthma Command, an interactive computer game (Rubin et al., 1986).

Evans and Mellins (1991) listed common elements of asthma self-management programs.

1. Families receive opportunities to learn new information, gain and rehearse skills, and discuss application of these skills at home.
2. Topics covered by programs are similar and consist of physiological mechanisms underlying asthma, identification of symptoms and triggers, management of symptoms and attacks, and adjustment to living with asthma.
3. Families obtain encouragement to become active participants, along with their physicians, in their children's asthma care.
4. Increasing compliance with medical regimens and coping with asthma-related problems at home and in school are goals of the programs.

Although these programs offer many similar features, they do differ with respect to several other aspects (Evans & Mellins, 1991; Lemanek, 1990). For instance, most programs focus on school-age children and their parents, but one program does exist for pre-school-age children (Mesters, Meertens, Crebolder, & Parcel, 1993). Programs have also tended to be for use mainly in private medical offices, outpatient clinics, hospitals, and, to a lesser extent, schools and community settings. Teaching sessions have typically been in a group format, but the length of each session differs (between 1/2 to 2 hours) as does the total number of sessions (four to eight). Although programs have focused on mild to severe asthma in educational sessions, few have really targeted difficult to control asthma. Finally, leaders of educational sessions have represented various disciplines, such as medicine, nursing, psychology, health education, and social work.

Researchers have obtained positive outcomes on select medical and psychological variables following participation in self-management programs; such variables include decreases in number of emergency room visits, hospitalizations, and days spent in the hospital; fewer school days missed; increased knowledge about asthma; and improved asthma-management behaviors (e.g., symptom discrimination, appropriate use of medications). However, the evidence regarding increases in knowledge is less straightforward.

Perrin, MacLean, Gortmaker, and Asher (1992) found a linear relationship between knowledge and daily activities, but Rubin, Bauman, and Lauby (1989) revealed a nonlinear relationship between knowledge and management behaviors. A threshold effect seemed to be operating in that knowledge evidenced less of a relationship with behavior after patients had obtained a certain level of information. Differences in knowledge questionnaires and the specific asthma behaviors examined could have accounted for the discrepancy between these studies.

Individual studies have also obtained outcomes similar to group self-management programs when investigating effects of intervention programs that incorporated many components of published asthma self-management programs. These interventions have focused on an individually tailored treatment package administered at home (Dahl, Gustafsson, & Melin, 1990), a combined education and stress management program (Perrin et al., 1992), and the addition of progressive muscle relaxation to a self-management program (Vazquez & Buceta, 1993a, 1993b, 1993c).

Results of these studies are less consistent than those from self-management programs discussed earlier with respect to measures of family stress and coping, pulmonary function measures, and self-perception profiles. However, some data suggest that inclusion of relaxation may be particularly beneficial for children who evidence emotionally triggered attacks. Additional research is necessary to determine the relevance of specific treatments geared toward psychological adaptation of patients (Vazquez & Buceta, 1993a).

Although asthma self-management programs have resulted in successful outcomes in different areas of functioning, they should be considered supplements to physician education and reliable medical care (Creer et al., 1990; Evans & Mellins, 1991). Positive improvements in children's asthma result not only from learning opportunities in these programs but also from maturation, taking medications correctly, and changes in medication (Barnett, Fatis, Sonnek, & Torvinen, 1992). In addition, difficulties evaluating efficacy of self-management programs in detail have been present due to the variability of asthma attacks (i.e., duration, frequency, and intensity) as well as methodological shortcomings of studies (Creer et al., 1990). For example, of the 19 programs reviewed, each used standardized assessment and treatment procedures, but one could question reliability and validity of the mostly paper-and-pencil measures employed. Medication effects could also have clouded individual findings.

Comprehensive care should, in any case, include a psychoeducational component that incorporates use of peak flow meters to assess status and to adjust medications in order to prevent and/or decrease severity of asthma attacks (Creer et al., 1992). Readings of peak expiratory flow rates have, in fact, improved the prediction of asthma attacks over and above medication compliance information and exercise data (Pinzone Carlson, Kotses, & Creer, 1991). Controlled studies evaluating effectiveness of self-management programs will need to conduct a task analysis of management behaviors and determine if skill acquisition leads to skill performance in the natural environment (Creer et al., 1990; Lemanek, 1990). Researchers will also need to remember the interdependence between compliance and self-management behaviors when they examine efficacy of asthma self-management programs (Creer et al., 1990).

Compliance

Rates of noncompliance with therapeutic regimens for asthma have ranged from 17 to 90 percent in children and adolescents (e.g., Baum & Creer, 1986; Coutts, Gibson, & Paton, 1992; Miller, 1982). For example, Coutts and colleagues (1992) found that children underused a Nebulizer Chronolog device, which administered corticosteroids, 55 percent of the study days; overuse occurred only 2 percent of the days.

Children and adolescents with asthma seem particularly susceptible to problems related to noncompliance due to the use of multiple medications on routine and as-needed (PRN) schedules, the long-term nature of the regimens, and varying periods when symptoms are not present (Rand & Wise, 1994).

The negative consequences resulting from noncompliance underscore the importance of complying with treatments for asthma. These negative consequences include, for instance, increased emergency-room (ER) visits and hospital admissions (Abduelrhman, & Loftus, 1993; Ashkenazi, Amir, Volovitz, & Varsano, 1993), escalating expenses from unused medications and unnecessary laboratory tests, and possibly death (Epstein & Cluss, 1982). Although asthma-related deaths are low compared to the number of deaths from other illnesses (e.g., cancer), the mortality rate may be as high as 1 to 2 percent (Strunk, Mrazek, Fuhrmann, & LaBrecque, 1985). Delineation of these negative consequences of noncompliance has prompted physicians, psychologists, and health educators to explore assessment and intervention issues related to asthma management in more detail than they have in the past.

Lemanek (1990) and Rand and Wise (1994) have provided comprehensive reviews of assessment and intervention issues related to compliance with asthma treatments, from which relevant data are summarized in this section. Methods employed to assess medical compliance in pediatric asthma are either direct or indirect. *Direct* methods include biochemical assay of blood, urine, and saliva samples and observation of correct use of metered-dose inhalers (MDI). Although biochemical assays provide an objective measure of compliance, theophylline-based compounds are currently the only drugs easily analyzed using this method. In addition, some assays can be invasive if performed on a regular basis (e.g., drawing blood) and may be inaccurate due to the effects of diet and other drugs. In terms of MDIs, only one standardized scale exists to accurately observe appropriate technique (Rand & Wise, 1994).

Indirect measures, more varied than direct measures, have consisted of physician judgments, self-report, self- or parent-monitoring of medication-taking behavior (e.g., dose) and asthma attacks (e.g., frequency of wheezing), parent/child interviews or questionnaires about compliance and knowledge, medication measurement (e.g., pill counts, weighing canisters), and, most recently, electronic medication monitors (e.g., release of eye drops, chronolog devices).

For illustration, Zora, Lutz, and Tinkelman (1989) studied compliance of 17 children (ages 5 to 13 years) with asthma who were on metaproterenol. The authors assessed compliance before and after a two-week or four-week period of treatment by way of canister weights. Results showed that 40 percent of children completing the two-week period were compliant, but only 8 percent ($N = 1$) were compliant during the four-week period. All of these methods have, of course, advantages and disadvantages. For example, self-reports and monitoring of compliance may be inexpensive and efficient means of data collection, but both are subject to falsification. Medication measurement and monitors may be appropriate for unobtrusively assessing compliance with long-term regimens, but they do not provide accurate estimates of the timing of medication administration.

The heterogeneous nature of asthma, including the variety and severity of symptoms across attacks and children, has made it difficult to assess compliance reliably (Lemanek, 1990). At this time, there is no "gold standard" for assessing compliance or therapeutic outcome in asthma (Lemanek, 1990; Rand & Wise, 1994). In addition, the correspondence between different methods of assessment tends to be low, further complicating the task of reliably assessing compliance. For example, Coutts and colleagues (1992) found differences between self-reported and Chronolog-recorded medication use by all children, with self-report indicating better compliance than the Chronolog.

Furthermore, data associating compliance with therapeutic outcome are lacking and difficult to ascertain because it is not uncommon for children to be, at times, compliant *and* symptomatic. Deaton (1985), in fact, found that parental adaptiveness about compliance decisions and accuracy of predictions of task performance correlated with better outcomes, but actual degree of compliance did not. Assessment of compliance with treatments for asthma will require development of standard and practical compliance criteria, examination of interrater reliability for individual methods, and detailed delineation of reasons

for noncompliance or erratic compliance (Rand & Wise, 1994).

Such factors as underdiagnosis and undertreatment, noncompliance by patients, inadequate education and understanding of asthma and its treatment, and poor self-management skills may all contribute to treatment failure (Ashkenazi et al., 1993; Donnelly, Donnelly, & Thong, 1989). Intervention strategies to improve compliance in pediatric asthma have tended to target one of these factors, thereby fitting into one of three categories: (1) educational, (2) organizational, or (3) behavioral strategies.

Educational strategies have centered on dispensing verbal or written instructions to inform children and their families about the nature of asthma and its management, as well as improving doctor/patient (parent) communication to enhance recall of these instructions. *Organizational strategies* have focused on clinic and regimen convenience to promote compliance, including extended supervision by physicians or other health care professionals and minimizing the complexity of medication schedules. Self-monitoring, visual reminders, and incentive systems have served as *behavioral strategies* to enhance compliance with asthma treatments. Unfortunately, many of these strategies, used alone or in combination, have not received rigorous empirical investigation.

Several investigators have proposed that educating children and their families about asthma within self-management programs will enhance compliance with therapeutic regimens and promote adequate treatment (e.g., Boner, 1989; Eiser, Town, & Tripp, 1988). However, research literature has not consistently revealed a positive relationship between education and/or skill acquisition and compliance. Ashkenazi and colleagues (1993) compared compliance rates of 100 consecutive referrals to a pediatric ER to those of 50 children seen in a hospital asthma clinic, where education and instruction about asthma and its treatment were part of their treatment. The compliance rate of the clinic group was 92 percent compared to 25 percent for the ER group; mean serum theophylline levels were also significantly different, with a reading of 11.4 ug/ml for the clinic group versus 6.8 ug/ml for the other children.

On the other hand, Baum and Creer (1986) examined effects of self-monitoring in comparison to a combined treatment package, consisting of self-monitoring, education, and a token system for symptom monitoring in two groups. Although children in the combined group evidenced greater skills in the areas taught in the education session, there were no group differences in medication compliance.

There is currently a need for randomized clinical trials in this area, not only in terms of documenting effective methods of improving compliance but also the most feasible means of implementing these methods in different health care settings. In addition, future research will need to address the question of how best to handle information from patients who apparently discard medications prior to compliance assessments (i.e., "dumpers") because their high compliance rates may conflict with poor therapeutic outcome data (Rand & Wise, 1994).

FUTURE DIRECTIONS

Research on the psychological, school, and medical adaptation of children and adolescents with asthma is in a preliminary stage of development. In general, studies indicate that children and adolescents with asthma appear to be at increased risk for emotional/behavioral problems, particularly anxiety and depression. Although current research on self-esteem and self-concept is inconclusive, the majority of studies suggest that asthma has little effect on how children and adolescents view themselves in comparison to their peers. Research on social competence, in general, and peer relationships, in particular, is lacking, although Spirito and associates (1991) listed several suggestions for possible avenues to pursue.

Most studies on family adjustment have focused on parent report of warmth, cohesion, and communication, revealing difficulties in heightened anxiety and overprotectiveness. Level of school adaptation seems to be variable and dependent on a combination of physiological aspects of asthma, psychological characteristics of the children, and the social environment of the family and community. In particular, effects of theophylline and corticosteroids on the academic performance and classroom behavior of children and adolescents with asthma is a matter of individual sensitivity to the medications. In terms of medical adaptation, self-management programs appear to be benefit children and their parents by de-

creasing utilization rates and increasing management skills.

Finally, compliance with treatments for asthma continue to be an area of concern due to adverse consequences resulting from noncompliance and the lack of direct correspondence between compliance and therapeutic outcome. Studies in these areas of adaptation are replete with differences in subject characteristics, measurement strategies, experimental designs, and, thus, conclusions. In addition, methodological flaws are present in most, if not all, studies. This analysis of the available literature on the adaptation of children and adolescents with asthma and their families should not detract, however, from the knowledge generated from these studies as well as their implications for working with patients and families. The studies' limitations may provide guidance in formulating future research questions and goals.

Future research must target psychological, school, and medical adaptation not only to decrease the risk of children with asthma developing difficulties in these areas but also to increase competencies. In the area of psychological adaptation, research needs to systematically document the impact of asthma on abilities of children and adolescents to achieve normal developmental tasks in terms of emotional/behavioral functioning, social relationships, and school performance (Creer et al., 1992). Children's and adolescents' perceptions of their reactions to and resources coping with disease-related and non-disease-related stress also needs to be a focus of future research. Studies employing a longitudinal approach would help examine developmental differences in adaptation as well as factors related to long-term outcome in children and their families.

To assess effects of asthma medications on behavior and learning, researchers need to utilize more direct measures of classroom performance (e.g., number of correct math problems completed, grammatical errors on writing assignment) and behavior (e.g., number of times out of seat and talking without permission in one class period) than currently employed. In addition, studies that delineate characteristics of children and adolescents who exhibit behavioral and learning effects following administration of different medications are necessary (Creer & Gustafson, 1989).

Controlled studies on self-management programs need to determine critical management skills requiring training and strategies to ensure generalization of these skills to the natural environment. Further delineation of the positive effects of these programs on specific variables and characteristics of families that may benefit most from them are additional topics for future investigations (Creer et al., 1992). Studies on the development of reliable and valid techniques for measuring compliance plus preventive and intervention strategies conducted across research and clinical settings are crucial to understanding the disorder (Rand & Wise, 1994).

Data generated from future research should aid in enhancing the comprehensive care of children and adolescents with asthma and their families. Comprehensive care must emphasize a family-centered approach that addresses physiological, psychological, and social aspects of asthma to foster adequate disease and psychosocial management (Davis & Wasserman, 1992). Future health care policies will need to take into consideration this family-centered approach in attempting to design and provide a comprehensive and effective service delivery system.

REFERENCES

Abduelrhman, E. M., & Loftus, B. G. (1993). Childhood asthma, can admissions be avoided? *Irish Medical Journal, 86,* 22–23.

Achenbach, T. M., & Edelbrock, C. (1983). *Manual for the Child Behavior Checklist and Revised Child Behavior Profile* (2nd ed.). New York: Wiley.

Ashkenazi, S., Amir, J., Volovitz, B., & Varsano, I. (1993). Why do asthmatic children need referral to an emergency room? *Pediatric Allergy and Immunology, 4,* 93–96.

Askildsen, E. C., Watten, R. G., & Faleide, A. O. (1993). Are parents of asthmatic children different from other parents? *Psychotherapy Psychosomatics, 60,* 91–99.

Barnett, T. E., Fatis, M., Sonnek, D., & Torvinen, J. (1992). Treatment satisfaction with an asthma management program: A "five"-year retrospective assessment. *Journal of Asthma, 29,* 109–116.

Baum, D., & Creer, T. L. (1986). Medication compliance in children with asthma. *Journal of Asthma, 23,* 49–59.

Bender, B. G., Lerner, J. A., Ikle, D., Comer, C., & Szefler, S. (1991). Psychological change associated with theophylline treatment of asthmatic children: A 6-month study. *Pediatric Pulmonology, 11,* 233–242.

Bender, B. G., Lerner, J. A., & Kollasch, E. (1988). Mood and memory changes in asthmatic children receiving corticosteroids. *American Academy of Child and Adolescent Psychiatry, 27,* 720–725.

Biederman, J., Milberger, S., Faraone, S. V., Guite, J., & Warburton, R. (1994). Associations between childhood asthma and ADHD: Issues of psychiatric comorbidity and familiality. *Journal of the American Academy of Child and Adolescent Psychiatry, 33,* 842–848.

Bennett, D. S. (1994). Depression among children with chronic medical problems: A meta-analysis. *Journal of Pediatric Psychology, 19,* 149–169.

Blessing-Moore, J., Landon, M., Miya, A., & Berman, A. (1981). Camp Wheeze: An educational/recreational program for asthmatic children and their parents. In *Self-management educational programs for childhood asthma* (pp. 151–198). Washington, DC: National Institute of Allergy and Infectious Diseases.

Boner, A. L. (1989). Therapy of asthma in children. *European Respiratory Journal, 2,* 545s–550s.

Bussing, R., & Burket, R. C. (1993). Anxiety and intrafamilial stress in children with hemophilia after the HIV crisis. *Journal of the American Academy of Child and Adolescent Psychiatry, 32,* 562–566.

Butz, A. M., & Alexander, C. (1993). Anxiety in children with asthma. *Journal of Asthma, 30,* 199–209.

Cadman, D., Boyle, M., Szatmari, P., & Offord, D. R. (1987). Chronic illness, disability, and mental and social well-being: Findings of the Ontario Child Health Study. *Pediatrics, 79,* 805–813.

Carson, D. K., & Schauer, R. W. (1992). Mothers of children with asthma: Perceptions of parenting stress and the mother-child relationship. *Psychological Reports, 71,* 1139–1148.

Celano, M. P., & Geller, R. J. (1993). Learning, school performance, and children with asthma: How much at risk? *Journal of Learning Disabilities, 26,* 23–32.

Christiaanse, M. E., Lavigne, J. V., & Lerner, C. V. (1989). Psychosocial aspects of compliance in children and adolescents with asthma. *Journal of Developmental and Behavioral Pediatrics, 10,* 75–80.

Clark, N. M., Feldman, C. H., Freudenberg, N., Millman, E. J., Wasilewski, Y., & Valle, I. (1980). Developing education for children with asthma through study of self-management behavior. *Health Education Quarterly, 7,* 278–296.

Coutts, J. A. P., Gibson, N. A., & Paton, J. Y. (1992). Measuring compliance with inhaled medication in asthma. *Archives of Diseases of Children, 67,* 332–333.

Creer, T. L., & Gustafson, K. E. (1989). Psychological problems associated with drug therapy in childhood asthma. *Journal of Pediatrics, 115,* 850–855.

Creer, T. L., Stein, R. E. K., Rappaport, L., & Lewis, C. (1992). Behavioral consequences of illness: Childhood asthma as a model. *Pediatrics, 90,* 808–815.

Creer, T. L., Wigal, J. K., Kotses, H., & Lewis, P. (1990). A critique of 19 self-management programs for childhood asthma: Part II. Comments regarding the scientific merit of the programs. *Pediatric Asthma, Allergy & Immunology, 4,* 41–55.

Dahl, J., Gustafsson, D., & Melin, L. (1990). Effects of a behavioral treatment program on children with asthma. *Journal of Asthma, 27,* 41–46.

Davis, J. K., & Wasserman, E. (1992). Behavioral aspects of asthma in children. *Clinical Pediatrics, 31,* 678–681.

Deaton, A. V. (1985). Adaptive noncompliance in pediatric asthma: The parent as expert. *Journal of Pediatric Psychology, 10,* 1–14.

diBlasio, P., Molinari, E., Peri, G., & Taverna, A. (1990). Family competence and childhood asthma: A preliminary study. *Family Systems Medicine, 8,* 145–149.

Donnelly, J. E., Donnelly, W. J., & Thong, Y. H. (1989). Inadequate parental understanding of asthma medications. *Annals of Allergy, 62,* 337–341.

Drotar, D., & Bush, M. (1985). Mental health issues and services. In N. Hobbs & J. M. Perrin (Eds.), *Issues in the care of children with chronic illness* (pp. 827–863). San Francisco: Jossey-Bass.

Easier, C., Havermans, T., Pancer, M., & Eiser, J. R. (1992). Adjustment to chronic disease in relation to age and gender: Mothers' and fathers' reports of their children's behavior. *Journal of Pediatric Psychology, 17,* 261–275.

Eiser, C., Town, C., & Tripp, J. H. (1988). Illness experience and related knowledge amongst children with asthma. *Child: Care, Health, and Development, 14,* 11–24..

Epstein, L. H., & Cluss, P. A. (1982). A behavioral medicine perspective on adherence to long-term medical regimens. *Journal of Consulting and Clinical Psychology, 50,* 950–971.

Evans, D., & Mellins, R. B. (1991). Educational programs for children with asthma. *Pediatrician, 18,* 317–323.

Feldman, C., & Clark, N. (1981). Development and evaluation of a self-management program for childhood asthma. In *Self-management educational programs for childhood asthma* (pp. 53–106). Washington, DC: National Institute of Allergy and Infectious Diseases.

Fowler, M. G., Davenport, M. G., & Garg, R. (1992). School functioning of US children with asthma. *Pediatrics, 90,* 939–944.

Freudenberg, N., Feldman, C. H., Clark, N. M., Millman, E. J., Valle, I., & Wasilewski, Y. (1980). The impact of bronchial asthma on school attendance and performance. *The Journal of School Health, 40,* 522–526.

Furrow, D., Hambley, J., & Brazil, K. (1989). Behavior problems in children requiring inpatient rehabilitation treatment for asthma. *Journal of Asthma, 26,* 123–132.

Gizynski, M., & Shapiro, V. B. (1990). Depression and childhood illness. *Child and Adolescent Social Work, 7,* 179–197.

Gortmaker, S. L., Walker, D. K., Weitzman, M., & Sobol, A. M. (1990). Chronic conditions, socioeconomic risks, and behavioral problems in children and adolescence. *Pediatrics, 85,* 267–276.

Gutstadt, L. B., Gillette, J. W., Mrazek, D. A., Fukuhara, J. T., LaBrecque, J. F., & Strunk, R. C. (1989). Determinants of school performance in children with chronic asthma. *American Journal of Diseases of Children, 143,* 471–475.

Hambley, J., Brazil, K., Furrow, D., & Chua, Y. Y. (1989). Demographic and psychosocial characteristics of asthmatic children in a Canadian rehabilitation setting. *Journal of Asthma, 26,* 167–175.

Hamlett, K. W., Pellegrini, D. S., & Katz, K. S. (1992). Childhood chronic illness as a family stressor. *Journal of Pediatric Psychology, 17,* 33–47.

Harper, D. C. (1991). Paradigms for investigating rehabilitation and adaptation to childhood disability and chronic illness. *Journal of Pediatric Psychology, 16,* 533–542.

Harter, S. (1985). *The Self-Perception Profile for Children: Revision of the Perceived Competence Scale for Children.* Manual, University of Denver.

Kaliner, M., Barnes, P., & Persson, C. (1991). *Asthma: Its pathology and treatment.* New York: Marcel Dekker.

Kashani, J. H., Konig, P., Shepperd, J. A., Wilfley, D., & Morris, D. A. (1988). Psychopathology and self-concept in asthmatic children. *Journal of Pediatric Psychology, 13,* 509–520.

Klinnert, M. D., Gavin, L. A., Wamboldt, F. S., & Mirazek, D. A. (1992). Marriages with children at medical risk: The transition to parenthood. *Journal of the American Academy of Child and Adolescent Psychiatry, 31,* 334–342.

Lemanek, K. L. (1990). Adherence issues in the medical management of asthma. *Journal of Pediatric Psychology, 15,* 437–458.

Lewis, C., Rachelefsky, G., & Lewis, M. A. (1981). ACT for Kids. In *Self-management programs for childhood asthma* (pp. 21–52). Washington, DC: National Institute of Allergy and Infectious Diseases.

Lewis, M. A., & Lewis, C. E. (1990). Consequences of empowering children to care for themselves. *Pediatrician, 17,* 63–67.

Lindgren, S., Lokshin, B., Stromquist, A., Weinberger, M., Nassif, E., McCubbin, M., & Frasher, R. (1992). Does asthma or treatment with theophylline limit children's academic performance? *The New England Journal of Medicine, 327,* 926–930.

MacLean, W. E., Perrin, J. M., Gortmaker, S., & Pierre, C. B. (1992). Psychological adjustment of children with asthma: Effects of illness severity and recent stressful life events. *Journal of Pediatric Psychology, 17,* 159–171.

Mascia, A., Frank, S., Berkman, A., Stern, L., Lampl, L., Davies, M., Yeager, T., Birmaher, B., & Chieco, E. (1989). Mortality versus improvement in severe chronic asthma: Physiological and psychological factors. *Annals of Allergy, 62,* 311–318.

McLoughlin, J., Nall, M., Isaacs, B., Petrosko, J., Karibo, J., & Lindsey, B. (1983). The relationship of allergies and allergy treatment to school performance and student behavior. *Annals of Allergy, 51,* 506–510.

Mesters, I., Meertens, R., Crebolder, H., & Parcel, G. (1993). Development of a health education program for parents of preschool children with asthma. *Health Education Research: Theory and Practice, 8,* 53–68.

Miller, B. D., & Wood, B. L. (1991). Childhood asthma in interaction with family, school, and peer systems: A developmental model for primary care. *Journal of Asthma, 28,* 405–414.

Miller, K. A. (1982). Theophylline compliance in adolescent patients with chronic asthma. *Journal of Adolescent Health Care, 3,* 177–179.

Moffitt, J. E., & Moffitt, J. L. (1989). Behavioral and cognitive effects of theophylline. *Pediatric Nursing, 15,* 277.

Morey, P., & Jones, K. (1993). Past maternal experiences of asthma, childhood morbidity, and the psychosocial impact of the disorder. *Journal of Asthma, 30,* 271–276.

National Asthma Education Program. (1991). *Guidelines for the diagnosis and management of asthma* (NIH Publication No. 91-3042). Bethesda, MD: National Institute of Health.

Nelms, B. C. (1989). Emotional behaviors in chronically ill children. *Journal of Abnormal Child Psychology, 17,* 657–668.

Parcel, G. S., Gilman, S. C., Nader, P. R., & Bunce, H. A. (1979). A comparison of absentee rates of elementary school children with asthma and non-asthmatic school mates. *Pediatrics, 64,* 878–881.

Parcel, G. S., Nader, P. R., & Tiernan, K. (1980). A health education program for children with asthma. *Developmental and Behavioral Pediatrics, 1,* 128–132.

Patterson, J. M., & Geber, G. (1991). Preventing mental health problems in children with chronic illness or disability. *Children's Health Care, 20,* 150–161.

Peri, G., Molinari, E., & Taverna, A. (1991). Parental perceptions of childhood illness. *Journal of Asthma, 28,* 91–101.

Perrin, E. C., Ayoub, C. C., & Willett, J. B. (1993). In the eyes of the beholder: Family and maternal influences on perceptions of adjustment of children with a chronic illness. *Journal of Developmental and Behavioral Pediatrics, 14,* 94–105.

Perrin, J. M., & MacLean, W. E. (1988). Children with chronic illness. The prevention of dysfunction. *The Pediatric Clinics of North America, 35,* 1325–1337.

Perrin, J. M., MacLean, W. E., Gortmaker, S. L., & Asher, K. N. (1992). Improving the psychological status of children with asthma: A randomized controlled trial. *Developmental and Behavioral Pediatrics, 13,* 241–247.

Pinzone, H. A., Carlson, B. W., Kotses, H., & Creer T. L. (1991). Prediction of asthma episodes in children using peak expiratory flow rates, medication compliance, and exercise data. *Annals of Allergy, 67,* 481–485.

Pless, I. B., & Roghmann, K. J. (1971). Chronic illness and its consequences: Observations based on three epidemiological surveys. *Journal of Pediatrics, 79,* 351–359.

Rachelefsky, G. S., Wo, J., Adelson, J., Mickey, M. R., Spector, S. L., Katz, R. M., Siegel, S. C., & Rohr, A. S. (1986). Behavior abnormalities and poor school performance due to oral theophylline use. *Pediatrics, 78,* 1133–1138.

Rand, C. S., & Wise, R. A. (1994). Measuring adherence to asthma mediation regimens. *American Journal of Respiratory and Critical Care Medicine, 149,* S69–S76.

Rappaport, L., Coffman, H., Guare, R., Fenton, T., DeGraw, C., & Twarog, F. (1989). Effects of theophylline on behavior and learning in children with asthma. *American Journal of Diseases of Children, 143,* 368–372.

Richards, W., Church, J. A., Roberts, M. J., Newman, L. J., & Garon, M. R. (1981). A self-help program for childhood asthma in a residential treatment center. *Clinical Pediatrics, 7,* 453–457.

Roth, R. M. (1980). *The mother-child relationship evaluation.* Los Angeles, CA: Western Psychological Services.

Rubin, D. H., Bauman, L. J., & Lauby, J. L. (1989). The relationship between knowledge and reported behavior in childhood asthma. *Developmental and Behavioral Pediatrics, 10,* 307–312.

Rubin, D. H., Leventhal, J. M., Sadock, R. T., Letovsky, E., Schottland, P., Clemente, I., & McCarthy, P. (1986). Educational intervention by computer in childhood asthma: A randomized clinical trial testing the use of a new teaching intervention in childhood asthma. *Pediatrics, 77,* 1–10.

Schlieper, A., Alcock, D., Beaudry, P., Feldman, W., & Leikin, L. (1991). Effect of therapeutic plasma concentrations of theophylline on behavior, cognitive processing, and affect in children with asthma. *The Journal of Pediatrics, 118,* 449–455.

Schobinger, R., Florin, I. Reichbauer, M., Lindemann, H., & Zimmer, C. (1993). Childhood asthma: Mothers' affective attitude, mother-child interaction and children's compliance with medical requirements. *Journal of Psychosomatic Research, 37,* 697–707.

Schwam, J. S. (1987). Assisting the parent of a child with asthma. *Journal of Asthma, 24,* 45–54.

Seigel, W. M., Golden, N. H., Gough, J. W., Lashley, M. S., & Sacker, I. M. (1990). Depression, self-esteem, and life events on adolescents with chronic disease. *Journal of Adolescent Health Care, 11,* 501–504.

Spirito, A., DeLawyer, D. D., & Stark, L. (1991). Peer relations and social adjustment of chronically ill children and adolescents. *Clinical Psychology Review, 11,* 539–564.

Strunk, R. C., Mrazek, D. A., Fuhrmann, G. S. W., & La-Brecque, J. F. (1985). Deaths from asthma in childhood. Can they be predicted? *Journal of the American Medical Association, 254,* 1193–1198.

Suess, W. M., Stump, N., Chai, H., & Kalisker, A. (1986). Mnemonic effects of asthma medication in children. *Journal of Asthma, 23,* 291–296.

Townsend, M., Feeny, D. H., Guyatt, G. H., Furlong, W. J., Seip, A. E., & Dolovich, J. (1991). Evaluation of the burden of illness for pediatric asthmatic patients and their parents. *Annals of Allergy, 67,* 403–408.

Vazquez, M. I., & Buceta, J. M. (1993a). Effectiveness of self-management programmes and relaxation training in the treatment of bronchial asthma: Relationships with trait anxiety and emotional attack triggers. *Journal of Psychosomatic Research, 37,* 71–81.

Vazquez, M. I., & Buceta, J. M. (1993b). Psychological treatment of asthma: Effectiveness of a self-management program with and without relaxation training. *Journal of Asthma, 30,* 171–183.

Vazquez, M. I., & Buceta, J. M. (1993c). Relaxation therapy in the treatment of bronchial asthma: Effects on basal spirometric values. *Psychotherapy Psychosomatics, 60,* 106–112.

Vazquez, M. I., Fontan-Bueso, J., & Buceta, J. M. (1992). Self-perception of asthmatic children and modification through self-management programs. *Psychological Reports, 71,* 903–913.

Weinberger, M., Lindgren S., Bender, B., Lerner, J. A., & Szefler, S. (1987). Effects of theophylline on learning and behavior: Reason for concern or concern without reason? *The Journal of Pediatrics, 111,* 471–474.

Wigal, J. K., Creer, T. L., Kotses, H., & Lewis, P. (1990). A critique of 19 self-management programs for childhood asthma: Part I. Development and evaluation of the programs. *Pediatric Asthma, Allergy, & Immunology, 4,* 17–39.

Zora, J. A., Lutz, C. N., & Tinkelman, D. G. (1989). Assessment of compliance in children using inhaled beta adrenergic agonists. *Annals of Allergy, 62,* 406–409.

PART III

ISSUES IN ADDICTION

Although estimates of drug use among adolescents had been declining for many years, recent governmental indices have revealed that the declining trend may be reversing somewhat. The disturbing statistics indicate larger numbers of users at younger ages than was previously the case, along with some indication of more frequent use. This is problematic and of concern because of the potential health consequences of drug use and the fact that a large percentage of adult drug users and those with addictions indicate their initial drug exposure and use was during childhood or adolescence.

The four chapters in this section address four classes of substances that are subject to abuse and addiction: alcohol (Chapter 11), tobacco (Chapter 12), illicit drugs (Chapter 13), and food (Chapter 14). The last of these (i.e., food) rarely gets included among the addictions. However, because it shares some of the same characteristics (e.g., substances often taken in larger amounts than intended, numerous attempts to quit), it is included here. Each of the four chapters addresses identification of the etiological factors as a primary issue. The various authors recognize the multifactorial nature of the problems, but each author places different emphasis on different factors. For example, the smoking chapter (12) emphasizes peer influence and the obesity chapter (14) hypothesizes a developmental perspective whereby environmental factors (especially social ones) take over what were initially biological drives. The multifactorial nature of these problems poses a difficult challenge for clinicians and researchers.

CHAPTER 11

DRUG ABUSE IN ADOLESCENCE

Susan F. Tapert, JOINT DOCTORAL PROGRAM IN CLINICAL PSYCHOLOGY,
SAN DIEGO STATE UNIVERSITY AND UNIVERSITY OF CALIFORNIA, SAN DIEGO

David G. Stewart, JOINT DOCTORAL PROGRAM IN CLINICAL PSYCHOLOGY,
SAN DIEGO STATE UNIVERSITY AND UNIVERSITY OF CALIFORNIA, SAN DIEGO

Sandra A. Brown, VETERANS ADMINISTRATION MEDICAL CENTER
AND UNIVERSITY OF CALIFORNIA, SAN DIEGO

Adolescent drug involvement is a significant social and public health problem in the United States. A 1994 University of Michigan study found that illicit drug use among teens has increased by 3 percent overall in the past year (Johnston, Bachman, & O'Malley, 1994), with a marked increase in marijuana and inhalant use among young adolescents. Adolescent drug use peaked in the late 1970s, stabilized in the late 1980s, and appears again to be on the rise. This chapter presents an overview of effects of the most commonly abused drugs, research suggesting risk factors for development of drug problems in the teenage years, and summaries of assessment, prevention, and intervention strategies.

PREVALENCE

National estimates of drug use prevalence vary markedly by inclusion criteria. Most prevalence estimates consider frequency of use of particular drugs. The broadest estimates, based on school samples, under-estimate drug involvement because drug-involved teens are often truant or not on the enrollment (Brown, Vik, & Creamer, 1989). The National Institute on Drug Abuse conducts an Annual Household Survey on Drug Abuse that provides a population estimate of illicit drug use. The National Institute on Drug Abuse surveyed students from U.S. high schools, selected to be representative on demographic variables, from 1975 to 1992 (Johnston, Bachman, & O'Malley, 1993).

Tables 11.1 and 11.2 show the daily and past month prevalence of drug use. In 1992, 17 percent of adolescents (ages 12 to 17) reported having used illicit drugs at least once in their lives, and 6 percent reported use in the past month. The figures are higher for young adults: 52 percent reported lifetime use of illicit drugs, and 13 percent reported using in the past month. As exemplified by Table 11.2, the overall percentage of high school students who use illicit drugs appears to have decreased or stabilized for most drugs in recent years.

Table 11.1 Trends in Prevalence (%) of Daily Use of Drugs for Twelfth-Graders

SUBSTANCE	1976	1978	1980	1982	1984	1986	1988	1990	1992
Cannabis	8.2	10.7	9.1	6.3	5.0	4.0	2.7	2.2	1.9
Inhalants	—	0.1	0.2	0.2	0.2	0.4	0.3	0.3	0.2
Hallucinogens	0.1	0.1	0.2	0.2	0.2	0.3	—	0.3	0.1
Cocaine (incl. crack)	0.1	0.1	0.2	0.2	0.2	0.4	0.2	0.1	0.1
Opiates (incl. heroin)	0.1	0.1	0.1	0.1	0.1	0.1	0.1	0.1	—
Stimulants (incl. crystal meth/ice)	0.4	0.5	0.7	0.7	0.6	0.3	0.3	0.2	0.2
Sedatives	0.2	0.2	0.2	0.2	0.1	0.1	0.1	0.1	0.1
Tranquilizers	0.2	0.1	0.1	0.1	0.1	—	—	0.1	—

— = less than .05 percent.
Source: L. D. Johnston, P. M. O'Malley, & J. G. Bachman, *National survey results on drug use from Monitoring the Future Study, 1975–1992.* Rockville, MD: National Institute on Drug Abuse, 1993.

Table 11.2 Trends in Past Month Prevalence (%) of Drugs for Twelfth-Graders

SUBSTANCE	1976	1978	1980	1982	1984	1986	1988	1990	1992
Any illicit drug	34.2	38.9	37.2	32.5	29.2	27.1	21.3	17.2	14.4
Any illicit drug other than marijuana	13.9	15.1	18.4	17.0	15.1	13.2	10.0	8.0	6.3
Cannabis	32.2	37.1	33.7	28.5	25.2	23.4	18.0	14.0	11.9
Inhalants	0.9	1.5	2.7	2.5	2.6	3.2	3.0	2.9	2.5
Hallucinogens	3.4	3.9	4.4	4.1	3.2	3.5	2.3	2.3	2.3
Cocaine (incl. crack)	2.0	3.9	5.2	5.0	5.8	6.2	3.4	1.9	1.3
Opiates (incl. heroin)	2.2	2.4	2.6	2.0	2.1	2.2	1.8	1.7	1.5
Stimulants (incl. crystal meth/ice)	7.7	8.7	12.1	10.7	8.3	5.5	4.6	3.7	2.8
Sedatives	4.5	4.2	4.8	3.4	2.3	2.2	1.4	1.4	1.2
Tranquilizers	4.0	3.4	3.1	2.4	2.1	2.1	1.5	1.2	1.0

Source: L. D. Johnston, P. M. O'Malley, & J. G. Bachman, *National survey results on drug use from Monitoring the Future Study, 1975–1992.* Rockville, MD: National Institute on Drug Abuse, 1993.

Gender

Sex differences do exist in the prevalence of adolescent drug use. Overall, boys are more likely to use most types of illicit drugs and to use them more often than girls. However, the most striking difference is in the use of nonprescription diet pills. Although use of diet pills has decreased in the past decade, 23 percent of female high school seniors, compared to only 6 percent of male high school seniors, reported ever using nonprescription diet pills in 1992. Also, more girls than boys reported use of stimulants and tranquilizers during high school. Sex differences in use prevalence are smaller in the earlier grades than in the later

grades, and at least one group of investigators has suggested that girls who use drugs at a young age often date older boys (Johnston, Bachman, & O'Malley, 1993).

Age of Onset

Adolescents who start using drugs at an earlier age have a poorer prognosis than those who initiate drug use at a later age (Newcomb & Bentler, 1989). Age of first use of illicit drugs became earlier throughout the 1970s and peaked in 1982, when 52 percent of students surveyed had used some illicit drug by the end of grade 10. Encouragingly, the age of onset appears to have risen again since 1982 for most substances, with the exception of inhalants; current estimates indicate that 17 percent of eighth-graders have used inhalants at least once (Johnston, Bachman, & O'Malley, 1993).

Ethnic Differences

Although the overall sequence of initiation of substances appears relatively comparable across ethnic groups (Adler & Kandel, 1982), some differences do exist. White students appear to use more drugs at all age levels than black students. Marijuana use rates are equivalent for white and Hispanic students. More Hispanic students than students from other ethnic groups report use of the dangerous substances of cocaine and heroin in the senior year of high school (Johnston, Bachman, & O'Malley, 1993). Regional ethnic differences in drug use patterns also exist; for example, in a sample of 847 Los Angeles middle school students, Maddahian, Newcomb, and Bentler (1988) found that white students use significantly more cannabis than Asian American students.

ABUSE AND DEPENDENCE

Any substance whose administration leads to changes in mood, sensory perception, or brain functioning can become a drug of abuse (Schuckit, 1989). Most commonly abused illicit drugs produce highly reinforcing effects, and many are physically addictive after repeated use. Individuals may begin using drugs for social reasons but may eventually become physically dependent or unable to control their increased desire for the effects of the drug. This shift from use to abuse to dependence often includes specific behavioral components, such as using the drug in isolation or as the primary reason for social interaction with other drug abusers. Concurrently, antisocial behaviors often increase with efforts to acquire drugs.

As tolerance develops, more of the drug is necessary to obtain the desired effects, and use becomes more frequent. In addition, drugs of the same class, based on similar nervous system effects, often show cross-tolerance. Cross-tolerance arises when tolerance to one drug has developed and can be applied to other drugs of the same class so that more of those drugs are necessary to produce the same central nervous system effects. If a user simultaneously administers multiple drugs of the same class, potentiating effects occur, which can lead to overdose. Abusing adolescents commonly use several drugs in concert, and effects of drug potentiation are an important concern (Brown, Vik, & Creamer, 1989).

Physical dependence usually includes drug withdrawal, a syndrome of symptoms that appear upon cessation of drug administration following heavy, prolonged drug use. Symptoms are, to some degree, drug class specific.

The Diagnostic and Statistical Manual of Mental Disorders, Fourth Edition (American Psychiatric Association, 1994) differentiates between substance abuse and substance dependence. A diagnosis of substance abuse applies to maladaptive patterns of substance use that do not meet the more severe criteria for substance dependence. This distinction may be particularly important for adolescent drug users who have a brief history of use and different major role functions than adults. Although adolescents in treatment typically meet dependence criteria (Stewart & Brown, 1995), the substance abuse criteria may better capture typical adolescent use patterns.

It is important to note that adult abuse and dependency symptoms are the basis of *DSM-IV* criteria. Patterns of dependency symptoms, however, are different for adolescents than for adults. Stewart and Brown (1995) found, for example, that adolescents were likely to experience preoccupation with drugs and loss of control over their use as well as reckless behavior when using drugs, but were not likely to have used drugs for relationship or medical problems, which are common dependency symptoms among adults.

Stewart and Brown (1995) found that the majority of substance-abusing adolescents studied reported significant withdrawal symptoms for at least two psychoactive substances of abuse. The most prevalent of the psychoactive substance withdrawal symptoms reported by adolescents were mood-related symptoms (e.g., depression, anger, and anxiety), although a majority of adolescents also reported physiological and cognitive symptoms. Concurrent heavy use of alcohol as well as cigarettes correlated with an elevation in withdrawal symptoms. In the same study, most adolescents met *DSM-IV* substance dependence criteria for at least two drugs, and half also met dependency criteria for alcohol.

DRUGS OF ABUSE

Alcohol and tobacco are the most common substances used by adolescents and these substances serve as the gateway to marijuana and other drug use (Kandel, Yamaguchi, & Chen, 1992; Kandel & Yamaguchi, 1993). Tobacco and alcohol are not the focus of this chapter; reviews of these substances appear in Chapters 12 and 13, respectively, of this volume. The following section details the properties of individual substances; however, teens often use multiple drugs, and it is not easy to ascertain the purity and content of illicit drugs, thereby complicating accurate diagnoses.

Cannabis

Marijuana is the most commonly used illicit drug in the United States. The potency of marijuana has increased by as much as 15 percent in the past two decades (American Psychiatric Association, 1994) because growers have cultivated plants specifically to increase the primary psychoactive substance in cannabinoids, THC. Users ingest THC by smoking marijuana leaves ("pot," "weed"), smoking resin ("hashish"), or eating cannabinoids mixed with food.

Although its use involves less physiological and psychological changes than most other drugs of abuse, it is important to emphasize the potential dangers that may result from acute and chronic cannabis use (Brown, Mott, & Stewart, 1992). Intoxication effects include relaxation, euphoria, altered perceptions, impaired motor coordination, sensation of slowed time, impaired judgment, and social withdrawal. Sometimes anxiety, paranoia, concentration and memory impairment, panic, and hallucinations occur. Physical symptoms include increased appetite, dry mouth, bloodshot eyes, and tachycardia. Chronic use presents risk for lung damage, impaired sperm production, decreased testosterone secretion, decreased size of prostrate and testes in males, blocked ovulation in females, amotivational syndrome (Cohen, 1981; McGlothlin & West, 1968), and suppressed immune function.

Stimulants

Central nervous system (CNS) stimulants include caffeine and nicotine (discussed elsewhere in this vol-

ume), but the major intoxicating stimulants of abuse are cocaine and amphetamines. Drugs of this class typically produce physiological arousal, euphoria, reduction in appetite, insomnia, and sometimes sexual arousal.

Cocaine

Users can insuflate (snort) cocaine in powdered form, smoke it in powdered form (sometimes sprinkled on a tobacco or marijuana cigarette), smoke it in cooked form ("crack" or "rock"), or inject it in dissolved form. Crack is more potent than powdered cocaine, with intense effects experienced immediately after smoking and diminishing more rapidly than powdered cocaine. Because the content of any drug obtained on the street is difficult to specify, injectors are at particular risk for vein deterioration and endocarditis as well as for other risks associated with injection.

Cocaine use produces euphoria, sense of well-being, restlessness, mood swings, irritability, aggression, insomnia, and sometimes panic attacks, loss of control, paranoia, and hallucinations. Common physical effects include elevated heart rate, dry mouth, sweating, numbness of the mucous membranes, and hand tremors. Tolerance develops rapidly, usually within days of continued use. Withdrawal symptoms include depression, cravings, agitation, fatigue, and sometimes physical aggression.

Amphetamines

Amphetamines include pharmaceutically prepared substances (e.g., Benzedrine, Dexedrine, Ritalin, and some other drugs prescribed for obesity, attention deficit/hyperactivity disorder, and narcolepsy) as well as substances produced illegally, such as methamphetamine ("crystal meth," "speed," or "ice"). Users can powder and snort these drugs, dissolve and inject them, smoke them, or ingest them orally. Users experience euphoria, sociability, hypervigilance, anxiety, stereotyped behaviors, and impaired judgment. As with cocaine, smoked and injected forms are more intense and behaviors are more dramatically altered than with use of the other forms. Physical effects include increased heart rate, pupil dilation, and psychomotor agitation. Withdrawal symptoms involve depression, irritability, loss of energy, and sometimes physical aggression or hallucinations. Withdrawal-related depression can last several weeks.

Opiates

This drug class includes derivatives of the opium poppy (opium, morphine), semisynthetics (heroin), compounds synthesized to have morphine-like properties (codeine, hydromorphone [Dilaudid], methadone, oxycodone [Percodan], meperidine, and fentanyl), and medications with both opiate agonist and antagonist properties (buprenorphine, pentazocine). Some of these substances get prescribed for pain relief, for cough suppression, or to alleviate opiate withdrawal symptoms. Users commonly inject opiates but can also snort or smoke them; they experience euphoria (especially during the "rush" immediately following administration), apathy, dysphoria, impaired judgment, and relaxation. Physical effects of intoxication include suppressed respiratory functioning, slurred speech, psychomotor retardation, impairment of attention and memory, constricted pupils, and constipation.

Opiate tolerance develops rapidly, and, in dependent individuals, daily activities tend to revolve around obtaining and administering opiates. Opiate withdrawal can be very unpleasant, involving nausea, vomiting, diarrhea, muscle aches, tremor, fatigue, insomnia, fever, dysphoric mood, and cravings, and can last up to eight days. In addition, a study indicated an association between prolonged opiate use and depression (Kosten & Rounsaville, 1988). Administration of street opiates poses a particular risk for overdose because purity levels remain unknown to the user. Death from opiate overdose results from respiratory depression or cardiac arrest. Because many opiate users inject, additional risks of HIV infection, hepatitis, cellulitis, endocarditis, and tuberculosis are present. Opiate dependence is not common in early adolescence, and dependence usually develops in late adolescence or young adulthood.

Hallucinogens

These drugs produce dramatic alterations in sensation and perception. Drugs in this class include lysergic acid diethylamide (LSD), psilocybin (found in certain mushrooms), mescaline (found in the peyote cactus), dimethyltryptamine (DMT), 2,5-dimethoxy-4-methylamphetamine (STP), methylene dioxyamphetamine (MDA), and methylene dioxymethamphetamine (MDMA, "ecstasy," "E," or "X"). Certain

Native American cultures use psilocybin and mescaline as part of their established religious practices.

Hallucinogens are usually taken orally. Users experience intensification of perceptions, visual hallucinations, derealization, euphoria, alertness, and emotional lability. Sometimes confusion, paranoia, panic, loss of control, and depression result, and the most imminent risk of hallucinogen intoxication is acting on delusional beliefs (e.g., ability to fly). Physical effects include pupillary dilation, tachycardia, tremors, nausea, and sweating. Incorrect chemical synthesis of MDMA and MDA can produce substances that cause severe Parkinsonian symptoms (e.g., MTPT). Hallucinogenic effects tend to be more intense for younger users than for older users. Tolerance can develop with frequent use.

Phencyclidine (PCP)

PCP (Sernylan, "angel dust") and related compounds (Ketalar, Ketaject, TCP), developed as anesthetics, became street drugs in the 1960s. Users can smoke them, snort them, take them orally, or inject them. Because it is relatively inexpensive, manufacturers often substitute PCP for more expensive street drugs, and users may combine PCP with other drugs (particularly marijuana) to intensify effects. Intoxication effects often include marked behavioral change, assaultiveness, belligerence, unpredictability, impaired judgment, euphoria, hallucinations, intensified perceptions, heightened emotions, and sometimes hyperactivity, panic, paranoia, and confusion. Physical effects include numbness and diminished response to pain, psychomotor agitation and incoordination, tachycardia, slurred speech, and sometimes catatonia, convulsions, respiratory depression, coma, and death.

Inhalants

Inhalants of abuse include industrial and household compounds, such as glues, aerosol sprays, gasoline, paints, paint thinners, nail polish remover, correction fluid, certain cleaning solvents, and nitrous oxide ("poppers," "rush"). Children and young adolescents, especially youth in economically disadvantaged areas, are the most common users of inhalants, partly due to the availability and low cost of these drugs. Use of inhalants is more common among males than females. Users generally sniff inhalants from a rag soaked in the compound and experience euphoria, floating sensations, apathy, ringing in the ears, temporal distortion, and sometimes visual hallucinations, confusion, irritability, assaultiveness, and panic. Physical effects include loss of coordination, dizziness, headache, slurred speech, lethargy, psychomotor retardation, tremor, blurred vision, and sometimes coma. Inhalant abuse can lead to serious physiological problems, including respiratory damage, eye, nose, and throat damage, as well as kidney, liver, heart, gastrointestinal, and nervous system damage (Morton, 1990). Death can occur from heart arrhythmias or suffocation by the plastic bag containing the inhalant.

Depressants

These substances, which depress the central nervous system, include alcohol (discussed in chapter 13 of this volume) and sedative-hypnotics. Sedative-hypnotics include barbiturates (e.g., phenobarbital, secobarbital), benzodiazepines (e.g., Valium, Librium, Ativan), methaqualone (e.g., Quaalude), glutethimide (e.g., Doriden), and chloral hydrate (e.g., Noctec). Effects experienced after ingestion include euphoria, disinhibition, cognitive impairment, loss of motor coordination, and slurred speech. High doses can produce hallucinations or paranoia, ataxia, sedation, and increased risk for accidents (e.g., vehicular). Very high doses can produce decreased heart rate, respiratory failure, coma, or death. These drugs show cross-tolerance, presenting a high risk for lethal overdose if used simultaneously with combinations of different CNS depressants (e.g., alcohol used with barbiturates). A "paradoxical reaction" of excitability, fear, anger, and panic is sometimes evident in children under the influence of sedative-hypnotics (Schuckit, 1989). Withdrawal from CNS depressants entails anxiety, insomnia, headaches, tremors, muscle aches, increased heart and respiratory rates, fatigue, and sometimes disorientation, hallucinations, depression, and convulsions.

Polysubstance Use

Use of multiple substances complicates the acute effects and clinical course of substance use. Recent pop-ulation-based studies have found that use of multiple drugs (including alcohol) is common among adolescents (Stein, Newcomb, & Bentler, 1987). Martin, Arria, Mezzich, and Bukstein (1993) found that the majority of teens entering treatment for alcohol abuse concurrently used one or more other psychoactive substances. In a series of studies of clinical samples, Brown and colleagues have reported that teens in inpatient alcohol and drug treatment programs almost uniformly use multiple substances, with the average teen using three to four drugs other than alcohol during his or her lifetime (e.g., Brown, Mott, & Myers, 1990; Brown, Vik, & Creamer, 1989; Stewart & Brown, 1995).

ETIOLOGY OF ADOLESCENT DRUG ABUSE PROBLEMS

Research on development of drug problems in adolescence indicates that multiple factors set the stage for potential drug abuse in the teenage years. Biological, environmental, and intrapersonal factors each play a role in the initiation of drug use and progression to drug abuse.

Biological Factors

The role of genetics in development of substance abuse problems has become evident in twin, adoption, and other family studies (Cloninger, Bohman, & Sigvardsson, 1981; Cotton, 1979; Goodwin, 1979; Goodwin et al., 1974; Schuckit, 1985a; Sher, 1987). Although most of these studies have documented the genetic link between parental and offspring alcoholism, a variety of problems, including drug abuse, are more prevalent among offspring of alcoholics than among offspring of nonalcoholics (Sher, 1987). For example, Cadoret, Troughton, O'Gorman, and Heywood (1986) found that adopted individuals with drug abuse problems were significantly more likely than adopted individuals without drug problems to have biological relatives with alcohol problems. However, the genetic role in the etiology of drug abuse is less consistent than in the alcohol literature.

Although the influence of genetics appears to be significant, it is important to note that not all individuals with genetic risk for substance abuse go on to develop substance abuse problems. Environmental and personal factors also influence development of drug problems.

Comorbidity

Little research is available to date on the role of psychiatric symptomatology and drug use progression among adolescents. One recent study documented that 59 percent of adolescents evaluated during inpatient alcohol/drug treatment met criteria for one or more *DSM III-R* Axis I diagnoses in addition to their substance use diagnoses (Westermeyer, Specker, Neider, & Lingenfelter, 1994). Development of substance abuse problems and psychiatric problems involves reciprocal relationships (Brown, Mott, & Myers, 1990; Hansell & White, 1991; Johnson & Kaplan, 1990). Adolescents may use drugs to cope with psychological distress or psychiatric symptoms; however, use of drugs may create or contribute to psychiatric symptomatology and distress (Sadava, 1987; Sadava, 1990; Sadava & Pak, 1993).

Westermeyer and colleagues' (1994) study of 100 inpatient adolescents found that older adolescents (ages 15 to 18) were more likely to report depressive symptoms than younger adolescents (ages 12 to 15), perhaps because they may be experiencing more distress as a results of their drug involvement. However, the association between psychological distress and drug use has received mixed results. Hansell and White studied the relationship between drug use, psychological distress, and physical symptoms in 432 adolescents and found no evidence that psychological and physical distress caused drug use, but they did find support for the notion that drug use contributed to psychological problems. This effect may result from alterations in the maturational process, such as reduced participation in activities, school, employment, and other sources of positive social support, as well as direct physiological effects of drug use (Johnson & Kaplan, 1990; Vaillant, 1983).

Both internalizing and externalizing disorders are common among teens in treatment for substance abuse (Bukstein, Glancy, & Kaminer, 1992). For example, Brown and colleagues (Mott, Myers, Tammariello, & Brown, 1992; Stewart & Brown, 1994) found a high incidence of conduct disorder among adolescent substance abusers in treatment, poorer treatment outcome for substance-abusing adolescents with an independent diagnosis of conduct-disorder, a cluster of aggressive conduct-disorder behaviors that reliably discriminate between primary conduct-disorder teens with a substance abuse problem and teens whose conduct disorder appears secondary to substance use, and a 50 percent rate of antisocial personality disorder diagnosis among primary conduct-disorder teens at two years after treatment.

Environmental Factors

Family

Components of teens' environments may result in substance involvement independently or in interaction with biological factors (e.g., Sher, 1987). The family environment appears to have a significant role in the etiology of teen drug problems with positive, loving parent/child bonds associated with reduced risk for children to use drugs (Hundleby & Mercer, 1987; Kandel, 1978). Conversely, high levels of parent/adolescent conflict (Needle, Glynn, & Needle, 1983) and lack of familial cohesion (Hundleby & Mercer, 1987) correlate with increased risk for teen drug use.

In general, three family characteristics correlate with elevated risk for adolescent substance abuse: (1) parental deviance, including antisocial behaviors, alcoholism, and drug abuse; (2) minimal parental involvement with their children; and (3) dearth of affectionate, supportive parent/child interactions (Sadava, 1987). Parental monitoring and attitudes affect teen drug use indirectly by influencing peer selection (Brown, Mott, & Stewart, 1992; Chassin, Pillow, Curran, Molina, & Barrera, 1993; Dishion, Patterson, & Reid, 1988). Teens with substance-abusing parents have a significantly increased risk for using drugs above and beyond genetic risks because substance use is often a common coping response modeled to these teens (Chassin et al., 1993; Holden, Brown, & Mott, 1988).

Peers

The influence of peers increases during all stages of adolescent development and is the most consistent and strongest risk factor for adolescent drug use (Bentler, 1992). The desire to "fit in" with group norms is very strong in early adolescence (Costanzo & Shaw, 1966). Peers influence exposure and access to drugs, model use or abstinence, and act as powerful reinforcers regarding substance use decisions. Teens select their peer group and are selected by peers based largely on shared values and interests (Dishion, Patterson, & Reid, 1988).

Social support provided by peers may result in either increases or reductions in risk of teen drug use. For example, teens without social supports that model and reinforce coping strategies other than substance use are more likely to use drugs (Holden, Brown, & Mott, 1988; Tucker, 1982) or continue to abuse drugs (Myers & Brown, 1990; Richter, Brown, & Mott, 1991). In addition, teens with social networks composed of drug users will likely assume beliefs and values consistent with a drug use life-style (Brown, Mott, & Stewart, 1992). Hence, risk of drug use and abuse increases in concert with peer drug use. Furthermore, presence of positive social support during adolescence offsets potential problems (including problems often caused by teenage drug use) in young adulthood, even when controlling for possible confounding effects (Newcomb & Bentler, 1988b).

Ethnic Differences

Ethnicity and culture influence initiation of drug use and development of drug dependency through several societal and historical factors, including history of racial oppression; socioeconomic, educational, and employment disadvantage; geographic instability; and underutilization of community services (Office for Substance Abuse Prevention, 1992). Welte and Barnes (1987) found that the number of problems experienced per ounce of ethanol consumption was higher for African American adolescents than for adolescents from other ethnic backgrounds despite lower overall use. This suggests that socio-cultural environment may play an independent role in the development of substance use problems.

Some studies have noted differences across ethnic groups in terms of factors involved in development of drug use (Huba, Wingard, & Bentler, 1980; Zucker & Gomberg, 1986). Maddahian, Newcomb, and Bentler (1988) found ethnic differences in intentions to use drugs in the future. In particular, early intentions to use drugs related highly to subsequent hard drug use among white youth and related modestly to subsequent drug use among African American and Asian American youth, but intentions to use drugs did not relate to later actual use for Hispanic American youth. The researchers therefore concluded that childhood intentions to use drugs differentially relate to subsequent drug use depending on ethnicity.

Life Stress

Researchers have associated a variety of stressful life circumstances with the onset and progression of drug involvement. Life adversity—such as relationship problems, familial difficulties, legal troubles, and academic failure—appear to be risk factors for adolescent substance abuse (Pandina & Schuele, 1983). Furthermore, life stress is higher in families with histories of alcoholism (Brown, 1989; Sher, 1991). Teens with an alcoholic parent subjectively rate life stressors more negatively than do teens without an alcoholic parent (Brown, 1989). McCubbin, Needle, and Wilson (1985) found that stressful life events reported by families relate to adolescent offspring substance use, and Duncan (1977) found that high stress levels may precipitate drug use in some teens.

Intrapersonal Factors

Personality

A number of personality characteristics appear related to adolescent drug use: rebelliousness, autonomy striving, liberalism, willingness to try new experiences, and independence (Segal, Huba, & Singer, 1980). Similarly, research has linked sensation seeking (Cloninger, Sigvardsson, & Bohman, 1988; Kohn & Annis, 1977; Zuckerman, 1994), low self-esteem (Kaplan, 1977), impulsivity (Vistor, Crossman, & Eiserman, 1973), low self-efficacy (Schinke, Botvin, & Orlandi, 1991), and nonconventionality (Brook, Whiteman, & Gordon, 1983) to high rates of substance involvement. Labouvie and McGee (1986) found that these personality factors relate to early drug use and are risk factors for rapid development of substance abuse problems during adolescence.

Longitudinal research has also uncovered some personality characteristics associated with late adolescence development of frequent drug use. For example, in a study of 101 San Francisco-area youth, those who went on to use drugs in later adolescence frequently exhibited childhood personalities characterized by deviance, emotional lability, inattention, lack of involvement in activities, and stubbornness (Shedler & Block, 1990).

Drug Expectancies

Adolescents' drug outcome expectancies appear related to substance involvement and mediate initiation of use and progression to problematic use (Brown, 1993a; Christiansen, Goldman, & Brown, 1985; Schafer & Brown, 1991). Expectancies develop from both direct and vicarious experiences with substances and reflect culturally held beliefs as well as personal learning about drugs in school, in the media, and from peers and family (see Goldman, Brown, Christiansen, & Smith, 1991, for review). Research has also linked family history of alcoholism with increased positive expectancies of certain substance effects (Brown, Creamer, & Stetson, 1987; Sher, 1993).

Expectancies are generally substance specific, but some expectancies (e.g., relaxation/tension-reduction effects) are common to several different substances. Overall, youth who believe drugs produce positive effects are more likely than youth who do not hold this belief to use drugs frequently and develop drug-related problems. In contrast, expectancies of negative drug effects may act as deterrents to the initiation of drug use (Brown, 1993a).

Emotional and Behavioral Problems

Adolescent substance abuse also relates to behavioral problems and emotional disorders (Brown, Gleghorn, & Schuckit, 1989; Donovan & Jessor, 1985), which may operate as risk factors, exacerbating features, and consequences of youthful drug involvement. For example, research has linked drug use with prior conduct disorder, illegal activities, and aggression (Brown, Gleghorn, & Schuckit, 1989; Rydelius, 1983).

Additionally, involvement in delinquent behaviors both precipitates drug involvement (Johnston, O'Malley, & Eveland, 1978; Moffitt, 1993; Robins, 1986; Stewart & Brown, 1994) and follows from a drug-involved life-style. In particular, teens are more likely to engage in delinquent acts as a means of obtaining drugs or because they experience behavioral disinhibition during intoxication. The interplay of drug use and conduct-disordered behaviors may manifest differently in girls than in boys, with boys exhibiting more problem behaviors through criminal activities and aggressive acts and girls displaying more running away, sexual promiscuity, lying, truancy, and shoplifting (Robins, 1986).

Drug-abusing teens often display symptoms of mood disorders, including depression, suicidal ideation, anxiety, and anger. This emotional dysfunction can result from drug use (substance induced mood disorders; Brown & Schuckit, 1988; Schuckit, Irwin, & Brown, 1990). Mood dysfunction symptoms can result from drug intoxication (particularly CNS depressants, hallucinogens, PCP, opiates) or drug withdrawal (especially withdrawal from CNS depressants, cocaine, amphetamines, or opiates). To make a valid psychiatric diagnosis, drugs of abuse must not be present in the central nervous system, and the length of time required for the withdrawal-related effects to dissipate varies by drug type, although most drugs cease to have any direct impact on mood after four weeks of abstinence (Brown & Schuckit, 1988).

It appears that individuals with certain psychiatric problems, such as anxiety or depression, may select certain substances to alleviate psychiatric symptoms or "self-medicate" (Millman & Botvin, 1983). For example, individuals with anxiety disorders may find that central nervous system depressants or opiates may reduce anxiety. These individuals might experience certain drugs as more reinforcing than would individuals without psychiatric problems (Brown, Mott, & Stewart, 1992).

DEVELOPMENT AND PROGRESSION OF SUBSTANCE ABUSE

This section describes several theories of the trajectory toward drug problems in adolescence. Drug use can be a form of rebellion, an instrument toward cohesion with a peer group, or an attempt to appear grown-up (Hawkins, 1982). In the teenage years, many individuals experiment with different life-styles, some of which include drug use. This "normal" experimentation—especially with alcohol, cigarettes, and marijuana—can be part of the natural process of establishing identity independent from that of the parents (Schinke, Botvin, & Orlandi, 1991).

For example, in a longitudinal examination of the relationship between marijuana use and psychological health, Shedler and Block (1990) found that 18-year-olds who had experimented with marijuana had better social skills and a higher level of adjustment than both frequent users of marijuana and abstainers.

These subjects also had better maternal parenting. These results do not suggest that experimentation will lead to better adjustment but that some experimentation with marijuana may be normal and common in the present historical and cultural context and that in late adolescence, occasional experimentation with marijuana is not necessarily destructive. However, drug problems may develop for some of these individuals.

Newcomb and Bentler (1988a, 1988b) reported findings that suggested experimentation with alcohol is also a normal part of current adolescent development. In an eight-year follow-up of 654 adolescents into young adulthood, Newcomb and Bentler found that alcohol use in adolescence actually related to positive self-feelings, stable social relationships with family, and secure romantic attachments in young adulthood. Adolescents with life-styles of heavy drug use (e.g., cocaine, heroin) had more problems in young adulthood—including more health and family problems, dysphoric emotional functioning, and troubled romantic relationships—than young adults who had not abused hard drugs during teenage years. These results suggest a problematic life trajectory at least partially attributed to adolescent involvement with hard drugs.

Longitudinal studies have revealed some extended or delayed consequences of adolescent drug use that occur in young adulthood, such as physical problems, psychological maladjustment, unstable employment patterns, and higher divorce rates (Kandel, Davies, Karus, & Yamaguchi, 1986; Newcomb & Bentler, 1988b). Some authors have suggested that drug involvement during adolescence may impede psychosocial maturation and impair accomplishment of normative tasks of adolescent development (Baumrind & Moselle, 1985). Alternatively, adolescent drug misuse may also produce accelerated transition to new developmental stages and circumvention of the typical developmental sequence; that is, drug-abusing teens transition prematurely into adult roles without sufficient developmental preparation for success at adult roles and tasks (Newcomb, 1987; Newcomb & Bentler, 1988a, 1988b).

The relevance of various risk factors for drug abuse fluctuates with developmental stage and across and within ethnic-cultural groups. For example, the influence of peer behaviors and attitudes on substance involvement during adolescence appears greater than during other developmental stages. Personality traits and drug expectancies may stabilize with maturity and may therefore play a more powerful role in the perpetuation of drug involvement in later adolescence than in early adolescence (Brown, Mott, & Stewart, 1992).

Problem Behavior Theory

Problem behavior theory seeks to explain adolescent deviance as a single factor of unconventionality. Donovan and Jessor (1985) found, in a high school sample, that drug use in adolescence occurred frequently with other problem behaviors, such as delinquency and sexual precociousness, and that a single factor could account for the majority of variance in all of these behaviors. Discriminant validity for this theory is evident in negative associations of problem behaviors with conventional behaviors, such as church attendance. Implications of problem behavior theory are that intervention and prevention efforts must target multiple deviant behaviors and the social and personal factors that influence them rather than specific types of drugs or drug use exclusively.

Gateway Theory

Kandel and colleagues (Kandel, Yamaguchi, & Chen, 1992; Kandel & Yamaguchi, 1993) studied over 1,000 high school students through young adulthood and consistently found that drug involvement in adolescence follows a predictable sequence from use of substances that are legal for adults (i.e., alcohol or cigarettes), to use of marijuana, to use of hard drugs (most commonly cocaine), and finally to use of prescribed psychoactives as adults.

Alcohol use appears to have a stronger link to progression in this drug-involvement sequence for males than for females, and cigarette use has a stronger link for females than for males. The use of a drug at a particular stage in the sequence does not necessarily infer subsequent use of drugs in the next stage. Many teens stop at a certain stage without progressing farther. Rather, entry into a certain stage is essentially a prerequisite for the next stage.

Another aspect of the stage theory is the pattern of vulnerability or proneness that characterizes teens who use different classes of drugs. Young people who use a particular type of drug commonly exhibit other behavioral problems that may result from the same risk factors generally associated with drug use. This theory is particularly useful for identifying populations that are at risk for progression to a more serious stage of drug involvement from a less serious one and allocating intervention resources to those populations.

Neurological Factors and Risks

Research has identified some neurological deficits among adolescents who chronically abuse drugs. Because of the neuropsychological development that occurs during adolescence, teens may have a better chance of recovering function than do adults. However, drug abuse may impede development of some neurocognitive skills.

The relationship between adolescent drug use and neuropsychological functioning appears to be bidirectional. Protracted heavy drug use could cause neuropsychological impairment in certain domains of functioning. These impairments, if found to exist, could have differential rates of improvement with abstinence. It is also possible that cognitive deficiencies may be a risk factor for the development of drug abuse problems, or perhaps for the conduct problems that lead to drug abuse.

Yeudall, Fromm-Auch, and Davies (1982) found 84 percent of juvenile delinquents studied had abnormally greater anterior than posterior cerebral dysfunction. Another study (Pontius & Ruttiger, 1976) found delinquent adolescents less able to alter plans of ongoing activity, which suggested a maturational lag in the frontal system. Furthermore, sons of alcoholics have skill deficits in certain areas as well as an increased risk for substance abuse (Moss, Kirisci, Gordon, & Tarter, 1994).

Tapert and Brown (1994) evaluated the relationship between neuropsychological functioning and drug and alcohol use among a sample of adolescents recruited from inpatient substance abuse treatment programs four years posttreatment. Significant differences existed in attentional performance between chronic substance abusers and those who had abstained from alcohol and drugs posttreatment, with the abstainers performing better. Adolescents

who abused drugs throughout the four years exhibited deficits on tasks of concentration and attention. This suggests that poor neuropsychological performance may increase teens' vulnerability to continued drug and alcohol abuse, which may in turn exacerbate neurocognitive problems.

In addition, teens who reported experiencing more drug withdrawal symptoms, relative to teens who reported few withdrawal symptoms, performed more poorly on tasks of visuo-perceptual performance, memory, attention, and executive/inhibitory functioning above and beyond the effects accounted for by recent drug use (Tapert & Brown, 1994). This finding suggests that possibly the physical effects experienced by individuals may be more relevant to cognitive functioning than other factors related to drug and alcohol consumption for this age group. Drug withdrawal symptoms may be an indicator of heavy, potentially damaging drug use. Because neuropsychological deficits due to substance use are more difficult to detect in adolescents than in adults (Brandt & Doyle, 1983; Moss et al., 1994), it is reasonable to assume that deficits may become detected among adolescents only when they abuse substances severely enough to experience physiological repercussions.

ASSESSMENT

The recent development of standardized instruments that tap the multidimensional nature of adolescent drug involvement has facilitated assessment of adolescent drug use. For example, the Personal Experience Inventory (PEI; Winters, 1992) assesses problem severity on five scales: personal involvement, effects from drug use, social benefits of drug use, personal consequences of drug use, and poly-drug use. Researchers validated the PEI by comparing scores to *DSM* diagnoses as well as referral outcomes. This instrument may therefore be useful for diagnosing substance use disorders and determining treatment referral (e.g., outpatient vs. inpatient) as part of a comprehensive assessment framework.

Tarter (1990) developed a multiphasic system for evaluation and treatment of substance abuse in adolescents. He proposed three phases of assessment (screening, diagnosis, and treatment planning) across 10 domains of functioning, which include substance use, behavioral problems, health, psychiatric disorders, social skills, family systems, school, work, peer relationships, and leisure activities. The first phase uses the Drug Use Screening Inventory (Tarter & Hegedus, 1991) to identify problem areas, and the second phase of Tarter's assessment strategy utilizes standardized instruments such as the Child Behavior Checklist (Achenbach & Edelbrock, 1983), Wide Range Achievement Test (Jastak & Wilkinson, 1984) and Kiddie-SADS (Chambers et al., 1985) to assess each domain. Finally, treatment planning follows problems identified in each domain.

In terms of substance involvement and consequences, Brown has developed the Customary Drinking and Drug Use Record (CDDR; Brown, Creamer, & Stetson, 1987) to assess current and lifetime alcohol and other drug use patterns, withdrawal and dependency symptoms, and negative consequences for teens. The CDDR includes *DSM-III-R*-criteria-based questions for substance abuse, dependence, and withdrawal (American Psychiatric Association, 1987), and Lu's Drug Indulgence Index (Lu, 1974). The Alcohol Dependence Scale (ADS; Skinner, 1984), alcoholism life problem criteria (Schuckit, 1985b), and adolescent alcohol or drug related life problem items (Donovan & Jessor, 1985; Stein, Newcomb, & Bentler, 1988) are also part of the CDDR.

Interviewers using the CDDR gather substance use history for cigarettes, alcohol (i.e., beer, wine, liquor), marijuana, amphetamines, hallucinogens, cocaine, opiates, barbiturates, and inhalants. Age of first use, onset of weekly (regular) use, lifetime use episodes, and quantity and frequency of current use (i.e., previous three months) are evaluated separately for each substance. Intensity of use (e.g., frequency of intoxication) is also an evaluation component. Brown designed the CDDR to be sensitive to changes over time regarding drug use and consequences.

PREVENTION

Botvin and Botvin (1992) provide a thorough review of prevention strategies for adolescent drug use. They categorize prevention strategies as traditional, personal social skills, and social influence. *Traditional* approaches to substance use prevention focus on providing information about the negative consequences of drug use. However, these approaches have not been effective in changing substance use patterns (Botvin & Botvin, 1992). *Personal social skills* approaches are comprehensive attempts at increasing self-esteem, enhancing coping, and developing social and assertiveness skills. The *social influence* model attempts to strengthen a child's skills in identifying and resisting social pressure to use drugs.

Ellickson, Bell, and McGuigan (1993) found that junior high students given training in recognizing and resisting social pressure to use drugs showed short-term behavior change as well as long-term attitudinal change. Because behavioral changes brought about by the prevention program were not present by the twelfth grade, however, continuous or intermittent prevention efforts may be necessary for sustained behavioral effects. In general, prevention programs that delay onset of use of gateway substances may have an important effect on the sequence and outcome of drug use (Kandel & Yamaguchi, 1993).

TREATMENT

In a national survey, 20 percent of all drug treatment patients were adolescents, although only 5 percent of treatment programs were specific to adolescent treatment, with most adolescents treated in outpatient settings (Beschner & Friedman, 1985). Many of the treatment approaches used in adolescent substance abuse treatment are identical to those used with adults (Brown, Mott, & Myers, 1990; Kaminer, 1994). Abstinence is the primary goal of most adolescent treatment programs. Complicating attempts to encourage abstinence, however, is the adolescents' string of identification with drug-using peers and intense conflict with authority figures (Obermeier & Henry, 1985).

Adolescents often present at intake with problems other than substance abuse. Legal or academic problems, family conflict, conduct problems, and affective symptoms are common precipitants of substance abuse treatment (Williams, Feibelman, & Moulder, 1989). Thus, teens are seldom fully cognizant of the severity of their drug and alcohol problems but instead focus on the precipitating crisis.

Although intensive medical detoxification is seldom necessary for adolescents (Kaminer, 1994), withdrawal symptoms are common (Stewart & Brown, 1995). The first stage of treatment typically consists of a detoxification and problem identification phase, followed by rehabilitation efforts (Brown, Mott, & Stewart, 1992). Treatment activities, both inpatient and outpatient, typically include group and individual therapy, behavioral management through token economies or contracting, psychoeducational groups, involvement in 12-step programs, coping skills training, and written assignments (Brown, Mott, & Stewart, 1992; Kaminer, 1994). Because of legal requirements, treatment programs usually offer educational classes. Because of high relapse rates following substance abuse treatment (Brown, Vik, & Creamer, 1989), aftercare is critically important, as well as involvement in community support, such as Alcoholics or Narcotics Anonymous.

Relapse Prevention

Relapse prevention (RP) is a cognitive-behavioral strategy designed to prevent return to harmful use of the previously abused substance (Marlatt & Gordon, 1980, 1985). Practitioners can apply RP techniques to a wide range of behaviors, and RP is particularly popular in the treatment of addictive behaviors. These strategies have proven successful regardless of the methods used to initiate abstinence (Marlatt & George, 1984).

RP teaches patients to identify and anticipate high-risk situations in which an individual's sense of control becomes threatened and the risk of relapse to drugs is high. Assessment of individual high-risk situations involves daily self-monitoring of the addictive behavior. RP then works to teach coping skills for managing the high-risk situation without violating treatment goals. Coping strategies may include behavioral strategies (avoiding high-risk locations, engaging in alternative activities) and cognitive strategies (using imagery and self-talk).

By predicting difficult situations and learning how to cope with them, the individual's self-efficacy for maintaining treatment goals increases. RP also works to modify outcome expectancies for use of the drug, as positive expectancies for drug effects highly relate to drug use (Brown, 1993a). The RP program attempts to teach realistic expectations about the drug.

The RP model differentiates between a *lapse* and a *relapse*. A *lapse* is a limited return to drug use with a rapid cessation of use. Reframing the lapse as a learning experience helps individuals carefully assess the situation and coping responses and construct a strategy for coping effectively in the future. This process also serves to minimize feelings of guilt and decreased self-efficacy that often occur following return to drug use. A *relapse* is a prolonged return to drug use, usually with negative consequences.

Marlatt and Gordon also describe an Abstinence Violation Effect (AVE), in which an individual in the midst of a lapse experiences a decrease in self-efficacy and passively gives in to harmful use of the substance. The RP approach also emphasizes a balanced life-style between "shoulds" (i.e., responsibilities) and "wants" (pleasurable activities) to decrease the risk of relapse. The development of "positive addictions" that are incompatible with a drug-using life-style—such as exercise, meditation, and relaxation practices—are encouraged as part of the RP approach.

Adolescent relapse rates are relatively comparable to those for adults (Brown, Vik, & Creamer, 1989). The greatest risk for relapse is in the first six months following treatment, in which approximately two-thirds of teens relapse (Brown, Mott, & Myers, 1990), and up to 85 percent may relapse in the first year posttreatment (Brown, 1993b). There is considerable fluctuation in substance involvement for teens after treatment. For example, approximately half of the teens studied improved with time despite some time-limited use following treatment (Brown, Myers, Mott, & Vik, 1994).

The precursors to adolescent relapse appear somewhat different than for adults. Direct and indirect social pressure seem to be the most prominent and immediate precipitants of relapse among teens, whereas negative emotional states and interpersonal conflict commonly precipitate relapses for adults. One study found that 90 percent of adolescent substance abuse relapses occurred in the presence of other people, and in 73 percent of these situations, no abstinent model was present (Brown, Vik, & Creamer, 1989). Clearly, relapse prevention programs that help teens identify personal high-risk situations and teach effective coping strategies and life-styles are necessary to help teens maintain treatment goals long after they leave the inpatient treatment setting.

Harm Reduction

Harm reduction prevention and intervention techniques have received increasing attention in recent
years. Harm reduction strategies include those that
normalize rather than marginalize substance users,
focus attention on reducing the harmful consequences
of drug use, and refrain from making services contingent on the user's commitment to change. Harm reduction places substance use on a continuum, and reductions in harm can occur in steps. Although
abstinence from drug use may be the ultimate objective, significant reductions in personal and societal
harm can occur on the way to this goal. Therapists encourage any degree of positive change, and this attitude reduces negative reactance by participating users
(Marlatt, Somers, & Tapert, 1993).

Harm reduction approaches are particularly
promising for young people because the focus is on
practical concerns, and the techniques aim to avoid
creating negative reactance. An example of this strategy exists in the Netherlands, where marijuana and
other cannabis products are available in coffee shops
and youth centers. Although not legalized, the Dutch
have decriminalized and learned to tolerate possession of small amounts of marijuana for personal use.
The Dutch make a distinction between "soft drugs"
(alcohol and cannabis) and "hard drugs" (cocaine,
heroin, and other drugs) because scientific literature
indicates that use of hard drugs is riskier from a health
perspective than use of soft drugs.

Two benefits occur from this policy: The credibility of educational programs geared toward youth
increases, and markets for the sales of both types of
drugs remain separate; thus, cannabis users do not become tempted to buy stronger drugs because they are
not available in designated coffee shops. Despite the
implementation of decriminalization in 1976, the
prevalence of cannabis use in the Netherlands remains low. For youth in the Netherlands between the
ages of 10 and 18, only 4.2 percent have ever used
cannabis, and the number of daily users is less than 0.1
percent (Marlatt & Tapert, 1993). Empirical analysis
of these strategies with drug-abusing adolescents has
not yet transpired, but the theoretical framework
holds promise for teens who remain recalcitrant to
other treatment formats.

CONCLUSION

This chapter has provided an overview of the prevalence, etiology, course, and treatment of adolescent
drug abuse. The most striking fact of adolescent drug
involvement is its heterogeneity. No single theory or
approach can suffice in explaining the problem. Some
of the important sources of diversity highlighted here
are developmental considerations, psychiatric comorbidity, and cultural and gender differences. In addition, the tendency of adolescents to use multiple
substances complicates the diagnosis and assessment
of drug abuse. Clinicians, whether screening for or intervening in adolescent drug abuse, must be aware of
its heterogeneous nature, be ready to use multiple
methods of assessment, and be willing to tailor interventions to teen-specific needs.

REFERENCES

Achenbach, T. M., & Edelbrock, C. (1983). *Manual for the Child Behavior Checklist and Revised Child Behavior Profile.* Burlington, VT: University of Vermont Department of Psychiatry.

Adler, I., & Kandel, D. B. (1982). A cross-cultural comparison of sociopsychological factors in alcohol use among adolescents in Israel, France, and the United States. *Journal of Youth & Adolescence, 11,* 89–113.

American Psychiatric Association (1987). *Diagnostic and statistical manual of mental disorders* (3rd ed., rev.). Washington, DC: Author.

American Psychiatric Association. (1994). *Diagnostic and statistical manual of mental disorders* (4th ed.). Washington, DC: Author.

Baumrind, D., & Moselle, K. A. (1985). A developmental perspective on adolescent drug use. *Advances in Alcohol and Substance Use, 5,* 41–67.

Bentler, P. M. (1992). Etiologies and consequences of adolescent drug use: Implications for prevention. *Journal of Addictive Diseases, 11,* 47–61.

Beschner, G. M., & Friedman, A. S. (1985). Treatment of adolescent drug abusers. *International Journal of the Addictions, 20,* 971–993.

Botvin, G. J., & Botvin, E. M. (1992). Adolescent tobacco, alcohol, and drug abuse: Prevention strategies, empirical findings, and assessment issues. *Journal of Developmental & Behavioral Pediatrics, 13,* 290–301.

Brandt, J., & Doyle, L. F. (1983). Concept attainment, tracking, and shifting in adolescent polydrug abusers. *Journal of Nervous and Mental Disease, 171,* 559–563.

Brook, J. S., Whiteman, M., & Gordon, A. S. (1983). Stages of drug use in adolescence: Personality, peer, and family correlates. *Developmental Psychology, 19,* 269–277.

Brown, S. (1989). Life events of adolescents in relation to personal and parental substance abuse. *American Journal of Psychiatry, 146,* 484–489.

Brown, S. A. (1993a). Drug effect expectancies and addictive behavior change. *Experimental and Clinical Psychopharmacology, 1,* 55–67.

Brown, S. A. (1993b). Recovery patterns in adolescent substance abuse. In J. S. Baer, G. A. Marlatt, & R. J. McMahon (Eds.), *Addictive behaviors across the life span* (pp. 161–183). Newbury Park, CA.: Sage.

Brown, S. A., Creamer, V. A., & Stetson, B. A. (1987). Adolescent alcohol expectancies in relation to personal and parental drinking patterns. *Journal of Abnormal Psychology, 96,*117–121.

Brown, S. A., Gleghorn, A., & Schuckit, M. (1989). Conduct disorder among adolescent substance abusers. Unpublished manuscript.

Brown, S. A., Mott, M. A., & Myers, M. G. (1990). Adolescent alcohol and drug treatment outcome. In R. R. Watson (Ed.), *Drug and alcohol abuse prevention* (pp. 373–403). Totowa, NJ: Humana.

Brown, S. A., Mott, M. A., & Stewart, M. A. (1992). Adolescent alcohol and drug abuse. In C. E. Walker & M. C. Roberts (Eds.), *Handbook of clinical child psychology* (2nd ed., pp. 677–693). New York: John Wiley.

Brown, S. A., Myers, M. G., Mott, M. A., & Vik, P. W. (1994). Correlates of success following treatment for adolescent substance abuse. *Applied & Preventive Psychology, 3,* 61–73.

Brown, S. A., & Schuckit, M. A. (1988). Changes in depression among abstinent alcoholics. *Journal of Studies on Alcohol, 49,* 412–417.

Brown, S., Vik, P., & Creamer, V. (1989). Characteristics of relapse following adolescent substance abuse treatment. *Addictive Behaviors, 14,* 291–300.

Bukstein, O. G., Glancy, L. J., & Kaminer, Y. (1992). Patterns of affective comorbidity in a clinical population of dually diagnosed adolescent substance abusers. *Journal of the American Academy of Child & Adolescent Psychiatry, 31,* 1041–1045.

Cadoret, R. J., Troughton, E., O'Gorman, T. W., & Heywood, E. (1986). An adoption study of genetic and environmental factors in drug abuse. *Archives of General Psychiatry, 43,* 1131–1136.

Chambers, W. J. et al. (1985). The assessment of affective disorders in children and adolescents by semistructured interview: Test-retest reliability of the Schedule for Affective Disorders and Schizophrenia for School-Age Children, *Archives of General Psychiatry, 42,* 696–702.

Chassin, L., Pillow, D. R., Curran, P. J., Molina, B. S. G., & Barrera, M. (1993). Relation of parental alcoholism to early adolescent substance use: A test of three mediating mechanisms. *Journal of Abnormal Psychology, 102,* 3–19.

Christiansen, B. A., Goldman, M. S., & Brown, S. A. (1985). The differential development of adolescent alcohol expectancies may predict adult alcoholism. *Addictive Behaviors, 10,* 299–306.

Cloninger, C. R., Bohman, M., & Sigvardsson, S. (1981). Inheritance of alcohol abuse: Cross-fostering analysis of adopted men. *Archives of General Psychiatry, 38,* 861–868.

Cloninger, C R., Sigvardsson, S., & Bohman, M. (1988). Childhood personality predicts alcohol abuse in young adults. *Alcoholism: Clinical and Experimental Research, 12,* 494–505.

Cohen, S. (1981). Adolescence and drug abuse: Biomedical consequences. *National Institute on Drug Abuse Research Monograph, 38,* 104–112.

Costanzo, P., & Shaw, M. (1966). Conformity as a function of age level. *Child Development, 37,* 967–975.

Cotton, N. S. (1979). The familial incidence of alcoholism: A review. *Journal of Studies on Alcohol, 40,* 89–116.

Dishion, T. J., Patterson, G. R., & Reid, J. R. (1988). Parent and peer factors associated with drug sampling in early adolescence: Implications for treatment. *NIDA Research Monograph, 77,* 69–93.

Donovan, J. E., & Jessor, R. (1985). Structure of problem behavior in adolescence and young adulthood. *Journal of Consulting and Clinical Psychology, 53,* 890–904.

Duncan, D. F. (1977). Life stress as a precursor to adolescent drug dependence. *International Journal of the Addictions, 12,* 1047–1056.

Ellickson, P. L., Bell, R. M., & McGuigan, K. (1993). Preventing adolescent drug use: Long-term results of a junior high program. *American Journal of Public Health, 83,* 856–861.

Goldman, M. S., Brown, S. A., Christiansen, B. A., & Smith, G. T. (1991). Alcoholism and memory: Broadening the scope of alcohol-expectancy research. *Psychological Bulletin, 110,* 137–146.

Goodwin, D. W. (1979). Alcoholism and heredity: A review and hypothesis. *Archives of General Psychiatry, 36,* 57–61.

Goodwin, D. W., Schulsinger, F., Moller, N., Hermansen, L., Winokur, G., & Guze, B. (1974). Drinking problems in adopted and nonadopted sons of alcoholics. *Archives of General Psychiatry, 31,* 164–169.

Hansell, S., & White, H. R. (1991). Adolescent drug use, psychological distress, and physical symptoms. *Journal of Health and Social Behavior, 32,* 288–301.

Hawkins, R. O. (1982). Adolescent alcohol abuse: A review. *Developmental and Behavioral Pediatrics, 3,* 83–87.

Holden, M. G., Brown, S. A., & Mott, M. A. (1988). Social support network of adolescents: Relation to family alcohol abuse. *American Journal of Drug and Alcohol Abuse, 14,* 487–498.

Huba, G. J., Wingard, J. A., & Bentler, P. M. (1980). Framework for an interactive theory of drug use. In D. J. Lettieri, M. Sayers, & H. W. Pearson (Eds.), *Theories on drug abuse* (pp. 95–101). Rockville, MD: National Institute on Drug Abuse.

Hundleby, J. D., & Mercer, G. W. (1987). Family and friends as social environments and their relationship to young adolescents' use of alcohol, tobacco, and marijuana. *Journal of Marriage and the Family, 49,* 151–164.

Jastak, S., & Wilkinson, G. S. (1984). *The Wide Range Achievement Test-Revised administration manual.* Wilmington, DE: Jastak Associates.

Johnson, R. J., & Kaplan, H. B. (1990). Stability of psychological symptoms: Drug use consequences and intervening processes. *Journal of Health and Social Behavior, 31,* 277–291.

Johnston, L. D., Bachman, J. G., & O'Malley, P. M. (1993). *National survey results on drug use from Monitoring the Future Study, 1975–1992, Vol. 1: Secondary school students.* Rockville, MD: U.S. Department of Health and Human Services.

Johnston, L. D., Bachman, J. G., & O'Malley, P. M. (1994). *National survey results on drug use from Monitoring the Future Study, 1975–1993, Vol. 1: Secondary school students.* Rockville, MD: U.S. Department of Health and Human Services.

Johnston, L. D., O'Malley, P. M., & Eveland, L. (1978). Drug and delinquency: A search for causal connections. In D. B. Kandel (Ed.), *Longitudinal research on drug use: Empirical findings and methodological issues* (pp. 137–156). Washington, DC: Hemisphere-John Wiley.

Kaminer, Y. (1994). Adolescent substance abuse. In M. Galanter & Herbert Kleber (Eds.), *The American Psychiatric Press textbook of substance abuse treatment.* Washington, DC.: American Psychiatric Press.

Kandel, D. (1978). Convergences in prospective longitudinal surveys of drug use in normal populations. In D. Kandel (Ed.), *Longitudinal research in drug use: Empirical findings and methodological issues.* Washington, DC: Hemisphere-John Wiley.

Kandel, D. B., Davies, M., Karus, D., & Yamaguchi, K. (1986). The consequences in young adulthood of adolescent drug involvement. *Archives of General Psychiatry, 43,* 746–754.

Kandel, D. B., & Yamaguchi, K. (1993). From beer to crack: Developmental patterns of drug involvement. *American Journal of Public Health, 83,* 851–855.

Kandel, D. B., Yamaguchi, K., & Chen, K. (1992). Stages of progression in drug involvement from adolescence to adulthood: Further evidence for the gateway theory. *Journal of Studies on Alcohol, 53,* 447–457.

Kaplan, H. B. (1977). Antecedents of deviant responses: Predicting from a general theory of deviant behavior. *Journal of Youth and Adolescence, 7,* 253–277.

Kohn, P. M., & Annis, H. M. (1977). Drug use and four kinds of novelty-seeking. *British Journal of Addiction, 72,* 135–141.

Kosten, T. R., & Rounsaville, B. J. (1988). Suicidality among opioid addicts. *American Journal of Drug and Alcohol Abuse, 14,* 357–369.

Labouvie, E. W., & McGee, C. R. (1986). Relation of personality to alcohol and drug use in adolescence. *Journal of Consulting and Clinical Psychology, 54,* 289–293.

Lu, K. H. (1974). The indexing and analysis of drug indulgence. *International Journal of the Addictions, 9,* 785–804.

Maddahian, E., Newcomb, M. D., & Bentler, P. M. (1988). Adolescent drug use and intention to use drugs: Concurrent and longitudinal analysis of four ethnic groups. *Addictive Behaviors, 13,* 191–195.

Marlatt, G. A., & George, W. H. (1984). Relapse prevention: Introduction and overview of the model. *British Journal of Addiction, 79,* 261–273.

Marlatt, G. A., & Gordon, J. R. (1980). Determinants of relapse: Implications for maintenance of behavior change. In P. Davidson & S. Davidson (Eds.), *Behavioral medicine: Changing health lifestyles* (pp. 410–452). New York: Brunner/Mazel.

Marlatt, G. A., & Gordon, J. R. (1985). *Relapse prevention.* New York: Guilford Press.

Marlatt, G. A., & Tapert, S. F. (1993). Harm reduction: Reducing the risks of addictive behaviors. In J. S. Baer, G. A. Marlatt, & R. J. McMahon (Eds.), *Addictive behaviors across the lifespan* (pp. 243–273). Newbury Park, CA: Sage.

Marlatt, G. A., Somers, J. M., & Tapert, S. F. (1993). Harm reduction: Application to alcohol abuse problems. In L. S. Onken, J. D. Blaine, & J. J. Boren (Eds.), *Behavioral treatments for drug abuse and dependence.* Rockville, MD: National Institute on Drug Abuse.

Martin, C. S., Arria, A. M., Mezzich, A. C., & Bukstein, O. G. (1993). Patterns of polydrug use in adolescent alcohol abusers. *American Journal of Drug and Alcohol Abuse, 19,* 511–521.

McCubbin, H. I., Needle, R. H., & Wilson, M. (1985). Adolescent health risk behaviors: Family stress and adolescent coping as critical factors. *Family Relations, 34,* 51–62.

McGlothlin, W. H., & West, L. J. (1968). The marijuana problem: An overview. *American Journal of Psychiatry, 125,* 1126–1134.

Millman, R. B., & Botvin, G. J. (1983). Substance use, abuse, and dependence. In M. D. Levine, W. B. Carey, A. C. Crocker, & R. T. Gross (Eds.), *Developmental-*

behavioral pediatrics (pp. 683–708). Philadelphia: W. B. Saunders.

Moffitt, T. E. (1993). The neuropsychology of conduct disorder. *Development & Psychopathology, 5,* 135–151.

Morton, H. G. (1990). Occurrence and treatment of solvent abuse in children and adolescents. In D. J. K. Balfour (Ed.), *Psychotropic drugs of abuse* (pp. 431–451). New York: Pergamon.

Moss, H. B., Kirisci, L., Gordon, H. W., & Tarter R. E. (1994). A neuropsychologic profile of adolescent alcoholics. *Alcoholism: Clinical and Experimental Research, 18,* 159–163.

Mott, M. A., Myers, M. G., Tammariello, C. F., & Brown, S. A. (1992). *Conduct disorder diagnosis is related to long-term adolescent drug treatment outcome.* Presented at the annual convention of the American Psychological Society, San Diego, CA.

Myers, M. G., & Brown, S. A. (1990). Coping responses and relapse among adolescent substance abusers. *Journal of Substance Abuse, 2,* 177–189.

Needle, R., Glynn, T., & Needle, M. (1983). Drug abuse: Adolescent addictions and the family. In R. Figley & H. McCubbin (Eds.), *Stress and the family* (pp. 37–52). New York: Brunner/Mazel.

Newcomb, M. (1987). Consequences of teenage drug use: The transition from adolescence to young adulthood. *Drug and Society, 1* (4), 25–60.

Newcomb, M., & Bentler, P. (1988a). *Consequences of adolescent drug use: Impact on the lives of young adults.* Newbury Park, CA: Sage.

Newcomb, M., & Bentler, P. (1988b). Impact of adolescent drug use and social support on problems of young adults: A longitudinal study. *Journal of Abnormal Psychology, 97,* 64–75.

Newcomb, M. D., & Bentler, P. M. (1989). Substance use and abuse among children and teenagers. *American Psychologist, 44,* 242–248.

Obermeier, M. S., & Henry, P. (1985). Inpatient treatment of adolescent alcohol and polydrug abusers. *Seminars in Adolescent Medicine, 1,* 293–297.

Office for Substance Abuse Prevention. (1992). *Cultural competence for evaluators.* Rockville, MD: U.S. Department of Health and Human Services.

Pandina, R., & Schuele, J. (1983). Psychosocial correlates of alcohol and drug use of adolescent students and adolescents in treatment. *Journal of Studies on Alcohol, 44,* 950–973.

Pontius, A. A., & Ruttiger, K. F. (1976). Frontal lobe system maturational lag in juvenile delinquents shown in narratives test. *Adolescence, 11,* 509–518.

Richter, S. S., Brown, S. A., & Mott, M. A. (1991). The impact of social support and self-esteem on adolescent substance abuse treatment outcome. *Journal of Substance Abuse, 3,* 371–385.

Robins, L. (1986). The consequences of conduct disorder in girls. In J. B. Olweus & M. Radke-Yarrow (Eds.), *Development of antisocial and prosocial behavior.* Orlando, FL: Academic Press.

Rydelius, P. A. (1983). Alcohol-abusing teenage boys: Testing a hypothesis on the relationship between alcohol abuse and social background factors, criminality and personality in teenage boys. *Acta Psychiatrica Scandinavia, 63,* 368–380.

Sadava, S. W. (1987). Interactionist theories. In H. T. Blane & K. E. Leonard (Eds.), *Psychological theories of drinking and alcoholism* (pp. 90–130). New York: Guilford Press.

Sadava, S. W. (1990). Problem drinking and alcohol problems: Widening the circle of covariation. In M. Galanter (Ed.), *Recent developments in alcoholism, Vol. 8: Combined alcohol and other drug dependence* (pp. 173–201). New York: Plenum Press.

Sadava, S. W., & Pak, A. W. (1993). Stress-related problem drinking and alcohol problems: A longitudinal study and extension of Marlatt's model. *Canadian Journal of Behavioural Science, 25,* 446–464.

Schafer, J., & Brown, S. A. (1991). Marijuana and cocaine effect expectancies and drug use patterns. *Journal of Consulting and Clinical Psychology, 59,* 558–565.

Schinke, S. P., Botvin, G. J., & Orlandi, M. A. (1991). *Substance abuse in children and adolescents: Evaluation and intervention.* Newbury Park, CA: Sage.

Schuckit, M. A. (1985a). Genetics and the risk for alcoholism. *Journal of the American Medical Association, 254,* 2614–2617.

Schuckit, M. A. (1985b). The clinical implications of primary diagnostic groups among alcoholics. *Archives of General Psychiatry, 42,* 1043–1049.

Schuckit, M. A. (1989). *Drug and alcohol abuse: A clinical guide to diagnosis and treatment* (3rd ed.). New York: Plenum.

Schuckit, M. A., Irwin, M., & Brown, S. A. (1990). The history of anxiety symptoms among 171 primary alcoholics. *Journal of Studies on Alcohol, 51,* 34–41.

Segal, B., Huba, G. J., & Singer, J. L. (1980). *Drugs, daydreaming, and personality: A study of college youth.* Hillsdale, NJ: Erlbaum.

Shedler, J., & Block, J. (1990). Adolescent drug use and psychological health. *American Psychologist, 45,* 612–630.

Sher, K. J. (1987, December). *What we know and do not know about COAs: A research update.* Paper presented at the MacArthur Foundation Meeting on Children of Alcoholics, Princeton, NJ.

Sher, K. J. (1991). *Children of alcoholics: A critical appraisal of theory and research.* Chicago: University of Chicago Press.

Sher, K. J. (1993). Children of alcoholics and the intergenerational transmission of alcoholism: A biopsychosocial perspective. In J. S. Baer, G. A. Marlatt, & R. J.

McMahon (Eds.), *Addictive behaviors across the life span* (pp. 3–33). Newbury Park, CA: Sage.

Skinner, H. A. (1984). Instruments for assessing alcohol and drug problems. *Bulletin of the Society of Psychologists in Addictive Behaviors, 3,* 21–33.

Stein, J., Newcomb, M., & Bentler, P. (1987). An 8-year study of multiple influences on drug use and drug use consequences. *Journal of Personality and Social Psychology, 53,* 1094–1105.

Stein, J., Newcomb, M., & Bentler, P. (1988). Structure of drug use behaviors and consequences among young adults: Multitrait-multimethod assessment of frequency, quantity, work site, and problem substance use. *Journal of Applied Psychology, 73,* 595–605.

Stewart, D. G., & Brown, S. A. (1994, August). Antisocial behavior and long-term outcome of adolescent substance abuse treatment. In S. A. Brown (Chair), *Long-term outcome among adolescents following alcohol and drug treatment.* Symposium presented at the annual convention of the American Psychological Association, Los Angeles.

Stewart, D. G., & Brown, S. A. (1995, in press). Withdrawal and dependency symptoms among adolescent alcohol and drug abusers. *Addictions.*

Tapert, S. F., & Brown, S. A. (1994, August). Neuropsychological correlates of adolescent drug and alcohol abuse. In S. A. Brown (Chair), *Long-term outcome among adolescents following alcohol and drug treatment.* Symposium presented at the annual convention of the American Psychological Association, Los Angeles.

Tarter, R. E. (1990). Evaluation and treatment of adolescent substance abuse: A decision tree method. *American Journal of Drug & Alcohol Abuse, 16,* 1–46.

Tarter, R. E., & Hegedus, A. M. (1991). The Drug Use Screening Inventory: Its applications in the evaluation and treatment of alcohol and other drug abuse. *Alcohol Health & Research World, 15,* 65–75.

Tucker, M. B. (1982). Social support and coping: Applications for the study of female drug abuse. *Journal of Social Issues, 38,* 117–137.

Vaillant, G. E. (1983). *The natural history of alcoholism: Causes, patterns, and paths to recovery.* Cambridge, MA: Harvard University Press.

Vistor, H. R., Crossman, J. C., & Eiserman, R. (1973). Openness to experience and marijuana use in high school students. *Journal of Consulting and Clinical Psychology, 41,* 78–85.

Welte, J. W., & Barnes, G. M. (1987). Alcohol use among adolescent minority groups. *Journal of Studies on Alcohol, 48,* 4, 329–336.

Westermeyer, J., Specker, S., Neider, J., & Lingenfelter, M. A. (1994). Substance abuse and associated psychiatric disorder among 100 adolescents. *Journal of Addictive Diseases, 13,* 67–89.

Williams, R. A., Feibelman, N. D., & Moulder, C. (1989). Events precipitating hospital treatment of adolescent drug abusers. *Journal of the American Academy of Child & Adolescent Psychiatry, 28,* 70–73.

Winters, K. C. (1992). Development of an adolescent alcohol and other drug abuse screening scale: Personal Experience Screening Questionnaire. *Addictive Behaviors, 17,* 479–490.

Yeudall, L. T., Fromm-Auch, D., & Davies P. (1982). Neuropsychological impairment in persistent delinquency. *Journal of Nervous and Mental Disorders, 170,* 257–265.

Zucker, R. A., & Gomberg, E. S. L. (1986). Etiology of alcoholism reconsidered: The case for a biopsychosocial process. *American Psychologist, 41,* 783–793.

Zuckerman, M. (1994). *Behavioral expressions and biosocial bases of sensation seeking.* New York: Cambridge University Press.

CHAPTER 12

SMOKING AND PEER INFLUENCE

Patrick West, MRC MEDICAL SOCIOLOGY UNIT, GLASCOW, SCOTLAND
Lynn Michell, MRC MEDICAL SOCIOLOGY UNIT, GLASCOW, SCOTLAND

Teaching kids who want to say "Yes" how to say "No" may be about as useful as teaching pyromaniacs how to use a fire extinguisher. (Kozlowski, Coambs, Ferrance, & Adlaf, 1989, p. 453)

Evidence of the adverse effects of smoking on health is incontrovertible. Since the 1950s, when the link with lung cancer first became established (Hammond & Horn, 1958; Doll & Hill, 1964) and widely publicized in the United Kingdom (Royal College of Physicians, 1962), the United States (Surgeon General, 1964), and elsewhere (World Health Organization [WHO], 1975), a succession of studies has attested to an association between smoking and disease, including various cancers, chronic obstructive airways disease, coronary heart disease, and stroke (*British Medical Journal,* 1994; Royal College of Physicians, 1983, 1992; Surgeon General, 1979).

Although the major impact of such smoking-related disease occurs toward the latter part of life, expressed as impairment, disability, and premature mortality, the young are not immune either as passive smokers exposed to the smoke of others (Couriel, 1994; Michell, 1990) or as active smokers themselves. Several studies have shown increased rates of respiratory problems among child and adolescent smokers even after relatively short smoking careers

(Adams, Lonsdale, Robinson, Rawbone, & Guz, 1984; Townsend, Wilkes, Haines, & Jarvis, 1991).

Despite the known risks, children and adolescents continue to start smoking. Smoking rates have declined in the population as a whole, but in most industrial countries (including the United Kingdom, Northern Europe, North America, and Australia), this has occurred principally because of increased numbers of adult smokers quitting the habit rather than fewer people beginning it (Amos & Hillhouse, 1991; Partridge, 1992). Among children of school age, rates of smoking have remained remarkably constant over the past two decades and may even be increasing. In Britain, for example, successive studies of secondary school children (ages 11 to 15), conducted for the Office of Population Censuses and Surveys (now the office of National Statistics) between 1982 (Dobbs & Marsh, 1983) and 1994 (Diamond & Goddard, 1995), have shown that some 30 percent of 11- to 12-year olds have tried smoking, a figure rising to 70 percent at ages 15 to 16. Corresponding rates of "regular" smoking (usually defined in school children as 1+ cigarettes per week) rise from around 2 percent at age 11 to 20 to 25 percent by the end of statutory education.

A WHO cross-national study, undertaken in 11 countries in 1985–1986, revealed that smoking prevalence rates were similar to those described earlier for Britain, with only Israel distinguished from other (European) countries as having lower rates (Aaro & Wold, 1990). The period after leaving school is also important for the uptake of smoking. Numbers of smokers continue to increase in mid to late adolescence so that by early adulthood, the prevalence of regular smoking is higher than at any other period in one's lifetime (West, 1993; West & Sweeting, in press). Although boys start smoking at an earlier age than girls, most recent studies have found the prevalence of smoking is higher among girls from about the age of 14 onward (Goddard, 1990; Thomas et al., 1993).

So, why in the face of the evidence, do children and adolescents continue to smoke? Certainly it is not that the facts are unknown to them. In survey after survey (Charlton, 1984; Goddard, 1990), it is clear that children and adolescents understand the health hazards. It is also the case that younger children, when asked their opinions of smoking, typically view it negatively (Michell, 1989; 1990); yet within the space of a few years, these views, held even by non-smokers, change and incorporate at least some positive images. These images relate not merely to the smoking agent (tobacco) but, through attractive and desirable role models, to identity—the type of person a smoker is or can be. Such images are present in tobacco advertisements (Smee, 1993), youth style magazines (Amos, 1993), and the media (Piepe et al., 1986; Amos & Hillhouse, 1992), and children know about and value these images (Aitken, Leathar, & O'Hagan, 1985; Amos & Hillhouse, 1992; Hastings, Ryan, Tees, & MacKintosh, 1994).

That a significant minority of children and adolescents begin a habit they know is bad for them and that they once viewed with disgust reveals how powerful these images can be. Thus, what may seem irrational from the perspective of the (adult) health educationalist may not be irrational from the perspective of the adolescent. To understand why children and adolescents smoke, we need to start from a perspective that gives their interests and priorities a central focus. In particular, we need to place that understanding against a background of knowledge about the peer group as the main arena for social interaction during this period and its influence in the shaping of attitudes and behaviors. Smoking as an isolated health risk may

have little meaning for adolescents, but as part of a repertoire of behaviors that define an individual's self-image or a peer group's identity, it may be very important indeed.

Within the voluminous literature on the causes of smoking in childhood and adolescence, the role of peers (often considered alongside that of the family) probably remains the most extensively investigated. Despite this, the processes underlying the research findings, particularly in respect of peer influence, remain poorly understood. It is an issue about which there is probably more conjecture by consensus than in any other area of smoking research. The underlying assumption is that peers *cause* smoking, typically via some kind of coercive pressure. In reality, much less is known about the origins, mechanisms, and consequences of peer influence on smoking, than one supposes.

This chapter focuses on these issues. It begins by taking a step back to consider what is known about friendships and peer groups in childhood and adolescence generally. In this literature, two perspectives on friendship formation dominate—pressure (influence) and choice (selection)—whereas a third—identity modeling—remains largely ignored. Until recently, research on smoking in childhood and adolescence did not incorporate a theoretical framework reflecting choice and identity modeling perspectives; the majority of studies assumed an influence model only.

After reviewing the three models, the chapter considers the evidence on smoking and the peer group. This ranges from evidence about the association between friends' smoking to children's and adolescents' own beliefs about the mechanisms involved. Each of these sets of evidence, when considered separately, in one way or another presents a limited perspective, yet in combination, they suggest how researchers and clinicians may develop, relative to what is currently available, a more comprehensive understanding of the processes involved.

Finally, discussion focuses on prevention programs and an assessment of their effectiveness. Most of them, the authors believe, remain limited by exactly the same assumption that underpins most research—namely, that children and adolescents smoke because of coercive peer pressure. In common with others (Hill, 1990; Newman, 1984), the authors view this concept of influence as being far too narrow and believe that without a more complete understanding of the range of processes involved in friendship formation and peer group dynamics than currently exists, programs to combat peer pressure will fail.

Inevitably, any review of this field cannot do justice to the full range of factors affecting peer-group processes, whether extrinsic or intrinsic to individuals. Among the former are broad social factors—such as socioeconomic status, family structure, and adolescent life-styles—that differentially expose children to smoking peers and shape the nature of peer influence. Evidence linking childhood smoking with lower socioeconomic status (Conrad, Flay, & Hill, 1992; Green et al., 1991), one-parent families (Goddard, 1990; Green, Macintyre, West, & Ecob, 1990), or life-styles characterized by a nonacademic and antischool orientation (Newcomb, McCarthy, & Bentler, 1989), truancy (Goddard, 1990) and other problem behaviors (Jessor & Jessor, 1977) are all indicative of ways in which this may occur.

With respect to intrinsic factors, their potential salience resides in the way some individuals may be at greater risk to smoke than others and by implication, therefore, more susceptible to peer pressure. These might include biological (or genetic) factors that not only differentiate smokers with respect to their dependence on nicotine (Russell, 1989) but also triers or experimenters with respect to their susceptibility to the addictive properties of tobacco (Jarvik, 1979); personality factors such as extroversion and neuroticism (Cherry & Kiernan, 1976), which may predispose one to smoking; and differential tolerance of stress to which smoking may be an adaptive behavior (Penny & Robinson, 1986). Although the evidence at present is inconclusive as to the importance of intrinsic factors, we cannot completely rule them out of the picture. The assumption throughout, however, is that any child or adolescent can become a smoker.

FRIENDS, PEERS, MODELS, AND MECHANISMS

Friends and peers are not one and the same thing, though authors often use the terms synonymously. *Friendship,* usually defined very broadly, is a social relationship that is neither consanguineous nor sexual in nature (Claes, 1992). As such, it includes relationships of varying intimacy from best or close friend to

friend, buddy, mate, or even acquaintance. Despite this variability, friendship conveys the notion of an essentially voluntaristic and nonhierarchical relationship emphasizing informality, sociability, and expressiveness between individuals engaged in reciprocal activities (Allan, 1989). Fundamental to any account of friendship, therefore, are the elements of choice, attraction, and similarity between individuals.

By contrast, following Epstein and Karweit (1983), an individual's *peer group* refers to an essentially involuntary population containing friends *and* nonfriends. This can include broad categories, such as a whole age group (e.g. teenagers in general), but is more commonly used to describe an immediate group, such as members of a school class. Either way, the distinction directs attention to a range of influences, other than those based on friendship, that arise from the wider peer group. Among these are influences reflecting the power structure of a group, expressed either as strong coercive pressure by a leader or, alternatively, one that might operate via processes of identification with powerful (and popular) individuals. Other influences are those emanating from the culture of a whole peer group, which itself constitutes an arena for the assimilation and subsequent behavioral expression of wider societal influences. Fundamental to any account of the peer group, therefore, is a recognition of influences beyond that of friendship, some of which may involve coercion.

The distinction between friends and peers draws attention to the diversity of processes involved in shaping a child's experience, identity, attitudes, and behavior. As children move away from their family of origin toward the independence of adulthood, the salience of friends, nonfriends, and the wider peer group may change. Although there is enormous variability, it is possible to elucidate some central features of this transition.

Among younger children, friendships are typically loose, fragmentary relationships arising in the context of shared activities, largely organized and controlled by parents and other adults (Wiist & Snider, 1991). As children enter and move through school or join clubs or other organizations, a child's immediate peer group begins to assume more importance. At this stage, friendships remain somewhat opportunistic and fleeting, and the importance of nonfriends (whose friendship they may desire) appears particularly strong. By age 12 or 13, young adolescents often have lots of friends, go around in large groups based on common interests, and continue to change friends fairly frequently. The number of friends is at a maximum in early adolescence and declines thereafter (Claes, 1992).

As they move through adolescence, children change friends less often, become more discriminating in their friendship choices, and remain loyal to a smaller number of friends with whom they have increasingly intimate relationships. These smaller groupings provide a mechanism through which adolescents may assimilate (and subsequently receive reinforcement) or resist wider peer influences. For those without friends, the loners or isolates, influences external to the immediate peer group may be particularly salient.

The relative importance of friends and peers, therefore, appears to shift as children move through adolescence. In very general terms, the salience of the immediate peer group and the potential impact of nonfriends within that group would seem to peak around early adolescence, thereafter declining in significance. Correspondingly, the salience of friendships, which may reflect wider peer influences, increases in mid- to late adolescence. This change in the balance of relationships also reflects a shift from an activity or context focus, often controlled by adults, to one emphasizing shared attitudes and behaviors increasingly determined by friends or group members themselves. Throughout, girls tend to develop closer and more intimate relationships than boys and offer more self-disclosure (Bernt, 1982).

Research evidence bearing on these issues is, however, less conclusive than suggested by this representation, possibly because there has not been enough attention given to the subtleties of change with age. Most studies have focused rather broadly on adolescents and reflect the diversity of influences operating throughout this period. Several key studies of adolescent friendship conclude that the strongest influence on behavior comes from those peers regarded as close friends rather than mere acquaintances or other known peers (Cohen, 1983; Coleman, 1980). Reciprocal friends may exert a particularly strong influence (Epstein, 1983).

Urberg and Deqirmencioglu (1990), in contrast, concluded that peers who do not reciprocate friendship have more influence on adolescents than those who do because the power asymmetry places pressure to change on the individual who wants the friendship. Others argue that cliques or self-defined reference groups, identifiable to adolescents themselves by their clearly defined styles, have a stronger influence than close friends (Mosbach & Leventhal, 1988). Hallinan (1980, 1983) identified both close friends and the wider peer group as important sources of influence.

In short, evidence suggests a range of influences operating in adolescence, with close friends on balance appearing to be the more significant influence. It is possible, however, that research has overestimated their importance because the evidence in this area typically involves individuals' reports of friendships rather than data about group structures as a whole. Studies that attribute influence to friends often fail to acknowledge the embedded nature of friendships in the wider peer group.

Whatever the relative importance of friends or peers, the particular significance of these relationships in childhood and adolescence resides in the way they both shape and reflect an individual's emergent sense of identity (Erikson, 1968). Newman and Newman (1976) described this as a process of identification and affiliation with a group that supports individuals as they move away from parents. It is fundamentally a two-way process, as children and adolescents use their friends as models and mirrors and try on and test out different selves (Cooley's [1902] concept of the "looking-glass self" is still valid here), and friends in turn mold, reinforce, and challenge one another's identities (Rubin, 1985).

Identity formation is therefore both a consequence of the influence of others to conform to particular images and the selection from a range of images of an identity that meets with approval, all of which takes place against a background of societal images, or putative identities, that are available as desirable models. The result of these processes is the formation of several different groups, some of which, like friendships, may be relatively tight, while others, like affiliations or liaisons between peers, are looser collections of individuals. The more stable of these groups tend to be distinct from one another, signaled perhaps by identifiable youth styles, whose members hold similar attitudes and values, such as music or fashion preferences.

This dynamic between self and other in the process of identity formation draws attention to different mechanisms by which children and adolescents form friendships and other peer relationships. In the friendship literature generally, authors refer to these mechanisms as the influence and selection models. Within these two broad perspectives, it is possible to identify several different processes and pressures, summarized here in Table 12.1.

Influence

The influence model implies that an individual's identity and behavior are shaped (or influenced) by others in a variety of ways. Thus, influence contributes to friendship or peer group homogeneity when individuals who join groups become similar to existing members. Within this *social* perspective, at least two types of influence may operate. The first, which corresponds closely to commonly held ideas of peer pressure, involves a concept of influence as directly coercive and includes strategies such as teasing, taunting, bullying, and the threatened exclusion of individuals from the group who fail to conform to established norms. The second type of influence is "softer" but potentially no less powerful and involves facilitative pressures in the form of exhortations, encouragement, and offers and rewards to individuals to behave in a way similar to other group members. These types of influence almost certainly merge into one another and to some extent reflect pressures to inhibit nonconformity and promote conformity, respectively.

Another set of processes refers to *normative influence*, which some writers (Fisher & Bauman, 1988; Friedman, Lichtenstein, & Biglan, 1985) classify as a form of social influence while others (e.g., Urberg, Shyu, & Liang, 1990) treat it separately. Normative influence has two components: (1) an individual's own appraisal of how normal and acceptable certain behaviors are among a salient group of friends or peers and (2) judgments about how important it is to adopt those behaviors in order for the individual to gain approval and acceptance from the group. This has parallels with Azjen and Fishbein's (1970) theory

Table 12.1 Processes Linking Peers

MECHANISM	TYPE	EXAMPLES
Influence (pressure)	*Social* 1. Coercive	Teasing Taunting Bullying Threats/Bribes
	2. Facilitative	Exhortations Encouragement Offers/Rewards
	Normative 1. Normality	Perceived frequency
	2. Reaction of others	Perceived approval
Selection (choice)	*Acquisition*	Similarity of characteristics
	Rejection	Dissimilarity of Characteristics
Modeling (choice/pressure)	*Role models*	Identification

of behavioral intention in which expectations about the reactions of others is one of two key components predicting intention. Each of these approaches emphasizes the way individuals act in terms of the other, and, as such, they involve subjectively perceived pressures.

Selection

In complete contrast, the selection model of friendship formation assumes that individuals purposefully choose and keep friends whom they perceive as having attitudes and behaviors similar to their own (Cohen, 1977). This view, therefore, emphasizes the elements of choice, attraction, and similarity implicit in general theories and common-sense understandings of friendship. Evidence from several studies shows how important similarity is in determining friendship formation and maintenance (Berscheid & Walster, 1969; Hallinan & Tuma, 1978; Newcomb, 1962, 1964). Similarity of attitudes, interests, and values oil the wheels of social interaction within a group by providing the basis for approval (Newcomb, 1964), validating fragile adolescent identities and reducing the possibility of conflict within the group (Sherif & Sherif, 1964). Selection operates in two ways: individuals acquire friends who are similar to themselves, and they reject or drop friends whose identity or behavior proves to be dissimilar to their own (Fisher & Bauman, 1988).

The relative importance of the influence (including normative influence) and selection models for an individual's behavior and attitudes has been the subject of some research. Fisher and Bauman (1988) reviewed three studies that used longitudinal designs to differentiate and compare the different processes in relation to different behaviors and found quite marked differences between them. Thus, Cohen (1977) concluded that "homophilic selection" accounted for much of the groups' similarity in behavior, whereas "conformity pressures" accounted for very little. Kandel (1978) found the processes of peer influence and selection to be equal for marijuana use, educational aspirations, political orientation, and participation in minor delinquency. Billy and Udry's (1985) study of adolescent friendships and sexual behavior concluded that the selection model provided the best description for both black and white groups, while the

influence model only contributed to explaining behavior in white females. It seems clear, then, that both processes are important, though each may be more so in different circumstances and with respect to different behaviors.

Modeling

The distinction between influence and selection models is undoubtedly useful in identifying different sets of processes involved in friendship formation, but as conventionally formulated, they exclude another type of process altogether. This process, which is particularly relevant to children and adolescents in their development of identity, is modeling. In social psychology generally, as represented by Bandura's (1969) social learning theory, modeling is typically classified as a major type of influence within socialization, most clearly seen with respect to the parent/child dyad wherein young children imitate or pattern their behavior on a model (the parent). In the case of a friendship, where a central feature of modeling, identification, is being like, or wanting to be like, a friend or would-be friend, modeling may be more appropriately categorized as selection rather than influence. It is equally clear, however, that models constitute influences, albeit chosen influences, and it is for this reason that it appears separately in Table 12.1.

Furthermore, the particular significance of modeling resides in the fact that it provides a link with the broader society. Identification does not occur in a social vacuum but rather via socially constructed (and usually highly gendered) identities encapsulated in and by friendships and available in the wider peer group as a series of possible repertoires. From this perspective, the distinction between influence and selection disappears.

It is clear from this brief overview of the friendship literature that much remains unknown about the processes involved in friendship formation and peer-group dynamics generally. It is equally clear, however, that these processes are extremely complex and involve several different kinds of mechanism, of which coercive peer pressure is only one expression. A comprehensive account must include both coercive and facilitative pressures, subjectively perceived pressures, modeling, and those aspects of friendship formation based on choice, attraction, and similarity. It is also probable that the significance of these processes varies both across childhood and adolescence; between sexes; and between friendships, other groupings like cliques or liaisons, and the wider peer group as a whole.

Although the evidence is far from conclusive, it seems plausible that the significance of the immediate peer group diminishes through adolescence as that of friendship increases. This, in turn, suggests that the impact of social influences, including coercive pressure, is greater earlier on and that the selection of friends with characteristics similar to oneself gradually replaces such influences. Modeling appears to be important throughout childhood and adolescence, though the source of identification almost certainly widens beyond the immediate peer group to incorporate broader societal images as one ages.

SMOKING AND PEERS: THE EVIDENCE

Against this background, one can now consider the evidence relating to peer influence and smoking. Before doing so, however, it is important to recognize one simple and basic feature of smoking in childhood and adolescence. One is not dealing with a behavior defined simply as smoking or not. As evidenced by the fact that only a relatively small proportion of children who try smoking go on to smoke regularly, it refers to a complex process by which the behavior becomes established. Therefore, it is useful to distinguish between different stages in the process of becoming a smoker because different influences may be apparent at each stage.

In a major review of research on childhood and adolescent smoking, Flay, D'Avernas, Best, Kersell, and Ryan (1983) argued that much of the inconsistency in findings resulted from conflation of the different stages of smoking, with comparisons typically made between nonsmokers and smokers who could be at any stage in a smoking career from experimental to long-term regular smoker. These authors argued that it is important to distinguish between five stages of smoking: preparation and anticipation, initiation (trying), learning and becoming (experimentation), habituation, and maintenance (regular smoking). It is likely that different influences operate at each stage.

Drawing on a wide range of research on social correlates of smoking, Flay and colleagues (1983) proposed that (1) family influences were most important during the preparation stage, thereafter declining in importance; (2) peer pressure and selection of friends with similar attitudes was most important for initiation and experimentation; and (3) although peer pressure and the social reinforcements obtained from smoking remain important during habituation and maintenance, the later stages of smoking increasingly involve internal influences and the pharmacological effects of nicotine rather than external influences. A decade later, in another major review, Conrad, Flay, and Hill (1992) reiterated the importance of distinguishing between stages of smoking and noted that most investigators have continued to conflate them.

Despite the importance of these two reviews, neither of them gives much attention to the different kinds of peer influence that might operate at different stages of smoking. In Figure 12.1, in a tentative model representing a typical smoking career from around age 11 to 16, some possible connections are suggested. The first stage of preparation and anticipation probably involves normative influences, particularly perceived approval or disapproval of friends and peers and expectations about peer pressure. At this time, views expressed by adults (particularly parents) and older children may be especially important. The authors believe many children *expect* to experience coercive peer pressure to smoke.

At the stage of initiation and experimentation, the model suggests that the experience of both coercive and facilitative pressures, perhaps in the form of exhortations to smoke or offers of cigarettes, is particularly important. Here, the salience of the immediate peer group, including the role of nonfriends, might be at a maximum. The model also suggests an increasing role for the selection of friends who smoke at later stages of experimentation and particularly in the transition to regular smoking. Here, societal images of the smoker, as they become incorporated into and solidify friendships, might be especially salient.

Because the process of becoming a smoker is only partially age dependent, there is bound to be considerable variation in the influences occurring at any stage, but there is a clear connection between the early stages, particularly experimentation, and a variety of peer influences, including that of coercive pressure.

Figure 12.1   Possible Model of Peer Processes in Relation to Stages of Smoking

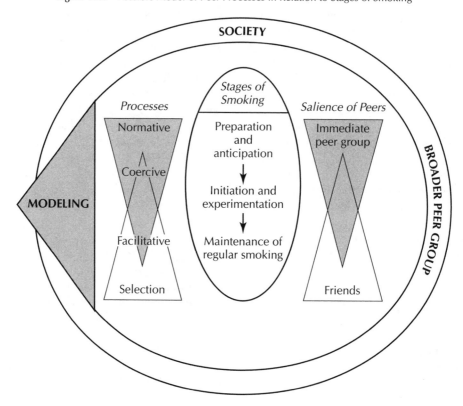

Because boys tend to start smoking at an earlier age than girls, the model suggests that boys are more likely to experience such pressures, with girls being more subject to modeling influences.

Friends Smoking

The key evidence in relation to peer influence and smoking in childhood and adolescence relates to associations between the smoking behavior of friends. The considerable research endeavor in this area consists of three types of investigations: cross-sectional studies, which still constitute the great majority; the many fewer studies with longitudinal designs; and sociometric studies, which at present represent no more than an embryonic research tradition. This last approach is the only one that gives any attention to the immediate peer group as a whole.

Cross-Sectional Studies

Cross-sectional studies of smoking collect information at one time point only. Typically, study subjects themselves provide data relating to friends' smoking. A common approach is to ask subjects to estimate how many of their friends smoke, using categories such as "none," "some," "half," "most," or "all." In these studies, there is usually a striking relationship found between subjects' and friends' smoking behavior. For example, in Bynner's (1966) seminal study of British schoolboys (ages 11 to 15), the prevalence of regular smoking (1 or more cigarettes a week) increased steadily from 0 percent among those who said none of their friends smoked to 62 percent among those who reported all of their friends smoked. Among those classified as "triers," the pattern differed, with the highest proportion (46 percent) occurring in the "half" group—a finding interpreted by

Bynner as indicative of the pressures on triers to become regular smokers.

Several studies of school children in the United States (Flay, D'Avernas, Best, Kersell, & Ryan, 1983; Hover & Gaffney, 1988; Hunter, Baugh, Webber, Sklov, & Berenson, 1982; Palmer, 1970) and Canada (Van Roosmalen & McDaniel, 1989), and more recently among older adolescents (ages 15 and 18) in Scotland (West & Sweeting, in press), have found results similar to Bynner. In one study (Flay, Koepke, Thomson, Santi, Best, & Brown, 1989), the pattern for quitters was much closer to that of the never-smokers than to either experimenters or regular smokers. There is evidence that these findings hold within sociodemographic categories. For example, the Bogalusa heart study (Hunter, Webber, & Berenson, 1980) revealed similar patterns of smoking in different age, sex, and race groups that were similar to those found in the other cross-sectional studies reviewed here.

Another equally prevalent approach involves asking subjects about their best friend's smoking behavior. Most usually, studies report strong associations. For example, in a study of Norwegian 12- to 15-year-olds (Aaro, Hauknes, & Berglund, 1981) just 5 percent of boys and girls whose best friend did not smoke were daily smokers compared to 46 percent of boys and 54 percent of girls whose best friend was a smoker. Several other studies (Byckling & Sauri, 1985; Charlton & Blair, 1989) have reported differences similar to Aaro, Hauknes, and Berglund, but some have found the relationship restricted to same-sex friends (Gottlieb, 1982), opposite-sex friends (Van Roosmalen & McDaniel, 1989), or smoking in boy/girlfriends (Banks, Bewley, Bland, Dean, & Pollard, 1978).

It is evident, therefore, that on a range of measures, a consistent finding in the literature is the strong relationship between the smoking behavior of friends. Although the methodology of these studies is open to the criticism that it results in an exaggerated association because smokers overestimate (and nonsmokers underestimate) the proportion (or number) of friends who smoke (Kandel, 1980), in the few studies with data on friends' actual smoking (Eiser, Morgan, Gammage, Brooks, & Kirby, 1991; Hunter, Croft, Vizelberg, & Berenson, 1987; Urberg, Shyu, & Liang,

1990), the findings are similar to those based on subjective estimates or reports.

The relationship also appears to hold at different ages and stages of smoking, though there is some suggestion, mainly from British studies (Banks, Bewley, Bland, Dean, & Pollard, 1978; Bewley, Bland, & Harris, 1974; Bewley, & Bland, 1977), of a smaller association with friends' smoking among experimenters compared to regular smokers and in younger compared with older children. Such a finding is compatible with the conclusion drawn by Flay, D'Avernas, Best, Kersell, and Ryan (1983) that family influences are relatively important in young children and at early stages in the process of becoming a smoker, and that these influences diminish as the influence of peers increases in adolescence.

By itself, this relationship between friends' smoking, based as it is on cross-sectional data, means nothing more than that smokers tend to associate with smokers and nonsmokers tend to associate with nonsmokers. Even though it may be tempting to interpret this as evidence of peer influence, one cannot legitimately draw inferences either about the direction of causality or the underlying mechanisms involved. This is a widely acknowledged problem in the literature; the evidence is compatible with either a selection or influence model of the uptake of smoking. Do smokers select friends who smoke or does having smoking friends make it more likely children or adolescents will smoke? To answer this question, longitudinal research is needed.

Longitudinal Studies

To date, the potential afforded by longitudinal studies to sort out the direction of causality has not been fully realized for several reasons. These relate to methodological and conceptual problems. Among the former is the failure of investigators to capitalize on the longitudinal design of their studies to analyze *change* between one stage in a smoking career and another. The inclusion of time 1 smokers in the analysis conflates effects on uptake and maintenance of smoking between time 1 and time 2, possibly leading to an overestimate of the influence of friends on uptake. With respect to conceptual problems, researchers have increasingly recognized that demonstrating friends' smoking to be antecedent to that of subjects' smoking does not by itself reveal much about the processes involved. It is therefore more appropriate to refer to predictors rather than causes of smoking (Conrad, Flay, & Hill; 1992; Hill, 1990).

One of the main conclusions of longitudinal studies is that the size of the effect of most predictors, including that of friends' smoking, is not as large as that observed in cross-sectional studies. For example, in a German study (Semmer, Lippert, Cleary, Dwyer, & Fuchs, 1987), 4 percent of nonsmokers with a "few" smoking friends became smokers a year later compared with 16 percent with "many" such friends. Similarly, in a study of Australian 10- to 12-year-olds also reassessed 12 months later, 22 percent of subjects whose friends smoked at time 1 had taken up smoking compared to 7 percent of those whose friends did not smoke (Alexander et al., 1983). Findings similar to these appear in studies using measures of any friend's smoking (Mittlemark et al., 1987), number of friends smoking (Ary & Biglan, 1988; McCaul & Glasgow, 1982; Flay et al., 1994), closest friends' smoking (Chassin, Presson, Sherman, Corty, & Olshavsky, 1984), best friend's smoking (Krohn, Naughton, & Lauer, 1987) and boy/girl friend's smoking (McNeill et al., 1988).

Therefore, there is evidence of a significant, if modest, effect of friend's smoking on the uptake of (any) smoking, though the effect may diminish with time. In one recent Norwegian study (Oygard, Klepp, Tell, & Vellar, 1995) involving 11- to 14-year-olds followed up 2 and 10 years later, an effect of friends' smoking on uptake observed at time 2 had diminished considerably at time 3 and, in a multivariate analysis with family smoking variables, this effect was not a significant predictor of subjects' adult smoking at all.

The very few studies that have examined the effect of friends' smoking on different smoking transitions have produced a rather inconsistent picture. In one study (Flay et al., 1994), the direct effect of friends' smoking was entirely confined to initiation; only indirect efforts (e.g., perceived friends' approval of smoking) were related to escalation to higher levels of smoking. In two others (Chassin, Presson, Sherman, Corty, & Olshavsky, 1984; Krohn, Naughton, & Lauer, 1987), similar results were found with friends' smoking being a much stronger predictor of initiation than the transition from experimental to regular smoking.

By contrast, Ary and Biglan (1988) found friends' smoking to be more strongly predictive of continued smoking than initiation, and, in two others (Chassin, Presson, Sherman, Montello, & McGrew 1986; West & Sweeting, in press), the effect was similar for each smoking transition. In the latter study, which focuses on older adolescents, the likelihood of becoming an experimental smoker and a regular smoker between the ages of 15 and 18 each increased about threefold among those with "most" friends compared with no friends smoking at time 1. However, the same study, which collected data about friends' smoking at both time points, also found that those subjects with "most" friends smoking at time 1 but no friends smoking at time 2 had *low,* not high, rates of smoking. This suggests that changes in friendship and smoking behavior are linked in a much more dynamic way than a simple model of peer influence would predict.

The accumulating evidence from longitudinal studies of smoking in childhood and adolescence presents a rather complex picture. It is certainly the case that the smoking behavior of friends is antecedent to that of subjects, though the size of the effect is substantially lower than that observed in cross-sectional studies, and it may apply as much to the maintenance of smoking as initiation. The evidence rules out a *simple* model of selection as a complete explanation for the association between friends' smoking. However, the finding that friends' smoking is predictive of the uptake and/or maintenance of smoking is not the same as inferring that friends "cause" smoking, whatever the mechanism by which this might occur. The finding is also compatible with a model in which individuals choose friends who happen to smoke and in time choose to take up the habit themselves. Thus, although longitudinal findings appear to resolve the problem of causality and provide evidence for peer influence on smoking, in reality researchers are not much closer to understanding the processes involved.

Sociometric Studies

The third source of data about friends' smoking comes from a small number of studies using sociometric techniques. In this approach, the emphasis switches from the individual as the unit of analysis to that of the relationship of individuals to groups. By collecting information from all group members about who they like (and less often who they do not like), it is possible to classify individuals into various categories, such as dyads, cliques, liaisons, or isolates. In the simplest case, and the only one used to date in the smoking literature, children nominate (usually up to three) other children they consider their best friends. This permits an analysis based on reciprocated friendships, which goes beyond what individuals simply report about best friends. As such, it enables an examination of what characteristics (including smoking) individuals actually share and with what magnitude. In as much as friendships suggest influences other than coercive pressures, this is an important source of evidence about the role of peers in smoking.

One study that utilized this approach is the Avon study of smoking among 11- to 16-year-olds in England (Eiser, Morgan, Gammage, & Gray, 1989; Eiser et al.; 1991; McNeill et al.; 1988; Nelson, Budd, Eiser, Morgan, Gammage, & Gray 1985). In an important paper, Eiser, Morgan, Gammage, Brooks, and Kirby (1991) described the findings of a subsample of the study that included data on the actual (not perceived) smoking behavior of the subjects' three best friends. In common with other studies, there were significant correlations in 12 age/sex groups between the smoking status of friends, but in addition, this pattern held with respect to several other characteristics, such as parental socioeconomic status, school performance, spending money, or (dis)approval of smoking.

Furthermore, after controlling for smoking status, the correlations between friends on issues other than smoking persisted, being as high for nonconformists (not sharing smoking habit) as for conformists (sharing smoking habit). In other words, smoking was simply one of several characteristics shared by friends, a picture not commensurate with a simple model of peer pressure. The authors concluded by proposing an alternative view emphasizing the role of choice in friendship formation in which "in an important sense young people choose the influences they experience." (Eiser, Morgan, Gammage, Brooks, & Kirby, 1991, pp. 3–6). Despite the plausibility of this conclusion, it goes beyond what can be legitimately inferred from evidence based on cross-sectional data and restricted to an analysis of friendship pairs.

To the authors' knowledge, only one study, conducted by Ennett and Bauman (1993) on ninth-grad-

ers in North Carolina, has examined the relationship between smoking and *peer-group structure* beyond that of nonsmoking dyads. Based on "best friend" data, the investigators used social network theory to distinguish between cliques, liaisons, and isolates, and examined current smoking rates of individuals in these categories after controlling for sociodemographic characteristics. Contrary to expectations, the highest rate of smoking occurred among the isolates who, ironically, nominated more friends who were smokers than did clique members. Indeed, the majority of cliques were nonsmoking.

In a related analysis (Ennett & Bauman, 1994), these investigators examined longitudinal changes (over one year) in peer affiliations and smoking behavior to ascertain the relative importance of influence and selection. Among nonsmokers at time 1 who remained in smoking cliques over the year period, 23 percent had become smokers at time 2 compared with only 2 percent in nonsmoking cliques. Conversely, among clique members and isolates who changed or joined cliques between time 1 and time 2, there was evidence of selection according to the smoking characteristics of the time 2 group. The investigators concluded that selection and influence contributed about equally to peer-group homogeneity in adolescent smoking. Most smoking, however, continued to occur among the isolates, who were not subject to peer-group influence contingent on clique or liaison membership.

This study, then, does provide evidence of *influence* operating through clique membership, albeit balanced by selective processes of the sort implied by Eiser and associates (1991), but, more importantly, it also shows that friends' smoking is not a proxy for peer-group structure. The clearest demonstration of this is the paradoxical finding that isolates have the highest rates of smoking. This paradox becomes resolved when one realizes that influences to smoke need not derive, as is usually assumed, from (immediate) peer-group pressure.

As Ennett and Bauman (1993) observed, isolates might smoke for reasons related to their marginal peer-group position, by, for example, modeling desirable clique members' (smoking) characteristics, or their more salient peer groups may be outside the school context. The fact that most cliques and liaisons are nonsmoking further diminishes the significance of the immediate peer-group. Overall, the findings are not consistent with the assumption implicit in much of the literature that smoking in childhood and adolescence is largely the result of peer-group influence or indeed that of best friends.

Initial Smoking Situations

One reason why the evidence about the role of friends' smoking remains so inconclusive may be that even when research demonstrates an *influence* rather than *selection* effect, little or nothing is known about the underlying processes involved. A second set of evidence relating to the occasion of first smoking, and specifically the role played by friends, promises to get researchers closer to these processes. Certainly, authors often cite the findings of studies in this area to support the claim that peer pressure is a central element in the onset of smoking, the (mainly implicit) assumption appearing to be that on a first occasion choosing to smoke is not an option, even if it may be on the second or subsequent occasions.

In general, studies that have addressed this issue do suggest that friends are important, but, unfortunately, what the actual mechanisms are is once again less than clear. Almost all of these studies have utilized retrospective reports of first smoking experiences, sometimes well after that event, and have typically referred to whom subjects were with on that occasion and/or the source of cigarettes.

With regard to the former, most studies find that friends, and particularly same-sex friends, are the most frequently reported companions on first smoking occasions. For example, in a study of junior high school students (Palmer, 1970), among experimental and regular smokers, around half reported being with friends, with only about 1 in 10 smoking their first cigarette alone. A British study of younger children, aged 10 to 11½, found results similar to the Palmer study, with 56 percent of boys (girls were not in the analysis) reporting being with friends compared to 11 percent with a parent, 10 percent with a sibling, and 9 percent alone (Bewley, 1974). Another study (Baugh, Hunter, Webber, & Berenson, 1982) also suggested that family members may figure more in first smoking occasions among children who start smoking earlier than among those who start smoking at a later age,

though even in this study friends were the most frequently mentioned companions.

With regard to the source of cigarettes, most studies have found that friends are most frequently cited. For example, in Bynner's (1969) study, 57 percent said they had received their first cigarette from a friend, a much higher percentage than any other source. That about three-quarters of all boys also said they had smoked because they wanted to know what it was like is not, however, consistent with a simple model of coercive pressure. Rather, it suggests an element of volition and that whatever peer pressures are present are more indirect than direct.

Surprisingly, perhaps, given the emphasis on the importance of refusal skills in antismoking programs, rather little research has examined initial smoking situations in any detail. An exception is a study by Friedman, Lichtenstein, and Biglan (1985), who used a semistructured interview to question 157 adolescents aged 12 to 19 about their first three smoking occasions or, for nonsmokers, the first three occasions they either considered smoking or felt pressured to smoke. In common with other studies, same-sex friends were the most frequent companions on smoking occasions. When asked about pressures to smoke, in only 30 percent of occasions was there any recollection of either external pressures (e.g. teasing) or internal pressures (e.g., the need to feel accepted by others)—a picture that applied as much to nonsmokers as to smokers. Subjects, however, recalled that most smoking occasions involved suggestions by others to smoke (76 percent), offers of cigarettes (63 percent), and, less often, overt encouragement to smoke or teasing if the subject refused or hesitated (36 percent). To complicate the picture further, a significant minority reported planning to smoke prior to the smoking occasion (22 percent) and taking a cigarette without hesitation (38 percent).

This study, then, provides evidence both for and against peer pressure in initial smoking situations. The authors accounted for the paradox as the inability of adolescents to perceive influences in the form of suggestions or offers as pressure. In adopting this view, they chose not to believe their subjects' versions of the situation and, in their advocacy of refusal training, implicitly identified those influences as coercive pressures. An alternative version, which they partially acknowledged, is that adolescents may not feel pressured because for most of them, smoking with friends is a chosen activity.

Peer Pressure and Peer Approval

Further evidence on the nature of peer influence beyond the first smoking occasion is available from several studies, though given the centrality of the issue, it is surprising that there is not more. The first set of studies, principally associated with British research and reflecting common assumptions about the nature of peer influence, focuses on the experience of peer pressure. The second set of studies refers to peer approval, which is conceptualized here as a type of normative influence. In combination, a few studies suggest a possible role for modeling.

Those studies that have attempted to measure peer pressure have typically done so by giving subjects Likert-type statements to which they indicate their agreement or disagreement. A few, including Bynner's (1969) study, have found quite strong evidence of peer pressure. In his sample, on the basis of answers to two items relating to teasing ("if you don't smoke other boys make fun of you") and encouragement to smoke ("others are often trying to encourage me to smoke"), around half of the subjects reported experiencing coercive and facilitative peer pressure. Higher levels of agreement with these statements were present among nonsmokers and triers compared to smokers, suggesting more coercion to start smoking than to maintain it.

Most studies have not, however, found as much evidence of peer pressure as the Bynner study did; nor have they found that peer pressure relates particularly to uptake. For example, in the MRC/Derbyshire Smoking survey (Banks, Bewley, Bland, Dean, & Pollard, 1978; Murray, Swann, Bewley, & Johnson, 1983; Swann, Murray, & Jarrett, 1991), a 10-year follow-up study of 11-to 12-year-olds, there were considerably lower levels of felt pressure, even though the authors used items similar to those used by Bynner. In addition, these investigators found nonsmokers were much less likely to have experienced pressure than smokers, particularly with respect to the apparently strongly coercive item ("you have to smoke when you're with friends"), where only 2 per-

cent of non-smoking boys and girls compared with 26 percent of boy and 36 percent of girl smokers endorsed the statement (Banks, Bewley, & Bland, 1981; Murray & Cracknell, 1980). This finding, in direct contrast to Bynner's, suggests a greater influence of peers in maintenance rather than initiation of smoking.

The MRC/Derbyshire study (Swann, Murray, & Jarrett 1991), however, found a small, but persisting, effect of peer pressure on initiation at all follow-ups to age 21, though inclusion in the peer-pressure measure of one item ("most of my friends smoke") makes it difficult to evaluate the significance of coercion on smoking initiation. It is also interesting that, in a related analysis, the majority of subjects (68 percent) reported they had tried smoking *before* experiencing peer pressure, but the reverse was the case for the maintenance of regular smoking (Swan, Murray, & Jarrett, 1991). Several other investigators (Aitken, 1980; de Vries & Kok, 1986; Van Roosmalen & McDaniel, 1989) have reported findings similar to those found in the MRC study. The cumulative evidence suggests that peer pressure to smoke is not more than a minor influence, though the evidence results from items that are crude to say the least.

The second perspective on peer influence stems from Azjen and Fishbein's (1970) theory of behavioral intention. This theory postulates that behavior (smoking) results from behavioral intention, which is itself a function of two components: attitudes toward the behavior (e.g., positive and negative images) and expectations about the reactions of others to engage in the behavior (e.g., disapproval).

Adopting this approach, one British study (Eiser, Morgan, Gammage, Brooks, & Kirby, 1991; Eiser, Morgan, Gammage, & Gray, 1989) examined the relationships between friends' approval of smoking (how much their best friends would mind) and both intention to smoke and the uptake of regular smoking. The findings revealed only a relatively small relationship with intention but a larger one with actual smoking. Those subjects feeling their best friends would approve were nearly twice as likely to become regular smokers than those expecting disapproval. However, in a multivariate analysis, and taking into account other variables (including intention to smoke), the effect was substantially lower, only barely remaining statistically significant. The authors argued that the difference in the findings in relation to intention and the uptake of regular smoking reflects the greater salience of choice over peer influence regarding intention to smoke.

Other studies have reported findings similar to those in the Eiser and colleagues' (1989, 1991) studies. In a study of Dutch 10- to 15-year-olds, De Vries and Kok (1986), found a small effect of positive subjective norms (items reflecting friends' and classmates' approval) on smoking, which was more apparent among regular than initial smokers. Chassin, Presson, Sherman, Montello, and McGrew (1986) also found an effect of peer attitudes ("my friends think that I should smoke cigarettes") on the transition from experimental to regular smoking but for girls only, and no effect on initiation of experimental smoking.

In a related analysis (Chassin, Presson, Sherman, Corty, & Olshavsky, 1984), these investigators tested the relative importance of sets of variables representing various theoretical perspectives on different smoking transitions, including the Azjen/Fishbein model. Although the attitudes of others (including friends) did significantly discriminate between groups at each transitional stage, it was a more important discriminator of becoming a regular smoker than of earlier stages. Variables representing Jessors' (1977) problem behavior theory, including expectations for academic success and tolerance of deviance, were more important in explaining experimental smoking.

Reflecting the different focuses of research in this area, very few studies have collected data that permit assessment of the relative importance of peer pressure and peer approval in the same analytic model. An exception is a study of eighth- and eleventh-graders conducted by Urberg, Shyu, and Liang (1990). These investigators used structural equation modeling (LISREL) to examine the effect of direct (coercive) and normative pressure to smoke and *not* to smoke, together with actual and perceived smoking behavior of friends. The results of this study showed almost no support for direct pressure to smoke. Only normative pressure to smoke and direct pressure *not* to smoke had significant paths to subjects' smoking, though the effects were moderate compared to that attributable to both actual and perceived friends' smoking behavior.

The investigators concluded that although the normative dimension appears more important than direct peer pressure, overall the climate is one in which friends do not so much encourage smoking as not discourage it. They also noted, however, that they based the estimate of the effect of direct peer pressure on just one item, which might not adequately represent the dimension.

The fact that friends' smoking (actual and perceived) was the most important variable in this study raises the intriguing question as to what such an effect might mean over and above peer pressure and approval. The interpretation offered by these authors is that it is evidence of the process of modeling. In this respect, and in common with the few other studies using similar analytic techniques (Chassin, Presson, Sherman, Corty, & Olshavsky, 1984; Flay et al., 1994), the assumption is that after testing for other kinds of peer influence, any remaining effect must be modeling. The assumption is implicit in Flay and associates' recent study where the direct effects of friends' smoking on smoking initiation are seen as confirmation of a modeling hypothesis compared to that of normative influence. In this case, the assumption is made even though there was no measure of peer pressure.

Although this emerging body of research is to be applauded because it is theoretically grounded, it is clearly the case that any influence attributable to modeling has been demonstrated by omission rather than commission. The size of the effect could be quite large but no study to date in this tradition has incorporated any measure of identification with friends that would allow a direct test of the hypothesis in conjunction with others.

Overall, then, the evidence about the role of peer pressure and approval with regard to smoking is less than convincing, and it remains to be demonstrated that modeling is related to smoking. Acknowledging the limitations of the data, however, it appears that both peer pressure and approval may play a small part, with normative influences possibly being more significant than coercive pressure. It also seems that the effects of each type of influence is more apparent with respect to regular compared to experimental smoking. This is precisely the reverse of what the model outlined in Figure 12.1 would predict and most commentators would expect. Along with the evidence about the relationship between subjects' and friends' smoking behavior, it shows that researchers have inadequately specified the processes salient to the smoking behavior of children and adolescents. In an arena dominated by ideas of coercive peer pressure, this is perhaps not surprising.

PREVENTION PROGRAMS

This part of the chapter focuses on programs designed to prevent children and adolescents from becoming smokers. Particular interest resides in the extent to which the effectiveness or ineffectiveness of these programs reveals how adequate the knowledge is about the meaning of smoking in the lives of children and adolescents and its relationship to friendships and the wider peer group. It is therefore important to identify the assumptions underlying prevention programs. Over the past two decades, the majority of such programs have been premised on the same assumption that has underpinned most research—namely, that nonsmoking children yield to the influence of their smoking peers and that they must therefore learn the social skills to resist such powerful pressures to smoke (Michell, 1994).

Most smoking intervention programs have consisted of relatively short-term school-based packages or modules embedded in the general curriculum and led by teachers. The earlier programs concentrated on health messages about the long-term consequences of smoking and used scare tactics to shock children into not starting to smoke or quitting (Thompson, 1978). As evidence accumulated that children were continuing to smoke, researchers began to question the effectiveness of this approach, not the least because of the realization that from a child's or adolescent's viewpoint, the risk of cancer in old age is potentially meaningless. Following two key studies (Evans, 1976; Evans, Rozelle, Mittlemark, Hansen, Bane, & Havis, 1978), an alternative approach evolved, focusing on programs designed to promote an awareness of the social pressures to smoke.

Earlier, naive approaches, such as the Just Say No campaign, have given way to more sophisticated techniques that encourage children in the secure environment of the classroom to acquire and practice the skills needed to resist pressures from peers to begin smoking. Programs have become increasingly interactive, involving pupils in varying levels of participation from discussion to role-play to peer-led sessions. Some aim to build general confidence and social skills, whereas others focus on specific strategies for resisting pressures to smoke. Other programs, acknowledging normative pressures to smoke, aim to correct false assumptions about the prevalence and acceptability of smoking among peers (Botvin & Dusenburg, 1992). Thus, adolescents receive assertiveness training to increase self-esteem and resistance to drug use (Strasburger, 1989). In short, for well over a decade, children and adolescents have been recipients of increasingly sophisticated programs to resist peer pressure.

Despite the often excellent quality of the materials, these programs (like the earlier scare tactics) do not appear to have resulted in any downward shift in smoking prevalence among children and adolescents in general. Obviously, one could argue that it takes time for the effects to filter through to measurable population statistics and that it is difficult to isolate an intervention effect, but this argument is rather more hopeful than convincing. Much more pertinently, the findings of specific evaluation studies suggest that intervention programs have only minimal impact.

Although there may be some discernible effect in delaying the onset of smoking (Garcia, D'Avernas, & Best, 1988; Murray, Pirie, Leupker, & Pallonen, 1989; Reid, Killoran, McNeill, & Chambers, 1992; Tobler, 1986), several well-designed longitudinal trials from the United States (Flay, D'Avernas, Best, Kersell, & Ryan 1983; Murray, Pirie, Leupker, & Pallonen, 1989; Perry, Kelder, Murray, & Klepp, 1992) and Scandinavia (Vartiainen, Fallonen, McAlister, & Puska, 1990) suggest that any initial benefits gradually dissipate with time. Indeed, some reviewers even disagree about the short-term benefits, arguing that they yield only a 5 to 10 percent reduction in the onset of experimental smoking (Kozlowski, Coambs, Ferrance, & Adlaf, 1989; Reid, Killoran, McNeill, & Chambers, 1992). A recent British study evaluating the effect of two school smoking education programs found no effect of either program, or even both in sequence, in delaying initiation of smoking (Nutbeam, Macaskill, Smith, Simpson, & Catford, 1993). The unfortunate conclusion from these evaluation studies is that a decade of widely implemented school programs, based on the assumption that adolescents need to learn to resist peer pressure, have proved ineffective in persuading children and adolescents not to smoke.

In light of these findings, there has been a shift away from isolated curriculum packages to community-based and communitywide programs that include a school-based component (Baudier et al., 1991; Perry, Kelder, Murray, & Klepp, 1992; Vartiainen, Fallonen, McAlister, & Puska, 1990). The point of this broader approach is to avoid isolating health messages within an educational context and to reduce the blatantly contradictory messages about smoking that children receive in and outside the classroom. The aim is to promote an antismoking climate and ethos within a community, not just in school. In the first major out-of-school initiative in the United Kingdom, the Scottish Grampian "Smokebusters" Club (Teijlingen & Friend, 1993a), the results are disappointing. The relatively positive findings at 22 months have not been sustained after four years, with little or no difference in smoking prevalence between members, ex-members, and those who had never been members (Teijlingen & Friend, 1993b). It is possible, however, that the community focus is still not wide enough in this club-based approach. An even broader approach may be necessary.

The Minnesota Heart Health Program (Perry, Kelder, Murray, & Klepp, 1992) is an example of such an approach. Designed to operate at policy, community, and educational levels, it has as its primary concern the promotion of healthy life-styles across all age groups. It is the only study to date to report significant long-term reductions in smoking prevalence. The risk of a student being a smoker at graduation was 40 percent lower in the intervention group than in the community as a whole. In a recent review, Reid, Killoran, McNeill, and Chambers (1992) argued strongly in support of this "all-out" approach, including use of the media, restrictions on smoking in public places, provision of cessation clinics and quit lines, and fiscal action to raise the price of tobacco products, as well as implementation of youth programs.

As promising as this broader community approach may be, it simply serves to underline the limi-

tations of the more conventional prevention programs. There are several possible reasons for their failure, including the fact that they are typically adult (usually teacher) led and school based. Not only do they exclude adolescents most disaffected with the educational system, and who, in consequence, might feel even more motivated to smoke, but both the establishment values and adult authority associated with the school may fundamentally conflict with what adolescents themselves value and view as relevant. Prevention programs are also competing with powerful messages about the desirability of smoking contained in advertising, sports sponsorship, and the media in general, all of which work against the small influence offered by even the best-designed curriculum package. Perhaps the single most important reason for their ineffectiveness, however, resides in the fact that these programs have their basis in unfounded assumptions about the nature of peer influence. In assuming that children and adolescents smoke because of coercive peer pressure, these programs may have fundamentally missed the mark. The problem with adult-led programs that do not correspond with the reality of children's lives is that children (the target audience) will not believe the messages.

CONCLUSION

In this review of peer influence and smoking, it is impossible to avoid one simple and rather depressing conclusion: Despite a considerable volume of research and a considerable investment in prevention programs, remarkably little is known about the processes by which friends, the wider peer group, and society in general influence children and adolescents to smoke. The conceptual framework offered by theories of friendship has not informed the area; studies of smoking often have significant design limitations and inadequately specify the processes involved; measures remain limited, and interpretation of findings, which is fraught with difficulty, has run way ahead of what the studies have really justified. Furthermore, because research in this area has now spanned almost three decades, it is extremely difficult to know how much the findings are period specific. What may appear as inconsistent findings may simply reflect diverse historical circumstances with different images of smoking and consequences in terms of peer approval or pressure.

If all of this seems a harsh judgment, the authors fully recognize that this is a difficult area that addresses issues at the heart of social psychology, such as that relating to identity formation. It involves consideration, too, of the relationships between individuals and society, between choice and constraint, between perceived and actual pressure, the meanings of influence, and so on. Addressing those issues has been more difficult because of the pervasive assumption, which has dominated the literature, that children and adolescents smoke because they are pressured by others to do so, typically via some form of coercion.

Despite these problems, it is possible to draw some central findings from research in this area, which increasingly points to the need to reconceptualize the ideas of influence. What do researchers know? First, they know from cross-sectional studies alone that friends are in one way or another important in relation to smoking behavior. Although this does not say anything about the direction of causality, longitudinal evidence does show friends' smoking to be antecedent to subject's smoking, though the effect is much lower when compared to that found in cross-sectional research. Thus, friends' smoking behavior is predictive of initiation, though there is clearly a strong selection effect. However, the fact that friends' smoking *predicts* subsequent smoking among others is not the same as inferring that friends "cause" others to begin smoking. The finding is still compatible with a model in which children choose both their friends and the influences they experience, including smoking.

Longitudinal studies, then, do not reveal much about the underlying processes involved. Examination of these underlying processes in relation to initial smoking situations or by reference to reports about peer pressure or normative influence shows a somewhat complementary picture. The findings of studies into these processes show how important friends are as smoking companions and as sources of cigarettes, but there is little evidence of either the need to gain friends' approval or coercive peer pressure. This absence of coercive influence is particularly apparent in the earlier experimental stages of smoking, precisely the point at which one would expect it to most likely occur. If there are constraining influences operating at

this stage, it seems more likely they are of the facilitative rather than coercive kind.

Though the evidence is far from conclusive, it also appears that girls are more likely than boys to report coercive and normative pressure to smoke. In short, the model outlined in Figure 12.1 seems quite inadequate in specifying the peer processes involved in both the initiation of smoking and transition from experimental to regular smoker. The cumulative evidence of research to date strongly suggests that researchers have underestimated the role of choice, particularly its involvement in friendship formation and maintenance, and have grossly overestimated the role of coercive pressures.

In reaching such an assessment, however, there is one major reservation, which relates to the adequacy of the methods used to investigate the extremely complex processes involved. Typically, studies have addressed the issue of peer pressure using the survey method with a very limited range of questionnaire items. Sometimes, items phrased overtly in terms of pressure (as Friedman, Lichtenstein, & Biglan, 1985 observed) raise the question as to what children and adolescents mean by the term. Is it the same as bullying, teasing, or taunting, or is it something different? One does not know. It is possible that the finding that only a small minority appear to experience pressure to smoke is an artifact of the measures used and that items with a greater degree of specificity and meaningfulness would reveal more evidence of coercion. It is also possible that "better" items would not fully resolve the issue because children and adolescents may find it difficult to admit to experiences of a hurtful or undermining nature. Alternatively, they may simply affirm accepted and stereotypical knowledge about coercive pressure.

Another issue concerns the focus on friends as the source of pressure in these items rather than that of the wider peer group. If smoking with friends is least likely to involve coercion, as the evidence suggests, then the items that focus on pressure from friends would underestimate coercive pressures arising from either other immediate peers or from wider peer groups. In this connection, it is interesting to note that the only study reporting high levels of peer pressure is that of Bynner (1969), where the items referred to "others" rather than "friends." More generally, the almost complete lack of attention to the wider peer group means that there is no evidence about the role of coercion from nonfriends. It is possible, therefore, that the evidence suggesting only a minor role for coercive peer influence simply reflects bad items coupled with a much too restricted focus. There is clearly a need for more research here, both quantitatively via sociometric techniques and qualitatively to explore the meaning of smoking, friendship, and group dynamics.

Although interpretation of the relationship between friends' smoking is typically in terms of the selection/influence dichotomy outlined earlier, a third process, identity modeling, has until recently received almost no attention whatsoever. In only a few studies (Ennett & Bauman, in press; Flay et al., 1994; Friedman, Lichtenstein, & Biglan, 1985) is there any reference to modeling effects, and in each case, it remains either undefined or assumed as an effect in the relationship between friends' and subjects' smoking. The effects could be quite large but the modeling hypothesis remains to be directly tested. This is extremely surprising, given widespread references in the scientific literature and the popular media to the potential importance of role models, such as sports stars or rock singers, to young people. Its potential significance resides in the way both selection and influence mechanisms link in processes of identification within the immediate peer group and the wider society. With respect to the immediate peer group, it invites investigation not merely of the characteristics shared and mutually valued by friends (such as smoking) but also of the characteristics of nonfriends, particularly strong peer leaders who children value and with whom they identify.

Although the implications may differ for individuals according to their position in the group, in each case modeling is occurring. The identities constructed in these processes do not remain bounded by the peer group but, to a large extent, reflect models available in the wider society. With respect to smoking, reference is made to those images contained in advertising, TV programs, and teenage magazines that portray smokers in a desirable way (Amos, 1993). In the process of modeling, there is a connection between identity formation in the peer group and social representations of identity. This connection might, in part, make sense of one of the major paradoxes in the literature—namely,

the high levels of smoking found among isolates. One possible explanation is that such individuals engage in what they perceive is a desirable social identity in order to gain acceptance in the peer group. Alternatively, it might consciously express an individual's espousal of a deviant identity within a group. All of these processes merit much closer investigation.

One of the reasons investigators may have largely overlooked modeling in research on peer influence and smoking is that, to date, they have restricted the framework within which they have conducted almost all the studies to the immediate peer group, or more precisely to the even smaller grouping of friendship. One result of this is that researchers have focused their conceptualization of the mechanisms involved on influence and selection processes occurring between individuals in small groups. The way the wider society affects those processes has gone largely ignored.

The only way this issue has been even partially addressed is by examining whether relationships between variables such as peer pressure or approval and subjects' smoking varies between individuals with different characteristics. The very few studies that have tested for interaction effects with respect to factors such as gender, socioeconomic status, or ethnicity have not yet produced conclusive findings. That girls may be more vulnerable to peer influence than boys is, however, illustrative of the potential of this approach. Theoretically, there is no reason why quite different types of influence, of quite different magnitude, should not operate in different social contexts or by characteristics as fundamental as gender.

In reformulating the issue to take account of the broader social context, attention should focus on the social meanings of smoking as constructed and used by children and adolescents in the development of individual and group identity. From this perspective, it is not so much that friends "cause" smoking (though this may be part of the picture), nor even that children select nonsmokers as friends, but that the images represented by smoking become incorporated in and signify friendship or other peer-group relations.

Smoking is simply part of a particular adolescent life-style, reflecting both who an individual is and with which group he or she identifies. Evidence linking smoking with particular youth styles, such as punks or hippies (West & Macintyre, 1990), or with types of music (Teijlingen & Friend, 1993a) shows in rather extreme form how young people associate smoking with identity and life-style. This may also be a component of one of the more consistently observed associations between smoking and social deviance, whether expressed in disaffection from school (Newcomb, McCarthy, & Bentler, 1989) or a range of problem behaviors (Jessor & Jessor, 1977). More generally, it may also be part of the explanation for the increase in smoking among girls and young women, who display through that behavior a particular social identity.

In one way or another, then, a focus on the wider social context allows one to see how societal images of smoking permeate friendships and peer relations. Within the orthodox conceptualization of mechanisms, such a process becomes entirely obscured and understandable only as selection rather than influence. Broadening the focus, however, blurs that distinction because selection is not a matter of unlimited choice but of choice between a limited number of possibilities. With respect to smoking, the construction of desirable images through tobacco advertising and other means effectively influences choice and as such constitutes pressure. In this view, one gets a much broader perspective about the pressures on individuals and specifically those that have an impact on children's and adolescents' decision making about smoking.

Based on the evidence currently available, the role of coercive peer pressure is relatively slight, particularly (and against expectation) in relation to the early stages of experimentation. There is now a generation of children and adolescents who have taken part in prevention programs based on that assumption. It is entirely plausible, therefore, that there is a widespread expectation among those anticipating smoking that they will be subject to pressures like bullying, teasing, or exclusion. This may lead to avoidance of situations where they perceive such pressures are likely to occur, and, ironically, it may heighten smoking as a characteristic that children use to select their friends.

By comparison, there is evidence that those influences regarded as facilitative, such as offers or encouragement to smoke, are a component of initial and subsequent smoking situations. These may not initially appear as pressures, but they are influences nonetheless. With respect to normative influence, the

evidence is equivocal, though the authors believe that perceived peer approval plays a part in children's and adolescents' smoking behavior. Each of these processes, however, is small compared with that attributable to various types of modeling. Modeling may occur between friends, between nonfriends, within groups, and between individuals, groups, and the broader society. Its fundamental power resides in the process of identification with a desirable model that creates and solidifies individual and group identity. In its link with broader social images, modeling redefines the origins, nature, and consequences of peer influences on smoking.

This shift in emphasis away from peer-group dynamics to the way society permeates the peer group also has consequences for programs and policies designed to prevent children and adolescents from initiating smoking. The challenge, then, is not to develop increasingly sophisticated refusal skills programs. Not only is it likely they will be unsuccessful but, because the basis of their assumption does not correspond with the reality of children's and adolescents' experiences, the target population (children and adolescents) will not believe or accept these programs, and they may even be counterproductive. The challenge now is to refocus attention on the broader societal influences on peer groups and specifically the images of smoking used by peer members in establishing individual and group identity. This means identifying what is attractive to children and adolescents in the portrayal of smoking and smokers in tobacco advertising, youth-style magazines, and the media in general, and developing policies to counter their appeal.

Some of this may be achieved by an extension of bans and controls on tobacco advertising and sports sponsorship, together with a redefinition of smoking images in the media, but there is a real risk that children and adolescents will perceive such policies as yet another adult ploy to prevent them from doing something they want to do. The significance of smoking in the lives of many children and adolescents goes much deeper than this and reflects who they are or might become, together with the identity of their friends or group. Until researchers begin to identify what smoking means to this age group, society will not be able to develop policies that have any real chance of reducing current levels of smoking among children and adolescents.

NOTE

The authors would like to thank Mary Robins for her help in searching for references, Sally Macintyre and Helen Sweeting for comments on earlier drafts, and Jacqui Irwin, Jean Money, and Louise O'Neill for typing various versions of the manuscript. Patrick West receives financial support from the Medical Research Council of Great Britain, and Lynn Michell receives financial support from the Scottish Office Home and Health Department.

REFERENCES

Aaro, L. E., Hauknes, A., & Berglund, E. L. (1981). Smoking among Norwegian schoolchildren 1975–80. *Scandinavian Journal of Psychology, 22,* 279–309.

Aaro, L., & Wold, B. (1990). *Health behaviour in schoolchildren: A WHO cross-national survey.* University of Bergen, Research Center for Health Promotion: World Health Organization Regional Office for Europe.

Adams, L., Lonsdale, D., Robinson, M., Rawbone, R., & Guz, A. (1984). Respiratory impairment induced by smoking in children in secondary schools. *British Medical Journal, 288,* 891–895.

Aitken, P. P. (1980). Peer pressure, parental controls and cigarette smoking among 10 to 14 year olds. *British Journal of Social and Clinical Psychology, 19,* 141–146.

Aitken, P. P., Leathar, D. S., & O'Hagan, F. J. (1985). Children's perceptions of advertisements for cigarettes. *Social Science and Medicine, 21* (7), 785–797.

Alexander, H. M., Callcott, R., Dobson, A. J., Hardes, G. R., Lloyd, D. M., O'Connell, D. L., & Leeder, S. R. (1983). Cigarette smoking and drug use in schoolchildren: IV—factors associated with changes in smoking behavior. *International Journal of Epidemiology, 12* (1), 59–66.

Allan, G. (1989). *Friendship: Developing a sociological perspective.* New York: Harvester Wheatsheaf.

Amos, A. (1993). Youth and style magazines: Hooked on smoking? *Health Visitor, 66*(3), 1–93.

Amos, A., & Hillhouse, A. (1991). *Tobacco use in Scotland.* Edinburgh: ASH Scotland.

Ary, D. V., & Biglan, A. (1988). Longitudinal changes in adolescent cigarette smoking behavior: Onset and cessation. *Journal of Behavioural Medicine, 11* (4), 361–382.

Azjen, I., & Fishbein, M. (1970). The prediction of behaviour from attitudinal and normative variables. *Journal of Experimental Social Psychology, 6,* 466–487.

Bandura, A. (1969). Social-learning theory of identificatory processes. In D. A. Goslin (Ed), *Handbook of socialization theory and research* (pp. 213–262). Chicago: Rand McNally.

Banks, M. H., Bewley, B. R., & Bland, J. M. (1981). Adolescent attitudes to smoking: Their influence on behav-

iour. *International Journal of Health Education, 24,* 39–44.

Banks, M. H., Bewley, B. R., Bland, J. M., Dean, J. R., & Pollard, V. (1978). Long term study of smoking by secondary schoolchildren. *Archives of Diseases in Children, 53,* 12–19.

Baudier, F., Henry, Y., Marchais, M., Dorier, J., Lombardet, A., Llaona, P., & Pinochet, C. (1991). The "Besancon Smoke-free" programme. *Hygiene, 10* (4), 18–24.

Baugh, J. G., Hunter, S. M., Webber, L. S., & Berenson, G. S. (1982). Developmental trends of first cigarette smoking experience of children: The Bogalusa heart study. *American Journal of Public Health, 72* (10), 1161–1164.

Bernt, T. (1982). The features and effects of friendship in early adolescence. *Child Development, 53,* 1447–1460.

Berscherd, E., & Walster, E. H. (1969). *Interpersonal attraction.* Reading MA: Addison-Wesley.

Bewley, B. R., & Bland, J. M. (1977). Academic performance and social factors related to cigarette smoking by schoolchildren. *British Journal of Preventive and Social Medicine, 31,* 18–24.

Bewley, B. R., Bland, J. M., & Harris, R. (1974). Factors associated with the starting of cigarette smoking by primary school children. *British Journal of Preventive and Social Medicine, 28,* 37–44.

Billy, J. O. G., & Udry, J. R. (1985). Patterns of adolescent friendship and effects on sexual behaviour. *Social Psychology Quarterly, 48,* 27–41.

Botvin, G. J., & Dusenburg, L. (1992). Smoking prevention among urban minority youth: Assessing effects on outcome and mediating variables. *Health Psychology, 11* (5), 290–299.

British Medical Journal. (1994, October 8). A 44 year campaign, but the epidemic is growing (Editorial), p. 309.

Byckling, T., & Sauri, T. (1985). Atherosclerosis precursors in Finnish children and adolescents. XII. Smoking behaviour and its determinants in 12-18 year old subjects. *Acta Paediatrica Scandinavia Supplement, 318,* 195–203.

Bynner, J. M. (1969). *The young smoker,* London: HMSO.

Charlton, A. (1984). The Brigantia smoking survey: A general review. *Public Education about Cancer.* (UICC Technical Report Series ,Vol. 77, pp. 92–102). Geneva, Union Internationale Contre le Cancer.

Charlton, A., & Blair, V. (1989). Predicting the onset of smoking in boys and girls. *Social Science and Medicine, 29* (7), 813–818.

Chassin, L., Presson, C. C., Sherman, S. J., Corty, E., & Olshavsky, R. W. (1984). Predicting the onset of cigarette smoking in adolescents: A longitudinal study. *Journal of Applied Social Psychology, 14* (3), 224–243.

Chassin, L., Presson, C. C., Sherman, S. J., Montello, D., & McGrew, J. (1986). Changes in peer and parent influence during adolescence: Longitudinal versus cross-sectional perspectives on smoking initiation. *Developmental Psychology, 22* (3), 327–334.

Cherry, N., & Kiernan, K. (1976). Personality scores and smoking behaviour: A longitudinal study. *British Journal of Preventive and Social Medicine, 30,* 123–131.

Claes, M. E. (1992). Friendship and personal adjustment during adolescence. *Journal of Adolescence, 15,* 39–55.

Cohen, J. (1977). Sources of peer group homogeneity. *Sociology of Education, 50,* 227–241.

Cohen, J. (1983). Commentary: The relationship between friendship selection and peer influence. In J. L. Epstein & N. Karweit (Eds.), *Friends in school: Patterns of selection and influence in secondary school* (pp. 163–174). New York: Academic Press.

Coleman, J. C. (1980). *The nature of adolescence.* London: Methuen.

Conrad, K. M., Flay, B. R., & Hill, D. (1992). Why children start smoking cigarettes: Predictors of onset. *British Journal of Addiction, 87,* 1711–1724.

Cooley, L. (1902). *Human nature and the social order.* New York: Scribners.

Couriel, J. M. (1994). Passive smoking and the health of children. *Thorax, 49,* 731–734.

De Vries, H., & Kok, G. J. (1986). From determinants of smoking behaviour to the implications for a prevention programme. *Health Education Research, 1* (2), 85–94.

Diamond, A., & Goddard, E. (1995). *Smoking among secondary school children in 1994.* London: HMSO.

Dobbs, J., & Marsh, A. (1983). *Smoking among secondary schoolchildren.* London: HMSO.

Doll, R., & Hill, A. B. (1964). Mortality in relation to smoking: 10 years observation of British doctors. *British Medical Journal,* 1399–1460.

Douvan, E., & Adelson, J. (1966). *The adolescent experience.* New York: John Wiley & Sons.

Eiser J. R., Morgan, M., Gammage, P., Brooks, N., & Kirby, R. (1991). Adolescent health behaviour and similar attraction: Friends share smoking habits (really) but much else besides. *British Journal of Social Psychology, 30,* 339–348.

Eiser, J. R., Morgan, M., Gammage, P., & Gray, E. (1989). Adolescent smoking: Attitudes, norms and parental influence. *British Journal of Social Psychiatry, 28,* 193–202.

Ennett, S. T., & Bauman, K. E. (1993). Peer group structure and adolescent cigarette smoking: A social network analysis. *Journal of Health and Social Behaviour, 34,* 226–236.

Ennett, S. T., & Bauman, K. E. (1994). The contribution of influence and selection to adolescent peer group homogeneity: The case of adolescent cigarette smoking. *Journal of Personality and Social Psychology, 6,* 653–663.

Epstein, J. L. (1983). Examining theories of adolescent friendship. In J. L. Epstein & N. Karweit (Eds.), *Friends in school: Patterns of selection and influence in secondary school* (pp. 39–61). New York: Academic Press.

Epstein, J. L., & Karweit, N. L. (Eds.). (1983). *Friends in school: Patterns of selection and influence in secondary schools.* New York: Academic Press.

Erikson, E. (1968). *Identity, youth and crisis.* New York: Norton.

Evans, R. I. (1976). Smoking in children: Developing a social psychological strategy of deterrence. *Preventive Medicine, 5,* 122–127.

Evans, R. I., Rozelle, R. M., Mittelmark, M. B., Hansen, W. B., Bane, A. L., & Havis, J. (1978). Deterring the onset of smoking in children: Knowledge of immediate physiological effects and coping with peer pressure, media pressure, and parent modeling. *Journal of Applied Social Psychology, 8,* 126–135.

Fisher, L. A., & Bauman, K. E. (1988). Influence and selection in the friend-adolescent relationship: Findings from studies of adolescent smoking and drinking. *Journal of Applied Social Psychology, 18,* 289–314.

Flay, B. R., D'Avernas, J. R., Best, J. A., Kersell, M. W., & Ryan, K. B. (1983). Cigarette smoking: Why young people do it and ways of preventing it. In P. J. McGrath & P. Firestone (Eds.), *Pediatric and adolescent behavioural medicine: Issues in treatment* (pp. 132–183). New York: Springer.

Flay, B. R., Hu, F. B., Siddiqui, O., Day, L. E., Hedeker, D., Petraitis, J., Richardson, J., & Sussman, S. (1994). Differential influence of parental smoking and friends' smoking on adolescent initiation and escalation of smoking. *Journal of Health and Social Behaviour, 35,* 248–265.

Flay, B. R., Koepke, D., Thomson, S. J., Santi, S., Best, J. A., & Brown, K. S. (1989). Six-year follow-up of the first Waterloo School Smoking Prevention Trial. *American Journal of Public Health, 79,* 207–218.

Friedman, L., Lichtenstein, E., & Biglan, A. (1985). Smoking onset among teens: An empirical analysis of initial situations. *Addictive Behaviours, 10,* 1–13.

Garcia, J., D'Avernas, J. R., & Best, J. A. (1988). Smoking prevention for Ontario school children: We know what works, now let's make it happen. *Canadian Journal of Public Health, 79,* S55–S60.

Goddard, E. (1990). *Why children start smoking.* London: HMSO.

Gottlieb, N. H. (1982). The effects of peer and parental smoking and age on the smoking career of college women: A sex-related phenomenon. *Social Science and Medicine, 16,* 595–600.

Green, G., Macintyre, S., West, P., & Ecob, R. (1990). Do children of lone parents smoke more because their mothers do? *British Journal of Addiction, 85,* 1497–1500.

Green, G., Macintyre, S., West, P., & Ecob, R. (1991). Like parent like child? Associations between drinking and smoking behaviour of parents and their children. *British Journal of Addiction, 86,* 745–758.

Hallinan, M. T. (1980). Patterns of cliquing among youth. In H. C. Foot (Ed.), *Friendship and social relations in children* (pp. 321–342). New York: Wiley.

Hallinan, M. T. (1983). New directions for research on peer influence. In J. L. Epstein & N. L. Karweit (Eds.), *Friends in school: Patterns of selection and influence in secondary school* (pp. 219–231). New York: Academic Press.

Hallinan, M. T., & Tuma, N. (1978). Classroom effects on change in children's friendships. *Sociology of Education, 51,* 270–282.

Hammond, E. C., & Horn, D. (1958). Smoking and death rates—Report on forty-four months of follow-up of 187,783 men. *Journal of American Medical Association, 166,* 1294–1308.

Hastings, G. B., Ryan, H., Tees, P., & MacKintosh, A. M. (1994). Cigarette advertising and children's smoking: Why Reg was withdrawn. *British Medical Journal, 309,* 933–937.

Hill, D. (1990). Causes of smoking in children. In B. Durston & K. Jamrozik (Eds.), *Tobacco and health: The global war: Proceedings of the Seventh World Conference on Tobacco and Health* (pp. 205–209). Perth: Health Dept. of Western Australia.

Hover, S. J., & Gaffney, L. R. (1988). Factors associated with smoking behaviour in adolescent girls. *Addictive Behaviours, 13,* 139–145.

Hunter, S. M., Baugh, J. G., Webber, L. S., Sklov, M. C., & Berenson, G. S. (1982). Social learning effects on trial and adoption of cigarette smoking in children: The Bogalusa heart study. *Preventive Medicine, 11,* 29–42.

Hunter, S. M., Croft, J. S., Vizelberg, B. A., & Berenson, G. S. (1987). Psychosocial influences on cigarette smoking among youth in a Southern community: The Bogalusa heart study. In *Psychosocial predictors of smoking among adolescents* (Morbidity Mortality Weekly Report, Vol. 36, No. 4S, pp. 17–24). Atlanta, U.S. Department of Health and Human Services.

Hunter, S. M., Webber, L. S., & Berenson, G. S. (1980). Cigarette smoking and tobacco usage behaviour in children and adolescents: The Bogalusa Heart Study. *Preventive Medicine, 11,* 29–42.

Jarvik, M. E. (1979). Biological influences on cigarette smoking. *Smoking and health.* Rockville, MD: U.S. Dept. of Health, Education & Welfare.

Jessor, R., & Jessor, S. L. (1977). *Problem behaviours and psychosocial development: A longitudinal study of youth.* New York: Academic Press.

Kandel, D. B. (1978). Similarity in real-life adolescent friendship pairs. *Journal of Personality and Social Psychology, 36,* 306–312.

Kandel, D. (1980). Drug and drinking behaviour among youth. *Annual Reviews of Sociology, 6,* 235–285.

Klepp, K. I., Tell, G. S., & Vellar, O. D. (1993). Ten year follow-up of the Oslo Youth Study. *Preventive Medicine, 22* (4), 453–462.

Kozlowski, L. T., Coambs, R. B., Ferrance, R. G., & Adlaf, E. M. (1989). Preventing smoking and other drug use: Let the buyers beware and the interventions be apt. *Canadian Journal of Public Health, 80,* 452–456.

Krohn, M. D., Naughton, M. J., & Lauer, R. M. (1987). Adolescent cigarette use: the relationship between attitudes and behaviour. In *Psychosocial predictors of smoking among adolescents* (Morbidity Mortality Weekly Report, Vol. 36, No. 4S, pp. 25–34). Atlanta: U.S. Dept. of Health and Human Services.

McCaul, K., & Glasgow, R. (1982). Predicting adolescent smoking. *Journal of School Health, 52,* 342–346.

McNeill, A. D., Jarvis, M. J., Stapleton, J. A., Russell, M. A. H., Eiser, J. R., Gammage, P., & Gray, E. M. (1988). Prospective study of factors predicting uptake of smoking in adolescents. *Journal of Epidemiology and Community Health, 43,* 72–78.

Michell, L. (1989). Clean-air kids or ashtray kids—Children's views about other people smoking. *Health Education Journal, 48* (4), 57–161.

Michell, L. (1990). *Growing up in smoke.* London: Pluto Press.

Michell, L. (1994). *Smoking prevention programmes for adolescents: A literature review.* Directorate of Health Policy and Public Health, Anglia & Oxford Regional Health Authority with The National Adolescent & Student Health Unit.

Mittlemark, M. B., Murray, D. M., Luepker, R. V., Pechacek, T. F., Pirie, P. L., & Pallonen, N. E. (1987). Predicting experimentation with cigarettes: The childhood antecedents of smoking study (CASS). *American Journal of Public Health, 77* (2), 206–208.

Mosbach, O., & Leventhal, H. (1988). Peer group identification and smoking: Implications for intervention. *Journal of Abnormal Psychology, 97,* 238–245.

Murray, M., & Cracknell, A. (1980). Adolescents' views on smoking. *Journal of Psychosomatic Research, 24,* 243–251.

Murray, D. M., Pirie, P., Leupker, R. V., & Pallonen, U. (1989). Results from a state-wide approach to adolescent tobacco use. *Preventive Medicine, 21* (4), 449–472.

Murray, M., Swan, A. V., Bewley, B. R., & Johnson, M. R. D. (1983). The development of smoking during adolescence—The MRC/Derbyshire smoking study. *International Journal of Epidemiology, 12* (2), 185–192.

Nelson, S. C., Budd, R. J., Eiser, J. R., Morgan, M. J., Gammage, P., & Gray, E. (1985). The Avon prevalence study: A survey of cigarette smoking in secondary schoolchildren. *Health Education Journal, 44* (1), 12–14.

Newcomb, M. D., McCarthy, W. J., & Bentler, P. M. (1989). Cigarette smoking, academic lifestyle and social impact efficacy: An eight-year study from early adolescence to young adulthood. *Journal of Applied Psychology, 19* (3), 251–281.

Newcomb, T. (1962). Student peer-group influence. In N. Sanford (Ed.), *The American college: A psychological and social interpretation of leaving* (pp. 469–488). New York: Wiley.

Newcomb, T. (1964). *The acquaintance process.* New York: Holt, Rinehart and Winston.

Newman, I. M. (1984). Research into health behaviour and the prevention of smoking: Pressures affecting teenage health behaviour. In G. Campbell (Ed.), *Health education and youth: A review of research and development* (pp. 173–193) London: Falmer.

Newman, P. R., & Newman, B. M. (1976). Early adolescence and its conflict: Group identity vs. alienation. *Adolescence, 11,* 261–274.

Nutbeam, D., Macaskill, P., Smith, C., Simpson, J. M., & Catford, J. (1993). Evaluation of two school smoking education programmes under normal classroom conditions. *British Medical Journal, 306,* 102–107.

Oygard, L., Klepp, K. I., Tell, G. S., & Vellar, O. D. (1995). Parental and peer influences on smoking among young adults: Ten year follow-up of the Oslo youth study participants. *Addiction, 90,* 516–569.

Palmer, A. B. (1970). Some variables contributing to the onset of cigarette smoking among junior high school students. *Social Science and Medicine, 4,* 359–366.

Partridge, M. (1992). Smoking and the young. *British Medical Journal, 305,* 2.

Penny, G. N., & Robinson, J. O. (1986). Psychological resources and cigarette smoking in adolescents. *British Journal of Psychology, 77* (3), 351–357.

Perry, C. L., Kelder, S. H., Murray, D. M., & Klepp, K. I. (1992). Communitywide smoking prevention: Long-term outcomes of the Minnesota Heart Health Program and the Class of 1989 Study. *American Journal of Public Health, 82* (9), 1210–1216.

Piepe, T., Cattermole B., Charlton P., Morey F., Morey, J., & Yerrell, P. (1988). Girls smoking and self-esteem—The adolescent context. *Health Education Journal, 47* (2/3), 83–85.

Reid, D. J., Killoran, A. J., McNeill, A. D., & Chambers, J. (1992). Choosing the most effective health promotion options for reducing a nation's smoking prevalence. *Tobacco Control, 1,* 185–197.

Royal College of Physicians. (1962). *Smoking and health: A report on smoking in relation to lung cancer and other disease.* London: Pitman Medical.

Royal College of Physicians. (1983). *Health or smoking: A follow-up report.* London: Pitman Medical.

Royal College of Physicians. (1992). *Smoking and the young.* London: Royal College of Physicians.

Rubin, L. B. (1985). *Just friends: The role of friendship in our lives.* New York: Harper and Row.

Russell, M. A. H. (1989). The Addiction Research Unit of the Institute of Psychiatry, University of London—II,

The work of the unit's smoking section. *British Journal of Addiction, 84,* 853–863.

Semmer, N. K., Lippert, P., Cleary, P. D., Dwyer, J. H., & Fuchs, R. (1987). Psychosocial predictors of adolescent smoking in two German cities: The Berlin-Bremen Study. In *Psychosocial predictors of smoking among adolescents* (Morbidity Mortality Weekly Report, Vol. 36, No. 4S, pp. 3–10). Atlanta: U.S. Dept. of Health and Human Services.

Sherif, M., & Sherif, C. W. (1964). *Exploration into conformity and deviance of adolescents.* New York: Harper and Row.

Skinner, W. F., Massey, J. L., Krohn, M. D., & Lauer, R. M. (1985). Social influences and constraints on the initiation and cessation of adolescent tobacco use. *Journal of Behavioural Medicine, 8* (4), 353–376.

Smee, C. (1993). *The European Commission's proposed directive on the advertising of tobacco products.* London: HMSO.

Strasburger, V. C. (1989). Prevention of adolescent drug abuse: Why "Just Say No" just won't work. *Journal of Pediatrics, 114* (1), 676–681.

Surgeon General. (1964). *Smoking and health: Report of the Advisory Committee to the Surgeon General.* Washington, DC: U.S. Dept. of Health, Education and Welfare.

Surgeon General. (1979). *Smoking and health: A report of the Surgeon General.* Rockville, MD: U.S. Dept. of Health, Education & Welfare.

Swan, A. V., Murray, M., & Jarrett, L. (1991). *Smoking behaviour from pre-adolescence to young adulthood.* Aldershot: Avebury.

Teijlingen, E. R. van., & Friend, J. A. R. (1993a). Smoking habits of Grampian school children and an evaluation of the Grampian Smoke Busters campaign. *Health Education Research Theory & Practice, 8* (1), 97–108.

Teijlingen, E. R. van., & Friend, J. A. R (1993b). *Smoking prevalence of Grampian schoolchildren: An evaluation of the Regional Smokebusters Club.* University of Aberdeen: Cancer Research Campaign.

Thompson, E. L. (1978). Smoking education programs 1960–1976. *American Journal of Public Health, 69* (3), 250–257.

Tobler, N. S. (1986). Meta-analysis of 143 adolescent drug prevention programs: Quantitative outcome results of programs participants compared to a control or comparison group. *Journal of Drug Issues, 56,* 537–567.

Townsend, J., Wilkes, H., Haines, A., & Jarvis, M. (1991). Adolescent smokers seen in general practice: Health lifestyle, physical measurements and response to anti smoking advice. *British Medical Journal, 303,* 947–950.

Urberg, K. A., & Deqirmencioglu, S. (1990). *Peer influence on adolescent values.* Paper presented at meeting of the American Psychological Association, Boston.

Urberg, K. A., Shyu, S-J., & Liang, J. (1990). Peer influence in adolescent cigarette smoking. *Addictive Behaviours, 15,* 247–255.

Van Roosmalen, E. H., & McDaniel, S. A. (1989). Peer group influence as a factor in smoking behaviour of adolescents. *Adolescence, 24* (96), 801–816.

Vartiainen, E., Fallonen, U., McAlister, A. L., & Puska, P. (1990). Eight-year follow-up results of an adolescent smoking prevention program: The North Karelia Youth Program. *American Journal of Public Health, 82* (9), 1210–1216.

West, P. (1993). Do Scottish schoolchildren smoke more than their English and Welsh peers? *Health Bulletin, 51* (4), 230–239.

West, P., & Macintyre, S. (1990). *Youth style and health behaviour.* Paper presented at Third Congress at European Society of Medical Sociology, Marburg, Germany.

West, P., & Sweeting, H. (in press). Family and friends' influences on smoking in mid to late adolescence. *Addiction.*

Wiist, W. H., & Snider, G. (1991). Peer education in friendship cliques: Prevention of adolescent smoking. *Health Education Research Theory and Practice, 6* (1), 101–108.

World Health Organization. (1975). *Smoking and its effects on health. Report of WHO Expert Committee* (WHO Technical Report Series No. 568). Geneva: World Health Organization.

CHAPTER 13

ALCOHOL ABUSE

Ralph E. Tarter, CENTER FOR EDUCATION AND DRUG ABUSE RESEARCH
UNIVERSITY OF PITTSBURGH MEDICAL SCHOOL
Timothy C. Blackson, CENTER FOR EDUCATION AND DRUG ABUSE RESEARCH
UNIVERSITY OF PITTSBURGH MEDICAL SCHOOL

Alcohol consumption among adolescents is benignly accepted, even though purchasing and drinking alcohol beverages are illegal. Unlike other easily obtainable drugs having addiction potential, especially tobacco, alcohol is considered to be a less serious problem, as indicated by the comparatively low level of media attention.

U.S. society tolerates alcohol consumption in a wide array of settings. Drinking is common, and even sometimes expected, at social events, holiday celebrations, religious rituals, and during business transactions. Because adolescence is the time when autonomy from parents is exercised and the behavior of adults emulated, it is to be expected that the incidence of alcohol consumption increases during the teenage years. Thus, high alcohol availability, combined with socialization and maturation, leads to an increasingly higher incidence of initiation of drinking during adolescence, defined herein as the period encompassing 13 to 18 years of age.

This chapter reviews the literature pertaining to the etiology, assessment, and treatment of adolescent alcoholism. This disorder is increasingly recognized as the outcome of disturbed or deviant development (Tarter & Vanyukov, 1994). As will be observed, this is an alarmingly prevalent disorder which, to date, remains poorly understood despite consensual agreement that there are enormous health, safety, legal, and economic consequences of alcohol abuse among adolescents.

EPIDEMIOLOGY

The *Monitoring the Future* epidemiological study is an annual survey of a representative sample of high school youths. The aim of this survey is to track the incidence and prevalence of alcohol and drug use among eighth-, tenth-, and twelfth-grade students (Johnston et al., 1994; NIDA Notes, 1995). The most recent survey indicates that approximately 56 percent of eighth-graders, 71 percent of tenth-graders, and 80 percent of 12th-graders have used alcohol at some time in their lives. Approximately 26 percent, 39 percent, and 50 percent, respectively, of youths in these grades report having used alcohol in the month prior to responding to the survey. At least one lifetime intoxication experience is reported by 26 percent, 47 percent, and 63 percent of eighth-, tenth-, and twelfth-grade students, respectively. Indeed, 28 percent of students in these grades report having been intoxicated between 1 and 5 times in their lifetimes. Daily alcohol consumption is reported by 1 percent, 1.7 percent, and 2.9 percent of students in grades 8, 10, and 12, respectively. These data illustrate that alcohol use is prevalent among adolescents. Also, there is a high level of alcohol involvement, as reflected by the frequency of intoxication and prevalence of daily alcohol consumption. Indeed, the observation that almost 3 percent of twelfth-graders are daily drinkers underscores the conclusion that alcoholism begins during adolescence for many individuals.

Table 13.1 demonstrates that female and male adolescents differ with respect to drinking behavior. Heavy use (5+ drinks) differentiates male from female adolescents. Specifically, there is a higher rate of heavy alcohol use among males compared to females across the eighth, tenth, and twelfth grades. In-

spection of Table 13.1 also indicates that males and females increasingly separate as they get older.

As shown in Table 13.2, there is a gradation of alcohol involvement across white, Hispanic, and African American youths. The highest rates are observed on all variables in white youths followed by Hispanic youths. African American youths have the lowest rate of alcohol involvement across all grades.

The descriptive epidemiological data presented in Tables 13.1 and 13.2 demonstrate that there is substantial heterogeneity of alcohol consumption behavior according to gender and ethnicity in the general population. Reasons underlying such heterogeneity have been the subject of much speculation and research; however, empirical investigations have not revealed the factors contributing to variation in drinking topography according to gender and ethnicity. For example, level of education of parents, population density of the respondent's location of residence,

Table 13.1 Gender Differences in Alcohol Consumption Behavior

GRADE	USE IN PAST YEAR, %		USE IN PAST MONTH, %		5 OR MORE DRINKS DURING THE PAST TWO WEEKS, %	
	M	F	M	F	M	F
8th	52	53	27	26	14.8	12.3
10th	69	70	43	39	26.5	19.3
12th	76	76	55	47	34.6	20.7

Source: L. Johnston, P. O'Malley, & J. Bachman, *National Survey results on drug use from the Monitoring the Future Study, 1975–1993* (Washington, DC: U.S. Department of Health and Human Services, 1994).

Table 13.2 Prevalence of Alcohol Consumption in White (W), African American (AA) and Hispanic (H) Youths

GRADE	USE IN PAST YEAR, %			USE IN PAST MONTH, %			5 OR MORE DRINKS DURING THE PAST TWO WEEKS, %		
	W	AA	H	W	AA	H	W	AA	H
8	56	43	57	27	20	32	13	11	21
10	72	60	70	43	29	40	23	15	24
12	80	64	77	56	32	51	31	13	27

Source: L. Johnston, P. O'Malley, & J. Bachman, *National Survey results on drug use from the Monitoring the Future Study, 1975–1993* (Washington, DC: U.S. Department of Health and Human Services, 1994).

and geographic region are not related to lifetime prevalence of alcohol consumption in adolescents (Johnston et al., 1994).

In contrast to alcohol use, there is almost no documentation as to the epidemiology of the disorders of alcohol abuse or alcohol dependence, defined according to standard taxonomic criteria. In one study employing *DSM-III-R* criteria, Reinherz and colleagues (1993) reported that 34.6 percent ($n = 66$ of 192) of adolescents qualified for a diagnosis of alcohol abuse or dependence among a community dwelling sample of youths drawn primarily from lower socioeconomic strata. Among youths selected from higher socioeconomic strata, the prevalence was 30.3 percent. Severity of disorder was also notable. Among those qualifying for a diagnosis of abuse or dependence, 62 percent were classified as moderately dependent on alcohol, whereas 12 percent were classified as severely dependent.

These findings suggest that alcoholism is the most prevalent psychiatric disorder among adolescents and is much more common than generally appreciated. However, this observation needs to be tempered by the fact that *DSM* criteria were not designed to be appropriate for adolescents. Thus, the rate of misclassification may be high. For example, Martin and colleagues (in press) reported that *DSM* criteria pertaining to tolerance, withdrawal, and medical problems are manifested differently in adolescents than adults. Furthermore, the category of abuse presents as a very heterogeneous pattern of symptoms, indicating perhaps that the *DSM* criteria for the diagnosis of abuse are too broad, thereby yielding the large prevalence rates observed by Reinherz and associates (1993). Moreover, the possibility remains that adolescents qualifying for a diagnosis of alcohol abuse may be manifesting a transient disorder, whereas in adults this diagnosis is a harbinger for the more severe and chronic disorder of alcohol dependence.

To date, research has not been conducted to address these issues. Nonetheless, it is important to emphasize that a diagnosis of alcohol abuse is not innocuous. In the Martin and colleagues' (in press) study, 26 percent and 10 percent of youths with this diagnosis report, respectively, blackouts and a history of alcohol-induced unconsciousness. Also, craving is described by 12%. Risky sexual behavior is reported by

12 percent of youths with a *DSM-IV* alcohol abuse diagnosis. Thus, although there is reason to be cautious about the validity of estimates of the prevalence of alcohol abuse, there is no doubt that individuals so classified manifest potentially severe and life-threatening consequences.

SUBTYPES OF ALCOHOLISM

Several classification schemas have been proposed to aggregate alcoholics into subtypes within this heterogeneous population (e.g., Cloninger and associates 1981, 1987; Schuckit et al., 1985). Based on a Swedish adoption study, Cloninger and associates (1981, 1987) classified alcoholics into two subtypes. Type 1 (milieu limited) alcoholism is featured primarily by adult onset, minimal criminality, age of onset after 25, guilt and fear about alcohol dependence, and psychological dependence. This variant of alcoholism is largely determined by environmental factors. Type 2 (male limited), in contrast, has high heritability. It is manifested as severe alcoholism accompanied by criminality that begins before age 25.

Problem involvement with alcohol is most likely present during adolescence. Recently, Babor and colleagues (1992) provided some confirmatory evidence for this dichotomy and demonstrated that treatment prognosis is poorer in the early age onset subtype. However, there is considerable variability in assigning diagnoses of Type 1 and Type 2, as well as overlap between the typology systems (Anthenelli et al., 1994). Moreover, Schuckit and associates (1994) found no reliable personality profile associated with risk for alcoholism except when a comorbid antisocial personality disorder is present.

Psychosocial research has also delineated two subtypes in which age of onset of alcoholism is the salient discriminating variable. The most notable taxonomy is the essential-reactive alcoholism dichotomy (Tarter, 1982). *Essential alcoholism* is a developmentally based disorder that is manifested primarily as psychosocial immaturity. This variant of alcoholism typically begins during adolescence. *Reactive* alcoholics, in contrast, develop problem involvement with alcohol concomitant to stress or personal crisis. Significantly, combined scores on the essential alcoholism questionnaire and a childhood hyperactivity checklist accounts for almost 50 percent of the variance on a scale measuring alcoholism severity (Tarter, 1992).

In summary, there is evidence pointing to an early age onset variant of alcoholism that is rather severe and culminates from deviant development (Tarter & Vanyukov, 1994). In this subtype, severe behavioral problems precede alcohol use, such that by the time of adolescence and early adulthood, the person qualifies for a diagnosis of substance use disorder—alcohol abuse or alcohol dependence. However, it is important to point out that adolescent alcoholism is not a unitary disorder. For example, in a recent study (Mezzich et al., 1993), it was found that adolescent alcoholics comprise two general subgroups. In the first subgroup, conduct disorder is the most salient feature, whereas the second subgroup is primarily featured by an affective disturbance. Approximately 75 percent of alcoholics are classifiable in the first group, which is also more heavily represented by males. Finally, it is important to emphasize that whereas an early age onset variant of alcoholism has been identified and appears to consist of two broad subtypes, there is nonetheless substantial heterogeneity with respect to etiology, natural history and clinical presentation.

ETIOLOGY OF ALCOHOLISM

Developmental Perspective

Alcoholism has a multifactorial etiology. Each factor can be considered as a trait (or dimension) such that deviations from the population norm independently contribute to the liability for alcoholism. As shown in Figure 13.1, these deviations can be conceptualized as vectors (V_1, V_2, etc.), in as much as they shape or bias the developmental trajectory to either a normal or alcoholism outcome. The person's overall liability consists of the interaction among all scores on the traits contributing to liability. This is depicted in Figure 13.1 as R, or the resultant vector of all traits contributing to liability.

During ontogeny, the person's position on the liability trait determines how he or she responds to the social environment as well as how he or she selects environments that influence subsequent developmental course. In effect, liability status at one time contributes to liability status in the future; however, changing circumstances can deflect the person toward either higher or lower liability status. As can be seen in Figure 13.1, the pathway linking liability status at the time of conception to outcome (*DSM-IV* diagnosis) is not linear. Thus, liability is not fixed; rather, it changes during development concomitant to changing circumstances. Depending on the person's unique and changing circumstances, the developmental trajectory can orient toward or away from an alcoholism outcome. In other words, liability can be increased or decreased, depending on the presence of factors that, in aggregate, augment or attenuate liability.

Numerous factors have been identified that increase or decrease liability to alcoholism (Tarter, Alterman, & Edwards, 1985). In the hypothetical example provided, the trajectory of development is liability augmenting and culminating in an alcoholism disorder. This is shown by the person manifesting a suprathreshold diagnosis, illustrated by the shaded area in the distribution at the bottom. For a more detailed description of the multifactorial model of alcoholism, the reader is referred to Tarter and Vanyukov (1994).

One paradigm that is useful for elucidating the contributors to liability is to compare children who are at high risk for alcoholism with children who are at low or average risk. Offspring whose parents are alcoholics are at high risk, as indicated by the fact that they are four to six times more likely to become alcoholic than children of parents who have no lifetime history of alcohol abuse or dependence (Cloninger et al., 1981; Goodwin et al., 1974). This elevated risk is observed even if children are reared away from their biological alcoholic parents. In other words, children of alcoholics are more likely to manifest the characteristics associated with high liability. Thus, by comparing and tracking prospectively the children of alcoholics and nonalcoholics, it is possible to delineate the contributors to liability and their mode of interaction. To date, numerous biological factors have been implicated to contribute to alcoholism liability (Alexopoulos et al., 1983; Schuckit et al., 1982, 1983; Begleiter et al., 1984). The biological aspects of liability will not, however, be reviewed in this discussion. In order to maintain focus, this discussion will be confined to an examination of liability from the perspective of psychosocial processes.

Figure 13.1 Conceptual Framework for Understanding the Etiology of Alcoholism

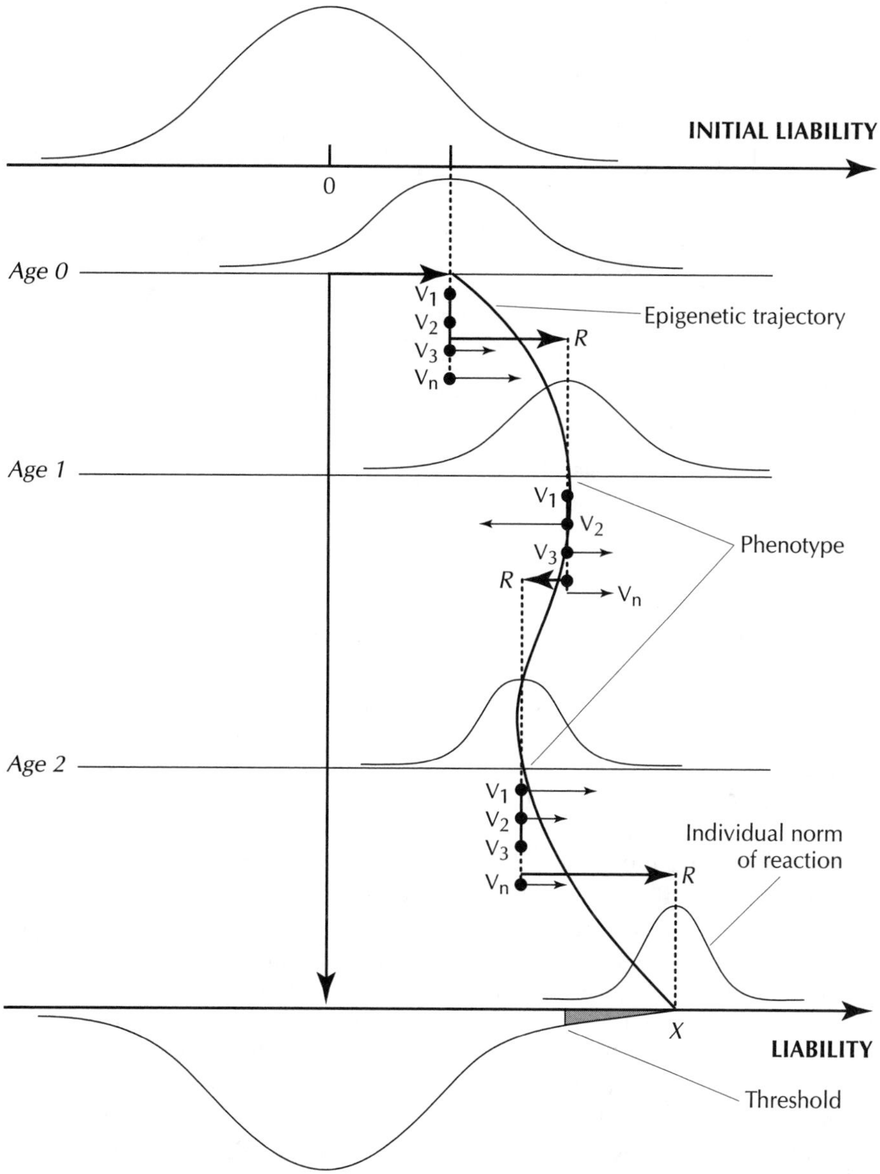

Determinants of Liability

Figure 13.2 depicts a framework for researching the relationship among individual, family, and peer variables that are salient to the development of alcoholism (Blackson, 1994a). Each variable, as noted previously in Figure 13.1, comprises a vector that, in aggregate, determines the person's liability status at a given point in time.

As can be seen, individual, family, and peer affiliation factors are conjointly predictive of prodromal outcomes. These prodromal disturbances—consist-

Figure 13.2 Relationship Among the Variables Integral to Etiology of Alcoholism

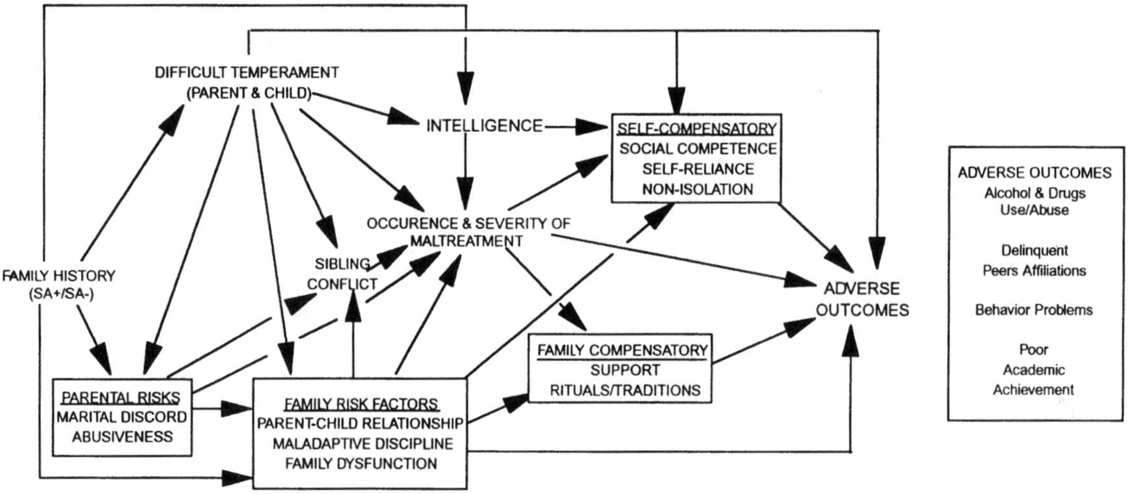

ing of behavioral maladjustment, academic underachievement, dysfunctional interactions in the family, and deviant peer affiliations—are commonly associated with early-age alcohol use. Furthermore, these prodromal disturbances, in turn, predispose to habitual and excessive alcohol use as part of a deviant life-style and increasing assumption of adult-like behavior as the youngster becomes older. Under facilitating circumstances, drinking and its consequences escalate such that the person qualifies for a *DSM* diagnosis of abuse or dependence. Hence, early-age alcohol exposure, deviancy, and chronological age interact to foster a habitual and excessive pattern of alcohol involvement. Prior to alcohol exposure, there are, however, several important factors that contribute to liability, thereby orienting the developmental trajectory to an alcoholism outcome. The following discussion succinctly reviews the factors that contribute to the liability of alcoholism.

Temperament

A major contributor to liability is a deviation in temperament. A theoretical definition proposed by Allport (1961) captures the meaning of *temperament:* "the characteristic phenomena of an individual's nature, including his customary strength and speed of response, the quality of his prevailing mood, and all the peculiarities of fluctuations and intensity of mood,

these being phenomena regarded as dependent on constitutional makeup, and therefore largely hereditary in origin" (p. 34). Because these characteristics are present within the first month or two after birth, they can be considered the building blocks for the acquisition of more complex psychological processes (e.g., habits, personality, etc.). Hence, temperament disposition provides the framework for understanding habitual alcohol use and a disorder of abuse or dependence within a developmental framework. Furthermore, recognizing that genetic factors contribute significantly to expression of temperament characteristics, it has been argued that these traits afford the opportunity to elucidate the etiology of alcoholism (and other types of drug abuse) within a behavior genetic framework (Tarter et al., 1985; Tarter et al., 1995).

Temperament in early childhood is an important determinant of behavioral and social adjustment. Deviations from the norm on temperament traits are associated with an increased risk for a variety of psychopathological disturbances (Maziade et al., 1990). Within particular contexts (e.g., family, peer, etc.), temperament deviations in childhood also predispose to alcohol use by the time of adolescence (Tarter et al., 1990; Blackson & Tarter, 1994). At this juncture, there is strong evidence indicating that deviations in several temperament traits augment alcohol abuse liability. These traits include high behavioral activity level, high emotionality, low sociability, and low attentional capacity (for reviews see Tarter et al., 1985; Tarter & Vanyukov, 1994).

In aggregate, individuals manifesting these characteristics are referred to as having a "difficult" temperament disposition (Chess & Thomas, 1984; Windle, 1992). Difficult temperament in childhood predisposes to alcohol and other substance use in adolescence (Lerner & Vicary, 1984). Indeed, magnitude of temperament deviations correlates with severity of alcohol and drug use among adolescents (Tarter et al., 1990; Windle, 1991).

Results of several studies demonstrate that temperament deviations are associated with maladaptive discipline practices by parents (Tarter et al., 1993a; Blackson et al., 1996a). Dysfunctional parent/child interaction increases risk for oppositional defiant behavior (Maziade et al., 1985; Maziade et al., 1989). Significantly, disruptive behavior commonly presages alcohol use (Lerner & Vicary, 1984; Robbins & McEvoy, 1990). The point to be made is that temperament disposition operates contextually; that is, the child's temperament evokes reactions from the social environment as well as influences the selection of environments. These ongoing reciprocal interactions, occurring during development, foster the acquisition of behaviors that either augment or diminish liability to alcohol use and alcoholism.

Difficult temperament, when manifest by both parents and their children, has a profound effect on the family environment (Blackson et al., 1994a). In effect, congruity between parent and child sets the stage for conflict due to the disruptiveness associated with this type of temperament disposition. In a recently completed study, it was found that temperament mediates the effects of family history of substance abuse on the child's behavioral characteristics (Blackson et al., 1994b). In other words, behavioral maladjustment of children in substance abuse families is partially transmitted through temperament disposition—namely, the dyadic concordance in difficult temperament between parents and children.

Concomitant to disruptive interaction with the social environment, a variety of adverse outcomes has been documented in children having a temperament deviation that increase the risk of alcohol (and drug) abuse. These intermediary outcomes include maladjustment at school (Martin, 1989; Maziade et al.,

1988) and deviant peer affiliations (Blackson et al., 1996b). Maladjustment at school and peer relationship disturbances are among the most significant problems reported among adolescents who abuse alcohol (Hawkins et al., 1992), as well as those who qualify for a diagnosis of alcoholism (Kirisci et al., 1995). In addition, children manifesting temperament deviations receive less parental supervision than children with normative temperament. These latter findings are important because low parental supervision predisposes to delinquency (Loeber et al., 1983), which is almost invariably associated with alcohol and drug abuse.

Intelligence

Juvenile delinquents have been observed to obtain, on average, lower IQ scores than nondelinquents (Moffitt & Silva, 1988; White et al., 1989). Sons of alcoholic fathers, as a group, also have been shown to have lower IQ scores compared to sons of nonalcoholics (Tarter et al., 1984). Furthermore, Kandel and colleagues (1987) found that higher intelligence protects against development of antisocial personality disorder. In contrast to these findings, Fleming and associates (1982) reported that high intelligence in first-grade students predicted subsequent alcohol use among inner-city African American adolescents. The reasons for this discrepant finding are not clear but may be due to greater sensitivity to environmental stress in disadvantaged youths (Luthar, 1991).

A recent study observed that intellectual capacity partially mediated the relationship between paternal history of substance abuse and reading levels in 10- to 12-year-old boys (Blackson, 1995). These results suggest that higher intelligence may be protective for children who have a substance-abusing father. This protective process may be exercised through a developmental pathway that provides opportunity for academic success, and accordingly, the opportunity to affiliate with normative peers and with adults who can serve as positive role models.

Family Dysfunction and Parental Discipline Practices

Family relationship patterns influence alcohol use behavior in adolescents (Johnson & Pandina, 1991). Studies attempting to disaggregate the specific intrafamilial processes have addressed several factors.

One potentially important factor that may influence a child's risk for alcohol use is the degree of relationship satisfaction between the parent and child. In this regard, Shedler and Block (1990) found that the quality of parent/child interactions, when the children were 5 years of age, was associated with marijuana use when the children attained 18 years of age. Another study observed that externalizing and internalizing maladaptive behavior in the child, co-occurring with mother/son mutual dissatisfaction, fosters disengagement from the parental sphere of influence to promote association with peers having a negative influence on behavior (Tarter et al., 1993b).

Another parental factor that may contribute to early-age alcohol use is deficient discipline practices. Maladaptive discipline practices—characterized by inconsistency, inordinate severity, and ineffectiveness—have been found to explain a significant amount of variance on a child's externalizing and internalizing behavior in substance abuse families (Tarter et al., 1993a). Blackson and colleagues (1996a) recently found that interaction between difficult temperament in children and their perceptions of maladaptive discipline by parents accounted for additional variance beyond main effects in explaining externalizing and internalizing behavior. The observation that maladaptive discipline by parents is associated with externalizing and internalizing behavior problems in the child suggests that, without offsetting protective resources, there is increased probability that the child will initiate alcohol use as one facet of generalized deviancy.

Previous studies buttress this conclusion by indicating that dysfunctional parental discipline practices predict initiation of substance use in children (Beschner & Friedman, 1985; Kandel & Andrews, 1987; Penning & Barnes, 1982). Moreover, conduct-disordered youth, who also typically consume alcohol as part of their deviancy, commonly have parents whose discipline skills are ineffective (Loeber & Dishion, 1983; McHale et al., 1995; Vuchinich et al., 1992).

Other studies have observed that incongruity in discipline practices by fathers and mothers (e.g., one parent being permissive and the other parent being overinvolved) is also associated with an increased risk for alcohol abuse in children (Kaufman & Kaufman, 1979; Ziegler-Driscoll, 1979). Moreover, Rutter (1987) observed that children with temperament devi-

ations were more likely than other children to be the target of parental hostility, criticism, and irritability. Considered together, these studies clearly indicate that familial dysfunction and ineffective parenting increase the risk for maladjustment and alcohol use at an early age. This risk is magnified when the temperament characteristics of the parents and children are conjointly considered. It is not surprising, therefore, that when temperaments clash, and the family is strife ridden, that the youngster is inclined at a young age toward, disengagement from the family sphere of influence to the peer sphere of influence (Wills, 1990). Such disengagement augments the risk for alcohol abuse due to absence of parental supervision and tendency to affiliate with deviant peers.

Child Abuse

Another important family interaction factor that appears to contribute to a child's risk for alcohol abuse is severe punishment. In the extreme, this behavior can be considered to reflect child abuse (Whitbeck & Simons, 1990). Specific behavioral characteristics in children (e.g., difficult temperament, hyperactivity, aggressivity) that challenge parenting skills augments the likelihood that the child will be physically punished (Ammerman, 1991), Studies have shown that there is a greater frequency of child abuse in sons of alcoholic fathers compared to sons of nonalcoholic fathers (Tarter et al., 1984a). In addition, it has been found that a history of child abuse is more common among delinquent adolescents (Burgess et al., 1987; Tarter et al., 1984b). This latter finding is especially noteworthy because delinquency is typically associated with alcohol and drug abuse. Thus, child abuse may bias the child's developmental trajectory toward generalized maladjustment and social deviancy. These disturbances predispose to early-age onset alcohol use and abuse.

Cognitive Misattributions

Besides familial influences on behavior, there are also familial influences on the development of cognitive style. Growing up in a disruptive family impedes the child's opportunity to learn how to normatively interpret the meaning, context, and intentions of others in social interactions. The cognitive distortions include unjustified self-blame and a tendency to personalize situations and events (Mazur et al., 1992). Children of alcoholic families make more attributional errors regarding self and others than children of normal parents (Giglio & Kaufman, 1990). In a dysfunctional family, cognitive misattributions may thus foster the development of maladjustment, including withdrawal from parents to affiliate with deviant peers (Brook et al., 1990; Loeber & Hay, 1995). This is especially likely to occur where the child has a discordant relationship with both mother and father. In effect, cognitive misattributions may contribute to liability to alcohol abuse among adolescents by producing a cognitive style that does not allow for accurate interpretation of social interactions.

Affiliation with Nonnormative Peers

Involvement in normative activities with peers is associated with tolerance of deviance (Moffitt, 1993). This, in turn, augments the likelihood of early-age alcohol and drug use (Brook et al., 1993). Furthermore, affiliation with peers involved in delinquent behaviors is featured by higher acceptance of deviancy, an inclination to interpret deviant behavior as normative (Loeber et al., 1991), and negative reciprocity in antisocial behavior (Dishion et al., 1995). It is also important to note, however, that children who get into trouble at school prefer to affiliate with peers who do not get into trouble (Gillmore et al., 1992). This finding suggests that friendships with conventional peers are more desirable than friendships with deviant peers, even though the latter may be the only available option to youths who are deviant.

Finally, results of several recent studies indicate that children having difficult temperament affiliate with peers who engage in fewer conventional activities and more delinquent behaviors (Blackson, 1994b; Blackson & Tarter, 1994; Blackson et al., 1996b; Tubman & Kindle, 1995). Alcohol use, therefore, reflects the culmination of parent/child and subsequent peer/peer interactions mediated to a significant degree by temperament makeup.

Factors That Reduce Liability

Factors such as self-efficacy, initiative, and humor can lower risk for adverse outcome (Werner & Smith, 1992). A close relationship with a significant other (Masten et al., 1991) and family rituals that lend sta-

bility to an otherwise disruptive home environment can also attenuate risk (Wolin et al., 1979).

Research conducted by Werner and Smith (1992) and Luthar and Ziegler (1992) have contributed to the growing recognition that high liability need not necessarily culminate in a negative outcome. Rather, outcome is determined by the interaction among liability-enhancing and liability-reducing factors ongoing throughout development. The point to be made is that liability is not a constant state, but rather is subject to change in response to environmental exposure and maturational processes.

Difficult temperament in children is commonly associated with low support from family and friends (Tubman & Windle, 1995; Windle, 1992). By evoking negative reactions in others, difficult temperament in children works against acquiring strong parental attachment and support. Lack of bonding between parent and child (Kandel, 1973; Brook et al., 1980) and low parental involvement or supervision in the activities of their children (Braucht et al., 1978; Loeber & Hay, 1995; Penning & Barnes, 1982) increase risk for alcohol use.

Based on the preceding discussion, it is apparent that risk can be potentially offset by liability-reducing factors. For example, results from the Kauai Longitudinal Study (Werner & Smith, 1992) demonstrate that children having an easy temperament disposition are more likely to develop effective coping strategies and form extrafamilial relationships that enable the youngster to obtain help and support to surmount adversity. To date, an intervention program has not been designed to help youths with difficult temperament learn how to access resources that can reduce their liability. Whereas children with easy temperament have a more facile task because the response to the child in the social environment is congenial, these potential resources are not available to the child having difficult temperament. For this reason, it is important to underscore the need for prevention programs that are tailored to the interpersonal problems of youths who have a difficult temperament.

ASSESSMENT OF ALCOHOL ABUSE IN ADOLESCENTS

Alcohol abuse is associated with a variety of problems among youths. These problems include the direct adverse biological consequences of drug toxicity, as well as encompass the indirect consequences of a life-style concomitant to habitual alcohol (and other drug) abuse. In addition, there are several other important sequelae that appear to have increasing incidence among youths, such as sexually transmitted disease, unplanned pregnancy, and HIV infection. Furthermore, social problems concomitant to alcohol and drug use commonly have egregious consequences (e.g. violence, school failure, expulsion from the home by parents). Thus, evaluation of adolescent alcohol abuse necessitates a multivariate approach encompassing health, behavior, and interpersonal processes.

The following discussion reviews the range of instruments appropriate for evaluation of adolescents having known or suspected problem involvement with alcohol or drugs.

Psychiatric Interviews

Several structured and semistructured interviews are used in research for the objective psychiatric diagnosis of adolescents. The most common are the Diagnostic Interview Schedule for Children (Costello et al., 1984), the Diagnostic Interview for *Children and Adolescents* (Wellner et al., 1987), and the Kiddie Schedule for Affective Disorders and Schizophrenia (Orvaschel et al., 1982). The purpose of these interview schedules is to formulate an objective diagnosis of the substance use disorders and other psychiatric disorders. Although objectivity for diagnosis is increased by structured psychiatric interviews, the range of problems covered, particularly the diversity of behavioral and psychosocial processes, is not comprehensively assessed by these latter interviews. For example, a *DSM-IV* diagnosis of a substance use disorder requires only that three of seven criteria are present to formulate a diagnosis. This information is inadequate for designing a treatment program.

Drugs and Alcohol Interviews

The Addiction Severity Index (ASI; McClellan et al., 1992) is the most widely used multidimensional assessment tool for evaluating severity of drug/alcohol problems. Increasingly, the ASI has been used for assessment, treatment planning, and determination of treatment effectiveness. A parallel adolescent version, the Teen-ASI (Kaminer et al., 1991), has been developed but has not yet been submitted to psychometric validation.

The Adolescent Drug Abuse Diagnosis (ADAD; Friedman, 1991) is a 150-item structured interview modeled on the ASL. Severity ratings are obtained in nine areas during and after treatment. The ADAD measures (1) the degree to which the client has been "troubled" by each type of problem, (2) the interviewer's rating of the client's need for treatment for each problem, (3) the level of motivation for treatment and (4) the degree of client's denial or misrepresentation of their behavior. Additionally, the ADAD allows for tracking changes and severity of problems over time.

Self-Administered Instruments

Several self-report instruments have been developed having varying degree of psychometric validation. The Personal Experience Inventory (PEI); (Winters &Henleg,1988) contains 33 scales and is appropriate for youths between ages 12 and 18 who can read at the fourth-grade level. The PEI consists of two sections. One section measures the severity of drug problems and the other evaluates psychosocial risk factors. Originally standardized on 1,200 youths in treatment, the PEI has been widely adopted and is recommended for use following screening assessment. It is one of the few self-report instruments having psychometric validity.

The Drug Use Screening Inventory (DUSI) was initially developed in 1990 (Tarter, 1990) and subsequently revised (DUSI-R) in 1992 (Tarter, 1992). The revision contains three separate versions for evaluating the person in different timeframes (past year, past month, past week). Additionally, the DUSIR contains a Lie Scale to detect invalid protocols.

The DUSI-R consists of 159 items organized into 10 domains of measurement: Substance Use, Health Status, Behavior, Psychiatric Status, Family, Work, Peer Relationship, Social Skill, School, and Leisure/ Recreation. A Lie Scale consists of 10 items scattered through the questionnaire. Each item is geared toward a minimum fifth-grade reading level and requires a yes or no response. In each domain, the raw score is converted to a standard "problem density score" ranging from 0 to 100 percent. To further facilitate interpretation through direct comparison of the 10 domains, the scores are graphically displayed as a histogram. An overall problem density index, expressed as a percent, is also obtained, which is the number of items endorsed divided by the total number of items in the inventory. In addition to quantification of problem severity in the 10 domains, the DUSI-R documents frequency of drug and alcohol consumption and drug preference across 20 different types of commonly abused substances.

The DUSI has well-established psychometric properties. Internal reliability, test-retest reliability, and construct validity have been documented using both classical psychometric and item response theory methods (Tarter et al,, 1994; Kirisci et al., 1994; Kirisci et al., 1995). Internal and test-retest reliability coefficients exceed 0.8 for each domain. Analyses between gender and comparisons between African-Americans and whites demonstrate its usefulness in different ethnic groups. Recently, factor analytic studies have revealed that the DUSI may yield several important subscale scores in addition to the 10 domain scores. For example, the School Adjustment domain appears to consist of separate factors measuring school adjustment and school performance (Tarter et al., in press). The Behavior domain also measures three dimensions: impulsive aggressive behavior, paranoid anger, and social withdrawal (Kirisci & Tarter, unpublished manuscript).

The DUSI-R can be administered in either a paper-and-pencil or computer-administered format. It was developed with several factors in mind: (1) the areas or domains of assessment are linked to drug abuse etiology and comprise the most common areas of disturbance requiring intervention; (2) severity across the 10 domains is quantified on an easily understood standard scale (0–100 percent), thereby enabling efficient prioritization of intervention modalities by allocating treatment resources commensurate with problem severity; (3) straightforward administration and scoring provides the opportunity to monitor and quantify status from pretreatment through active treatment and aftercare using a repeat testing format in the one-week, one-month, or one-year timeframe versions; (4) the screening function readily identifies the areas in need of more intensive comprehensive assessment; (5) the simple yes/no response format is appropriate

for persons of limited literacy and comprehension capacity; and (6) the use of easily understood percentage scores allows the DUSI-R to be accurately interpreted by paraprofessionals (e.g. drug/alcohol counselors, probation officers, etc.).

The DUSI-R is thus appropriate in practical settings where multivariate screening is required. Application of the DUSI-R is appropriate for (1) determining an intervention modality based on identified areas of disturbance, (2) monitoring change during the course of intervention, and (3) detection of youth with drug/alcohol and related problems (e.g., in school, juvenile court, primary medical settings, etc.). The rationale underlying development of the DUSI-R is that prognosis is maximized if the range of problems is delineated and quantified explicitly, thereby enabling implementation of specific and focused interventions.

From the standpoint of treatment, the DUSI-R enables ranking severity across 10 domains so that treatment resources can be prioritized. In effect, this results in the provision of treatment, with respect to consideration of both type and intensity that is commensurate with the magnitude of disturbances identified by the DUSI-R. This strategy of rationing and selective application of resources will in all likelihood become increasingly required in the emerging health service delivery environment.

Furthermore, the content areas of the 10 domains of the DUSI-R facilitates the coordination of health and social services available within a local community. For instance, individuals whose drug/alcohol involvement is comorbid to a psychiatric disorder would likely benefit most from a treatment facility where there is psychiatric expertise. On the other hand, treatment of individuals whose problematic involvement with drugs/alcohol emanates from family or school problems would accordingly benefit most from treatment at facilities which provide these types of specialized interventions. In effect, the 10 domains covered by the DUSI-R map to the range of services that are needed within a local community or by comprehensive organizations to provide multimodal intervention.

Finally, by tailoring treatment intervention to the specific problems (in contrast to the current accepted procedure of providing a standard program, where the same basic treatment is administered to all clients), the likelihood of relapse may be reduced. This individualized approach to treatment is fostered by an understanding of each person's unique configuration of problems. As previously noted, the DUSI was originally developed to uniquely characterize each person's problems within a 10-domain framework.

PREVENTION

Prevention of alcohol and drug use currently involves education, behavioral skill development (e.g., resistance skills), and the establishment of laws or policy to minimize exposure (e.g., regulation of advertising). To date, prevention practice has not extended to focused interventions in which the specific and unique liabilities of each individual are addressed. In effect, prevention practice does not currently encompass the crucial fact that everyone in the population is different. Thus, for prevention to be ultimately successful, individual differences must be recognized and addressed insofar as they contribute to risk for alcohol (and other drug) abuse.

As noted previously, temperament is the earliest expression of individual differences. Variation in temperament makeup, concomitant to interaction with the social environment, determines to large degree whether the person will experience a negative or positive developmental outcome. It follows, therefore, that interventions directed at modifying the quality of interpersonal interactions that take into consideration variation in temperament would be effective for prevention of alcohol abuse.

One innovative family-centered approach recently implemented by a major health care provider attempts to attenuate liability to an adverse outcome through temperament counseling (Kaiser-Permanente, 1994). Temperament counseling consists of psychoeducation in which parents and children are apprised of the reasons why children behave in certain ways. For example, a child that strongly manifests the temperament characteristics of rigidity, poor mood quality, and social withdrawal is prone to react to novel situations with negativism as well as oppositional or avoidant behavior. Having the parent and child appreciate the basis for these behavioral tendencies promotes acceptance that these response patterns are neither abnormal nor expressions of willful defiance. Awareness that temperament expression is

largely biologically determined and comprises the spectrum of normal variation provides the basis to modulate interpersonal interactions that are less conflictual. Temperament counseling provided to the parent and child may thus shape behavioral development to a more normative style of interpersonal interaction which, in turn, fosters bonding and effective communication.

TREATMENT

Controlled studies of treatment outcome of adolescent alcoholics have not been conducted. This is a significant issue inasmuch as substance abuse and associated problems, if not treated, are likely to sustain into adulthood (Benson, 1985; Bry & Krinsley, 1992; Keller et al., 1992). Several investigations have, however, identified a number of factors that appear to affect prognosis. Marshall and colleagues (1994) observed that getting high at a younger age and polydrug abuse were associated with poor prognosis. Parental alcoholism had no effect on duration of posttreatment sobriety or number of relapses, Myers and colleagues (1993) observed that a significant proportion of variance on a treatment outcome composite index was explained by coping style. Length of abstinence posttreatment and total days consuming alcohol were predicted by wishful thinking and social support.

Available evidence indicates that rate of relapse among adolescent alcoholics is approximately the same as for adults (Brown, 1993). This finding is somewhat surprising, considering that chronicity is much shorter in adolescents. It appears, therefore, that the greater range and severity of psychological and social problems manifest by adolescent alcoholics compared to adults (Brown, 1993; Kaminer, et al., 1991) offsets whatever advantage that may be afforded by shorter chronicity.

Preliminary evidence has been accrued indicating that amelioration of substance abuse problems is associated with improvement in other areas of psychosocial functioning (Brown et al., 1994). However, severity of behavior disturbance pretreatment correlates negatively with prognosis (Doyle et al., 1994). In an interesting study, Vik (1994) reported that severity of substance abuse predicts short-term treatment outcome but that long-term outcome is more contingent on the social environment and severity of risk contributing to the substance abuse.

Research on the factors contributing to relapse implicates social pressure as the most common factor (Brown et al, 1994). This is not surprising in view of findings demonstrating that peer pressure is reported by adolescents to be a cause of drinking. As noted previously in this chapter, by the time drinking is initiated, the adolescent has typically already established behavioral deviancy and affiliations with nonnormative peers.

SUMMARY

Clearly, systematic controlled studies are needed to clarify the factors that catalyze treatment seeking and treatment retention. Furthermore, the factors associated with good prognosis need to be delineated. In addition, investigations remain to be conducted that are aimed at devising innovative treatment methods that are tailored to the specific needs of the adolescent client rather than applying the same interventions to all clients as is currently the practice. Finally, it is important to recognize that adolescent alcoholism is manifest before biobehavioral maturation is completed. Consequently, treatment must encompass procedures to inculcate the behavioral, cognitive, and social skills that were not normally acquired as the result of habitual alcohol (and other drug) involvement. Thus, treatment should be directed at identifying disturbances that need to be ameliorated as well as developmental deficiencies that need to be overcome.

REFERENCES

Alexopoulos, G., Lieberman, K., & Francis, R. (1983). Platelet MAO activity in alcoholic patients and their first-degree relatives. *American Journal of Psychiatry, 140,* 1501–1504.

Allport, G. (1961). *Pattern and growth in personality.* New York: Holt, Reinhart and Winston.

Ammerman, R. (1991). The role of the child in physical abuse: A reappraisal. *Violence and Victims, 6,* 87–101.

Ammerman, R., Loeber, R., Kolko, D., & Blackson, T. (1994). Parental dissatisfaction with sons in substance abusing families: Relationship to child and parent dysfunction. *Journal of Child and Adolescent Substance Abuse, 3* (4), 23–37.

Anthenelli, R., Smith, T., Irwin, M., & Schuckit, M. (1994).

A comaprative study of criteria for subgrouping alcoholics: The primary/secondary diagnostic scheme versus variations of the type 1/type 2 criteria. *American Journal of Psychiatry, 151,* 1468–1474.

Babor, T., Hofmann, M., DeBoca, F., Hesselbrock, V., Meyer, R., Dolinsky, Z., & Rounsville, B. (1992). Types of alcoholics, 1. Evidence for an empirically derived typology based on indicators of vulnerability and severity. *Archives of General Psychiatry, 49,* 599–608.

Barron, A., & Earls, F. (1984). The relation of temperament and social factors to behavior problems in three-year-old children. *Journal of Child Psychology and Psychiatry, 25,* 23–33.

Begleiter, H., Porjesz, B., & Kissin, B. (1984). Event related brain potentials in children at risk for alcoholism. *Science, 255,* 1493–1496.

Benson, G., (1985). Course and outcome of drug abuse and medical and social condition in selected young drug abusers. *Acta Psychiatrica Scandinavica, 21,* 48–66.

Beschner, G., & Friedman, A, (1985). Treatment of adolescent drug use. *The International Journal of the Addictions, 20,* 971–993.

Blackson, T. (October 1994a). Temperament: Risk and resilience to psychosocial maladjustment. Paper presented at the International Occasional Temperament Conference, Berkeley, CA.

Blackson, T. (1994b). Temperament: A salient correlate of risk factors for alcohol and drug abuse. *Drug and Alcohol Dependence 36,* 205–214.

Blackson, T. (1995). Temperament and IQ mediate the effects of family history of substance abuse and family dysfunction on academic achievement. *Journal of Clinical Psychology, 51,* 113–122.

Blackson, T., & Tarter, R., (1994). Individual, family and peer affiliation factors predisposing to early age onset of alcohol and drug use. *Alcoholism: Clinical and Experimental Research, 18,* 813–821.

Blackson, T., Tarter, R., Loeber, R., Ammerman, R., & Windle, M. (1996b). The influence of paternal substance abuse and difficult temperament in fathers and sons on sons' disengagement from family to deviant peers. *Journal of Youth and Adolescence, 25,* 389–411.

Blackson, T., Tarter, R., Martin, C., & Moss, H. (1994a). Temperament induced father-son family dysfunction: Etiological implications for child behavior problems and substance abuse. *American Journal of Orthopsychiatry, 64,* 280–292.

Blackson, T., Tarter, R., Martin, C., & Moss, H. (1994b). Temperament mediates the effects of family history of substance abuse on externalizing and internalizing child behavior. *American Journal on Addictions, 3,* 58–66.

Blackson, T., Tarter, R., & Mezzich, A. (1996a). Interaction between childhood temperament and parental discipline practices on behavioral adjustment in preadolescent sons of substance abusing and normal fathers. *The American Journal of Drug and Alcohol Abuse, 22,* 335–348.

Braucht, G., Kirby, M., & Berry, G. (1978). Psychosocial correlates of empirical types of multiple drug abusers. *Journal of Consulting Psychology, 46,* 1463–1475.

Brook, J., Brook, D., Gordon, A., Whiteman, M., & Cohen, P. (1990). The psychosocial etiology of adolescent drug use: A family interactional approach. *Genetic, Social. and General Psychology Monographs 116* (Whole No. 2).

Brook, J., Lukoff, I., & Whiteman, M. (1980). Initiation into adolescent marijuana use. *Journal of Genetic Psychology, 137,* 133-142.

Brook, J., Whiteman, M., & Finch, S. (1993). Role of mutual attachment in drug use: A longitudinal study. *Journal of the American Academy of Child and Adolescent Psychiatry, 32,* 982–989.

Brown, S. (1993). Recovery patterns in adolescent substance abuse. In J. Baer, G. Marlatt, & R. McMahon (Eds.), *Addictive Behaviors Across the Life Span.* London: Sage.

Brown, S., Myers, M., Mott, M., & Vik, P. (1994). Correlates of success following treatment for adolescent substance-abuse. *Applied and Preventive Psychology, 3,* 61–73.

Bry, B., & Krinsley, K. (1992). Booster sessions and long-term effects of behavioral family therapy on adolescent substance use and school performance. *Journal of Behavior Therapy and Experimental Psychiatry, 23,* 182–189.

Burgess, A., Hartman, C., & McCormack, A. (1987). Abused to abuser: Antecedents of socially deviant behavior. *American Journal of Psychiatry, 144,* 1431–1436.

Buss, A., & Plomin, R. (1975). *A temperament theory of personality development.* New York: Wiley.

Chess, S., & Thomas, A. (1984). *Origins and evolution of behavior disorders from infancy to early adult life.* New York: Brunner/Mazel.

Cloninger, C. (1987). Neurogenetic adaptive mechanisms in alcoholics. *Science, 236,* 410–416.

Cloninger, C., Bohman, M. & Sigvardsson, S. (1981). Inheritance of alcohol abuse: Cross fostering analysis of adopted men. *Archives of General Psychiatry, 38,* 861–868.

Costello, J., Edelbrock, C., & Costello, A. (1984). *The validity of the NIMH Diagnostic Interview Schedule for Children: A comparison between pediatric and psychiatric referrals.* Unpublished manuscript, Department of Psychiatry, University of Pittsburgh Medical School, Pittsburgh, PA.

Dishion, T., Andrews, D., & Crosby, L. (1995). Antisocial boys and their friends in early adolescence: Relationship characteristics, quality, and interactional process. *Child Development, 66,* 139–151.

Doyle, H., Delaney, W., & Tobin, J. (1994). Follow-up study of young attenders at an alcohol unit. *Addiction, 89,* 183–189.

Fleming, J., Kellam, S., & Brown, C. (1982). Early predictors of age of first use of alcohol, marijuana, and cigarettes. *Drug and Alcohol Dependency, 9* (4), 285–303.

Friedman, A. S., Tomko, L. A., & Utada, A. (1991). Client and family characteristics that predict better family therapy outcome for adolescent drug abusers. *Family Dynamics of Addiction Quarterly, 1,* 77–93.

Giglio, J., & Kaufman, E, (1990). The relationship between child and adult psychopathology in children of alcoholics. *International Journal of the Addictions, 25,* 263–290.

Gillmore, M., Hawkins, D., Day, E., & Catalano, R. (1992). Friendship and deviance: New evidence on an old controversy. *Journal of Early Adolescence, 12* (1), 80–95.

Goodwin, D., Schusinger, F., Moller, N., Hermansen, L., Winoker, G., & Guze, S. (1974). Drinking problems in adopted and nonadopted sons of alcoholics. *Archives of General Psychiatry, 31,* 164–169.

Hawkins, J., Catalano, R., & Miller, J. (1992). Risk and protective factors for alcohol and other drug problems in adolescence and early adulthood: Implications for substance abuse prevention. *Psychological Bulletin, 112,* 64–105.

Johnston, L., O'Malley, P., & Bachman, J. (1994). *National survey results on drug use from the Monitoring the Future Study, 1975–1993.* U.S. Department of Health and Human Services, Public Health Service, National Institute of Health.

Johnson, V., & Pandina, R. (1991). Effects of the family environment on adolescent substance use, delinquency, and coping styles. *American Journal of Drug and Alcohol Abuse, 17,* 71–88.

Kaiser-Permanente. (1994). *Kaiser-Permanente temperament program.* Oakland, CA: Author.

Kaminer, Y., Tarter, R., & Bukstein, O. (1991). Teen Addiction Severity Index. Rationale and reliability. *International Journal of Addictions, 26,* 219–226.

Kandel, D. (1973). Adolescent marijuana use: Role of parents and peers. *Science, 181,* 1067–1070.

Kandel, D., & Andrews, K. (1987). Processes of adolescent socialization by parents and peers. *International Journal of the Addictions, 22,* 319–342.

Kaufman, E., & Kaufman, P. (1979). *Family therapy of drug and alcohol abuse.* New York: Gardner Press.

Kellam, S., Brown, H., Rubin, B., & Ensminger, M. (1991). Paths leading to teenage psychiatric symptoms and substance use: Developmental epidemiological studies at Woodlawn. In S. Guze, F. Earls, & J. Barrett (Eds.), *Child psychopathology and development.* New York: Raven Press.

Keller, M., Lavori, P., Beardslee, W., Wrender, J., & Hasin, D. (1992). Clinical course and outcome of substance abuse disorders in adolescents. *Journal of Substance Abuse Treatment, 9,* 1–14.

Kern, J., Hassett, C., Collipp, P., Bridges, C., Solomon, M.,

& Condren, R. (1981). Children of alcoholics: Locus of control, mental age, and zinc level. *Journal of Psychiatric Treatment and Evaluation, 3,* 169–173.

Kirisci, L., Hsu, T-C., & Tarter, R. (1994). Fitting a two parameter logistic item response model to clarify the Psychometric properties of the Drug Use Screening Inventory for adolescent alcohol and drug abusers. *Alcoholism: Clinical and Experimental Research. 18,* 1335–1341.

Kirisci, L., Mezzich, A., & Tarter, R. (1995). Norms and sensitivity of the adolescent version of the Drug Use Screening Inventory. *Addictive Behaviors, 20,* 149–157.

Kirisci, L., &,Tarter, R. (unpublished). *Psychometric characteristics of the Behavior Domain in the Drug Use Screening Inventory.* Department of Psychiatry, University of Pittsburgh Medical School, Pittsburgh, PA.

Lerner, I., & Vicary, J. (1984). Difficult temperament and drug use: Analysis from the New York Longitudinal study. *Journal of Drug Education, 14,* 1–8.

Loeber, R., & Dishion, T. (1983). Early predictors of male delinquency: A review. *Psychological Bulletin, 94,* 68–99.

Loeber, R., & Hay, D. (1995). Developmental approaches to aggression and conduct problems. In M. Rutter & D. Hay (Eds.), *Development through life: A handbook for clinicians* (pp. 488–516). Oxford, England: Blackwell Scientific Publications.

Loeber, R., Stouthamer-Loeber, M., Van Kammen, W., & Farrington, D. (1991). Initiation, escalation and desistance in juvenile offending and their correlates. *The Journal of Criminal Law & Criminology, 82,* 36–82.

Luthar, S. (1991). Vulnerability and resilience: A study of high risk adolescents. *Child Development, 62,* 600–616.

Luthar, S., & Ziegler, E. (1992). Intelligence and social competence among high-risk adolescents. *Development and Psychopathology, 4,* 287–299.

Marshall, M. J., Marshall, S., & Heer, M. J. (1994). Characteristics of abstinent substance abusers who first sought treatment in adolescence. *Journal of Drug Education, 24,* 151–162.

Martin, C., Kaczynski, N., Maisto, S., Bukstein, O., & Moss, H. (in press). Patterns of DSM-IV alcohol abuse and dependence symptoms in adolescent drinkers. *Journal of Studies on Alcohol.*

Martin, R. (1989). Activity level, distractibility, and persistence: Critical characteristics in early schooling. In G. Kohnstamm, J. Bates, & M. Rothbart (Eds.), *Temperament in childhood.* New York: John Wiley & Sons.

Masten, A., Best, K., & Garmezy, N. (1991). Resilience and development: Contributions from the study of children who overcame adversity. *Development and Psychopathology, 2,* 425–444.

Maziade, M., Caprara, P., LaPlante, B., Boudreault, M., Thiverge, J., Cote, R., & Boutin, P. (1985). Value of difficult temperament among 7-year olds in the general population for predicting psychiatric diagnosis at age 12. *American Journal of Psychiatry, 142,* 943–946.

Maziade, M., Caron, C., Cote, R., Merette, C., Bernier, H., Laplante, B., Boutin, P., & Thivierge, J. (1990). Psychiatric status of adolescents who had extreme temperaments at age 7. *American Journal of Psychiatry, 147,* 1531–1537.

Maziade, M., Cote, R., Thivierge, J., Boutin, P., & Berner, H. (1989). Significance of extreme temperament in infancy for clinical status in preschool years: Value of extreme temperament at 4–8 months for predicting diagnosis at 4.7 years. *British Journal of Psychiatry, 154,* 535–543.

Mazur, E., Wolchik, S., & Sandier, I. (1992). Negative cognitive errors and positive illusions for negative divorce events: Predictors of children's psychological adjustment. *Journal of Abnormal Child Psychology 20,* 523–542.

McHale, S., Crouter, A., McGuire, S., & Updegraff, K. (1995). Congruence between mothers' and fathers' differential treatment of siblings: Links with family relations and children's well-being. *Child Development, 66,* 116–128.

McClellan, A. T., Kushner, H., & Metzger, D., et al. (1992). The fifth edition of the Addiction Severity Index: Historical critique and normative data. *Journal of Substance Abuse Treatment, 9* (3), 199–213.

Mezzizh, A., Tarter, R., Kirisci, L., Clark, D., Bukstein, O., & Martin, C. (1993). Subtypes of early age onset alcoholism. *Alcoholism: Clinical and Experimental Research, 17,* 767–770.

Moffitt, T. (1993). Adolescent-limited and life-course-persistent antisocial behavior. *Psychological Review, 100,* 674–701.

Moffin, T., & Silva, P, (1988). IQ and delinquency: A direct test of the differential detection hypothesis. *Journal of Abnormal Psychology, 97,* 330–333.

Myers, M., & Brown, S. (1990a). Coping and appraisal in potential relapse situations among adolescent substance abusers following treatment. *Journal of Adolescent Chemical Dependency, 1,* 95–115.

Myers, M. G., Brown, S. A., & Mott. M. A. (1993). Coping as a predictor of adolescent substance abuse treatment outcome. *Journal of Substance Abuse, 5,* 15–29.

NIDA Notes. (1995). NIH Publication No. 95-3478. Rockville, MD: National Institute on Drug Abuse.

Orvaschel, H., Puig-Antich, J., Chambers, W., Fabrizi, M., & Johnson, R. (1982). Retrospective assessment of prepubertal major depression with the Kiddie-SADS-E. *Journal of the American Academy of Child Psychiatry, 2,* 392–397.

Penning, M., & Barnes, G. (1982). Adolescent marijuana use: A review. *International Journal of the Addictions, 17,* 749–791.

Reinherz, H., Ginconia, R., Lefkowitz, E., Pakiz, B., & Frost, A. (1993). Prevalence of psychiatric disorders in a community sample of older adolescents. *Journal of the American Academy of Child and Adolescent Psychiatry, 32,* 369–377.

Robins, L., & McEvoy, L. (1990). Conduct problems as predictors of substance abuse. In L. E. Robins & M. Rutter (Eds.), *Straight and devious pathways from childhood to adulthood.* Cambridge, England: Cambridge University Press.

Rutter, M. (1987). Psychosocial resilience and protective mechanisms. *American Journal of Orthopsychiatry, 57,* 316–331.

Schuckit, M., Klein, B., Twitchell, G., & Smith, T. (1994). Personality test scores as predictors of alcoholism, almost a decade later. *American Journal of Psychiatry, 151,* 1038–1042.

Schuckit, M., Parker, D., & Rossman, L. (1983). Ethanol-related prolactin responses and risk for alcoholism. *Biological Psychiatry, 18,* 1153–1159.

Schuckit, M., & Russel, J. (1983). Clinical importance of first drink in a group of young men. *American Journal of Psychiatry, 140,* 1221–1223.

Schuckit, M., Shaskan, F., Duby, J., Vega, R., & Moss, M. (1982). Platelet monoamine oxidase activity in relatives of alcoholics: Preliminary study with matched control subjects. *Archives in General Psychiatry, 39,* 137–140.

Schuckit, M., Zisook. S., & Mortola, J. (1985). Clinical implications of DSM-III diagnosis of alcohol abuse and alcohol dependence. *American Journal of Psychiatry, 142,* 1403–1408.

Shedler, J., & Block, J. (1990). Adolescent drug use and psychological health: A longitudinal inquiry. *American Psychologist, 45,* 612–630.

Tarter, R. (1992). Psychosocial history, minimal brain dysfunction and differential drinking patterns of male alcoholics. *Journal of Clinical Psychology, 38,* 867–873.

Tarter, R. (1990). Evaluation and treatment of Adolescent Substance Abuse: A decision tree method. *American Journal of Drug and Alcohol Abuse, 16,* 1–46.

Tarter, R. (1992). *Manual for the Revised Drug Use Screening Inventory.* Hartsville, SC: Gordian Group.

Tarter, R., Alterman, A., & Edwards, K. (1985). Vulnerability to alcoholism in men: A behavior genetic perspective. *Journal of Studies on Alcohol, 46,* 329–356.

Tarter, R., Blackson, T., Martin, C., Loeber, R., & Moss, H. (1993a). Characteristics and correlates of child discipline practices in substance abuse and normal families. *The American Journal on Addictions, 2,* 18–25.

Tarter, R., Blackson, T., Martin, C., Seilhamer, R., Loeber, R., & Pelham, W. (1993b). Mutual dissatisfaction between mother and son in substance abuse and normal families. *The American Journal on Addictions, 2,* 116–125.

Tarter, R., Hegedus, A., Goldstein, G., Shelly, C., & Alterman, A. (1984b). Adolescent sons of alcoholics: Neu-

ropsychological and personality characteristics. *Alcohol Clinical and Experimental Research, 8,* 216–222.

Tarter, R., Hegedus, A., Winsten, N., & Alterman, A. (1984a). Neuropsychological, personality and familial characteristics of physically abused juvenile delinquents. *Journal of the American Academy of Child Psychiatry, 23,* 668–674.

Tarter, R., Kabene, M., Escallier, E., Laird, S., & Jacobs, T. (1990). Temperament deviations and risk for alcoholism. *Alcoholism: Clinical and Experimental Research, 14,* 380–382.

Tarter, R., Kirisci, L., & Mezzich, A. (1996). The Drug Use Screening Inventory: School adjustment. *Measurement and Evaluation in Counselling and Development. 29,* 25–34.

Tarter, R., Laird, S., Kahene, M., Bukstein, O., & Kaminer, Y. (1990). Drug abuse severity in adolescents is associated with magnitude of deviation in temperament traits. *British Journal of Addictions, 85,* 1501–1504.

Tarter, R., & Mezzich, A. (1992). Ontogeny of substance abuse: Perspectives and findings. In M. Glantz and R. Pickens (Eds.), *Vulnerability to drug abuse.* Washington, DC: American Psychological Association.

Tarter, R., Mezzich, A., Kirisci, L., & Kaczynski, N. (1994). Reliability of the Drug Use Screening Inventory among adolescent alcoholics. *Journal of Child and Adolescent Substance Abuse, 3,* 25–36.

Tarter, R., Moss, H., & Vanyukov, M. (1995). Behavior genetic perspective of alcoholism etiology. In H. Begleiter & B. Kissin (Eds.), *Alcohol and alcoholism (Vol. 1) Genetic factors and alcoholism.* New York: Oxford University Press.

Tarter, R., & Vanyukov, M. (1994). Alcoholism: A developmental disorder. *Journal of Consulting and Clinical Psychology, 62,* 1096–1107.

Tubman, J., & Windle, M. (1995). Continuity of difficult temperament in adolescence: Relations with depression, life events, family support, and substance use across a one-year period. *Journal of Youth and Adolescence, 24,* 113–153.

Vik, P. (1994). *Adolescent substance abuse recovery: A path analysis.* Paper presented at the Annual Meeting of the American Psychological Association, Los Angeles, CA.

Vuchinich, S., Bank, L., & Patterson, G. (1992). Parenting, peers, and the stability of antisocial behavior in preadolescent boys. *Developmental Psychology, 28,* 510–521.

Wellner, Z., Reich, W., Herjanic, B., Jung, K., & Amado, K. (1987). Reliability, validity and parent-child agreement studies of the Diagnostic Interview for Children and Adolescents (DICA). *Journal of the American Academy of Child Psychiatry, 26,* 649–653.

Werner, E., & Smith, R. (1992). *Overcoming the odds: High-risk children from birth to adulthood.* Ithaca, NY: Cornell University Press.

Whitbeck, L., & Simons, R. (1990). Life on the streets: The victimization of runaway and homeless adolescents. *Youth and Society, 22,* 108–125.

White, J., Moffitt, T., & Silva, P. (1989). A prospective replication of the protective effects of IQ in subjects at high risk for juvenile delinquency. *Journal of Consulting and Clinical Psychology, 57,* 719–724.

Wills, T. (1990). Multiple networks and substance use. *Journal of Social and Clinical Psychology, 9,* 78–90.

Windle, M. (1991). The difficult temperament in adolescence: Associations with substance use, family support, and problem behaviors. *Journal of Clinical Psychology, 47,* 310–315.

Windle, M. (1992). Temperament and social support in adolescence: Interrelations with depressive symptoms and delinquent behaviors. *Journal of Youth and Adolescence, 21,* 1–21.

Winter, K. C., & Henly, G. A. (1988). *Personal Experience Inventory Test and manual.* Los Angeles, CA: Western Psychological Services.

Wolin, S., Bennett, L., & Noonan, L. (1979). Family rituals and the recurrence of alcoholism over generations. *American Journal of Psychiatry, 136,* 589–593.

Ziegler-Driscoll, G. (1979). The similarities in families of drug dependents and alcoholics. In E. Kaufman & P. Kaufman (Eds.), *Family therapy of drug and alcohol abuse.* New York: Gardner Press.

CHAPTER 14

A MODEL OF RISK FACTORS INVOLVED IN CHILDHOOD AND ADOLESCENT OBESITY

Carole J. Vogt, PSYCHOLOGIST

Childhood and adolescent obesity is a widely recognized problem. Obesity occurs when there is food intake that is consistently beyond energy expenditure (Epstein, 1985; Epstein & Wing, 1987). In general, the standard definition of *obesity* is weight that is 20 percent over ideal body weight based on age, height, and gender (Epstein & Wing, 1987).

For most children and adolescents, as they gain weight they also increase the amount of fat on their bodies. Accurate estimates of ideal body weight typically result from height to weight ratios. An exception may be a person who has an extraordinary amount of lean body mass, such as an adolescent who participates in sports. In such cases, it may be inaccurate to estimate ideal body weight by height to weight ratios (Epstein, 1985). When obesity is the accurate description of a person's weight status, either amount of food intake, energy expenditure, or both may be the cause.

The Health and Nutrition Examination Surveys (HANES) conducted by the National Center for Health Statistics estimated that over the past 20 years, the rate of obesity among 6- to 11-year-old children in the United States has increased by 54 percent, and among the 12- to 17-year-old age group, the obesity

rate has increased by 39 percent (cited by Kolata, 1986). One estimate of obesity in preschool children suggested that approximately 5 to 10 percent are obese (Maloney & Klykylo, 1983). Other reports estimate that between 15 to 25 percent of U.S. children are obese (Brownell & Stunkard, 1978). Clearly, obesity in childhood and adolescence is a considerable problem with many health-related and psychological consequences.

HEALTH RISK FACTORS

There is evidence of a variety of medical risk factors associated with childhood and adolescent obesity. Physical activity of obese children and adolescents and their family/parental relationships also have effects on health risk factors.

Medical Risk of Obesity

In addition to the risk of becoming heavy adults, medical complications of obesity in children include physiologic and behavioral factors (Epstein, 1985). Obese children and adults have many of the same medical risks (Berenson, 1980). Cardiovascular risk factors, including elevated blood pressure and blood lipid levels, correlate with obese weight status of children (Berenson, 1980). Cardiovascular risk factors "track over time," indicating that young children with high blood pressure or elevated lipids are likely to continue to have elevated levels into adulthood (Epstein, 1985). Not surprisingly, obese children have greater amounts of fat (adipose tissue) deposits on their bodies than do nonobese children; these fat deposits occur as a result of hyperplasia and cellular enlargement (Kannel, 1983).

Preadolescence may be the final opportunity for obese children to control their body composition before long-term effects of overloading the cardiorespiratory and musculoskeletal organs occur during adolescence and adulthood (Hills & Parker, 1988). Treatment of obesity by early adolescence may be critical because of increased risk of atherosclerosis and diabetes in addition to increased risk of hypertension (Hoerr, Nelson, & Essex-Sorlie, 1988). Hoerr and colleagues also noted that a high percentage of adolescent girls are dieting, and they have the "poorest diets qualitatively of any age and sex group."

Effect of Activity on Health Risk

Physical activity relates to health risk in children, but this relationship is not as strong for children as it is for adults (Montoye, 1985). Most children need encouragement to participate in the amount and intensity of active play necessary to receive health benefits from their exercise (Baranowski, Hooks, Tsong, Cieslik, & Nader, 1987). School-aged children are likely to have lower than normal blood pressure as a result of active physical exercise (Panico et al., 1987).

Family Coping and Health Risk

Health risk factors can change, as shown in five family-based studies of preadolescents (Epstein, 1985). Blood pressure change was one of the dependent measures in four studies, and serum lipids served as the dependent measures in two studies. Epstein noted that initial risk levels significantly related to the degree of blood pressure or lipid change following weight loss, increased exercise, and improvement in coping skills. With regard to coping skills, there seems to be a relationship between an avoidant coping style in mothers

and high blood pressure and obesity in their children. In addition, obese children with avoidant-coping mothers had higher blood pressure than obese children whose mothers did not use avoidant coping (Hanson, Klesges, Eck, Cigrang, & Carle, 1990).

Summary of Health Risk Factors

Two of the most common health risks that are stable over time in obese children and adults are elevated blood pressure and increased fat deposits on the body. Other noted health risks include diabetes, cardiovascular disease, and atherosclerosis. Health risk factors tend to extend from childhood into adulthood if left untreated. Adolescence may be a critical time for reducing health risks through weight loss. Children and adolescents who have increased their physical activity have found it was an effective means for decreasing health risks related to obesity. Obese families who have increased their coping skills have noted a decrease in blood pressure in their obese children.

UNDERSTANDING CHILDHOOD/ADOLESCENT OBESITY

Given the incidence and seriousness of childhood and adolescent obesity, understanding, preventing, and treating its development would improve the lives of innumerable youth and potentially save millions of dollars in related health care costs. There is sufficient evidence about the etiology of childhood/adolescent obesity to build an integrated model of how children/adolescents become obese. There is also sufficient evidence to suggest an adequate model of treatment for childhood and adolescent obesity using a behavioral family/parental treatment approach or a behavioral individual approach. Posttreatment maintenance of weight loss appears difficult, but has been successfully addressed in behaviorally based family treatment. However, there is not sufficient understanding based on present knowledge about weight loss maintenance concerning prevention of relapse. In addition, public health professionals have not consistently applied knowledge about child and adolescent obesity toward development of primary prevention of this problem.

ETIOLOGY OF CHILDHOOD/ ADOLESCENT OBESITY

As Figure 14.1 shows, there are multiple etiological factors that contribute to development of child and adolescent obesity (Brone & Fisher, 1988; Carey, Hegvik, & McDevitt, 1988; Klesges, Eck, Hanson, Haddock, & Klesges, 1990; Woolston, 1987). Genetic factors, environmental influences, and developmental changes in eating interact and contribute to childhood obesity (Birch, 1991; Epstein, 1985; Garn, LaVelle, & Pilkington, 1984). There is enough evidence available to construct an integrated model that explains how children and adolescents become obese. The model integrates the factors involved in development of childhood/adolescent obesity. Genetic factors that contribute to obesity demonstrate a family predisposition for obesity. Children from obese families are at

risk for becoming obese as genetic factors interact with environmental influences during the normal process of childhood development. Family eating habits and activity preferences as well as social "norms" influence the developmental process of why children eat for reasons other than "hunger only." Social eating in young children develops because families reward and encourage eating, and obese families may excessively reward and encourage eating behaviors.

In summary, genetic predisposition interacts with family and social environment factors as children mature from "hunger only" eating (depletion driven) to eating when they are hungry as well as eating for a variety of social and psychological reasons. Eating for reasons other than hunger, in addition to genetic predisposition, leads to the development of childhood and adolescent obesity.

Figure 14.1 Model of Risk Factors Involved in Child/Adolescent Obesity

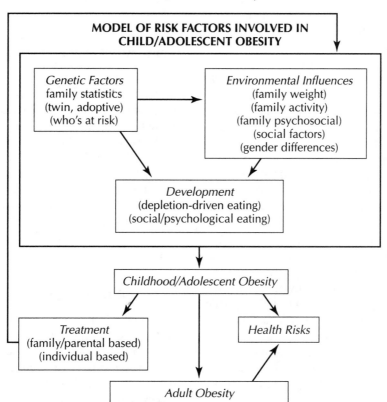

GENETIC FACTORS

One of the heterogeneous factors clearly involved in the onset of childhood obesity is a genetic predisposition (Epstein & Cluss, 1986). Hereditary factors may affect food preferences, calorie consumption, and metabolic rate as well as amount of energy expended (Epstein & Cluss, 1986). Stunkard and associates (1986) emphasized that the benefit of behavioral genetic studies are to determine who is at risk for becoming obese adults. Genetic factors that contribute to obesity in children and adolescents are evident in research on family statistics, twin studies, and adoptive studies.

Family and Adoptive Studies

Obesity tends to occur within families (Epstein & Cluss, 1986). Deutscher, Epstein, and Kjelsberg (1966) determined that 52 percent of the children of two obese parents were obese, whereas 23 percent of the children of one obese parent were obese and 10 percent of children with normal-weight parents were obese. In addition, obese children and adolescents are likely to have obese siblings (Garn, Bailey, Solomon, & Hopkins, 1981).

Both twin and adoption studies have suggested a genetic component to the development of childhood obesity. Epstein and Cluss (1986) found that monozygotic twin pairs have a greater concordance for obesity than do dizygotic pairs or nontwin pairs of siblings. Brook, Huntley, and Slack (1975) found that obesity (20 percent overweight for height and age) in twins over age 10 had a concordance of 0.91, whereas twins under age 10 had a concordance of 0.71. Feinleib and colleagues (1977) found obesity correlated at 0.71 in twins.

Another investigation found no concordance between adopted children and their adoptive parents but did find a concordance of 0.31 for obesity between biologic parents and their children living in the same family (Biron, Mongeau, & Bertrand, 1977). Genetic factors also influence the weight of adults (Stunkard, Foch, & Hrubec, 1986), In a study of 540 adult adoptees, there was a stronger weight relationship between adult adoptees and their biologic parents than between adult adoptees and their adoptive parents (Stunkard et al., 1986).

Evidence of How Risk May Lead to Obesity

There is evidence that genetic factors influence children's activity levels and energy expenditures as well as diet-induced thermogenesis and metabolic rates (Epstein & Cluss, 1986). Griffiths and Payne (1976) studied two groups of children with the same body weight: One group was thin children with thin parents; the second group was thin children who had heavy parents. They found evidence of diet-induced and exercise-induced thermogenesis, which is the body's ability to burn available energy more efficiently. The metabolic rate for the thin children with thin parents in this study was 181 greater calories per day than the rate of the thin children with heavy parents, who used 184 calories less per day. This implies that thin children of thin parents eat and burn more than their thin peers of obese parents. This raises the question whether thin low-risk children are more active or whether their metabolic rate is more efficient than higher risk children who weigh the same amount. Research has not provided an answer to this question thus far.

Summary of Genetic Factors

What researchers do know about genetic factors thus far is that children have a greater risk of becoming obese if their biologic parents or siblings in their family are obese than if obesity does not occur in their family. This effect is due, at least in part, to the role of genetic vulnerability. Specifically, obese parents and their children likely have lower metabolic rates than thin parents and thin children, though how this actually affects obesity is still an unanswered question. Children who have lower than normal metabolic rates are likely to become overweight when they eat for reasons other than hunger.

ENVIRONMENTAL FACTORS

Environmental influences on development of childhood and adolescent obesity are primarily apparent within families. Obese families are likely to involve themselves in sedentary activities, and they may have poor psychosocial adjustment. Evidence exists of social environmental influences that affect peer acceptance and self-concept in obese children and adolescents. In addition, cultural environmental influences are apparent in gender differences between obese girls and obese boys.

Family Environment

The family environment regarding food and activity plays a significant role in childhood and adolescent obesity. One of the familial factors that contributes to childhood and adolescent obesity is parental weight (Charney, Goodman, McBride, Lyon, & Pratt, 1976; Epstein, 1985; Garn & Clark, 1976). Metabolic rate, activity-related caloric expenditure, and caloric intake are all significantly different for children of lean parents versus children of obese parents (Griffiths & Payne, 1976). Parents may use sedentary activities or foods as rewards, which affect activity and food preferences (Birch, Marlin, & Rotter, 1984). Also, family environments tend to increase the family's exposure to certain types of exercise and foods that contribute to preferences (Birch & Marlin, 1982). Thus, children at risk for obesity may have a family environment that reinforces participation in sedentary activities such as watching television, and in overeating while watching television.

Preschool-age children with normal-weight parents are more active than children with one or two obese parents, and children with two obese parents are less active than children with one obese parent (Klesges et al., 1990). An unexpected finding from Klesges and associates' study was that children with normal-weight parents are not as active at high levels of active family interaction (activities that required active participation by parents and children together) as were children with either one or two obese parents. Possibly, children at higher risk for obesity are more sedentary than average when they are not urged by their parents to actively participate in family interactions.

Family Psychosocial Influences

It appears there are specific psychosocial factors that are characteristic in families with obese children and adolescents. Banis and associates (1988) found that families of obese children were similar to distressed families and significantly different from nondistressed families in several areas of family psychoso-

cial functioning. Families of obese children and distressed families were more apt than nondistressed families to have a low opinion of themselves in the areas of competence and self-perception. Both family types reflected distressed family environments (i.e., a great deal of tension among family members) and experienced more than average behavior problems in their children.

Mothers of children with different chronic physical disorders (including childhood obesity) reported their children as having significantly more internalizing behavior problems and lower social competence than expected when compared to nonclinic children from the community (Wallander et al., 1989). Obese children did not differ significantly from other types of chronically ill children in the types of adjustment problems they developed. Results from this study suggest that children with chronic disorders are at risk for having psychosocial adjustment problems and that they are confronted with similar challenges regardless of which specific chronic disorder they have.

Social Influence

Obese adolescent females have more of an external locus of control and feel they have limited control over a variety of factors in their lives than do obese adult females (Mills, 1990). Obese adult females showed significantly higher internal locus of control than adolescent females undergoing weight reduction. Obese adults in this study who felt they had an internal locus of control were likely to seek help regarding their weight problem. An external locus of control may have an effect on development of obesity in childhood and adolescence. Such children and adolescents are more likely influenced by family and social pressure as it relates to eating and choice of activities.

Obese girls had more somatic complaints and obese boys had more social withdrawal when compared to a mental health clinic population of children (Israel & Shapiro, 1985). In another study (Banis et al., 1988), obese girls were similar to a mental health clinic population but different from a normal nonobese population in the areas of somatic complaints and social activities. Boys were similar in the areas of school performance, social competence, social withdrawal, obsessive-compulsive behavior, social activities, somatic complaints, and schizoid-anxious tendencies.

It appears there are differences in peer acceptance for obese children versus nonobese children. In comparison to normal-weight children, obese elementary-aged children feel more rejected and less liked by their peers (Strauss, Smith, Frame, Forehand, 1985). In addition, Strauss and colleagues found that obese children feel more depressed and have lower self-concepts than nonobese children. Parents communicate stereotypic attitudes of physical attractiveness to children as young as preschool age (Adams, Hicken, & Salehi, 1988). Parents asked to tell stories about either obese, disabled, or "normal" children to their own children portray obese children as having poor self-esteem and self-concept and receiving negative reactions from peers (Adams et al., 1988).

Gender Differences

There are gender differences in obese and nonobese families (Kinston, Miller, Loader, & Wolff, 1990), especially in the area of psychosocial functioning of the family. In families of obese girls, hostility and ambivalence were overt. Families of obese girls blamed the girl for her obesity but were not supportive of efforts to reduce her weight. There was criticism around weight, food, and meals. In families of obese boys, there was a less intense and more supportive, positive attitude toward the boys' obesity than toward the girls' obesity. The findings of this study support the view that obesity in girls relates to a conflicted role in families. Martin and associates (1968) found a relationship between adolescent girls' self-esteem and their weight, with self-esteem decreasing as the "obesity index" (weight divided by height squared) increased. For both boys and girls, being overweight relates to worries about weight, figure, and physique. Also, boys worry about their health (Wadden, Brown, Foster, & Linowitz, 1991).

Summary of Environmental Influences

It is apparent that families are an important influence in the development of childhood and adolescent obesity. Parental weight and life-style toward activity and food preference are crucial in determining children's subsequent attitudes toward activity and eating

habits. Families of obese children have a higher rate of low self-perception and higher distress levels in their families than in nonobese families. They also have more adjustment problems, behavior problems, and are less liked by their peers than are nonobese families.

Family environment and, to a lesser extent, social environment affect developmental processes that lead to dysfunctional eating and obesity. Obese families may reward with food, console with food, or use food to distract themselves from boredom. Families set their own standards and habits of eating. Obese families may eat for reasons other than hunger and children learn these reasons at a very young age.

DEVELOPMENTAL FACTORS

Childhood developmental changes are evident in how and why children eat. Infants begin life eating only when they are hungry. By preschool age, however, children eat for a variety of reasons other than hunger. Parental and family influence affect when and why children eat. It appears that as children develop, their reasons for eating become increasingly complex and socially influenced.

Developmental Data

Data regarding the course of obesity in children at different developmental stages is contradictory (Woolston, 1987). The most accepted view is that early-onset obesity (obesity that develops prior to adolescence) is a progressive and chronic condition (Woolston, 1987). Charney and colleagues (1976) reported that 36 percent of infants who weighed over the 90th percentile became overweight adults; this compared to 14 percent of normal-weight or less-than-normal-weight infants. In a related study, Poskitt (1980) found that out of a group of 203 children, 40 percent were obese or overweight as infants, but only 13.5 percent were overweight and 2.5 percent were obese at age 5. At present, it thus appears there is a correlation between infant obesity and later childhood and adolescent obesity.

Types of Obesity

Woolston (1987) made the distinction between two types of infantile obesity based on etiology: endogenous or organic obesity versus exogenous or nonorganic obesity. *Endogenous* obesity, although quite rare, is an important diagnosis for physicians to consider as a possible cause of infantile obesity. Some of the forms of endogenous obesity include Frohlich's Klinefelter's, Klein-Levin, Lawrence Mood Biedl, and Mauriac syndromes (Woolston, 1987). *Exogenous* forms of obesity are further subclassified into obesity caused by familial factors, psychogenic problems, excessive caloric intake, and mixed etiologies. One distinction between exogenous and endogenous obesity is that children with endogenous obesity are usually below the 25th percentile in height and have delayed bone age, and children with exogenous obesity are typically above the 50th percentile in height and do not have delayed bone age (Woolston, 1987).

Depletion-Driven Eating

As infants, almost all humans begin life receiving nourishment from the same food: milk. It appears that only infants and very young children are solely depletion driven in their approach to eating, that is, they eat only when they are hungry (Birch, 1991). A review of studies of depletion-driven eating provides evidence that young children respond to internal satiety cues by regulating how much and how often they eat (Birch, 1991). Six-week-old infants drink a larger amount of diluted formula than concentrated formula (Fomon, 1974).

Preschoolers who received a preload of high or low calorie food followed by an "ad-lib" exposure to additional food responded to energy density of the preload by eating less ad-lib food if preload was high and more ad-lib food if preload was low (Birch & Deysher, 1985). Children not only decreased the amount of ad-lib food they ate following an energy-dense preload, but in this condition, they also limited their ad-lib foods to "preferred" foods (Birch, McPhee, & Sullivan, 1989).

When preschool children received a choice of high-density versus low-density food, they learned to prefer the taste associated with the high-density version of the food (Birch, McPhee, Steinberg, & Sullivan, 1990). However, children also learned to modify the amount of food eaten over time in response to the food's density level (Birch, McPhee, Shoba, Steinberg, & Krehbiel, 1987). Therefore, children adjust the amount and density of food they eat in relation to

their internal satiety cues when they have the choice to do so.

Early Childhood Eating

In contrast to the depletion-driven eating of infants, early childhood eating is mostly contingent on environmental cues. Birch (1991) demonstrated conditioned initiation of eating in response to contextual cues in sated children. Children are affected by many internal and external cues available to them regarding food intake. Birch and colleagues (1987) conducted a study with an "internal cues" context and an "external cues" context. Internal cues included such situations as adults discussing their feelings about hunger and satiety; external cues included such situations as adults focusing children's attention on eating when a bell rang and on how much food remained on their plate or on earning stickers for eating. Both the internal and external feeding contexts simulated child-feeding practices.

Results indicated that only the internal cues group responded to energy density prior to learning and had evidence of conditioning. In other words, the internal control group of children were more responsive to their internal feedback regarding energy intake. The external cues group showed effects of reinforcement (i.e., they ate more high-density food in response to the contingency than the internal cues group), but there was no indication that they were responding to energy density as a gauge for intake. It appears from these data that children can learn whether to respond to internal feedback cues in regulating their food intake.

Childhood Socialized Eating

Because humans need food as energy to stay alive, children have repeated opportunities to develop food preferences and to learn when to eat (Birch, McPhee, Sullivan, & Johnson, 1989) and which foods to eat at particular times (Birch, Billman, & Richards, 1984). Children learn cues to control the "initiation, maintenance, and termination of eating" (Birch, 1991). Obviously, children are dependent on adults for food, and adult attitudes influence children's eating behaviors. Approaches used by adults to "convince" children to eat include bribery, trickery, and threats. Adult approaches toward child feeding generally backfire because children learn to dislike the food that their parents reward them for eating (Birch, Marlin, & Rotter, 1984).

Summary of Developmental Factors

Evidence suggests that as children develop, they begin to expand the variety of foods they include in their diet. Cultural norms influence food customs as do complex interactions of social factors and family beliefs about good health and nutrition (Birch, 1991). It seems at some point children lose touch with purely physiological cues for eating and instead focus on sociocultural feedback for how, when, and why to eat.

Results of developmental changes in eating have substantial implications for childhood and adolescent obesity. When children start eating for reasons other than hunger, they are essentially not paying attention to internal cues that inform them of how much to eat and when to stop eating. Children frequently receive reinforcements for attending to external cues, such as eating at certain times of the day rather when they are hungry, finishing food on their plate even when they are full, and earning high fat/high calorie "treats" for behavioral compliance. Children who have obese parents are especially at risk for losing touch with physiologic reasons for eating because their parents may model an "obese life-style" of sedentary activities and eating out of boredom or for pleasure, as opposed to eating to satisfy a physiological need.

Summary of Childhood/Adolescent Obesity Risk Model

As children develop, their reasons for eating change. They begin life eating only when they are hungry and stopping when they are sated. Children become socialized to pay attention to external cues regarding when, where, and why to eat instead of paying attention to internal hunger cues. By the time they are preschool-age, they learn that food is able to satisfy many social and psychological needs, such as a sense of belonging, boredom, and loneliness. Nonobese families seem better able to modulate eating for reasons other than hunger, but obese families tend to model a lifestyle that is sedentary and adapted to overeating.

Genetic factors contribute to childhood obesity, as well. When children have obese parents or obese

siblings, they are at increased risk for obesity. Children with genetic risk for obesity are likely to have lower metabolisms than children who are not genetically at risk and may therefore be eating an excess number of calories from an early age. As children grow and become sociable, they are exposed to family, peer, and cultural influences regarding eating, and obesity may be the result.

There are no simple reasons why children become obese, but rather there is an interaction between genetic factors and environmental influences that lead to obesity. The cost (emotionally and physically) for obese children is high if they do not have effective prevention/intervention that teaches them how to modify their environment and reduce their risk of lifelong obesity. Obese children are at risk for becoming obese adults, with all the ensuing health problems associated with adult obesity. Given this model of how obesity in children and adolescents develops, the next issue to address is what to do about the problem of obesity after it has developed in children and adolescents.

REVIEW OF TREATMENT STUDIES

A review of recent literature indicated that researchers use two general approaches to study treatment of obesity in children and adolescents: interventions that involve parents and/or families and those that involve obese children alone. Parental and/or family treatment, studies have examined aspects of eating and exercise behaviors, adherence to treatment, and impact of child weight loss on other family members. Studies in which obese children and adolescents received treatment alone investigated obese children's choices of activities, an after-school behavior modification treatment program, and effects of an exercise program on obese boys.

PARENTAL AND FAMILY TREATMENT

Behavioral Studies of Family/Parental Treatment

A review of family-based treatment for childhood obesity indicates the relative effectiveness of behavioral treatment. Behavioral treatment addresses changing unhealthy behaviors and attitudes that maintain a person's obese life-style. For example, behavioral treatment for weight loss was more successful than a health education program for 5- to 8-year-old obese children and their families (Epstein et al., 1985). Children in the behavioral treatment lost approximately twice the amount of weight as children in the health education program. Subjects maintained effects of behaviorally based family treatment (Epstein, McCurley, Wing, & Valoski, 1990).

There was evidence that four targeted variables predicted a child's weight loss success: low-calorie snacks, weight graphing, eating less high-calorie/low-nutrient foods than children ate in the control group, and parent praise. Additionally, parents' percent weight loss related to their child's long-term outcome (Epstein et al., 1990). Five years following family-based treatment for obese children, children who had at least one obese parent were likely to be more obese than obese children who had normal-weight parents (Epstein & Wing, 1987). Success of family-based treatment is likely due in part to the influence parents have over what foods are available for children to eat.

Effect of Parental Training on Weight-Loss Treatment

Behavioral-based treatment that includes a parental training component has proven successful. In one study (Graves, Meyers, & Clark, 1988), three groups of parents participated in a behavioral weight loss program for childhood obesity. One group received training in problem solving in addition to the weight loss program. The other two groups in this study were given instruction only and behavioral intervention only. The problem-solving group of parents showed the greatest increase in problem-solving skills at the end of treatment, and at six-month follow-up, their children showed the greatest decrease in weight reduction (Graves et al., 1988). Children in both the problem-solving and the behavioral-intervention treatment group significantly decreased their intake of high-calorie/high-fat food. In addition, increase in healthy eating correlated with weight loss. Significant weight loss that was evident in children of problem-solving parents indicated the importance of learning strategies that help children maintain their weight in the face of problems that develop.

There was no significant difference after 8 weeks between a group given weight reduction plus two hours of parental training in general child management skills and a group given weight reduction with no additional parental training (Israel, Stolmaker, & Andrian, 1985). However, after one year, the group that received two hours of parental training in general child management skills had maintained their weight loss, whereas the group with no extra training did not maintain weight loss. In addition, parents with the extra training showed increased knowledge of social learning principles at both eight weeks and one year.

Effects of Parental "Role" in Family-Based Treatment

Another significant variable in family-based treatment of childhood obesity is whether parents have active involvement in weight loss along with their children or whether they are in more of a supportive role. There is a relationship between child weight loss and parental weight loss (Epstein, 1985). It appears that obese children whose parents participate in some way in their children's weight loss program are more likely to maintain weight loss than those whose parents do not participate. After 21 months posttreatment, children whose parents were working on their own weight loss weighed less than when they started and were less likely to remain obese than were parents who were not working on their own weight loss (Epstein, 1985).

Epstein offered two explanations: Parents may provide continued support for weight loss in their children depending on whether they themselves have long-term weight loss success and/or the children may have learned coping skills that enabled them to continue to support their own weight loss independent of their parents, support. In addition, Epstein reported that children of thin parents lost more weight over time than did children of heavy parents.

A "helper" role compared with a "weight-loss" role in parental participation in obesity treatment for 9- to 13-year-old children indicated that the helper role and the weight loss role were both effective in supporting weight loss during an initial phase of treatment (weeks 4 to 8) (Israel, Solotar, & Zimand, 1990). However, a helper role was slightly more effective during an extended phase of treatment (weeks 9 to 26), and there was no significant difference between the effects of roles at one-year follow-up. Results from this study suggest an alternative strategy by parents; in lieu of active weight loss, participation in their child's treatment may consist of taking the role of a helper. Either active or supportive participation by parents in their children's weight loss efforts demonstrates the importance of parental influence on long-term weight management.

INDIVIDUAL TREATMENT

Diet and Exercise Studies

In individual treatment studies of childhood and adolescent obesity, the two components that are consistently part of treatment include diet and exercise. A multidisciplinary after-school program for weight loss was effective in helping 12 obese adolescent girls lose an average of 3 percent of body weight at the conclusion of three-month twice-weekly classes and an average of 11 percent body weight at nine-month follow-up (Hoerr, Nelson, & Essex-Sorlie, 1988). Treatment components included aerobic dance, behavior modification of food and exercise habits, and food modeling activities for weight reduction. Subjects maintained lean tissue throughout their weight loss. Outcome data suggested that maintenance of lean tissue was a result of continued exercise.

A 16-week exercise and diet program for obese prepubertal subjects, who were in an experimental group or a control group, resulted in average weight loss amounts of 5.5 kilograms for experimental subjects who exercised at home in addition to weekly exercise at the clinic (Hills & Parker, 1988). Experimental subjects also showed a reduction in body fat in comparison with the control group. Although body fat decreased in experimental subjects, lean body mass did not decrease.

Obese children thus seem to improve their body composition through exercise and diet changes. Results of a study that examined exercise-induced energy expenditure in obese, dieting 5- to 8-year-old girls showed that exercise-induced energy expenditure increased as subjects increased their activity levels (Epstein, Woodall, Goreczny, Wing, & Robertson, 1984). Exercise and diet changes in childhood weight loss programs are clearly important components for increasing lean body mass while decreasing

body fat and increasing exercise-induced energy expenditure.

Exercise-Only Studies

Reinforcement is effective in persuading many obese children to increase exercise. Nonobese and moderately obese children will choose a vigorous activity when a sedentary activity is on a lower schedule of reinforcement, but very obese children will choose a sedentary activity regardless of the rate of reinforcement (Epstein, Smith, Vara, & Rodefer, 1991). Implications for obesity treatment are that a moderately obese child will respond to reinforcement for exercise, whereas very obese children will likely not respond until they decrease their weight to within a moderately obese category.

Adults are able to maneuver obese children toward activities that will help facilitate weight loss. For example, three obese and three nonobese 11-year-old boys treated behaviorally with an exercise program based on a variable rate of reinforcement with changing criteria increased the length of exercising to the maximum time of 30 minutes when they used a token economy as reinforcement (DeLuca & Holborn, 1992).

Summary of Treatment of Obesity

Individual behavioral treatment is effective when the focus is on diet and exercise or on exercise alone. Although diet and exercise or exercise-alone intervention methods are successful in helping children and adolescents achieve weight loss, a question that remains is whether these methods are effective in helping children and adolescents maintain their decreased weight following treatment.

MAINTENANCE OF WEIGHT LOSS

Children and adolescents who participated in family-based treatments were most successful in maintaining weight loss following treatment (Epstein & Wing, 1987; Graves, Meyers, Clark, 1988). Although some studies have shown effective weight loss maintenance of five years, the majority of studies highlight the difficulty of weight loss maintenance. Children maintained 13.6 percent weight reduction after five years when both parents and children focused on weight loss (Epstein, 1985). Similarities in weight loss between parent and child may be due to modeling, common instruction, and sharing the same environment.

Parent and child weight changes may be different over time due to changing support (parents support child weight loss but children do not support parent weight-loss) (Epstein, 1985). Obese children with one or two obese parents regained weight faster five years following behaviorally based treatment than obese children with nonobese parents (Epstein et al., 1987). This suggests that parent weight may affect long-term treatment outcome. There are several possible explanations: There may be individual differences in metabolic rate, calorie intake, and activity patterns; there may be differences in adherence over time; or both may interact. Obese children with obese parents may lose less weight than children of normal-weight parents and have difficulty with maintenance which would cause them to become discouraged with future weight loss attempts (Epstein et al., 1987).

Maintaining weight loss by children and adolescents requires that they practice the new skills and behaviors they learned while in treatment. As the model of risk factors for obesity describes, there is an interaction between environmental influences and genetic factors. This makes maintenance of changes in eating and exercising very difficult for children in families with obese parents when their environment at home is pulling them back into old eating/exercising habits.

Maintenance Summary

Behaviorally based treatments are most effective for maintenance of weight loss in obese children and adolescents when parents/families are involved in initial weight loss. There are several long-term (five-year) follow-up studies that indicate maintenance of weight loss is most likely to occur when both parents and children target weight loss maintenance as a goal and when they reinforce each other for weight loss maintenance.

CONCLUSION

Childhood and adolescent obesity is a serious problem for both the medical/health risk complications it causes and for the emotional/psychological toll it has on children and adolescents. Although researchers have identified several significant risk factors that place children and adolescents at risk for developing obesity, questions still remain about how the risk factors combine and interact resulting in obesity. There is still a great deal that researchers do not know about childhood and adolescent obesity. What is known about obesity has not previously been formulated into a comprehensive model for identifying children at risk, primary prevention of obesity, and/or early intervention treatment.

This chapter contains a model that addresses the major risk factors and influences involved in the development of obesity in children and adolescents. Children who have obese parents are at an increased risk for becoming obese. Genetic factors seem to affect metabolism and energy expenditure in obese families. Obese children are at an increased risk of developing health-related problems and may become obese adults. Family and other social environmental influences interact with genetic predisposition in childhood obesity. The third component of the risk model is the effect of developmental changes in eating (from depletion-driven eating to eating for a variety of social and psychological reasons) in combination with environment and genetic predisposition.

Some of the major findings from childhood and adolescent obesity research are in the area of family influence. Family involvement in treatment, whether in a supportive or active role, is effective in helping obese children lose weight in treatment. Parents who are especially effective are those committed to weight loss themselves. Effective treatments focus on diet and exercise change. However, life-style exercise is most effective in helping children maintain weight loss. Finally, there is a need for further research, and intervention efforts are needed in the area of primary prevention of obesity.

REFERENCES

Adams, G. R., Hicken, M., & Salehi, M. (1988). Socialization of the physical attractiveness stereotype: Parental expectations and verbal behaviors. *International Journal of Psychology, 23,* 137–149.

Banis, H. T., Varni, J. W., Korsch, B. M., Jay, S. M., Adler, R., Garcia, E. A., & Negrete, V. (1988). Psychological and social adjustment of obese children and their families. *Child: Care, Health and Development, 14,* 157–173.

Baranowski, T. B., Hooks, P., Tsong, Y., Cieslik, C., & Nader, P. R. (1987). Aerobic physical activity among third- to sixth-grade children. *Journal of Development and Behavioral Pediatrics, 8,* 203–206.

Berenson, G. S. (1980). *Cardiovascular risk factors in children: The early natural history of atherosclerosis and essential hypertension.* New York: Oxford University Press.

Birch, L. L. (1991). Obesity and eating disorders: A developmental perspective. *Bulletin of the Psychonomic Society, 29* (3), 265–272.

Birch, L. L., Billman, J., & Richards, S. (1984). Time of day influences food acceptability. *Appetite, 5,* 109–112.

Birch, L. L., & Deysher, M. (1985). Conditioned and unconditioned caloric compensation: Evidence for self-regulation of food intake by young children. *Learning & Motivation, 16,* 341–355.

Birch, L. L., & Marlin, D. W. (1982). I don't like it; I never tried it: Effects of exposure on two-year old children's food preference. *Appetite: Journal of Intake Research, 3,* 353–360.

Birch, L. L., Marlin, D. W., & Rotter, J. (1984). Eating as the "means" activity in a contingency: Effects on young children's food preference. *Child Development, 55,* 431–439.

Birch, L. L., McPhee, L., Shoba, B. C., Steinberg, L., & Krehbiel, R. (1987). "Clean up your plate": Effects of child feeding practices on the conditioning of meal size. *Learning and Motivation, 18,* 301–317.

Birch, L. L., McPhee, L., Steinberg, L., & Sullivan, S. (1990). Conditioned flavor preferences in young children. *Physiology & Behavior, 47,* 501–505.

Birch, L. L., McPhee, L., & Sullivan, S. (1989). Children's food intake following drinks sweetened with sucrose or aspartame: Time course effects. *Physiology & Behavior, 45,* 387–396.

Birch, L. L., McPhee, L., Sullivan, S., & Johnson, S. (1989). Conditioned meal initiation in young children. *Appetite, 13,* 105–113.

Biron, P., Mongeau, J. G., & Bertrand, D. (1977). Familial resemblance of body weight and weight/height in 374 homes with adopted children. *Journal of Pediatrics, 91,* 555–558.

Bray, G. A. (1986). Effects of obesity on health and happiness. In K. D. Brownell & *J.* P. Foreyt (Eds.), *Handbook of eating disorders* (pp. 3–44). New York: Basic Books.

Brone, R. J., & Fisher, C. B. (1988). Determinants of adolescent obesity: A comparison with anorexia nervosa. *Adolescence, 23* (89), 155–169.

Brook, C., Huntley, A., & Slack, J. (1975). Influence of heredity and environment in determination of skinfold thickness in children. *British Medical Journal, 2,* 719–721.

Brownell, K. D., & Stunkard, A. J. (1978). Behavioral treatment of obesity in children. *American Journal of Disease of Children, 132,* 403–412.

Carey, W. B., Hegvik, R. L., & McDevitt, S. C. (1988). Temperamental factors associated with rapid weight gain and obesity in middle childhood. *Developmental and Behavioral Pediatrics, 9* (4), 194–198.

Charney, E., Goodman, H. C., McBride, M., Lyon, B., & Pratt, R. (1976). Childhood antecedents of adult obesity: Do chubby infants become obese adults? *New England Journal of Medicine, 295,* 6–9.

DeLuca, R. V., & Holborn, S. W. (1992). Effects of a variable-ratio reinforcement schedule with changing criteria on exercise in obese and non-obese boys. *Journal of Applied Behavior Analysis, 25,* 671–679.

Deutscher, S., Epstein, F., & Kjelsberq, M. (1966). Familial aggregation of factors associated with coronary heart disease. *Circulation, 33,* 911–924.

Dietz, W. H. (1988). You are what you eat: What you eat is what you are. *Journal of Adolescent Health Care, 11* (1), 76–81.

Epstein, L. H. (1985). *Advances in developmental and behavioral pediatrics, Vol 6. Family-based treatment for preadolescent obesity* (pp. 1–39). Greenwich, CT: JAI Press.

Epstein, L. H., & Cluss, P. A. (1986). Behavioral genetics of childhood obesity. *Behavior Therapy, 17,* 324–334.

Epstein, L. H., McCurley, J., Wing, R. R., & Valoski, A. (1990). Five-year follow-up for family-based behavioral treatments for childhood obesity. *Journal of Consulting and Clinical Psychology, 58* (5), 661–664.

Epstein, L. H., Smith, J. A., Vara, L. S., & Rodefer, J. S. (1991). Behavioral economic analysis of activity choice in obese children. *Health Psychology, 10* (5), 311–316.

Epstein, L. H., Valoski, A., Wing, R. R., Perkins, K. A., Fernstrom, M., Marks, B., & McCurley, J. (1989). Perception of eating and exercise in children as a function of child and parent weight status. *Appetite, 12,* 105–118.

Epstein, L. H., & Wing, R. R. (1987). Behavioral treatment of childhood obesity. *Psychological Bulletin, 101,* 91–95.

Epstein, L. H., Wing, R. R., Valoski, A., & Penner, B. C. (1987). Stability of food preferences during weight control. *Behavior Modification, 11* (1), 87–101.

Epstein, L. H., Wing, R. R., Woodall, K., Penner, B. C., Kress, M. J., & Koeske, R. (1985). Effects of family-based behavioral treatment on obese 5-8 year old children. *Behavior Therapy, 16,* 205–212.

Epstein, L. H., Woodall, K., Goreczny, A. J., Wing, R. R., & Robertson, R. J. (1984). The modification of activity patterns and energy expenditure in obese young girls. *Behavior Therapy, 15,* 101–108.

Feinleib, M., Garrison, R. J., Fabsitz, R., Christian, J. C., Hrubec, Z., Borhani, N. O., Kannel, W. B., Rosenman,

R., Schwartz, J. T., & Wagner, J. O. (1977). The NHLBI twin study of cardiovascular disease risk factors: Methodology and summary of results. *American Journal of Epidemiology, 106,* 284–295.

Fomon, S. J. (1974). *Infant nutrition* (2nd ed.). Philadelphia: W. B. Saunders.

Garn, S. M., Bailey, S. M., Solomon, M. A., & Hopkins, P. J. (1981). Effects of remaining family members on fatness prediction. *American Journal of Clinical Nutrition, 34,* 148–153.

Garn, S. M., & Clark, D. C. (1976). Trends in fatness and the origins of obesity. *Pediatrics, 57,* 443–456.

Garn, S. M., LaVelle, M., & Pilkington, J. J. (1984). Obesity and living together. *Marriage and Family Review, 7* (1), 33–47.

Graves, T., Meyers, A. W., & Clark, L. (1988). An evaluation of parental problem-solving training in the behavioral treatment of childhood obesity. *Journal of Consulting and Clinical Psychology, 56* (2), 246–250.

Griffiths, M., & Payne, P. R. (1976). Energy expenditure in small children of obese and non-obese parents. *Nature, 260,* 696–700.

Hanson, C. L., Klesges, R. C., Eck, L. H., Cigrang, J. A., Carle, D. L. (1990). Family relations, coping styles, stress, and cardiovascular disease risk factors among children and their parents. *Family Systems Medicine, 8* (4), 387–399.

Hills, A. P., & Parker, A. W. (1988). Obesity management via diet and exercise intervention. *Child: Care, Health, and Development, 14,* 409–416.

Hoerr, S. L. M., Nelson, R. A., & Essex-Sorlie, D. (1988). Treatment and follow-up of obesity in adolescent girls. *Journal of Adolescent Health Care, 9,* 28–37.

Israel, A. C., & Shapiro, L. S. (1985). Behavior problems of obese children enrolling in a weight reduction program. *Journal, of Pediatric Psychology, 10,* 449–460.

Israel, A. C., Solotar, L. C., & Zimand, E. (1990). An investigation of two parental involvement roles in the treatment of obese children. *International Journal of Eating Disorders, 9* (5), 557–564.

Israel, A. C., Stolmaker, L., & Andrian, C. A. (1985). The effects of training parents in general child management skills on a behavioral weight loss program for children. *Behavior Therapy, 16,* 169–180.

Javernick, E. (1988). Johnny's not jumping: Can we help obese children? *Young Children, 43* (2), 18–23.

Kannel, W. B. (1983). In E. A. De Felice & P. Kuo (Eds.), *Health and obesity.* New York: Raven Press.

Kinston, W., Miller, L., Loader, P., & Wolff, O. (1990). Revealing sex differences in childhood obesity by using a family systems approach. *Family Systems Medicine, 8* (4), 371–386.

Klesges, R. C., Eck, L. H., Hanson, C. L., Haddock, C. K., & Klesges, L. M. (1990). Effects of obesity, social interactions, and physical environment on physical activity in preschoolers. *Health Psychology, 9* (4), 435–449.

Kolata, G. (1986, April). Obese children: A growing problem. *Science,* 21–22.

Maloney, M. J., & Klykylo, W. M. (1983). An overview of anorexia nervosa, bulimia, and obesity in children and adolescents. *Journal, of American Academy of Child Psychiatry, 22,* 99–107.

Martin, S., Housley, K., McCoy, H., Greenhouse, P., Stigger, F., Kenney, M., Shoffner, S., Fu, V., Korlund, M., Ercanli-Huffman, F. G., Carter, E., Chopin, L., Hegsted, M., Clark A. J., Disney, G., Moak, S., Wakefield, T., & Stallings, S. (1988). Self-esteem of adolescent girls as related to weight. *Perceptual and Motor Skills, 67,* 879–884.

Mills, J. K. (1990). Differences in locus of control between obese adult and adolescent females undergoing weight reduction. *The Journal of Psychology, 125* (2), 195–197.

Mogan, J. (1986). Prevention of childhood obesity. *Issues in Comprehensive Pediatric Nursing, 9* (1), 33–38.

Montoye, H. J. (1985). Risk indicators for cardiovascular disease in relation to physical activity in youth. In R. A. Binkhorst, H. C. Kemper, & W. A. Saris (Eds.), *Children and exercise* (Vol. 11, pp. 3–25). Champaign, IL: Human Kinetics.

Morrill, C. M., Leach, J. N., Radebaugh, M. R, & Shreeve, W. C. (1991). Adolescent obesity: Rethinking traditional approaches. *School Counselor, 38* (5), 347–351.

Panico, S., Celentano, E., Krogh, V., Jossa, F., Farinaro, E., Trevisan, M., & Mancini, M. (1987). Physical activity and its relationship to blood pressure in school children. *Journal of Chronic Disease, 40,* 925–930.

Piscano, J. C., Lichter, H., Ritter, J., & Siegal, A. P. (1978). An attempt at prevention of obesity in infancy. *Pediatrics, 61,* 360–364.

Poskitt, E. M. E. (1980). Obese from infancy: A reevaluation. *Topics in Paediatrics, 2,* 81–89.

Price, J. H., Desmond, S. M., Ruppert, E. S., & Stelzer, C. M. (1989). Pediatricians, perceptions and practices regarding childhood obesity. *American Journal of Preventive Medicine, 5* (2), 95–103.

Strauss, C. C., Smith, K., Frame, C., & Forehand R. (1985). Personal and interpersonal characteristics associated with childhood obesity. *Journal of Pediatric Psychology, 10,* 337–343.

Stunkard, A. J., Foch, T. T., & Hrubec, Z. (1986). A twin study of human obesity. *Journal of the American Medical Association, 256,* 51–54.

Stunkard, A. J., Sorenson, T. I. A., Hanis, C., Teasdale, T. W., Chakraborty, R., Schull, W. J., & Schulsinger, F. (1986). An adoption study of human obesity. *New England Journal of Medicine, 314,* 193–198.

Wadden, T. A., Brown, G., Foster, G. D., & Linowitz, J. R. (1991). Salience of weight-related worries in adolescent males and females. *International Journal of Eating Disorders, 10* (4), 407–414.

Wallander, J. L., Varni, J. W., Babani, L., Banis, H. T., & Wilcox, K. T. (1988). Children with chronic physical disorders: Maternal reports of their psychological adjustment. *Journal of Pediatric Psychology, 13* (2), 197–212.

Woolston, J. L. (1987). Obesity in infancy and early childhood. *Journal of the American Academy of Child and Adolescent Psychiatry, 26* (2), 123–126.

PART IV

HEALTH PROMOTION

A key component of health psychology is the promotion of health through changing life-style patterns to increase health-promoting behaviors and decrease health-endangering behaviors. This may be one of the most important medical challenges as we enter the twenty first century. The reason for this is that the primary killers in the United States and other similar countries involve a large life-style component. One finding that is common among the health promotion literature is that changing and maintaining health-promoting behaviors is a difficult task. Although short-term treatments generally meet with some success, long-term adherence to changes has proven to be evasive. Clients often revert to their previously learned habits, behaviors they overlearned as children and for which treatments have only minimally reduced long-term habit strength. In addition, the literature is scant as to whether a change in life-style factors affects risk for development of disease. This is especially true for the area of childhood health promotion. Nonetheless, there have been some advances, and the area of health promotion remains a critical area for future study.

The five chapters in this section all address positive, health-enhancing behaviors. The first three chapters relate to traditional health-promotion activities (e.g., cardiovascular health promotion, nutrition, and exercise). The last two chapters focus on areas that do not relate to development of life-threatening disorders but promote health directly through adherence to proper dental regimen and learning techniques to successfully endure a surgery with minimal postsurgical complications.

CHAPTER 15

CARDIOVASCULAR HEALTH PROMOTION

Gregory A. Harshfield, UNIVERSITY OF TENNESSEE MEDICAL SCIENCES CENTER
Phyllis A. Richey, UNIVERSITY OF TENNESSEE MEDICAL SCIENCES CENTER
Gregory L. Austin, UNIVERSITY OF TENNESSEE MEDICAL SCIENCES CENTER
Frances Tylavsky, UNIVERSITY OF TENNESSEE MEDICAL SCIENCES CENTER

This chapter is divided into four sections. The first section provides a brief review of the structure and function of the cardiovascular system. This review is intended to present basic information on the cardiovascular system that will be helpful in reading this chapter. A physiology textbook should be consulted for more detailed information. The second section reviews the prevalence and consequences of cardiovascular disease (CVD) and demonstrates the magnitude of the problem and the need for preventive strategies. The third section discusses risk factors for CVD that are not modifiable or controllable by changes in lifestyle or treatment, including age, sex, race, and heredity. The fourth section discusses risk factors for CVD that are modifiable or controllable by changes in lifestyle or treatment. Many of these risk factors are the result of behavioral patterns established in childhood and adolescence. These include smoking, high blood pressure, poor diet, and low physical fitness. Recommendations will be provided for each of these risk factors.

STRUCTURE AND FUNCTION OF THE CARDIOVASCULAR SYSTEM

The cardiovascular system is composed of the heart, the pulmonary circulation, and the systemic circulation. The function of the cardiovascular system is to provide the cells with nutrients and oxygen and to remove waste by-products. Blood is pumped through the pulmonary circulation to become oxygenated in the lungs and then returned to the heart. It is then delivered to the remaining organs and tissues via the systemic circulation. The systemic circulation is a high pressure system that forces blood from larger arteries to increasingly smaller arteries, and finally into the arterioles, the smallest arteries. From there the blood is forced into the capillaries, where the exchange of oxygen and nutrients occurs. Blood returns to the heart via the venules, which collect the blood from the capillaries into a series of increasingly larger veins. Cardiac output is the amount of blood pumped from the left ventricle into the systemic circulation per minute. This is often indexed by body size, which is referred to as cardiac index. The resistance to the ejection of blood into the circulation is called the total peripheral resistance.

At any one time, the vast majority of the blood is contained in the venous system, with 39 percent in the large veins and 25 percent in the small veins. Only 8 percent of the blood is in the large arteries, 5 percent is in the smaller arteries, 2 percent is in the arterioles, 5 percent is in the capillaries, and 7 percent is in the heart. The remaining 9 percent of the blood is in the pulmonary circulation.

PREVALENCE AND CONSEQUENCES OF CARDIOVASCULAR DISEASE

The information provided in the next three sections was obtained from a variety of sources. These include data for 1985 from the National Center for Health Statistics, U.S. Public Health Service, DHHS; data for 1976–1980 from the National Health and Nutrition examination Survey II; data complied and presented in 1988 by the American Heart Association; data from the Framingham Heart Study (Kannel, 1983; Stokes, Kannel, Wolf, D'Agostino, & Cupples, 1989); and data from individual research studies. The Framingham Heart Study was a unique study that in all likelihood will never be duplicated. A total of 5,070 men and women between the ages of 35 and 64 years from the small town of Framingham, Massachusetts, comprised the original cohort of subjects. They were free of CVD when first examined between 1948 and 1952 and were followed for 30 or more years. Subsequently, many of these individuals developed various forms of CVD and suffered various morbid events. Much of what researchers know of the epidemiology of CVD is due to the efforts of the investigators from Framingham and the people who participated in this monumental study.

Prevalence

According to a report from the American Heart Association (1988), an estimated 65 million Americans (i.e., approximately one in four Americans) had one or more forms of CVD in 1988. The term *CVD* en-

compasses several different diseases and disorders resulting from inadequate regulation of the cardiovascular system. A selected list of these with definitions are presented in Figure 15.1.

Essential hypertension (i.e. hypertension with no known etiology) is the most prevalent form of CVD, afflicting approximately 58 million Americans. Coronary heart disease is the second most prevalent form, afflicting approximately 5 million Americans. Other major forms of CVD include rheumatic heart disease (afflicting approximately 2.1 million Americans), angina pectoris (afflicting 2.4 million), and atherosclerosis (American Heart Association, 1988).

Consequences

Cardiovascular disease (see Figure 15.2) is unquestionably the leading cause of death in the United

Figure 15.1 Definition of Selected Cardiovascular Disorders

Hypertension   High blood pressure

Coronary heart disease   Disease of vessels to the heart

Rheumatic heart disease   Heart valves damaged by rheumatic fever

Angina pectoris   Chest pain

Atherosclerosis   Thickening of the arteries

Vasculitis   Inflammation of the blood vessels

Congestive heart failure   Condition in which the output of the heart does not meet the demands of the body

Peripheral vascular disease   Narrowing of the vessels to the leg

Intermittent claudication   Intermittent blockage of the leg arteries

Arrhythmias   Irregular heart beats

Transient ischemic attacks   Temporary blockage of the blood to the brain

Left ventricular hypertrophy   Enlarged left ventricle

Figure 15.2 Definition and Consequences of Cardiovascular Disease

Myocardial infarction   Heart attack

Cerebral thrombosis and cerebral embolism   Stroke caused by blood clot

Cerebral hemorrhage and subarachnoid hemorrhage   Stroke caused by ruptured blood vessel

End-stage renal disease   Kidney failure

States and many other countries. According to the National Center for Health Statistics, CVD was responsible for an estimated 1 million deaths in 1985 alone. That was almost as many as all other causes *combined*, including cancer, accidents, and lung disease. To view this from another perspective, heart disease was responsible for 1 death approximately every 32 seconds. That is about 350,000 more deaths than in the Korean War, Vietnam, World War I, and World War II combined. Heart attacks accounted for the largest percentage of the deaths (54.6 percent), followed by strokes (15.4 percent), hypertensive disease (3.1 percent), and heart disease from rheumatic fever (0.6 percent). Other CVD combined accounted for the remaining 26.3 percent.

CVD takes a toll from an economic perspective, also. The estimated expenditure for 1988 from all forms of CVD was $83.7 billion (American Heart Association, 1988). The vast majority of these costs was due to hospital and nursing home services. The remaining costs (in order) were due to lost work output, physician and nursing services, and a small amount to medications. Coronary heart disease accounted for the largest percentage of the expenditure ($36.8 billion), followed by stroke ($12.9 billion), hypertension ($11.3 billion), and all other CVD ($22.7 billion).

NONMODIFIABLE RISK FACTORS FOR CARDIOVASCULAR DISEASE

Age and Sex

Age and sex are risk factors for CVD that are not modifiable. Estimates from the National Center for Health Statistics for 1985 demonstrated a progressive increase in the prevalence of coronary heart disease from approximately 114 million men between the ages of 25 and 34 years to 1.03 billion men between the ages of 55 and 64 years, and then declining thereafter. The pattern in women is similar, but at a lower level. The prevalence of coronary heart disease in 1985 in women between the ages of 25 to 34 was approximately 35 million, reaching a peak between ages 65 to 74 years and then declining thereafter. Similar trends have been demonstrated for other forms of cardiovascular disease and consequences, including hypertension, atherosclerosis, heart attacks, and strokes.

Race

African Americans have a greater prevalence of many forms of CVD, as shown in Figure 15.3. More importantly, the consequences of CVD are greater for African Americans than for whites. Data from 1979 to 1981 (U.S. Department of Health and Human Services, 1986) showed the average annual death rate from heart disease was 319.4 per 100,00 for African American males compared to 274.4 per 100,000 for white males. African American females had an average annual death rate from heart disease of 194.4 per 100,000 compared to 131.0 per 100,000 for white females during this same period.

Similar results were observed for strokes. The average annual death rate was 76.0 per 100,000 for African Americans compared to 41.2 per 100,000 for white males. For females, the rate was 60.2 per 100,000 for African Americans compared to 34.7 per 100,000 for whites. Furthermore, African Americans compared to whites have 3 to 5 times greater incidence of heart failure and 10 to 18 times greater incidence of kidney failure. Therefore, it is very important for African Americans to establish good cardiovascular health habits early in life.

Heredity

It is also important for children with a family history of CVD to establish good health habits. The heredity of different forms of CVD has been demonstrated, including hypertension, coronary heart disease, and atherosclerosis (Ward, 1990). The studies have employed a variety of techniques to demonstrate a genetic component to the disease (Figure 15.4). In each case, a significant genetic component was observed.

Figure 15.3 Cardiovascular Diseases with Greater Prevalence among African Americans

- Hypertension (Saunders, 1991)
- Coronary heart disease (Curry, 1991)
- Left ventricular hypertrophy (Savage, 1991)
- Heart attack (U.S. Department of Health and Human Services, 1986)
- Stroke (U.S. Department of Health and Human Services, 1986)
- End-stage renal disease (U.S. Department of Health and Human Services, 1986)

Figure 15.4 Studies Demonstrating the Influence of Heredity on Cardiovascular Disease

- *Family History*   There is greater prevalence among individuals with a positive family history.
- *Twins*   Higher correlations are found among identical as compared to fraternal twins.
- *Adoption*   Parents have higher correlations with natural as compared to adopted children (Annest, Sing, Biron, & Mongeau, 1979).
- *Siblings*   Children of the same parents have higher correlations than children of different parents.

Source: Adapted from R. Ward, "Familial aggregation and genetic epidemiology of blood pressure" in J. H. Laragh and B. M. Brenner (Eds.), *Hypertension: Pathophysiology, diagnosis, and management* (New York: Raven Press, 1990).

MODIFIABLE RISK FACTORS FOR CARDIOVASCULAR

Smoking

For most people, the habit of smoking begins in adolescence. Smoking is one of the major risk factors for different forms of CVD and the consequences of CVD (see Figure 15.5). Peripheral vascular disease occurs almost exclusively in smokers, leading to amputation. Data from the Framingham study (Stokes et al., 1989) found that cigarette smoking was an independent risk factor for coronary heart disease, congestive heart failure, angina pectoris, and overall CVD and strokes in men aged 35 to 64 years. For women of the same age, smoking was an independent risk factor for coronary heart disease and overall CVD. The risk of a heart attack is double in smokers compared to nonsmokers. Also, a smoker has between two and four times the risk of dying from a heart attack in the first hour following the attack. This is the bad news. The good news is that the deleterious effects of smoking are reversible. The risk begins to decline rapidly as soon as the smoker quits, and is

similar to that of individuals who never smoked within 10 years. Smoking is the only risk factor for which this true.

Blood Pressure

As stated previously, high blood pressure, or hypertension, is one of the most prevalent forms of CVD. However, this statement is somewhat misleading because hypertension is not a *disease* in the classic sense of the word. Blood pressure is normally distributed, and there is not a fixed level of blood pressure at which a person can be said to be "hypertensive" and therefore need treatment. The deleterious effects of blood pressure are related to the level of blood pressure in both men and women. Because of the nature of this relationship, it has been necessary to define a level of blood pressure at which the beneficial effects of treatment outweigh the risk and side effects associated with taking medication to control the blood pressure. The most recent guidelines are presented in Figure 15.6.

A multitude of studies have demonstrated the significance of high blood pressure in the development of CVD and its consequences (Lew, 1990). Perhaps the most convincing data are from the Framingham Heart Study (Stokes et al., 1989). Systolic blood pressure was a significant risk factor for coronary heart disease, transient ischemic attacks, intermittent

Figure 15.6 Definition of Hypertension among Adults (U.S. Department of Health and Human Services Public Health Service National Institutes of Health, 1988)

Diastolic Blood Pressure (mm Hg)

< 85	Normal
85–89	High normal
90–104	Mild hypertension
105–114	Moderate hypertension
≥115	Severe hypertension

Systolic Blood Pressure (mm Hg) (when diastolic blood pressure is < 90 [mm Hg])

< 140	Normal
140–159	Borderline isolated systolic hypertension
≥ 160	Isolated systolic hypertension

Source: U.S. Department of Health and Human Services Public Health Service National Institutes of Health, *The 1988 report of the Joint National Committee on detection, evaluation, and treatment of high blood pressure* (NIH Publication No. 88-1088), 1988.

Figure 15.5 Cardiovascular Risk Factors and Consequences Associated with Smoking

- *Peripheral vascular disease*   Occurs almost exclusively in smokers
- *Coronary heart disease*   Greater prevalence among smokers
- *Congestive heart failure*   Greater prevalence among smokers
- *Heart attack*   Greater prevalence among smokers

claudication, angina pectoris, congestive heart failure, and overall CVD in both men and women. Furthermore, systolic blood pressure predicted morbid cardiovascular events, including both heart attacks and strokes (see Figure 15.7).

The prevalence of essential hypertension is low in children and adolescents. Most hypertension in this age group is the result of a known etiology, such as renal artery stenosis (narrowing of the artery that supplies the kidney). However, a greater recognition of the scope and significance of blood pressure in youths has occurred in the last two decades, with publications of the First and Second Task Force Reports on Blood Pressure Control in Children (National Heart, Lung, and Blood Institute, 1977, 1987). Furthermore, studies have demonstrated evidence of blood pressure-induced target organ changes in children prior to development of clinical hypertension, including left ventricular hypertrophy (Culpepper, Sodt, Meserli, Ruschaupt, & Aecilla, 1983; Schieken, Clarke, & Lauer, 1981) and early atherosclerosis (Newman et al., 1986).

Additional interest in the investigation of childhood blood pressure has been generated by tracking studies that have demonstrated that children generally maintain their level of blood pressure relative to their peers as they age into adolescence and adulthood (Gillman et al., 1991; Kuller et al., 1980; Munger, Prineas, & Gomez-Marin, 1988; Seorge, Williams, & Silva, 1990; Webber, Cresanta, Voors, & Berenson, 1983; Woynarowska, Mukherjee, Roche, & Siervogel, 1985). This suggests that children at the high end of the blood pressure distribution will become hypertensive as adults.

The decision to treat is more difficult in children and adolescents. It is unknown what impact a lifetime of medication may have on these individuals. Furthermore, guidelines for the definition of hypertension in children and adolescents have yet to be established. The Second Task Force has provided normative data for these individuals, with the suggestion that individuals greater than the 95th percentile (see Table 15.1) be watched carefully for the development of adult hypertension.

Diet

Salt Intake

Establishment of good eating habits with well-balanced meals in youth is perhaps the best method of insuring cardiovascular health in childhood and on into adulthood. This is particularly true for those at risk, including African Americans and individuals with a family history of CVD. Several dietary factors are known to play an important role in the development of CVD. The effects of many of these act through their influence on blood pressure. Excessive intake of salt is the best known of the dietary factors. The blood pressure of a significant percentage of the population changes with salt intake, a condition known as "salt sensitivity." Estimates of the prevalence of salt sensitivity among hypertensives range between 40 and 60 percent, which makes it the most prevalent form of

Figure 15.7 Cardiovascular Risk Factors and Consequences Associated with High Blood Pressure

- Coronary heart disease
- Transient ischemic attacks
- Intermittent claudication
- Angina pectoris
- Congestive heart failure
- Heart attack
- Stroke
- End-stage renal disease

Table 15.1 The 95th Percentile of Blood Pressure in Children and Adolescents (National Heart, Lung, and Blood Institute, 1987)

AGE	≥ 95TH PERCENTILE (mmHg)
7 days	Systolic blood pressure ≥ 96
8–30 days	Systolic blood pressure ≥ 104
≤ 2 years	Systolic blood pressure ≥ 112 Diastolic blood pressure ≥ 74
3–5 years	Systolic blood pressure ≥ 116 Diastolic blood pressure ≥ 76
6–9 years	Systolic blood pressure ≥ 122 Diastolic blood pressure ≥ 78
10–12 years	Systolic blood pressure ≥ 126 Diastolic blood pressure ≥ 82
13–15 years	Systolic blood pressure ≥ 136 Diastolic blood pressure ≥ 86
16–18 years	Systolic blood pressure ≥ 142 Diastolic blood pressure ≥ 92

Source: Reproduced by permission of *Pediatrics,* Vol. 79, pages 1–30, 1987.

hypertension (Campese, 1994; Hollenberg & Williams, 1989; Sullivan, 1991; Weinberger & Fineberg, 1991; Williams & Hollenberg, 1991).

Furthermore, the pioneering studies of Luft, Grim, Weinberger, and their colleagues demonstrated that salt sensitivity is common among the African American and older normotensive populations, individuals at high risk for the development of CVD. First, (Luft, Grim, Higgins, & Weinberger, 1977) reported that African Americans excreted significantly less salt over a 24-hour period following a two-liter saline load than white Americans, indicating they were unable to excrete a salt load as efficiently as whites. Second, they examined the responses to volume expansion produced by a 4-hour infusion of saline. African Americans and whites under age 40 had significantly less salt excretion at 10 and 24 hours following the infusion than whites under age 40 had. These subjects also had greater increases of blood pressure in response to the salt load.

Third (Luft et al., 1979), they compared responses to six different levels of dietary salt intake (one week each) ranging from 10 to 1,500 mEq/24 hours. African Americans and whites over age 40 had significant elevations in blood pressure at or above 800 mEq salt intake; Whites under age 40 did not have a significant elevation until 1,200 mEq. African Americans also had a high correlation between salt excretion and blood pressure ($r = 0.73$), while the correlation was lower ($r = 0.48$) for whites. Several other investigators have also demonstrated that salt intake is important in the control of blood pressure in both African Americans and whites, although in a higher percentage of African Americans than white persons. For example, studies by Sullivan and his colleagues in young adults (Sullivan, Prewitt, Ratts, Josephs, & Conner, 1987; Sullivan & Ratts, 1988; Sullivan et al., 1980) found that 27 percent of African American and 15 percent of white normotensives subjects, as well as 50 percent of African American and 24 percent of white borderline hypertensive subjects were salt sensitive.

Dustan and Kirk (1988) reported racial differences in blood pressure changes in response to three days each of salt loading and depletion. African Americans had greater changes than whites. In a study of 83 African Americans and 38 whites between the ages of 18 and 23, Falkner and colleagues (Falkner & Kushner, 1990) classified 37.3 percent of the African

Americans and 18.4 percent of the whites as salt sensitive. Recommended guidelines for daily salt intake in children and adolescents are provided in Table 15.2.

Potassium Intake

It is important for children to have an adequate intake of potassium. Studies have also demonstrated an effect of low potassium intake on CVD, primarily, although not exclusively, through its effects on blood pressure (Svetkey & Klotman, 1990). An examination of data from the first National Health and Nutrition Evaluation Survey (NHANES I)(McCarron, Morris, Henry, & Stanton, 1984) and the INTERSALT studies (Intersalt Study, 1986; Intersalt Research Group, 1988; Stamler, Rose, Stamler, Elliott, Dyer, & Marmot, 1989) all showed a negative relationship between potassium intake and blood pressure. Furthermore, a double-blind crossover trial by Khaw and colleagues (Khaw, 1982) showed that potassium supplementation (64 mEq/24 hours) reduced both systolic and diastolic blood pressure. Recommended guidelines for daily potassium intake in children and adolescents are provided in Table 15.2.

Calcium and Magnesium Intake

It is also important for children and adolescents to receive an adequate intake of calcium and magnesium. Several population studies have reported an inverse relationship between calcium intake and blood pressure. Among these are the Honolulu Heart Study of 6,558 Japanese American men aged 35 to 64 years (Reed, McGee, & Yano, 1982). In this study, the association between milk intake and both systolic and diastolic blood pressure was negative. A similar associ-

Table 15.2 Recommended Daily Intake of Salt and Potassium for Children and Adolescents

AGE	SALT (MG/DAY)	POTASSIUM (MG/DAY)
1	225	1,000
2–5	300	1,400
6–9	400	1,600
10–18	500	2,000

Source: Reprinted with permission. © American Society of Contemporary Medicine & Surgery. (Arlene Spark, EDD, RD, FACN. Children's Diet and Health Requirements: Preschool Age through Adolescence. *Comprehensive Therapy* 1992; 18 (10): 9–20).

ation was observed in the Rancho Bernado Study of 5,050 individuals in which milk intake was significantly higher among normotensive compared to hypertensive individuals (Ackley, Barrett-Conner, & Suarez, 1983), and the Netherlands study of 1,088 men (Kromhout, Bosschieter, & Coulander, 1985) in which blood pressure was negatively associated with milk intake. Furthermore, several studies have demonstrated a reduction in blood pressure with calcium supplementation (Harlan & Harlan, 1990).

Less is known about the relationship between magnesium intake and CVD. However, a retrospective study found that magnesium intake was lower among hypertensives relative to normotensives. Recommended guidelines for daily calcium and magnesium intake in children and adolescents are provided in Table 15.3.

Cholesterol Intake

Atherosclerosis begins in childhood. It is a condition characterized by irregularly distributed deposits in the intima (innermost) of large and medium-sized arteries. These deposits are associated with fibrosis (an abnormal formation of fibrous tissue as a reparative or reactive process) and calcification (the hardening of tissue as a result of precipitates or larger deposits of insoluble calcium salts). Cholesterol intake is an important determinant of atherosclerosis. Total serum cholesterol is comprised of high-density lipoprotein

cholesterol, low-density lipoprotein cholesterol, and very low-density lipoprotein cholesterol.

Several major studies demonstrated the significance of atherosclerosis for CVD and mortality from CVD. These are summarized in a 1990 joint statement of the American Heart Association and the National Heart, Lung, and Blood Institute (Gotto et al., 1990). They include the Foramina study, the Multiple Risk Factor Intervention Trial, the Coronary Primary Prevention Trial, the Slinky Heart Study, the Rancho Bernado Study, the Tecumseh Study, the Charleston Study, and the Gothenburg Study. In these studies, CVD and/or CVD mortality was either related to cholesterol intake or reduced with cholesterol reduction.

Evidence exists that atherosclerosis begins in childhood and continues into adulthood (National Cholesterol Education Program, 1992). The National Cholesterol Education Program has established guidelines for cholesterol levels to help physicians identify and treat hypertension in children and adolescents who may be at an increased risk for the development of CHD (see Table 15.4).

Physical Fitness

A landmark study of 16,000 alumni at Harvard Medical School by Paffenbarger and colleagues demonstrated the importance of physical fitness on cardiovascular health. The results demonstrated that habitual aerobic exercise over a period of nine or more months maintained cardiovascular health and consequently reduced CVD-related morbid events (Paffenbarger, Hyde, Wing, & Steinmetz, 1984). The study focused on two factors that explain the connection between habitual exercise and the reduced risk for CVD. These two factors are physical fitness and physiological fitness. *Physical fitness* is determined by an indi-

Table 15.3 Recommended Daily Intake of Calcium and Magnesium for Children and Adolescents

AGE	CALCIUM (MG/DAY)	MAGNESIUM (MG/DAY)
1–3	800	80
4–6	800	120
7–10	800	170
Boys		
11–14	1,200	270
15–18	1,200	400
Girls		
11–14	1,200	280
15–18	1,200	300

Source: Reprinted with permission. © American Society of Contemporary Medicine & Surgery. (Arlene Spark, EDD, RD, FACN. Children's Diet and Health Requirements: Preschool Age through Adolescence. *Comprehensive Therapy* 1992; 18 (10): 9–20.)

Table 15.4 Recommended Levels of Fat Intake for Children and Adolescents

CATEGORY	TOTAL CHOLESTEROL (MG/DL)	LOW-DENSITY CHOLESTEROL (MG/DL)
Acceptable	< 170	< 110
Borderline	170–199	110–129
High	≥ 200	≥ 130

Source: Reproduced by permission of *Pediatrics,* Vol. 89, pages 485, 1987.

vidual's cardiovascular endurance, muscular strength and endurance, flexibility, and body composition. *Physiological fitness* refers to the more specific biological systems of the body that relate to cardiovascular health. These include blood cholesterol, blood pressure, and glucose metabolism (Malina, 1988). As such, exercise contributes to reduction of risk associated with many of the risk factors described above.

Physical fitness of children and adolescents is primarily determined by physical activity habits. The American College of Sports Medicine (1988) issued a position statement on physical fitness programs for children that gives rationale for developing fitness programs and guidelines for their design: "It is the opinion of the American College of Sports Medicine that physical fitness programs for children and youth should be developed with the primary goal of encouraging the adoption of appropriate lifelong exercise behavior in order to develop and maintain sufficient physical fitness for adequate functional capacity and health enhancement."

When developing an exercise program for children and adolescents, it is extremely important that the appropriate duration, frequency, intensity, and type of exercise is prescribed to ensure that positive physical and physiological benefits result. It is also important to determine the goal of the exercise program. If the goal is to improve health status, the exercise program should emphasize increasing energy expenditure through regular exercise, placing minimal emphasis on intensity. This type of exercise program will improve both cardiovascular endurance and body composition.

On the other hand, if the goal of the exercise is to improve performance in a particular sport or event, as is often the case with adolescent athletes, greater emphasis should be placed on intensity and skill specific exercises. However, performance focused exercise programs for children and adolescents should be approached with caution, even if they seem commonplace. Specific precautions to exercise must be particularly emphasized when designing a performance focused exercise program. These precautions will be discussed in more detail later. Additionally, exercise guidelines provide boundaries in which an individual can exercise safely. The exercise guidelines of the American College of Sports Medicine (American College of Sports Medicine, 1991) for children and

adolescents to improve health status are provided in provided in Figure 15.8.

Muscular *strength* is a measure of the greatest force that can be produced by a group of muscles. Muscular *endurance* is the ability of a muscle to contract repeatedly. The American Academy of Pediatrics recommends that strength training programs for prepubescents be conducted by well-trained adults following strict guidelines as set forth by the American Academy of Pediatrics. Such training programs should emphasize a higher number of repetitions at low resistance with proper technique, muscle balance, and flexibility being stressed. For more information on developing strength training programs for children and adolescents, additional reference sources should be consulted (Zwiren, 1993).

Flexibility is an important component of overall physical fitness that is often overlooked. Flexibility exercises aid in the improvement and maintenance of range of motion in the joints and can help reduce the risk of lower back pain and associated complications which often develop in adulthood. Flexibility exercises should be performed at least three times a week, including before and after cardiovascular endurance and strength training exercise. Static stretches for all the major muscle groups should be sustained for 10 to 30 seconds with three to five repetitions (Zwiren, 1993).

Exercise Precautions

The safety of exercise should always be the first concern when a physical fitness program is designed for an adult or child. A greater concern for safety is needed when children are involved. Children and adolescents are anatomically, physiologically, and psychologi-

---

Figure 15.8 Exercise Guidelines for Children and Adolescents

Duration   Twenty to thirty minutes of vigorous exercise per day

Frequency   Three to five periods per week

Intensity   A level at which the exercise can be maintained for the entire prescribed duration

Type   Exercise that involves large muscle groups and requires moving the whole body mass (e.g., walking, jogging, swimming, cycling, cross-country skiing)

Source: Adapted from American College of Sports Medicine, *Guidelines for exercise testing and prescription, 4th ed.* (Philadelphia: Lea & Febiger, 1991).

cally immature. As such, special precautions must be instituted when designing their exercise programs, especially if the program is performance focused. Children are more prone to heat injury as well as hypothermia. Therefore, special precautions should be taken to ensure safe, moderate exercise, with proper fluid replacement in either extremely hot or cold environments. In addition, children and adolescents are more susceptible to overuse injuries, which can damage their growth plates. Excessive endurance exercise should be avoided and strength training programs should be approached with *extreme* caution. Finally, the quantity of exercise for children should increase gradually. The child must possess adequate muscular strength and flexibility for the exercise task being performed, proper body mechanics should always be stressed, and proper footwear should be worn (American College of Sports Medicine, 1991).

SUMMARY

CVD is the major health problem affecting the United States today. Many of the risk factors for CVD are the result of behavioral patterns established early in life, including smoking, blood pressure, diet, and physical fitness. Not smoking, controlling blood pressure, eating a well-balanced diet, and exercising can dramatically reduce the risk for the development of CVD and the associated consequences.

REFERENCES

Ackley, S., Barrett-Conner, E., & Suarez, L. (1983). Dairy products, calcium, and blood pressure. *American Journal of Clinical Nutrition, 38,* 457–461.

American College of Sports Medicine. (1988). Opinion statement on physical fitness in children and youth. *Medicine and Science in Sports and Exercise, 20,* 422–423.

American College of Sports Medicine. (1991). *Guidelines for exercise testing and prescription* (4th ed.). Philadelphia: Lea & Febiger.

American Heart Association, (1988). *1988 heart facts* (Issue No. 55–0351). Author.

Annest, J. L., Sing, C. F., Biron, P., & Mongeau, J. G. (1979). Familial aggregation of blood pressure and weight in adoptive families. II. Estimation of the relative contributions of genetic and common environmental factors to blood pressure correlations between family members. *American Journal of Epidemiology, 110,* 492–503.

Campese, V. M. (1994). Salt sensitivity in hypertension renal and cardiovascular implications. *Hypertension, 23,* 531–550.

Culpepper, W. S., Sodt, P. C., Meserli, F. H., Ruschaupt, D. G., & Aecilla, R. A. (1983). Cardiac status in juvenile borderline hypertension. *Annals of Internal Medicine, 98,* 1–7.

Curry, C. S. (1991). Coronary artery disease in African-Americans. *Circulation, 83,* 1474–1475.

Dustan, H. P., & Kirk, K. A. (1988). Relationship of sodium balance to arterial pressure in black hypertensive patients. *American Journal of the Medical Sciences, 31,* 378–383.

Falkner, B., & Kushner, H. (1990). Effect of chronic sodium loading on cardiovascular response in young blacks and whites. *Hypertension, 15,* 36–43.

Gillman, M. W., Rosner, B., Evans, D. A., Keough, M. E., Smith, L. A., Taylor, J. O., & Hennekens, C. H. (1991). Use of multiple visits to increase blood pressure tracking correlations in childhood. *Pediatrics, 87,* 708–711.

Gotto, A. M., LaRosa, J. C., Hunninghak, D., Grundy, S. M., Wilson, P. W., Clarkson, T. B., Hay, J. W., & Goodman, D. S. (1990). The cholesterol facts. A summary of the evidence relating dietary fats, serum cholesterol, and coronary heart disease. *Circulation, 81*(5).

Harlan, W. R., & Harlan, L. C. (1990). Blood pressure and calcium and magnesium intake. In J. H. Laragh & B. M. Brenner (Eds.), *Hypertension: Pathophysiology, diagnosis, and management* (pp. 229–240). New York: Raven Press.

Hollenberg, N. K., & Williams, G. H. (1989). Sodium-sensitive hypertension: Implications of pathogenesis for therapy. *American Journal of Hypertension, 2,* 809–815.

Intersalt Research Group. (1988). Intersalt: An international cooperative study on electrolytes and blood pressure. *British Journal of Medicine, 297,* 319–328.

Intersalt Study. (1986). An international co-operative study on the relation of blood pressure to electrolyte excretion in populations. I. Design and Methods. *Journal of Hypertension, 4,* 781–787.

Kannel, W. B. (1983). Prevalence and natural history of electrocardiographic left ventricular hypertrophy. *American Journal of Medicine, 75* (Suppl 3A), 4–11.

Khaw, K. T. (1982). Randomized double-blind cross-over trial of potassium on blood pressure in normal subjects. *The Lancet, 2,* 1127–1129.

Kromhout, D., Bosschieter, E. B., & Coulander, C. L. (1985). Potassium, calcium, and alcohol intake and blood pressure: the Zutphen Study. *American Journal of Clinical Nutrition, 41,* 1299–1304.

Kuller, L. H., Crook, M., Almes, M. J., Detre, K., Reese, G., & Rutan, G. (1980). Dormont high school (Pittsburgh, Pennsylvania) blood pressure study. *Hypertension, 2* (Suppl I), 1109–1116.

Lew, E. A. (1990). Hypertension and longevity. In J. H. Laragh & B. M. Brenner (Eds.), *Hypertension: Patho-physiology, diagnosis, and management* (pp. 175–202). New York: Raven Press.

Luft, F. C., Grim, C. E., Higgins, J. T., & Weinberger, M. H. (1977). Differences in response to sodium administration in normotensive white and black subjects. *Journal of Laboratory and Clinical Medicine, 90,* 555–562.

Luft, F. C., Rankin, L. I., Bloch, R., Weyman, A. E., Willis, L. R., Murray, R. H., Grim, C. E., & Weinberger, M. H. (1979). Cardiovascular and humoral responses to extremes of sodium intake in normal black and white men. *Circulation, 60,* 697–706.

Malina, R. M. (1988). Growth, exercise, fitness, and later outcomes. In C. Bouchard, R. J. Shephard, T. Stephens, J. R. Sutton, & B. D. McPhearson (Eds.), *Exercise, fitness, and health: A consensus of current knowledge* (pp. 637–654). Champaign: Human Kinetics.

McCarron, D. A., Morris, C. D., Henry, H. J., & Stanton, J. L. (1984). Blood pressure and nutrient intake in the United States. *Science, 224,* 1392–1398.

Munger, R. G., Prineas, R. J., & Gomez-Marin, O. (1988). Persistent elevation of blood pressure among children with a family history of hypertension: The Minneapolis children's blood pressure study. *Journal of Hypertension, 6,* 647–653.

National Cholesterol Education Program. (1992). Report of the export panel on population strategies for blood cholesterol reduction. *Pediatrics, 89* (3), 525–535.

National Heart, Lung, and Blood Institute (1977). Report of the Task Force on blood pressure control in children. *Pediatrics, 59* (No. 5 Suppl.), 797–820.

National Heart, Lung, and Blood Institute (1987). Report of the Second Task Force on blood pressure control in children—1987. *Pediatrics, 79*(1), 1–25.

Newman, W. P., Freedman, D. S., Voors, A. W., Gard, P. D., Srinivasan, S. R., Crewsanta, J. L., Williamson, G. D., Webber, L. S., & Berenson, G. S. (1986). Relation of serum lipoprotein levels and systolic blood pressure to early atherosclerosis: The Bogalusa Heart Study. *New England Journal of Medicine, 314,* 138–144.

Paffenbarger, R. S., Hyde, R. T., Wing, A. L., & Steinmetz, C. H. (1984). A natural history of athleticism and cardiovascular health. *Journal of the American Medical Association, 252* (4), 491–495.

Reed, D., McGee, D., & Yano, K. (1982). Biological and social correlates of blood pressure among Japanese men in Hawaii. *Hypertension, 4,* 406–414.

Saunders, E. (1991). Hypertension in African-Americans. *Circulation, 83,* 1465.

Savage, D. D. (1991). Hypertensive Heart Disease in African-Americans. *Circulation, 83,* 1472–1474.

Schieken, R. M., Clarke, W. R., & Lauer, R. M. (1981). Left ventricular hypertrophy in children with blood pressure in the upper quintile of the distribution: The Muscatine study. *Hypertension, 3,* 669–675.

Seorge, I. M. S., Williams, S. M., & Silva, P. A. (1990). Blood pressure level, trend, and variability in Dunedin children. *Circulation, 82,* 1675–1680.

Spark, A. (1992). Children's diet and health requirements: Preschool age through adolescence. *Comprehensive Therapy, 18,* 9.

Stamler, J., Rose, G., Stamler, R., Elliott, P., Dyer, A., & Marmot, M. (1989). INTERSALT study findings: Public health and medical care implications. *Hypertension, 14,* 570–577.

Stokes, J., Kannel, W. B., Wolf, P. A., D'Agostino, R. B., & Cupples, L. A. (1989). Blood pressure as a risk factor for cardiovascular disease. The Framingham Study-30 years of follow-up. *Hypertension, 13* (Suppl I), I13–I18.

Sullivan, J. M. (1991). Salt sensitivity: definition, conception, methodology, and long-term issues. *Hypertension, 17* (Suppl I), I61–I68.

Sullivan, J. M., Prewitt, R. L., Ratts, T. E., Josephs, J. A., & Conner, M. J. (1987). Hemodynamic characteristics of sodium-sensitive human subjects. *Hypertension, 9,* 398–406.

Sullivan, J. M., & Ratts, T. E. (1988). Sodium sensitivity in human subjects: Hemodynamic and hormonal correlates. *Hypertension, 11,* 717–723.

Sullivan, J. M., Ratts, T. E., Taylor, J. C., Kraus, D. H., Barton, B. R., Patrick, D. R., & Reed, S. W. (1980). Hemodynamic effects of dietary sodium in man: A preliminary report. *Hypertension, 2,* 506–514.

Svetkey, L. P., & Klotman, P. A. (1990). Blood pressure and potassium intake. In J. H. Laragh & B. M. Brenner (Eds.), *Hypertension: Pathophysiology, diagnosis, and management* (pp. 217–227). New York: Raven Press.

U.S. Department of Health and Human Services. (1986). Cardiovascular and Cerebrovascular Disease. *Report of the secretary's task force on black and minority health, IV* (Part 1). Author.

U.S. Department of Health and Human Services Public Health Service National Institutes of Health. (1988). *The 1988 Report of the Joint National Committee on detection, evaluation, and treatment of high blood pressure* (NIH Publication No. 88–1088). Author.

Ward, R. (1990). Familial aggregation and genetic epidemiology of blood pressure. In J. H. Laragh & B.M. Brenner (Eds.), *Hypertension: Pathophysiology, diagnosis, and management.* New York: Raven Press.

Webber, L. S., Cresanta, J. L., Voors, A. W., & Berenson, G. S. (1983). Tracking of cardiovascular disease risk factor variables in school-age children. *Journal of Chronic Diseases, 36,* 647–660.

Weinberger, M. H., & Fineberg, N. S. (1991). Sodium and volume sensitivity of blood pressure. Age and pressure change over time. *Hypertension, 18,* 67–71.

Williams, G. H., & Hollenberg, N. K. (1991). Non-modulating hypertension: A subset of sodium-sensitive hypertension. *Hypertension, 17* (Suppl I), I81–I85.

Woynarowska, B., Mukherjee, D., Roche, A. E., & Siervogel, R. M. (1985). Blood pressure changes during adolescence and subsequent adult blood pressure level.
Hypertension, 7, 695–701.

Zwiren, L. D. (1993). Exercise prescription for children. In
J. L. Durstine, A. C. King, P. L. Painter, J. L. Roitman,
L. D. Zwiren, & W. L. Kenney (Eds.), *Resource manual for guidelines for exercise testing and prescription*
(pp. 409–417). Philadelphia: Lea and Febiger.

CHAPTER 16

NUTRITION AND FOOD CHOICE BEHAVIOR AMONG CHILDREN AND ADOLESCENTS

Isobel R. Contento, TEACHERS COLLEGE, COLUMBIA UNIVERSITY
John L. Michela, UNIVERSITY OF WATERLOO

Studies of nutrition in childhood and adolescence may be divided into three broad categories: (1) descriptions of food intake and its consequences for child and adolescent health and development; (2) examinations of determinants of food intake, including studies that seek to apply theories developed for older populations; and (3) evaluations of interventions in communities and schools for improved nutrition.

This chapter contains a section corresponding to each of these categories. Coverage of studies in each area draws on the author's primary research and review of primary literature, plus other reviews that have appeared recently (Centers for Disease Control, 1995; Contento, Balch, Bronner, Lytle, Maloney, Olson, & Swadener, 1995). Because of space limitations, coverage is restricted to selected topics and populations. The topical coverage is intended to provide a broad perspective on current theoretical understanding of influences on food intake and on progress to date with intervention programs. Emphasis is on basic research that informs practice, and practice that illuminates understanding of basic processes in food choice. Related topics of obesity and eating disorders are not addressed, since these are covered in other

chapters in this book. Coverage of populations is limited to healthy young people in developed nations. That is, studies of nutritional needs or approaches connected with various medical conditions (e.g., cystic fibrosis) are not reviewed, nor are the many papers concerned with developing nations. The author's provide relatively extensive coverage of food intake in the following section because behavioral researchers—typical readers of this chapter—may not be fully aware of the immediacy of concerns for child and adolescent health and development that are connected with nutrition.

NUTRITIONAL STATUS AND EATING PATTERNS IN CHILDREN AND ADOLESCENTS

Healthy eating patterns during childhood and adolescence are important for optimal health and development. Childhood nutrition affects immediate health problems such as dental caries, iron deficiency anemia, obesity, hunger, cognitive performance, and behavior. Nutrition-related physiological processes and eating patterns begun in childhood and adolescence can also predispose individuals to chronic diseases in adulthood, such as coronary heart disease, stroke, osteoporosis, and some types of cancer and diabetes. In terms of eating practices, children are generally like adults. They are currently consuming too much fat and salt and too few fruits, vegetables, and whole grains.

Health and Development Risks Related to Food Intake

The Importance of Diet for Optimal Growth and Health

Dental caries is the most common diet-related disease in children, affecting about 50 percent of those ages 5 to 17 and about 84 percent of 17-year-olds (National Institute of Dental Research, 1989). Dental problems result in 50 million hours of lost school time each year (Gift, Reisine, & Larach, 1992). A diet high in sugar contributes to dental caries and gum disease by fostering growth of bacterial plaque. To promote dental health, children should eat sugary foods only in moderation and eat more high-fiber snack foods, such as fruits and vegetables. They should also eat adequate amounts of low-fat dairy products and proteins to build strong teeth.

Iron deficiency anemia reduces the body's capacity to carry oxygen in the blood, and this, in turn, can impair normal growth and weight gain in young children, reduce resistance to infection, decrease work capacity, and contribute to scholastic underachievement and behavioral disturbances by shortening attention span and increasing fatigue (Public Health Service [PHS], 1988; Pollitt, 1993). Although it has declined in the past two decades (Yip, Binkin, Fleshood, & Trowbridge, 1987), prevalence of anemia is still an estimated 3 percent in children (Institute of Medicine, 1993) and 7 percent in girls ages 15 to 19 (PHS, 1988). To prevent anemia deficiency, children's eating patterns should include adequate amounts of foods high in iron such as dry beans, meat, fish, peas, and dark green leafy vegetables.

Obesity appears to be increasing, with 27 percent of children ages 6 to 11 estimated to be obese (Gortmaker, Dietz, Sobol, & Wehler, 1987). Prevalence of overweight increased in adolescents, ages 12 to 19, from 15 percent to 22 percent for girls and from 16 percent to 21 percent for boys between 1978–80 and

1988–90 (Centers for Disease Control [CDC], 1994). Obesity results in immediate health problems, such as high blood pressure, elevated blood cholesterol levels, and orthopedic conditions (Clarke, Woolson, & Lauer, 1986; Dietz, 1981; Freedman, Burke, Harsha, Srinivasan, Cresanta, Webber, & Berenson, 1985; Resnicow & Morabia, 1990). Obesity in childhood and adolescence has been shown to track into adulthood, where obesity can contribute to health problems such as high blood pressure and diabetes (Casey, Dwyer, Coleman, & Valadian, 1992; Guo, Roche, Chumlea, Gardner, & Siervogel, 1994).

Childhood obesity has also been shown to correlate with increased mortality in adulthood, independent of adult weight (Must, Jacques, Dallal, Bajema, & Dietz, 1992). It also carries with it immediate social consequences. Obese children often experience rejection by peers, psychological distress, dissatisfaction with their bodies, and low self-esteem (Wadden & Stunkard, 1985). To facilitate weight control, children and adolescents should eat diets that are low in fat and high in fruits, vegetables, and whole grains. Their physical activity levels should also be increased.

Hunger or inadequate food intake may impair growth and development. Because children experience rapid growth, they are vulnerable to growth retardation. Growth retardation prevalence rates that were as high as 13 percent and 16 percent in 1988 for young children in certain low-income subgroups seem to have decreased to the Healthy People 2000 objective of 5 percent in most cases (PHS, 1994). However, undernourishment that is short of growth retardation may also be a problem. Children who are undernourished are more likely to be sick, to miss school, and thus to fall behind in school (American Dietetic Association [ADA], 1990). Undernourished children are more likely to be apathetic and to have difficulty concentrating—conditions that impair academic performance (Troccoli, 1993). In addition to school performance, inadequate nutrition may also affect children's cognitive development. Even moderate undernutrition in the early years may have lasting effects on cognitive development and behavior (Galler & Ramsey, 1989; Pollitt, 1988; Gorman, 1995; Wachs, 1995). Studies also show that merely skipping breakfast can make a difference. In one study, skipping breakfast impaired children's performance in problem-solving situations (Pollitt, 1981). In another study, low-income students who participated in the school breakfast program had greater improvements in standardized test scores as well as fewer absences than those who did not participate (Meyers, Sampson, Weitsman, Rogers, & Kaynes, 1989). One advocacy organization has estimated that as many as 5 million children in the United States under the age of 12 experience inadequate food intakes or hunger (FRAC, 1991). However, there is no scientific agreement on how to define or measure hunger. Still, all children should be encouraged to eat breakfast. To reduce risk of hunger, the school breakfast and lunch programs should be widely available and children should be encouraged to participate.

The Importance of Diet to Reduce Risk of Chronic Diseases in Later Life

Diet is a risk factor for the development of 4 of the nation's 10 leading causes of death: coronary heart disease, some types of cancer, stroke, and diabetes (PHS, 1988). Diet is also related to hypertension, obesity, and osteoporosis. Studies have shown that some of the physiological processes, such as fatty streaks in arteries, the precursor to heart disease, begin to appear in childhood, and these fatty streaks are related to blood cholesterols (Newman, Freedman, Voors, Gard, Srinivasan, Cresanta, Williamson, Webber, & Berenson, 1986; Newman, Watttigney, Berenson, 1991; Strong, 1986). Elevated blood cholesterol, high blood pressure, and obesity, which are diet-related risk factors for chronic diseases, are common in childhood (CDC, 1994; Gortmaker et al., 1987; NCEP, 1991). In addition, children with these risk factors, compared to their peers, are still more likely to have these risk factors when they become adults (Ernst & Obarzanek, 1994; Freedman et al., 1987; Garn & LaVelle, 1985; Guo et al., 1994; Lauer & Clarke, 1984; Porkka, Viikari, & Akerblom, 1991).

Osteoporosis is a disease in which the bone mass declines to such an extent that fractures easily occur. The condition develops gradually and is associated with a low intake of calcium (PHS, 1988). Thus, children and adolescents need adequate amounts of calcium, not only because they are forming bone for normal growth and physical development, but because it is during the first two to three decades of life that

bones reach their maximum density. Bone loss then occurs gradually thereafter (Matkovic, 1992; Sandler et al., 1985). Diets of children and adolescents should contain adequate amounts of foods high in calcium such as dairy products, sardines, and dark green vegetables.

Dietary Intakes and Eating Patterns of Children and Adolescents

The *Dietary Guidelines for Americans* published by the U.S. Departments of Agriculture and Health and Human Services (USDA & USDHHS, 1990) and the *Food Guide Pyramid* published by USDA (1992) provide guidance for healthy diets for all those over the age of 2. Studies show that children and adolescents are consuming too much fat and salt and too few fruits, vegetables, and whole grains compared to amounts recommended by these documents. As indicated earlier, such poor eating patterns have specific consequences for health and development.

National surveys show that the energy intake of children and adolescents has remained fairly constant during the past decade, with mean energy intakes as follows: approximately 1,600 calories for ages 3 to 5; 1,900 for ages 6 to 11; 2,200 for ages 12 to 15; and 2,500 for ages 16 to 19 (McDowell et al., 1994). Other studies found intakes of around 2,050 calories for teenage girls and 3,000 calories for teenage boys (Kenney et al., 1986; Witschi, Capper, & Ellison, 1990), and around 2,100 calories for 10-year-olds during the decade 1973–1982 (Farris et al., 1986). Although the data regarding physical activity are difficult to interpret, they suggest that both activity levels and fitness have declined in the past decade, thus probably accounting to some degree for the increased obesity that has been observed (CDC, 1991; USDHHS, 1986).

National surveys as well as several individual studies show that children and adolescents eat too much fat. A recent national survey showed that children and adolescents are getting 34 percent of their calories from total fat and 13 percent from saturated fat (McDowell, Briefel, Alaimo, Bischof, Caughman, Carroll, Loria, & Johnson, 1994) compared to the 30 percent and 10 percent, respectively, recommended by the *Dietary Guidelines*. Several individual studies have found similar percentages (e.g., Witschi et al.,

1990), while others have shown higher amounts, such as 38 percent (Farris et al., 1986) and 39 percent (Kenney et al., 1986) of calories from fat. Lower-income students appear to eat more fat (Devaney, Gordon, & Burghardt, 1995).

Studies with 10-year-old children showed that snacks supplied one-third of their daily energy, more than from any given meal (Frank, Berenson, & Webber, 1978) and one-third of their fat intake (Farris et al., 1986). A national survey found that eighth- and tenth-graders eat, on average, three or more snacks a day, with most of them being high in fat, sugar, or salt (American School Health Association et al., 1989). One study with teenagers showed that the major sources of energy and fat in the diet were foods of low nutrient density, such as sodas, desserts, and sweet and salty snacks, followed by foods from the meat group (Kenney et al., 1986). Another study found that the major sources of fat were meat and dairy foods for boys, and dairy and baked goods for girls (Witschi et al., 1990). Youths appear to show a distinct preference for sweet and salty foods compared to adults (Heald, 1992).

Surveys also show that children and adolescents do not eat the five daily servings of fruits and vegetables that are recommended by the National Cancer Institute (Butrum, Clifford, & Lanza, 1988) and by the *Food Guide Pyramid.* This recommendation is based on the research evidence indicating that higher intake of fruits and vegetables are consistently, although not universally, associated with a lower risk of cancer at most sites (Steinmetz & Potter, 1991). It has also been suggested that the antioxidant vitamins found in fruits and vegetables reduce the risk of coronary heart disease (Gey, 1990). While it is not clear which specific food components are responsible for the effects, the evidence is strong for a protective effect of a diet rich in fruits and vegetables (Block, Patterson, & Subar, 1992).

In one survey, only 15 percent of high school students and only 9 percent of African American high school students ate the five recommended servings on the day before the survey (CDC, 1995). In fact, 41 percent reported that they did not eat *any* vegetables and 19 percent did not eat *any* fruits on that day (CDC, 1995). A similar pattern was observed in a survey of school children in New York state: 40 percent did not eat vegetables, except potatoes or tomato sauce, and 29 percent did not eat fruit. (At the same time, 36 percent ate at least four different types of snack foods and 16 percent did not eat breakfast). Somewhat similar results were found in a USDA survey: 25 percent of school-aged children do not eat any vegetables and 35 percent of elementary school children do not eat any fruit (USDA, 1994).

Fiber intake is also less than optimal. The overall evidence suggests that there is an inverse relationship between dietary fiber intake and long-term mortality for both colon cancer and coronary heart disease (PHS, 1988). The *Dietary Guidelines* recommend 6 to 11 servings per day of breads, pasta, and cereals, preferably whole grain, depending on age. This represents a range of about 8 grams of fiber among children 3 years old to about 23 grams for those at age 18. (The adult recommendation is 20 to 35 grams). Several surveys show that for almost all children, with the possible exception of the very youngest groups, current dietary intakes are well below recommendations (Alaimo et al., 1994; Albertson, Tobelmann, Engstron, & Asp, 1992).

Although vitamin and mineral intakes are generally adequate regardless of income level, low-income students have lower intakes of some key vitamins and minerals (Devaney et al., 1995). In national surveys, calcium intakes have been found to be inadequate for children over the age of 11 (Alaimo et al., 1994). Females are particularly unlikely to meet the Recommended Daily Allowances (RDA) for calcium intake. Adolescent females also do not meet the RDA for intake of iron (Alaimo et al., 1994). The Bogalusa Heart study (Frank, Webber, Nicklas, & Berenson, 1988) found that only about half of the children age 6 months through age 4 met the RDA for calcium and 60 to 80 percent of adolescents ingested less than two-thirds the RDA. Girls had lower intakes than boys. At the same time, at age 6 months, 66 percent of the infants exceeded the recommended range for sodium intake. During the ages 1 to 10 years, the percentage exceeding the recommended range increased to 90 to 100 percent, and remained at 65 percent for teenagers between ages 13 to 17.

Dietary restraint and unhealthy eating patterns related to weight control are also common. For example, skipping meals, fasting, using laxatives, and vomiting after meals are used by nearly one-quarter of adolescents (American School Health Association et al., 1989). Chronic dietary restraint can impair growth and delay pubertal development (Mellin, 1988). Inadequate intakes of calcium can also impair deposition of calcium in bone and increase risk of osteoporosis, as noted earlier. In a society preoccupied with thinness, many normal-weight women consider themselves overweight. Concern about weight is accompanied by negative body image and inappropriate eating patterns and dieting, and seems to be occurring at an ever-younger age, particularly in young women (Davies & Furnham, 1986; Drewnowski & Yee, 1987; Garner, Garfinkel, Schwartz, & Thompson, 1980; Mellin, 1988; Wardle & Marsland, 1990).

Overall, then, the quality of diet is very important in children and adolescents for normal growth and development and for reducing the risk of chronic disease later in life. At the same time, diet-related behaviors of children and adolescents are less than optimal. There is some evidence that dietary behaviors remain consistent over time at least between the sixth and twelfth grades (Kelder, Perry, Klepp, & Lytle, 1994). The implications are clear: It is extremely important to assist children in acquiring healthful eating habits. The next section explores how children acquire the food acceptance patterns that they do and examines the social psychological factors influencing their food choices.

DETERMINANTS OF FOOD CHOICES BY CHILDREN AND ADOLESCENTS

What are the influences on the food choices of children and adolescents? These influences fall into three broad categories: food and physiological factors; cognitive and motivational factors; and environmental factors.

Food Exposure, Physiological Consequences, and Conditioning Processes

Contrary to popular belief based on "research" (see Story & Brown, 1987, for clarification), infants appear *not* to be born with the natural ability to choose a nutritious diet. Indeed, infants appear to be born with few genetically preprogrammed behavioral propensities: The only known innate preference is for the sweet taste, inferred from the eagerness with which newborn infants will consume sweet substances, and from their facial expressions in response to such substances (Desor, Maller, & Greene, 1977). Infants also show a negative response to bitter and sour tastes and a neutral response to the salty taste.

After considerable research in this area, Birch (1989) has concluded that what seems to be inherited primarily is the capacity to learn about the consequences of eating foods. That is, food acceptance patterns are learned. Thus, early experience with food and eating is crucial in the development of eating patterns, in terms of both the acquisition of food preferences and the regulation of intake. Experience with food influences the development of eating patterns of young children through both the quantity and quality of exposure to food.

Quantity of Exposure: Familiarity and Food Acceptance

Rozin (1988) has pointed out that humans, like other omnivores, experience the "omnivore's paradox": They need to seek variety in their diets to meet nutritional requirements, but ingesting new substances can be potentially dangerous. Not surprisingly, young children, like other young omnivores, demonstrate neophobia, or negative reactions toward new foods. Birch has also shown, though, that neophobia can be reduced by experience (Birch, 1989), probably through a "learned safety mechanism." That is, when ingestion is not followed by negative consequences, increased food acceptance results. This probably accounts for Birch's finding that familiarity as well as sweetness is associated with food preferences in 3- and 4-year-olds (Birch, 1979). Birch's studies with 2- to 6-year-olds showed that only those ages 2 and 3 showed neophobia, but that for all age groups preference increased with exposure. She found that a minimum of 8 to 10 exposures were needed, with clear increases in food acceptance or preference after 12 to 15 exposures. In addition, tasting or actual ingestion was found to be necessary—not just looking at or smelling the food (Birch, McPhee, Shoba, Pirok, & Steinberg, 1987a).

Other researchers have found that greater familiarity with foods was associated with a more complex and varied diet (Yperman & Vermeersch, 1979). It has also been suggested that one of the functions of

cultural rules of cuisine and the use of culturally specific flavor principles (e.g., soy sauce in Chinese cuisine and chili in Mexican cuisine) is to define certain
foods as acceptable and to make new foods taste familiar (Rozin, 1973).

The implications are clear. To enhance preference for nutritious foods, often lacking in youthful diets, parents and preschool child-care programs will
need to offer such foods more frequently and be prepared for children's repeated rejection of these foods
before possible acceptance. We suspect that adults are
too quick to capitulate to food rejection, in part because the number of required exposures is higher than
commonly believed.

Quality of Exposure: Learning Preferences by Association with Food Cues

Research has shown that food preferences are shaped
through the repeated association of foods with the
postingestive physiological consequences of eating
them and with the social context. This process is
called *associative conditioning*. To the extent that the
consequences and contexts are positive, children will
learn to like the foods involved (Birch, 1989; Rozin,
1988; Rozin & Fallon, 1981).

*Postingestive Consequences and Learned Prefer-
ences.* Young children can be sensitive to caloric
density differences between foods and adjust their intake accordingly. However, there is evidence that satiety, or the sense of feeling full, can be conditioned;
children can learn to associate food flavor cues with
caloric density cues. In one study (Birch & Deysher,
1985), preschool children were provided repeated opportunities to associate a distinctive flavor (chocolate
or vanilla) with a given amount of calories (in similar-
tasting high- or low-density preparations of a pud-
ding) and hence to learn how much to eat to feel full.
When the caloric content of that particular flavor was
changed, children continued to eat that particular flavor (e.g., chocolate) as if it had the same number of
calories as before. That is, the frequent pairing of a
food with the "fillingness" or satiety value of the food
led the children to anticipate the consequences of eating that food and to regulate their intake according to
their anticipations.

Children were also shown to develop enhanced
preferences for flavors associated with high-calorie
versions (whether through high starch or high fat) versus low-calorie versions of the same food because the
high-calorie versions were perceived as pleasantly
filling, particularly when the children were hungry
(Birch, 1992). Birch also found that those children
who were led to pay attention to their internal cues
(feelings of hunger and being full) were more likely to
be able to regulate their intake appropriately than
those who were asked to focus on externally oriented
cues such as the time of day or the amount of food remaining on the plate (Birch, McPhee, Shoba, Steinberg, & Krehbiel, 1987b).

Social-Affective Context and Food Preferences.
Research has examined the influence of social learning on eating patterns and preferences (Rozin, 1988;
Birch, 1989). Food is eaten many times a day, providing opportunities for a child's emotional responses to
the social context of eating to become associated with
the specific foods being eaten. Building on the work
of previous researchers, Birch (1980a) examined the
role of peer models by seating at lunch a "target" child
who preferred peas to carrots with three or four other
children who strongly preferred carrots to peas. Both
vegetables were offered. The target child showed a
significant shift toward the initially nonpreferred vegetable by the fourth day. The preference was still
present six weeks later. When it came to adult models,
familiar adults were found to be more effective than
unfamiliar ones; and having the adults themselves
sample the foods was more effective than when adults
offered the foods without eating them (Harper &
Sanders, 1975).

In examining the effects of the social affective
context of feeding on food acceptance, Birch, Zimmerman, and Hind (1980) found that after 20 exposures over several weeks, there was an increase in the
preference for foods presented as rewards as well as
for the foods presented paired with positive adult attention. No such changes in acceptability were found
for the foods presented in more neutral social contexts.

However, use of rewards is more complex
(Birch, Marlin, & Rotter, 1984). If a food is given as a
reward, there is a significant *increase* in preference

("You did a good job cleaning up the toys. Here, have some peanuts"). The opposite is true if the child is asked to eat a food in order to obtain a reward ("If you eat your spinach, you can watch TV"). In particular, requiring eating of a less preferred food in order to obtain a more preferred food ("You can have dessert if you eat your spinach") can *decrease* even further the liking for the initially less preferred food.

These findings are consistent with intrinsic motivation theory (Deci & Ryan, 1980; Lepper & Greene, 1978). Parents and child-care providers often use this childrearing practice to get children to eat foods they believe are nutritious. But it is likely that this practice will lead, paradoxically, to even less liking for the foods that are nutritious. In addition, because the foods used as rewards are typically those high in sugar, fat, and salt (e.g., desserts and salty snacks), such a practice may enhance even further the preference for these items.

Implications of these findings with preschool-aged children are numerous and have been summarized by Birch (1989, 1992). Because taste or preference appears to be shaped by experience with foods and eating, parents, teachers, and child-care providers should expose children repeatedly to nutritious foods in a positive social affective context so that children will come to like nutritious foods. Use of foods in positive contexts as rewards or treats will enhance preferences for those foods, whereas having children eat a food in order to obtain a reward is likely to produce a decline in preference in that food. Because foods high in fat, sugar, and salt are widely available, particularly in positive social affective contexts, parents and other adults should reduce the extent to which their childrearing practices enhance preference for such foods. To help children develop internal controls over eating, parents or child-care providers should view themselves as responsible for what foods are presented to the child and the manner in which they are presented, but acknowledge that it is the child's responsibility as to what and how much of that to eat, as has been strongly argued by Satter (1987).

It can be seen that acquisition of eating patterns in very young children is based on learning from the postingestive physiological consequences of foods, and the social affective or emotional context of eating rather than based on cognitive learning. Indeed, children of this age are not yet very well developed cognitively. Although children between the ages of 2 and 6 become less dependent than infants on their direct sensory-motor actions for direction of behavior and become increasingly able to think (Piaget & Inhelder, 1969), reasoning is partly magical and unsystematic and does not readily lead to abstract generalizations or formation of logical concepts. Children 3 to 5 years old can easily identify foods (Gorelick & Clark, 1985). Children 5 to 6 years old do not understand what happens to food after it enters the body (Contento, 1981) and understandings about nutrients in foods are rudimentary (Michela & Contento, 1984). Consequences of food intake on health is too remote to be salient (Bush & Ionnatti, 1990).

Cognitive-Motivational Influences on Food Choice

As children become older, however, cognitive-motivational processes, in addition to social environmental forces, come into play. A comprehensive study of 5- to 11-year-children sought to understand whether, at what age, and which cognitive-motivational processes influenced children's food choices (Michela & Contento, 1986). The study was based on a value-expectancy model of human motivation (e.g., Lewin, Dembo, Festinger, & Sears, 1944), which proposes that people would be expected to choose foods they believe will provide consequences they desire from foods, such as good taste, convenience, health, and so forth. The study thus sought to establish associations between motivationally relevant beliefs about the food (cognitive-motivational factor) and food choices (behavior). A within-person, across-foods correlational method (Michela, 1990) was used since individuals normally make choices from a variety of alternative foods. This method is able to detect whether, for each person, the foods eaten most often are the same ones believed to produce desired consequences. Cognitive-developmental level of each child was also assessed and children were classified into those using preoperational (or prelogical) and those using concrete (or early logical) reasoning patterns.

A sample of 107 children provided ratings for 15 foods and seven beliefs about the consequences of eating the food, such as *tastes good*, *is good for me*, *makes me fat,* and *has much sugar,* and four social environmental influences such as *costs a lot, is easy to get, my friends eat it,* and *my parents serve it.* These potential influences are referred to as "food choice criteria." Within-person correlations were then calculated between each food choice criterion and frequency of consumption of each of the 15 foods. An examination of these "correlational indices" of influences on food choice showed that the two healthful criteria had moderate positive associations with food choice, having median values of 0.3 for *good for me* and 0.4 for *good for teeth,* while two of the unhealthful criteria had small negative associations with food choice, having median values of –0.2 for *makes me fat* and –0.1 for *has much salt.* Although the median association for *has much sugar* was –0.2, a frequency distribution showed that, for some children, sugar was positively associated with food choice, whereas for others it was negatively associated. The judgments involving *tastes good* and *I like to eat it* were strongly associated with choosing those foods, having median correlations of 0.5 for both variables. Correlations between social environmental factors and food frequencies were generally positive, with median values of 0.4 for *easy to get,* 0.3 for *my friends eat it,* and 0.6 for *my parents serve it.* There was no association between the judgment *costs a lot* and reported consumption.

A cluster analysis was then conducted on these correlational indices and revealed five distinct subgroups in the sample. Children at the concrete operational level of development tended to be in one of three groups characterized by their orientation in food choices. There was a *health-oriented* group, where *my parents serve it* was also highly correlated with intake, so the group was labeled Healthful/Parents (H/P). Children in this group appeared to be especially motivated to choose healthful foods and to avoid fattening ones; at the same time, parents provided environmental support for health-oriented food choices.

For a second group, *taste* was most important, but *my friends eat it* was also highly correlated with intake, so the group was labeled Tasty/Friends (T/F). Children in this group chose food primarily on the basis of taste and perceived their friends as doing so, too. For the third group, multiple motives characterized the orientation to food choice, since the mean values

of the correlational indices for *health, taste, friends,* and *parents* were in the same range as either of the first two groups, but the correlation was significantly higher on *easy to get.* This group was labeled Multiple Personal/Environmental (MP/E).

Food intake data, as measured by an independent food frequency instrument, supported the validity of these group designations. For example, candy was eaten more frequently by children in the T/F group than in the H/P group, and whole wheat bread was eaten more frequently by children in the H/P group than in the T/F group. There was also an association between membership in a particular cluster group and quality of diets of the children as measured by another independent instrument, 24-hour dietary recalls. The MP/E group had the most children with good diets followed by the H/P group. The T/F group had the most children with poor diets.

Results for children in the prelogical level of cognitive development, generally those 5 to 7 years old, differed from the older children in that three-quarters of them fell into the fourth and fifth groups: the Undifferentiated High group, where correlations between judgments about all potential food choice criteria and food intake were high, and the Undifferentiated Low group, where the correlations between cognitions and behavior were low. It appears that in children who are less cognitively developed there is less of a link between beliefs and behavior.

Part of the explanation for preoperational children's undifferentiated responses may be methodological: They may have had more difficulty understanding the interviewer's questions, and reliabilities of their reports were lower. In any case, research on the cognitive understandings about food in children is consistent with the notion that sufficient cognitive development generally is required for logically consistent or substantial relations to be seen between food choices and beliefs about the consequences of these choices. Children who are 5 to 7 years old have little understanding that food is transformed in the body into nutrients to have an effect (Contento, 1981). As children become older, they have a better understanding of the effects of food in the body and their descriptions of nutrients in food also become more complex (Michela & Contento, 1984). Children ages 4 to 7 can comprehend simple concepts such as having energy, healthy foods keep germs out of the body, and low fat foods keep the heart healthy (Singleton, Achterberg, & Shannon, 1992).

The basis of the food classifications created by 115 children, aged 5 to 11, also increased in complexity with age (Michela & Contento, 1984). Multidimensional scaling analysis revealed that the common underlying dimensions of the children's classification schemes were "sweet versus nonsweet" foods (used heavily by the 5- to 6-year-old, prelogical children) and "meal entres versus drinks and breakfast foods," suggesting that perceptual, functional, and physical properties of foods influenced food classifications by children regardless of cognitive developmental level. However, the concrete operational or early logical children were also substantially influenced by dimensions involving degree of processing of food and origin of food in plants or animals.

Results from these studies strongly suggest that cognitive-motivational processes operate in children's food choices, at least in those over the age of about 6 or 7 who were beyond the preoperational level of cognitive development. Most children were found to select foods in a pattern consistent with various beliefs about foods that are motivationally relevant. That is, they selected foods based on whether eating the food would bring about desired outcomes, such as the food would be tasty, healthful, and so forth. Thus, a process of cognitive self-regulation appeared to be operating where behaviors are brought into alignment with beliefs and values about the consequences of those behaviors.

A follow-up study demonstrated similar cognitive-motivational processes in adolescents, as well. Participants were 355 students between the ages of 11 and 18 (Contento, Michela, & Goldberg, 1988) who were given ratings of 20 foods in terms of 8 potential food choice criteria. Five distinct subgroups of adolescents were identified as having distinct orientations to food choice, with a gradation in motivations from a highly Hedonistic group at one end, where taste and environmental factors were most important, through Social/Environmental, Personal Health, Peer-Supported Health groups to a Parent-Supported Health-Oriented group at the other end of the gradation. There was also an undifferentiated group. Again, the group classifications were corroborated by

other evidence in the study. For example, those in the Parent-Supported Health-Oriented groups were more likely to eat healthful foods and to avoid harmful food and to get more calcium and vitamin C and less sugar in their diets than those in the Hedonistic group.

The sample was large and diverse enough to examine these cognitive-motivational processes by the demographic variables of age, sex, and ethnicity (47 percent white, 21 percent African American, 20 percent Latino American, and 12 percent Asian American, Native American, and others). The only significant association was with age. Adolescents ages 13 to 18 were present in greater numbers than preadolescents in two groups, the Hedonistic and Parent-Supported Health group. Preadolescents were especially prevalent in the other groups. This seems to suggest that increasing age brings about increased differentiation in food choice motivations, so that by age 18, adolescents are more likely to be either hedonistic or health-conscious.

A related study with these adolescents examined the relation of weight status, dieting status, and associated variables to the food choice criteria (Contento, Michela, & Williams, in press). A similar picture emerged. In this case, those who provided higher self-reports on a simple measure of dieting also obtained higher within-person correlations, indicating higher use of the food choice criterion that food *not* be *fattening*. Indeed, compared to their low dieting counterparts, they ate fewer of the foods judged by nutrition experts to be fattening and, from 24-hour dietary recall data, ate fewer calories, less fat, and less sugar overall. They gave less importance to *taste* and *convenience* as food choice criteria, compared to low dieters, suggesting they were willing to forego taste and convenience to some degree in order to obtain less fattening food. That is, those adolescents who wanted to be thinner made food choices that they believed would help them to accomplish their goal.

This research also raised some general methodological and conceptual issues. First, because the foods that promote health also tend to promote weight control, disentangling these two corresponding motivations can be tricky, and associations involving one or the other motivation must be interpreted in light of this connection. Also correlated are higher weight-for-height levels and higher frequency of dieting.

Consequently, data analyses involving either of these variables should be controlled for the other.

Somewhat similar thinking about food was captured in a qualitative study on 93 young women, ages 11 to 18, examining the meanings of food in adolescent women's culture (Chapman & MacLean, 1993). This study, based on in-depth interviews, found that the young women tended to divide all foods into two categories: junk food and healthy food. Junk food was associated with pleasure, friends, being away from home, peers, and independence, whereas healthy food was linked with family meals and being at home. They found it difficult to stay away from junk food because of its good taste, its convenience, and its affordability. Eating junk food was perceived to be the norm for teenagers and those who liked healthy food were thought to be oddities or weird. However, they described experiencing conflict in choosing foods because they wanted to eat junk food to demonstrate independence from their family and adherence to their peer group. At the same time, they wanted to eat healthy food to demonstrate maintenance of family ties and to achieve the thin figure they perceived was required to be accepted by society, their peers, and men.

Thus, in both this study and that of Contento and colleagues (1988), which included both men (40 percent) and women (60 percent), similar themes emerged—choosing foods based on taste and in common with what friends eat versus making choices based on health and supported by what parents serve. The study by Contento and colleagues suggests that some subgroups of teenagers are more likely to emphasize the taste/friends criteria in food choices while other subgroups are more likely to emphasize health. The health-conscious in that study were also not oddities but constituted some 45 percent of the sample. In addition, within the health-conscious group, about half of them perceived their friends as eating that way, too. It was not clear whether such similarity in reported eating patterns of self and others was evidence of social-motivational influences (e.g., conformity to reference groups), falsely assumed consensus (Ross, Greene, & House, 1977) between own and others' eating, or other factors.

In another study of adolescents' views on food and nutrition, 900 high school students were polled using a small group discussion format and qualitative

survey methods (Story & Resnick, 1986). In this case, the adolescents seemed to be well informed about good health and nutrition practices, but felt that there were many barriers to eating healthfully—in particular, lack of time, the inconvenience and expense of eating healthful foods, and lack of a sense of urgency about health outcomes. A study that did not examine teenagers' thinking processes, per se, but instead examined the different factors in influencing food choice found the order of importance to be taste, satiety or sense of fillingness of food, tolerance, prestige, familiarity, and cost (Lau, Krondl, & Coleman, 1984).

Environmental Influences on Food Choices

Evidence for cognitive-motivational processes in food choice does not, of course, deny that social-environmental factors are powerful and possibly predominant in food selection. Evidence for the importance of these factors for children and adolescents comes from various sources, including the cognitively oriented studies of Contento and Michela described earlier. Several of these factors are reviewed next. The availability and accessibility of food, economic resources of the family, and other environmental forces that are crucial will not be discussed here.

Cultural and Social Influences

Culture is concerned with shared knowledge and shared meanings, where *meanings* implies some complexity of belief or knowledge and a connection of values or feelings with beliefs (D'Andrade, 1984). Cultural knowledge and values develop over time for the group or society in ways that promote its survival (LeVine, 1984). Consequently, it is not surprising that food, which is essential to survival, is very much part of culture. One's culture defines what should or should not be eaten and prescribes how to prepare food, among other food-relevant matters (Rozin, 1982).

Children acquire their cultures' beliefs and values directly and indirectly (Spiro, 1984). Direct influence occurs when the child is told explicitly about "facts," norms, values, and so forth (e.g., "We don't eat pork"). Indirect acquisition occurs through observation of what other people do (norms), whether in reality or through the media, (e.g., television), and making inferences from norms and cultural artifacts about the values of the culture. For example, if existing members of a culture spend a lot of time preparing healthful food (norms), or if their kitchens are specially equipped to maximize healthfulness of foods (artifacts), children growing up in the culture are likely also to value healthful food. This outcome is likely in part because there is a tendency for the descriptive understanding of one's culture—how things are—to become fused with a normative understanding—how things should be. LeVine (1984) comments: "The fusion of what is and ought to be in a single vision...gives distinctive cultural ideologies their singular psychological power, their intimate linkages with individual emotion and motivation" (p. 78).

Given these definitions and observations, culture is connected intimately with the cognitive-motivational factors in food choice that were discussed in the previous section of this chapter. That is, the beliefs and values discussed there are the same ones under discussion here; culture may be understood as their primary source. The relation of culture to the food and physiological factors discussed earlier has been explored by Rozin (1982). Rozin describes how mild social pressure may maintain consumption of initially unpalatable foods, until preference becomes internalized by liking for the taste (as with chili) or other factors (e.g., addiction to coffee).

Social pressure of this kind tends to be consistent with cultural or subcultural (e.g., adolescent) beliefs, values, and behavior patterns. Nevertheless, cultural and social influences are distinguishable to some degree through the concept of internalization. Culture involves beliefs and values that are internalized or "believed in" widely among members of the group; as children acquire these beliefs and values, we say they become acculturated. By contrast, two kinds of social influence have been distinguished by Deutsch and Gerard (1955). In *normative* social influence, people conform with others' wishes in order to gain social acceptance. The literature reviewed elsewhere in this chapter suggests that conformity to the family's wishes is of some importance earlier in life, and later the key reference group consists of one's peers. In *informational* social influence, people learn about reality from what others say and do. Such learning then

comes into play in combination with values, the task at hand, and so forth.

Culture influences food choice behavior in other ways. When members of a culture come to use a specific set of items in specific ways (as snacks, breakfast foods, etc.), these items become the most physically available (e.g., they become available in supermarkets, or one's parents are more likely to serve them) and psychologically acceptable. In the largest frame of reference, culture is, in this sense, the most important influence on food choice (Rozin, 1982). For example, American, Chinese, and Mexican people each have distinctive cuisines.

The Role of the Family

Cultural influences on children and adolescents are largely mediated by the family. For example, the family selects, and children are thus exposed to, a subset of culturally available foods (Birch, 1989). Also, family members' behaviors are salient sources for inferring cultural values and meanings. Parents are key sources of normative and social influences; siblings may be influential as well (Pliner & Pelchat, 1986).

Given these considerations, one would expect some degree of association between children's food preferences and those of their parents. Strong resemblances have been hard to demonstrate in both young children and older adolescents (Birch, 1980; Logue, Logue, Uzzo, McCarty, & Smith, 1988; Pliner, 1983; Rozin, 1991). This observation, *the family paradox* (Rozin, 1991), may result from several factors. There is often very low variance in preferences resulting from the high degree of commonality of preference among the subcultural groups from which samples for the studies are often drawn. Parents give mixed messages because they differ from each other in food preferences. Other methodological difficulties may be operating, as well.

Despite these difficulties, there are some similarities between the diets eaten by children and the diets eaten by their parents. The studies of Michela and Contento (1986) and Contento and associates (1988) found that the food choices of children of all ages were correlated with what they reported their parents to serve, suggesting that family meals are important even into adolescence. In one study with 106 families, an analysis of nine-day diet records on parents and their children found a statistically significant but modest correlation between parents' and children's intakes for most nutrients, with the highest being for saturated fat and cholesterol (Oliveria, Ellison, Moore, Gillman, Garrahie, & Singer, 1992).

The nature of the interaction between parents and their children during mealtimes is another source of family influence on what children eat. For example, in a food choice situation where children were observed, both the threat of parental monitoring of their selections and actual monitoring lowered the number of nonnutritious foods chosen by children and the total caloric content of the meal (Klesges, Stein, Eck, Isbell, & Klesges, 1991). In another observational study, parental encouragement to eat correlated both with the percent of time the child ate and with relative weight (Klesges, Malott, Boschee, & Weber (1986).

The value the family places on the health benefits of food choices can also have an impact on what children eat. For example, in one study with 218 mothers and their 4- to 5-year-old children, mothers were segmented into groups according to beliefs about the importance of healthfulness in selecting foods for their child (Contento, Basch, Shea, Gutin, Zybert, Michela, & Rips, 1993). Children of mothers in the "high health" group had better quality diets than children of mothers in the "high taste" group. The mothers' values for health was associated with their children's diets—even with knowledge controlled—although it also found that the mothers who valued health had greater knowledge about the health effects of different foods. These results are similar to those obtained in an earlier study where children of mothers with higher education and more positive attitudes about the importance of nutrition also had more complex diets (Yperman & Vermeersch, 1979).

The Impact of Television Viewing

No discussion of influences on food choices of children and adolescents would be complete without some mention of the impact of television viewing. Children spend more time watching television than they do in school, with an average of 27 hours per week for preschool children, 23.5 hours per week for children ages 6 to 12, and 22 hours for children 12 to 17 (Neilsen, 1990). Kotz and Story (1994) found that about 50 percent of the 564 food advertisements shown in 52.5 hours of Saturday morning television

were for items that would fit in the "fats, oils, and sweets" group of the *Food Guide Pyramid*. Another 43 percent as were for breakfast cereals. No ads were for fruits or vegetables. About one-third of the ads appealed to taste; 17 percent used free toys as an incentive; and another 24 percent described the foods as fun, cool, or hip. Only 2.4 percent of the ads emphasized nutrition as a reason to buy the product.

However, the effects of television on food preferences and consumption have been difficult to document. In an experimental study, Galst and White (1976) found that the number of purchase requests in the supermarket was related to the amount of television children watched in the lab. More recently, Taras, Sallis, Patterson, Nader, and Nelson (1989) surveyed mothers of children ages 3 to 8, and found that after viewing TV, their children requested foods paralleling the frequencies with which those items were advertised on TV. The hours of TV watched weekly were positively correlated with requests by children and purchases of parents as well as with children's caloric intake.

The ultimate effects of TV on children's food intake may depend on parents' behavior, not only in terms of whether parents comply with children's purchase requests but also in framing or supporting TV messages. This point is illustrated by an experiment reported by Galst (1980). With adults and children watching TV together, it was found that having adults comment positively on public service announcements for nutritious snacks was more effective in reducing children's selection of highly sugared snacks than when adults commented negatively on commercials for sugared products, or when adults made no comments.

The impact of TV viewing on older children and adolescents have also been the subject of a few studies. Adolescents are heavy users of television: Teenage boys watch an average of 21 hours and girls watch an average of 22 hours of television a week (Dietz & Strasburger, 1991). Since they spend 5 to 10 times more time watching TV in prime time than on Saturday morning, food messages presented on prime-time television (8:00 to 11:00 PM) were analyzed by Story and Faulkner (1990). They found that references to food in both programming and advertisements occurred an average of 4.8 times per 30 minutes of programming time. About 60 percent of food references in programs were for low-nutrient beverages, sweets, and salty snacks.

In addition, national surveys showed that the prevalence of obesity increased 2 percent for each additional hour of television adolescents viewed, controlling for prior obesity, geographic region, season, population density, ethnicity, and socioeconomic status (Dietz & Gortmacher, 1985). Dietz and Strasburger (1991) also reported that television viewing is associated with snacking and with requests to parents for advertised foods. Taken together, these studies show that television viewing has a powerful influence on the eating patterns of children and adolescents and must be considered in any nutrition education effort.

School Meals

An environmental factor of some importance for the food intakes of children is the school meal. Studies have shown that it is possible to change school lunches to make them lower in fat and salt (Lytle, Kelder, & Snyder, 1991). It has also been shown that such lunches can reduce the overall intake of fat by children; they do not compensate at other meals (Simons-Morton, Parcel, Baranowski, Forthofer, & O'Hara, 1991). Finally, it has been shown that such changes in school meals can reduce fat and salt intakes even without an educational component for students (Ellison, Capper, Goldberg, Witschi, & Stare, 1989).

Overall Scheme of Influences on Food Choice: A Cognitive Self-Regulation Integration

Summarizing the research findings described here and modifying a generalized model of food choice put forward by Shepherd (1989), the authors propose an overall scheme for influences on food choice in children and adolescents (see Figure 16.1). Food choice can be seen as influenced by preferences; by cognitive-motivational processes that involve beliefs, values, and decision-making; and by environmental factors such as culture and availability of food.

Preferences are important determinants of food choices for people of all ages but in young children it is primary. Preferences, apart from the sweet preference, are learned through experience with food, which, in turn, reflects exposure through the family,

society, and culture. Repeated exposure makes food more familiar and thus more acceptable or preferred. That is, taste is shaped to a large extent by exposure. In addition, preferences are learned through the association of food cues with both the physiological consequences of eating and through social learning from family and peers. Children eat what they like, but they also come to like what they eat.

Cognitive-motivational processes become important influences on food choice as well when children become older and more developed cognitively. Children and adolescents become more able to link cause and effect and to perceive the consequences of their actions. Thus, they can make food choices in light of their perceptions of anticipated consequences from eating particular foods: that the food will taste good, be healthful, have vitamins and minerals, be good for teeth, not be fattening, and so forth. Perceived social-environmental factors also influence food choice, such as whether friends eat it, it is convenient, and parents serve it. These beliefs and values come from perceptions based on factors arising from the foods themselves, such as aroma and texture; exposure and social learning from family and peers; ideations (ideas) and concepts children acquire about food (Rozin & Fallon, 1981); and perceptions of what is economically available and social-culturally acceptable.

Environmental factors are also crucial. Availability of food is, of course, the fundamental determinant of food choices, since without food, none of the other forces would have an opportunity to operate. Availability, however, can be both actual and perceived. Foods may be actually available but not economically affordable, culturally acceptable, considered appropriate for children, or readily accessible to children without the perquisite skills to prepare them into edible form.

A Cognitive Self-Regulation Integration

From a social-psychological perspective, the picture that emerges from research is that older children and adolescents want particular consequences from the food they eat and want to become increasingly able to align their food choice behaviors with their goals. They integrate motivations and cognitions in a self-regulatory process.

NUTRITION EDUCATION INTERVENTIONS

A major implication of the preceding discussion is that the issues involved in food choice behavior and consequently in nutrition education shift radically through the period of childhood to adolescence. In the beginning, the goal is one of getting parents and others who care for children to provide adequate and healthful food and to adopt parenting practices that encourage the acquisition of eating patterns that are healthful. Later, the primary task of nutrition education is one of instilling healthful food habits in a relatively autonomous adolescent. How successful, then, has nutrition education been in achieving these goals?

Several recent reviews have been conducted of nutrition education interventions conducted since 1980 that had good research designs (Contento et al., 1995; Contento, Manning, & Shannon, 1992; Centers for Disease Control, 1995; Lytle & Achterberg, 1995). These reviews also describe implications for nutrition education policy, programs/curricula, and research. These reviews showed that in about half of the studies, nutrition education did not achieve these goals, largely because curricula or programs focused on dissemination of nutrition information and skills. Such a highly cognitive focus was successful in achieving knowledge goals in almost all instances, but not in achieving behavioral or eating pattern goals.

An examination of the reviewed studies shows that nutrition education interventions were most likely to be effective in achieving behavioral or eating pattern goals when they specifically targeted all three categories of factors as important influences on food choices in children and adolescents: food preferences, cognitive-motivational processes, and environmental factors (see Figure 16.1).

Effectiveness of Nutrition Education with Preschool-Aged Children

The relative importance of influences on food choices in children changes with age or cognitive developmental level. Thus, for young children, the most important forces in shaping eating patterns are preferences, social learning, and environmental factors.

Indeed, the findings from recent reviews (e.g., Contento et al., 1995) suggest that factors contributing to the success of nutrition education are those that address these influences in age-appropriate ways.

A behaviorally focused approach that specifically targets children's behaviors has been shown to increase preference and consumption for specific foods and the development of eating patterns, as seen from numerous research studies described in a previous section (e.g., Birch, 1989). This approach includes selecting specific healthful meals and snacks to target and then offering them frequently to increase familiarity. It also includes social modeling of eating these foods by peers and adult role models, adults offering foods to children in a positive social environment, and using rewards appropriately. Stark, Collins, Ocnes, and Stokes (1986) found that stickers and praise increased healthy snacks choices but only in the school (where the intervention took place) not in the home, and only during the period of use of rewards. Perhaps the best use of contingent rewards is to induce consumption initially for familiarity. Thereafter, other factors seem to be necessary for maintenance of consumption.

Activities that increased the familiarity of foods—such as tasting parties, participation in food preparation, vegetable gardens, engaging the five senses with food, and eating healthy meals and snacks—have been successful in increasing children's food preferences (e.g., Berenbaum, 1986; Birch & Marlin, 1982; Birch, 1989; Byrd-Bredbenner, Marecic, & Bernstein, 1993). Such exposure makes healthful foods familiar and hence more acceptable to children. Thus, meals and snacks at childcare centers should be the centerpiece of nutrition education in these settings (Briley & Roberts-Gray, 1994).

Involvement of parents/families, either as major recipients of the program or in conjunction with the program offered to the preschool child, is extremely important for influencing eating patterns. As seen earlier, the way foods are used in the home influences the development of eating patterns (Birch, 1989), and the degree to which mothers value health is associated with the quality of diets of children (Contento et al., 1993). In studies involving families, it was found that home-only interventions need to be fairly intensive, based on activities that parents and children can do together (Singleton et al., 1992). Parents and teachers working together can make more of an impact than either alone through mutual reinforcement (Essa, Read, & Haney-Clark, 1988). In studies with Head Start parents (Gunn & Stevenson, 1985; Koblinsky & Phillips, 1987; Koblinsky, Guthrie, & Lynch, 1992), it was found that educating and encouraging parents were effective in increasing children's knowledge and reported consumption of more nutritious foods. These studies point to the importance of family-based interventions.

Use of developmentally appropriate learning experiences and materials is critical to success (e.g., Gorelick & Clark, 1985). Understanding of nutrients in foods and what happens to food in the body is quite rudimentary (Contento, 1981; Michela & Contento, 1984), although Lee, Schvaneveldt, and Sorenson (1984) found that using cards that displayed a picture of a food, its name in large type, and color-coded bar graphs for vitamins A and C and iron and calcium, preschool children were able, *upon instruction,* to report on the concepts of nutritive value, nutrient function, and the impact of nutrition on health.

Singleton and associates (1992), in a study with 60 children, found that 4- to 7-year-olds can comprehend such concepts as energy, a strong heart, "good foods keep germs out of the body," and "a low-fat diet keeps the heart healthy." They also found that a nutrition education intervention significantly increased the children's perception that health and nutrition are related concepts. Thus, preschoolers are developing some emerging understanding of relevant concepts. Programs need to be tailored to children's emotional and motor developmental levels, as well.

Activity-based teaching strategies that encourage interaction with real-world objects are essential. Preschool children learn by manipulation of the environment rather than by passive listening. They learn by exploring, questioning, comparing, and labeling. In addition, language is developing very quickly. Physical manipulation skills are being developed when children touch, feel, look, mix-up, turn over, and throw. Emotionally, exploration and the need to test independence seem to dominate during this time. They take on more initiative, are more purposeful, and are eager to learn, usually from other people. They observe parents, teachers, and other children, they role-play, and they start to accumulate and process information. Where interventions had an impact on knowledge and eating practices, activity-based teaching strategies in a nonthreatening environment were involved (e.g., Community Research Center, 1980; Turner & Evers, 1987; Byrd-Bredbenner et al., 1993). Activities included art projects, songs, jingles, role-playing, stories, puppets, and puzzles.

Effectiveness of Nutrition Education with School-Aged Children

Over 40 studies were reviewed by Centers for Disease Control (1995), Contento and associates (1995), and Lytle and Achterberg (1995). An examination of these studies indicates that as was observed for research with preschool-aged children, programs were most effective when they addressed all three of the categories of factors influencing food choices described in Figure 16.1.

A behaviorally focused approach that targets specific behaviors is most likely to be effective, as was found in studies with preschool children. The studies reviewed showed that about half of the nutrition education curricula/programs focused on specific diet-related behaviors, such as use of salt at the table or eating fruits and vegetables. These programs also taught a systematic process for enhancing behavioral change involving setting goals and monitoring change (e.g., Domel, Baranowski, Davis, Thompson, Leonard, Riley, Baranowski, Dudovitz, & Smyth, 1993; Perry, Mullis, & Maile, 1985). These were more likely to result in behavioral changes than nutrition education interventions that were general in nature. For example, 18 of 23 such studies resulted in behavior change at least on some measures such as consumption of targeted foods (Perry, Klepp, Halper, Dudovitz, Golden, Griffin, & Smyth, 1987), decreased fat intake (Walter, 1989), or use of salt (Parcel, Simons-Morton, O'Hara, Baranowski, & Wilson, 1989). Behaviorally based curricula are those that address all three categories of factors discussed in the last section, such as influencing the food choices of children, to bring about the desired goal of shaping or making changes in eating patterns.

Addressing preferences or the affective domain remains important for children of all ages. As discussed earlier, social learning from family and culture

Figure 16.1 Factors Influencing Food Choices by Children and Adolescents

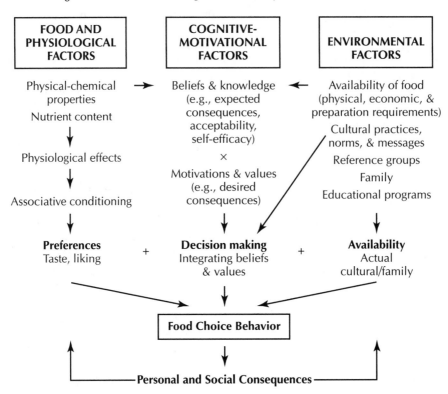

is the primary mode for acquisition of a repertoire of beliefs and behaviors related to food and health, long before children can deal with abstract concepts such as causality, prevention, or health (e.g., Birch, 1989; Rozin, 1988). Thus, it is not surprising that these beliefs and behaviors are so stable and are not easily amenable to change by cognitive means (Lewis & Lewis, 1982). Familiarity, taste, social learning, and reinforcements remain as important influences on food choices. Nutrition education curricula should provide opportunity for children to taste and enjoy a wide variety of healthful foods in positive social affective contexts, provide reinforcements, and increase availability of healthful foods.

Strategies for addressing cognitive-motivational processes are crucial for success. Results from studies described earlier demonstrate that cognitive-motivational processes begin to operate in children's food choices, at least in those over the age of about 6 or 7. Most children were found to select foods based on whether eating the food would bring about desired outcomes, such as the food would be tasty, healthful, and so forth. That is, evidence for a process of cognitive self-regulation was beginning to be seen where behaviors were brought into alignment with beliefs about the consequences of those behaviors.

As already discussed, children younger than age 11 deal in concrete experiences rather than abstract associations (Contento, 1980; Michela & Contento, 1984). Food classifications and understandings of the link between food and health are concrete. Self-assessments, using a food group approach, modeling by adults, beginning discussion on media and social influences, and practice of simple cognitive and behavioral skills should be stressed.

Children during the middle school years begin to place a value on health and can recognize connections between eating behavior and health consequences (Bush & Ionnatti, 1990; Contento et al., 1988; Michela & Contento, 1986; Mickalide, 1986). The behavioral strategies should target making food choices within a broader social and environmental context. More complex motivations can be explored, as well as emotional and functional meanings placed on food (e.g., appearance and body image concerns). The normative influences of peers and community become increasingly important. Students can learn to identify and practice strategies to resist social and media pressures. The teaching of decision-making skills and personal responsibility, as well as affective emotion-coping and behavioral skills, are appropriate content areas for older children.

At the middle and high school levels, more abstract concepts and causal relationships can be understood. Connections between food and present and future health can be made, as well as between dietary practices and the environment. Nutrition education can emphasize increasingly sophisticated critical thinking skills, including analysis of media and social influences and examination of the impacts of diet-related practices on health and the environment. Thus, nutrition education interventions should address the cognitive-motivational factors influencing food choices described earlier, but how these factors are addressed should be appropriate for each level of cognitive development.

Interventions for older children should include a self-evaluation or self-assessment and feedback component. Given the importance of cognitive-motivational processes, it is not surprising that effective programs emphasized self-assessment with personalized feedback, even sometimes without extensive other behavioral strategies. Examples are the "Secrets of Success" study with fifth-grade students that emphasized decision making and personal responsibility (Howison, Niedermeyer, & Shortridge, 1988), a study with high school students that used computer-assisted feedback letters (Burnett, Magel, Harrington, & Taylor, 1989), and another where high school students used three-day food records to identify problem vitamins and minerals in the diet (White & Skinner, 1988).

Interventions need to devote adequate time to nutrition education. Programs with longer durations and more contact hours achieve more positive results than shorter programs. The Know Your Body program, taught for 30 to 45 minutes per week over the entire school year, and usually for several consecutive

years, showed positive effects for both dietary intake and serum cholesterols. (Resnicow, Cohn, Reinhardt, Cross, Futterman, Kirschner, Wynder, & Allegrante, 1992; Walter, 1989) Most of the programs reviewed, however, involved only 10 to 15 hours of education over a 3- to 15-week period. When curricula were disseminated to teachers to use in real-world settings, even less time was spent on nutrition education (e.g., a median of 3 hours out of a potential 39 [Devine, Olson, & Frongillo, 1992] or an average 6 out 17 lessons [Lewis, Brun, Talmage, & Rasher, 1988]). In one case, only 12 percent of teachers were "high implementers" of the curriculum as planned (Resnicow et al., 1992). Yet the School Health Evaluation Study (Connell, Turner, & Manson, 1985) found that 15 hours could only be expected to bring about changes in knowledge, and 50 hours were required for changes in attitudes and behaviors, as well. Due to this time shortage, there is pressure for nutrition education to be integrated into other subject areas. However, nutrition education also needs to be implemented in such a way so as to preserve the coherence or integrity of the message.

Family involvement in programs for younger school-aged children can be effective. Several studies have shown the usefulness of including a family component for younger children. An example is the study by Kirks, Hendricks, and Wyse (1982) with children in grades K through 3 where the intervention lasted four months; the children were also followed up five years later (Kirks & Hughes, 1986). Another example is the Home Team program for grades 3 and 4 (Perry, Luepker, Murray, Kurth, Mullis, Crockett, & Jacobs, 1988), which involved not only a classroom component but also materials mailed home every week for five weeks. A third example is the family-based program of Nader, Sallis, Patterson, Abramson, Rupp, Senn, Atkins, Roppe, Morris, Wallace, and Vega (1989) and that of Baranowski, Henske, Simons-Morton, Palmer, Tiernan, Hooks, and Dunn (1990) conducted after school and involving both children and their families. The programs that were most effective were those of sufficient length and intensity. Also effective were those in which materials were mailed directly to homes and that involved activities for family members to carry out with their child, such as worksheets, games, and other activities, rather than newsletters. After-school meetings or phone calls were not preferred by parents, as indicated by the survey of Crockett and colleagues (1988) and by the low attendance rates in after-school programs in the Nader and Baranowski studies.

There is little evidence that family involvement is useful for middle or high school students, as has been shown in several studies (Coates, Barofsky, Saylor, Simons-Morton, Huster, Sereghy, Straugh, Jacobs, & Kidd 1985; Petchers, Hirsch, & Bloch, 1987; La Porte, Gibbons, & Cross, 1989). Peer involvement may be effective as shown in the "Slice of Life" study for tenth-graders (Perry, Klepp, Halper, Dudovitz, Golden, Griffin, & Smyth, 1987).

Programs that intervene on the school and larger environments are likely to enhance effectiveness. The United States Department of Agriculture, which provides funding for school meals, encourages a link between school meals and classroom education. Several of the school health promotion studies have included school lunch modifications as part of their overall programs. These have shown that school meals can be modified to make them more healthful (e.g., Simons-Morton et al., 1991) and that the combined effects of meal modifications and classroom education can have some positive effects (Arbeit, Johnson, Mott, Harsha, Nicklas, Webber, & Berenson, 1992; Parcel, Simons-Morton, O'Hara, Baranowski, & Wilson, 1989). In addition, making changes in the school meals themselves can modify dietary intakes even without an educational component (Ellison et al., 1989).

Several school-based studies were also part of larger community interventions. In the Class of 89 study, where a cohort of students was followed from grades 6 through 12, significant intervention effects for food choice behaviors were seen in both boys and girls and at most grades of the seven years of measurement (Lytle, Kelder, Perry, & Klepp, 1994). Since school-based interventions were rather minimal (one hour in grade 6 and 10 sessions in grade 10), the intervention effect must be at least partially due to the community intervention activities occurring concurrently.

Overall, then, effective programs are those that address all three categories that influence behavior summarized in Figure 16.1. The preferences/affective component focuses on providing opportunities to taste and enjoy healthful foods. The cognitive-motivational component of the programs focuses on exploring the motivations underlying food choice behaviors such as beliefs, values, and emotional meanings of foods to individuals. Cognitive understandings are also addressed, but the focus is on the concepts and cognitive skills that are needed to carry out targeted behaviors, including understanding the social, cultural, and environmental contexts of these behaviors, in addition to evaluation of these contexts. The successful programs also attempted to build normative support for desired change and to create more supportive environments.

Finally, effective nutrition education programs attempted to integrate these components in some way, usually by providing students practice in a systematic process of developing or changing behaviors (e.g., Coates, Jeffrey, & Slinkard, 1981). This process involves self-assessment of dietary intake or food-related practices in order to identify problem behaviors; understanding the motivational forces behind current behaviors; setting goals for change; observation of desired behaviors being modeled; enhancing self-efficacy through skill building; experiential, hands-on learning; and reinforcements and incentives for change.

SUMMARY

Various conditions of impaired health or developments in childhood and adolescence are associated with food choice behavior in this period of life. Risks for diseases that develop later in life, such as cancer and cardiac disease, also are linked with early nutrition, because early eating patterns persist to some degree and because some consequences of earlier nutrition only become evident much later in life (e.g., osteoporosis). Intakes of specific nutrients, such as calcium, and of types of foods, such as fruits and vegetables, are known to be generally deficient in these populations.

Influences on food choices by children and adolescents may be classified into three categories: food and physiological factors, cognitive-motivational factors, and environmental factors. Younger children's food choices are largely controlled by preferences or liking of foods, and by environmental factors, especially the family. Research has shed light on the development of food preferences and how food preferences may be shaped in the direction of a more healthful diet. With development, children and adolescents acquire beliefs and knowledge about food, which combine with values placed on consequences of food intake (e.g., to be healthy or slim) in a process of cognitive self-regulation in food choice. These beliefs and values are influenced by culture, reference groups, educational programs, and other environmental factors. Important environmental factors also include food availability and, possibly, television viewing.

Some success in changing children's and adolescents' food choice behaviors, nutrition knowledge, and attitudes has been reported in well-designed studies. Interventions for dietary improvement are more likely to be successful when they (1) address factors in all three categories of influences on food choices; (2) are appropriate to the developmental level of the participants, targeting influential factors for people at that developmental level in appropriate ways; (3) include family, school, or community components, as appropriate to the population, in addition to individually oriented cognitive and experiential learning; and (4) have sufficient duration.

NOTE

A research grant from National Institute of Child Health and Human Development, HD 16559, funded some of the research described in this chapter. In addition, sabbatical support to John Michela from the Universities of Amsterdam and Waterloo contributed to the preparation of this chapter.

REFERENCES

Alaimo, K., McDowell, M. A., Briefel, R. R., Bischof, A. M., Caughman, C. R., Loria, C. M., & Johnson, C. L. (1994). Dietary intake of vitamins, minerals, and fiber of persons ages 2 months and over in the United States: Third National Health and Nutrition Examination Survey, Phase 1, 1988–91. Advance data from vital and health statistics, no. 258. Hyattsville, MD: National Center for Health Statistics.

Albertson, A. M., Tobelmann, R. C., Engstron, A., & Asp, E. H. (1992). Nutrient intakes of 2 to 10 year old children: 10-year trends. *Journal of American Dietetic Association, 92,* 1492–1496.

American Dietetic Association. (1990). Position of the American Dietetic Association: Domestic hunger and inadequate access to food. *Journal of American Dietetic Association, 90,* 1437–1441.

American School Health Association, Association for the Advancement of Health Education, Society for Public Health Education. (1989). *The National Adolescent Student Health Survey: A report on the health of America's youth.* Oakland, CA: Third Party Publishing.

Arbeit, M. L., Johnson, C. C., Mott, D. S., Harsha, D. W., Nicklas, T. A., Webber, L. S., & Berenson, G. S. (1992). The Heart Smart cardiovascular school health promotion: Behavior correlates of risk factor change. *Preventive Medicine, 21,* 8–32.

Bandura, A. (1986). *Social foundations of thought and action:* Englewood Cliffs, NJ: Prentice-Hall.

Baranowski, T., Henske, J., Simons-Morton, B., Palmer, J., Tiernan, K., Hooks, P. C., & Dunn, J. K. (1990). Dietary change for cardiovascular disease prevention among Black-American families. *Health Education Research, 5,* 433–443.

Berenbaum, S. (1986). Evaluation of "Good Beginnings": A nutrition education program for preschoolers. *Journal of the Canadian Dietetic Association, 47,* 107–110.

Birch, L. L. (1979). Preschool children's food preferences and consumption patterns. *Journal of Nutrition Education, 11,* 189–192.

Birch, L. L. (1980a). Effects of peer models' food choices and eating behaviors on preschoolers' food preferences. *Child Development, 51,* 489–496.

Birch, L. L. (1980b). The relationship between children's food preferences and those of their parents. *Journal of Nutrition Education, 12,* 14–18.

Birch, L. L. (1989). Development aspects of eating. In R. Shepherd (Ed.), *Handbook of the Psychophysiology of Human Eating.* New York: Wiley.

Birch, L. L. (1992). Children's preferences for high-fat foods. *Nutrition Reviews, 50,* 249–255.

Birch, L. L., & Deysher, M. (1985). Conditioned and unconditioned caloric compensation: Evidence for self regulation of food intake by young children. *Learning and Motivation, 16,* 341–355.

Birch, L. L., & Marlin, D. W. (1982). I don't like it; I never tried it: Effects of exposure on two-year-old children's food preferences. *Appetite: Journal for Intake Research, 3,* 353–360.

Birch, L. L., Marlin, D. W., & Rotter, J. (1984). Eating as the "means" activity in a contingency: Effects on young children's food preferences. *Child Development, 55,* 431–439.

Birch, L. L., McPhee, L., Shoba, B. C., Pirok, E., & Steinberg, L. (1987a). What kind of exposure reduces children's food neophobia? *Appetite, 9,* 171–178.

Birch, L. L., McPhee, L., Shoba, B. C., Steinberg, L., & Krehbiel, R. (1987b). Clean up your plate: Effects of child feeding practices on the conditioning of meal size. *Learning and Motivation, 18,* 301–317.

Birch, L. L., McPhee, L., Steinberg, L., & Sullivan, S. (1990). Conditioned flavor preferences in young children. *Physiology & Behavior, 47,* 501–505.

Birch, L. L., Zimmerman, S. I., & Hind, H. (1980). The influence of social-affective context on the formation of children's food preferences. *Child Development, 51,* 856–861.

Block, G., Patterson, B., & Subar, A. (1992). Fruit, vegetables, and cancer prevention: A review of the epidemiologic evidence. *Nutrition & Cancer, 18,* 1–29.

Briley, M. E., & Roberts-Gray, C. R. R. (1994). Nutrition standards in child care programs: Technical support paper. *Journal of the American Dietetic Association, 94,* 324–328.

Burnett, K. F., Magel, P. E., Harrington, S., & Taylor, C. B. (1989). Computer-assisted behavioral health counseling for high school students. *Journal of Counseling Psychology, 36,* 63–67.

Bush, P. J., & Ionnotti, R. J. (1990). A children's health belief model. *Medical Care, 28,* 69–86.

Bush, P. J., Zuckerman, A. E., Taggart, V. S., Theiss, P. K., Peleg, E. O., & Smith, S. A. (1989). Cardiovascular risk factor prevention in black school children: The 'Know Your Body' evaluation project. *Health Education Quarterly, 16,* 215–227.

Butrum, R. R., Clifford, C. K., & Lanza, E. (1988). NCI dietary guidelines: Rationale. *American Journal of Clinical Nutrition, 48,* 888–895.

Byrd-Bredbenner, C., Marecic, M. L., & Bernstein, J. (1993). Development of a nutrition education curriculum for Head Start children. *Journal of Nutrition Education, 25,* 134–139.

Casey, V. A., Dwyer, J. T., Coleman, K. A., & Valadian, I. (1992). Body mass index from childhood to middle age: A 50 year follow-up. *American Journal of Clinical Nutrition, 56,* 14–18.

Centers for Disease Control. (1991). Participation in school physical education and selected dietary patterns among high school students - United States. *Morbidity and Mortality Weekly Report, 41.*

Centers for Disease Control. (1994). Prevalence of overweight among adolescents—United States. *Morbidity and Mortality Weekly Report, 43,* 818–821.

Centers for Disease Control. (1995). *Guidelines for nutrition education in school health programs.* Division of Adolescent and School Health, Center for Chronic Disease Prevention and Health Promotion, Centers for Disease Control and Prevention (CDC). Atlanta, GA: U.S. Department of Health and Human Services, Public Health Service.

Chapman, G., & MacLean, H. (1993). "Junk food" and "healthy food": Meanings of food in adolescent women's culture. *Journal of Nutrition Education, 25,* 108–113.

Clarke, W. R., Woolson, R. F., & Lauer, R. M. (1986). Changes in ponderosity and blood pressure in childhood: The Muscatine Study. *American Journal of Epidemiology, 124,* 195–206.

Coates, T. J., Barofsky, I., Saylor, K. E., Simons-Morton, B., Huster, W., Sereghy, E., Straugh, S., Jacobs, H., & Kidd, L. (1985). Modifying the snack consumption patterns of inner city high school students: The Great Sensations Study. *Preventive Medicine, 14,* 234–247.

Coates, T. J., Jeffrey, R. W., & Slinkard, L. A. (1981). Heart healthy eating and exercise: Introducing and maintaining changes in health behaviors. *American Journal of Public Health, 71,* 15–23.

Community Research Center. (1980). SPEAC for Nutrition: Preschool nutrition education project evaluation report. Report submitted to the Food and Nutrition Services, USDA, under contract 59-3198-8-28, Ausberg College, Minneapolis.

Connell, D. B., Turner, R. R., & Mason, E. F. (1985). Summary of findings of the School Health Education Evaluation: Health promotion effectiveness, implementation, and costs. *Journal of School Health, 55,* 316–321.

Contento, I. R. (1980). Kindergarten through sixth grade nutrition education. In *Teaching nutrition: A review of programs and research* (pp. 159–230). Cambridge, MA: Abt Books.

Contento, I. (1981). Children's thinking about food and eating—A Piagetian-based study. *Journal of Nutrition Education, 13(Suppl.),* S86–S90.

Contento, I. R., Balch, G. I., Bronner, V. L., Lytle, L. A., Maloney, S. K., Olson, C. M., & Swadener, S. S. (1995). The effectiveness of nutrition education and implications for nutrition education policy, programs and research. *Journal of Nutrition Education, 27,* forthcoming.

Contento, I. R., Basch, C., Shea, S., Gutin, B., Zybert, P., Michela, J. L. & Rips, J. (1993). Relationship of mothers' food choice criteria to food intake of preschool children: Identification of family subgroups. *Health Education Quarterly, 20,* 243–259.

Contento, I. R., Manning, A. D., & Shannon, B. (1992). Research perspective on school-based nutrition education. *Journal of Nutrition Education, 24,* 247–260.

Contento, I. R., Michela, J. L., & Goldberg, C. J. (1988). Food choice among adolescents: Population segmentation by motivations. *Journal of Nutrition Education, 20,* 289–298.

Contento, I. R., Michela, J. M., & Williams, S. S. (in press). Adolescent food choice criteria: Role of weight and dieting status. *Appetite.*

Crockett, S. J., Perry, C. L., & Pirie, P. (1988). Nutrition intervention strategies preferred by parents: Results of a marketing survey. *Journal of Nutrition Education, 21,* 90–94.

Crockett, S. J., & Sims, L. S. (1995). Environmental influences on children's eating. *Journal of Nutrition Education, 27,* forthcoming.

D'Andrade, R. G. (1984). Cultural meaning systems. In R. A. Shweder & R. A. LeVine (Eds.), *Culture theory: Essays on mind, self, and emotion* (pp. 88–119). Cambridge: Cambridge University Press.

Davies, E., & Furnham, A. (1986). The dieting and body shape concerns of adolescent females. *Journal of Child Psychology and Psychiatry, 27,* 417–427.

Deci, E. L., & Ryan, R. M. (1980). The empirical exploration of intrinsic motivational processes. In L. Berkowitz (Ed.), *Advances in experimental social psychology* (pp. 39–80). New York: Academic Press.

Desor, J. A., Maller, O., & Greene, L. S. (1977). Preference for sweet in humans: Infants, children, and adults. *Taste and Development: The Genesis of the Sweet Preference* (pp. 161–172). National Institute of Dental Research, DHEW Publ No. (NIH) 7-1068.

Deutsch, M., & Gerard, H. G. (1955). A study of normative and informational social influence upon individual judgement. *Journal of Abnormal and Social Psychology, 51,* 629–636.

Devaney, B. L., Gordon, A. R., & Burghardt, J. A. (1995). Dietary intakes of students. *American Journal of Clinical Nutrition, 61(suppl),* 205S–212S.

Devine, C. M., Olson, C. M., & Frongillo, E. A., Jr. (1992). Impact of the Nutrition for Life program on junior high students in New York State. *Journal of School Health, 62,* 381–385.

Dietz, W. H., Jr. (1981). Obesity in infants, children, and adolescents in the United States: I. Identification, natural history, and after-effects. *Nutrition Research, 1,* 117–137.

Dietz, W. H., & Gortmacher, S. L. (1985). Do we fatten our children at the TV set? Obesity and television viewing in children and adolescents. *Pediatrics, 76,* 807–810.

Dietz, W. H., & Strasburger, V.C. (1991). Children, adolescents, and television. *Current Problems in Pediatrics, 21,* 8–28.

Domel, S. B., Baranowski, T., Davis, H., Thompson, W. O. Leonard, S. B., Riley, P., Baranowski, J., Dudovitz, B., & Smyth, M. H. (1993). Development and evaluation of a school intervention to increase fruit and vegetable consumption among 4th and 5th grade students. *Journal of Nutrition Education, 25,* 345–349.

Drewnowski, A., & Yee, D. K. (1987). Men and body image: Are males satisfied with their body weight? *Psychosomatic Medicine, 49,* 626–634.

Ellison, R. C., Capper, A. L., Goldberg, R. J., Witschi, J. C., & Stare, F. J. (1989). The environmental component: Changing school food service to promote cardiovascular health. *Health Education Quarterly, 16,* 285–297.

Ernst, N. D., & Obarzanek, E. (1994). Child health and nutrition: Obesity and high blood cholesterol. *Preventive Medicine, 23,* 427–436.

Essa, E. L., Read, M., & Haney-Clark, R. (1988). Effects of parent augmentation of preschool children's knowledge scores. *Child Study Journal, 18,* 193–199.

Farris, R. P., Cresanta, J. L., Croft, J. B., Webber, L. S., Frank, G. C., & Berenson, G. S. (1986). Macronutrient intakes of 10-year-old children, 1973–1982. *Journal of the American Dietetic Association, 86,* 765–770.

FRAC. (1991). *Community Childhood Hunger Identification Project: A survey of childhood hunger in the United States. Executive Summary.* Washington, DC: Food Research and Action Center.

Frank, G. C., Berenson, G. S., & Webber, L. S. (1978). Dietary studies and the relationship of diet to cardiovascular disease risk factor variables in 10-year-old children—The Bogalusa Heart Study. *The American Journal of Clinical Nutrition, 31,* 328–340.

Frank, G. C., Webber, L. S., Nicklas, T. A., & Berenson, G. S. (1988). Sodium, potassium, calcium, magnesium and phosphorus intakes of infants and children: Bogalusa Heart Study. *Journal of the American Dietetic Association, 88,* 801–807.

Freedman, D. S., Burke, G. L., Harsha, D. W., Srinivasan, S. R., Cresanta, J. L., Webber, L. S., & Berenson, G. S. (1985). Relationship of changes in obesity to serum lipid and lipoprotein changes in childhood and adolescence. *Journal of American Medical Association, 25,* 515–520.

Freedman, D. S., Shear, C. L., Burke, G. L., Srinivasan, S. R., Webber, L. S., Harsha, D. W., & Berenson, G. S. (1987). Persistence of juvenile-onset obesity over eight years: The Bogalusa Heart Study. *American Journal of Public Health, 77,* 588–592.

Galler, J., & Ramsey, F. (1989). A follow-up study of the influence of early malnutrition on development: Behavior at home and at school. *Journal of the American Academy of Child and Adolescent Psychiatry, 28,* 254–261.

Galst, J. P. (1980). Television food commercials and pro-nutritional public service announcements as determinants of young children's snack choices. *Child Development, 51,* 935–938.

Galst, J. P., & White, M. A. (1976). The unhealthy persuader: The reinforcing value of television and children's purchase-influencing attempts at the supermarket. *Child Development, 47,* 1089–1096.

Garn, S. M., & LaVelle, M. (1985). Two-decade follow-up of fatness in early childhood. *American Journal of Diseases in Children, 139,* 181–185.

Garner, D. M., Garfinkel, P. E., Schwartz, D., & Thompson, M. (1980). Cultural expectations of thinness in women. *Psychological Reports, 47,* 483–491.

Gey, K. F. (1990). The antioxidant hypothesis of cardiovascular disease: Epidemiology and mechanisms. *Cardiovascular Dysfunction, 18,* 1041–1045.

Gift, H. C., Reisine, S. T., & Larach, D. C. (1992). The social impact of dental problems and visits. *American Journal of Public Health, 82,* 1663–1668.

Gorelick, M. C., & Clark, E. A. (1985). Effects of a nutrition program on knowledge of preschool children. *Journal of Nutrition Education, 17,* 88–92.

Gorman, K. S. (1995). Malnutrition and cognitive development: Evidence from experimental/quasi-experimental studies among the mild-to moderately malnourished. *Journal of Nutrition, 125* (Supplement): 2239–2244S.

Gortmaker, S. L., Dietz, W. H., Jr., Sobol, A. M., & Wehler, C. A. (1987). Increasing pediatric obesity in the United States. *American Journal of Diseases of Children, 141,* 535–540.

Gunn, B. S., & Stevenson, M. L. (1985). Food, fun and fitness: Nutrition education for a healthy heart. *Journal of Home Economics, 77,* 17–21.

Guo, S. S., Roche, A. F., Chumlea, W. C., Gardner, J. D., & Siervogel, R. M. (1994). The predictive value of childhood body mass index values for overweight at age 35. *American Journal of Clinical Nutrition, 59,* 810–819.

Harper, L. V., & Sanders, K. M. (1975). The effect of adults' eating on young children's acceptance of unfamiliar foods. *Journal of Experimental Child Psychology, 20,* 206–214.

Heald, F. P. (1992). Fast food and snack food: Beneficial or deleterious. *Society for Adolescent Medicine, 13,* 380–383.

Howison, D., Niedermyer, F., & Shortridge, R. (1988). Field testing a fifth-grade nutrition education program designed to change food-selection behavior. *Journal of Nutrition Education, 20,* 82–86.

Institute of Medicine. Food and Nutrition Board. (1993). In R. Earl & C. D. Woteki (Eds.), *Iron deficiency anemia: Recommended guidelines for the prevention, detection, and management among U.S. children and women of childbearing age.* Washington, DC: National Academy Press.

Johnson, S. L., McPhee, L., & Birch, L. L. (1991). Conditioned preferences: Young children prefer flavors associated with high dietary fat. *Physiology & Behavior, 50,* 1245–1251.

Kelder, S. H., Perry, C. L., Klepp, K.-I., & Lytle, L. A. (1994). Longitudinal tracking of adolescent smoking, physical activity, and food choice behaviors. *American Journal of Public Health, 84,* 1112–1126.

Kenney, M. S., McCoy, J. H., Kirby, A. L., Carter, E., Clark, A. J., Disney, G. W., Flyd, C. D., Glover, E. E., Korslund, M. K., Lewis, H., Liebman, M., Moak, W., Ritchey, S. J., & Stallings, S. F. (1986). Nutrients supplied by food groups in diets of teenaged girls. *Journal of The American Dietetic Association, 86,* 1549–1555.

Kirks, B. A., Hendricks, D. G., & Wyse, B. W. (1982). Parent involvement in nutrition education for primary grade students. *Journal of Nutrition Education, 14,* 137–140.

Kirks, B. A., & Hughes, C. (1986). Long-term behavioral effects of parent involvement in nutrition education. *Journal of Nutrition Education, 18,* 203–206.

Klesges, R. C., Malott, J. M., Boschee, P. F., & Weber, J. M. (1986). The effects of parental influences on children's food intake, physical activity and relative weight. *International Journal of Eating Disorders, 5,* 335–346.

Klesges, R. C., Shelton, M. L., & Klesges, L. M. (1993). Effects of television on metabolic rate: Potential implications for childhood obesity. *Pediatrics, 91,* 281–286.

Klesges, R. C., Stein, R. J., Eck, L. H., Isbell, T. R., & Klesges, L. M. (1991). Parental influence on food selection in young children and its relationship to childhood obesity. *American Journal of Clinical Nutrition, 53,* 859–864.

Koblinsky, S. A., Guthrie, J. F., & Lynch, L. (1992). Evaluation of a nutrition education program for Head Start parents. *Journal of Nutrition Education, 24,* 4–13.

Koblinsky, S. A., & Phillips, M. G. (1987). Special "Cooking Friends" add spice to Head Start programs. *Children Today, 16,* 26–29.

Kotz, K., & Story, M. (1994). Food advertising during children's Saturday morning television programming: Are they consistent with dietary recommendations? *Journal of the American Dietetic Association, 94,* 1296–1300.

La Porte, M. R., Gibbons, C. C., & Cross, E. (1989). The effects of a cancer nutrition education program on sixth grade students. *School Food Service Research Review, 13,* 124–129.

Lau, D., Krondl, M., & Coleman, P. (1984). Psychological factors affecting food selection. In J. R. Galler (Ed.), *Nutrition and behavior* (pp. 397–415). New York: Plenum Press.

Lauer, R. M., & Clarke, W. R. (1984). Childhood risk factors for high adult blood pressure: The Muscatine Study. *Pediatrics, 84,* 633–641.

Lee, T. R., Schvandeveldt, J. D., & Sorenson, A. W. (1984). Nutritional understanding of preschool children taught in the home or a child development laboratory. *Home Economics Research Journal, 13,* 52–60.

Lepper, M. R., & Greene, D. (1978). Overjustification research and beyond: Toward a means-ends analysis of intrinsic and extrinsic motivation. In M. R. Lepper & D. Green, (Eds.), *The hidden costs of reward.* Hillsdale, NJ: Erlbaum.

Lepper, M. R., & Greene, D. (Eds.). (1978). *The hidden costs of reward,* Hillsdale NJ: Erlbaum.

Lewin, K. T., Dembo, L., Festinger, L., & Sears, P. S. (1944). Level of aspiration. In L. M. Barker (Ed.), *Personality and the behavior disorders.* New York: Ronald.

Lewis, C. E., & Lewis, M. A. (1982). Determinants of children's health-related beliefs and behaviors. *Family and Community Health,* 85–97.

Lewis, M., Brun, J., Talmage, H., & Rasher, S. (1988). Teenagers and food choices: The impact of nutrition education. *Journal of Nutrition Education, 20,* 336–340.

LeVine, R. A. (1984). Properties of culture: An ethnographic view. In R. A. Shweder & R. A. LeVine (Eds.), *Culture theory: Essays on mind, self and emotion* (pp. 67-87). Cambridge: Cambridge University Press.

Logue, A. W., Logue, C. M., Uzzo, R. G., McCarty, M. J., & Smith, M. E. (1988). Food preferences in families. *Appetite, 10,* 169–180.

Lytle, L., & Achterberg, C. (1995, June). Changing the diet of America's children: What works and why? *Journal of Nutrition Education, 27,* 250–260.

Lytle, L. A. Kelder, S. H., Perry, C. L., & Klepp, K-I. (1995). Covariance of adolescent health behaviors: The Class of 1989 Study. *Health Education Research: Theory & Practice, 10,* 133–146.

Lytle, L. A., Kelder, S. H., & Snyder, M. P. (1991). A review of school foodservice research. *School Food Service Research Review, 16*, 7–14.

Matkovic, V. (1992). Calcium and peak bone mass. *Journal of Internal Medicine, 231*, 151–160.

McDowell, M. A., Briefel, R. R., Alaimo, K., Bischof, A. M., Caughman, C. R., Carroll, M. D., Loria, C. M., & Johnson, C. L. (1994). Energy and macronutrient intakes of persons ages 2 months and over in the United States: Third National Health and Nutrition Examination Survey, Phase 1, 1988–91. Advance data from vital and health statistics, no. 255. Hyattsville, MD: National Center for Health Statistics.

McPherson, R. S., Montgomery, D., & Nichaman, M. (1995). Nutrition in childhood: What do we know? *Journal of Nutrition Education, 27*, forthcoming.

Mellin, L. M. (1988). Responding to disordered eating in children and adolescents. *Nutrition News, 51*, 5–7.

Meyers, A. F., Sampson, A. E., Weitzman, M., Rogers, B. L., & Kayne, H. (1989). School breakfast program and school performance. *American Journal of Diseases of Children, 142*, 1234–1239.

Michela, J. L. (1990). Within-person correlational design and analysis. In C. Hendrick & M. Clark (Eds.), *Review of personality and social psychology* (vol. 11). Beverly Hills, CA: Sage.

Michela, J. L., & Contento, I. R. (1984). Spontaneous classification of food by elementary school-aged children. *Health Education Quarterly, 11*, 57–76.

Michela, J. L., & Contento, I. R. (1986). Cognitive, motivational, social, and environmental influences on children's food choices. *Health Psychology, 5*, 209–230.

Mickalide, A. D. (1986). Children's understanding of health and illness: Implications for health promotion. *Health values, 10*, 5–21.

Must, A., Jacques, P. F., Dallal, G. E., Bajema, C. J., & Dietz, W. E. (1992). Long-term morbidity and mortality of overweight adolescents. *New England Journal of Medicine, 327*, 1350–1355.

Nader, P. R., Sallis, J. F., Patterson, T. I., Abramson, I. S., Rupp, J. W., Senn, K. L., Atkins, C. J., Roppe, B. E., Morris, J. A., Wallace, J. P., & Vega, W. A. (1989). A family approach to cardiovascular risk reduction: Results from The San Diego Family Health Project. *Health Education Quarterly, 16*, 229–244.

National Cholesterol Education Program. (1991). *Report of the expert panel on blood cholesterol levels in children and adolescents*. Washington DC: US Department of Health and Human Services, Public Health Service, National Institutes of Health, National Heart, Lung, and Blood Institute; NIH Publication no. 91-2732.

National Institute of Dental Research. (1989). *Oral health of United States children: The national survey of dental cares in U.S. school children, 1986–87, national and regional findings*. Bethesda, MD: U.S. Department of Health and Human Services, Public Health Service; NIH publication no. 89-2247.

Neilsen, A. C. (1990). *Neilsen report of television*. New York: Nielsen Media Research.

Newman, W. P., Freedman, D. W., Voors, A. W., Gard, P. D., Srinivasan, S. R., Cresanta, J. L., Williamson, G. D., Webber, L. S., & Berenson, G. S. (1986). Relation of serum lipoprotein levels and systolic blood pressure to early atherosclerosis: The Bogalusa Heart Study. *New England Journal of Medicine, 313*, 138–144.

Newman, W. P., Wattingney, W., & Bereson, G. S. (1991). Autopsy studies in United States children and adolescents. *Annual New York Academy of Sciences, 623*, 16–25.

Oliveria, J. A. Ellison, R. C., Moore, L. L., Gillman, M. W., Garrahie, E. J., & Singer, M. R. (1992). Parent-child relationships in nutrient intake: The Framingham Children's Study. *American Journal of Clinical Nutrition, 56*, 593–598.

Parcel, G. S., Simons-Morton, B., O'Hara, N. M., Baranowski, T., & Wilson, B. (1989). School promotion of healthful diet and physical activity: Impact on learning outcomes and self-reported behavior. *Health Education Quarterly, 16*, 181–199.

Perry, C. L., Klepp, K. -I., Halper, A., Dudovitz, B., Golden, D., Griffin, G., & Smyth, M. H. (1987). Promoting healthy eating and physical activity patterns among adolescents: A pilot study of "Slice of Life." *Health Education Research: Theory and Practice, 2*, 93–103.

Perry, C. L., Luepker, R. V., Murray, D. M., Kurth, C., Mullis, R., Crockett, S., & Jacobs, D. J. (1988). Parent involvement with children's health promotion: The Minnesota Home Team. *American Journal of Public Health, 78*, 1156–1160.

Perry, C. L., Mullis, R. M., & Maile, M. C. (1985). Modifying the eating behavior of young children. *Journal of School Health, 55*, 399–402.

Petchers, M. D., Hirsch, E. A., & Bloch, B. A. (1987). The impact of parent participation on the effectiveness of a heart health curriculum. *Health Education Quarterly, 14*, 449–460.

Piaget, J., & Inhelder, B. (1969). *The psychology of the child*. New York: Basic Books.

Pliner, P. (1983). Family resemblance in food preferences. *Journal of Nutrition Education, 15*, 137–140.

Pliner, P., & Pelchat, M. L. (1986). Similarities in food preferences between children and their siblings and parents. *Appetite, 7*, 333–342.

Pollitt, E. (1988). Developmental impact of nutrition on pregnancy, infancy, and childhood: Public health issues in the United States. *International Review of Research on Mental Retardation, 15*, 33–80.

Pollitt, E. (1993). Iron deficiency and cognitive function. *Annual Review of Nutrition, 13*, 521–537.

Pollitt, E., Leibel, R. L., & Greenfield, D. (1981). Brief fasting, stress, and cognition in children. *American Journal of Clinical Nutrition, 34*, 1526–1533.

Porkka, K. V. K., Viikari, S. A., & Akerblom, H. K. (1991). Tracking of serum HDL-cholesterol and other lipids in children and adolescents: The cardiovascular risk in young Finns study. *Preventive Medicine, 20,* 713–724.

Public Health Service. (1988). *The Surgeon General's report on nutrition and health.* Washington, DC: U.S. Department of Health and Human Services; DHHS publication no. 88-50210.

Public Health Service. (1994). *Healthy People 2000 progress report on nutrition objectives.* Washington, DC: Author.

Resnicow, K. (1993). Evaluation of a school-site cardiovascular risk factor screening intervention. *Preventive Medicine, 22,* 838–856.

Resnicow, K., Cohn, L., Reinhardt, J., Cross, D., Futterman, R., Kirschner, E., Wynder, E. L., & Allegrante, J. P. (1992). A three-year evaluation of the Know Your Body program in inner-city school children. *Health Education Quarterly, 19,* 463–480.

Resnicow, K., & Morabia, A. (1990). The relation between body mass index and plasma total cholesterol in a multiracial sample of US school children. *American Journal of Epidemiology, 132,* 1083–1090.

Ross, L., Greene, D., & House, P. (1977). The "false consensus effect": An egocentric bias in social perception and attribution processes. *Journal of Experimental Social Psychology, 13,* 279–301.

Rozin, E. (1973). *The flavor principle cookbook.* New York: Hawthorne Books.

Rozin, E., & Fallon, A. E. (1981). The acquisition of likes and dislikes for foods. In J. Sohms & R. L. Hall (Eds.), *Criteria of food acceptance: How man chooses what he eats* (pp. 35–48). Zurich: Forster Verlag.

Rozin, P. (1982). Human food selection: The interaction of biology, culture, and individual experience. In. L. M. Barker (Ed.), *The psychobiology of human food selection.* Westport, CT: Avi Publishing.

Rozin, P. (1988). Social learning about food by humans. In T. R. Zengall & G. G. Bennett (Eds.), *Social learning: Psychological and biological perspectives* (pp. 165–187). Hillsdale, NJ: Erlbaum.

Rozin, P. (1991). Family resemblance in food and other domains: The family paradox and the role of parental congruence. *Appetite, 16,* 93–102.

Sandler, R. B., Slemenda, C. W., LaPorte, R. E., Cauley, J. A., Schramm, M. M., Barresi, M. L., & Kriska, A. M. (1985). Postmenopausal bone density and milk consumption in childhood and adolescence. *American Journal of Clinical Nutrition, 42,* 270–274.

Satter, E. (1987). *How to get your kid to eat . . . but not too much.* Palo Alto, CA: Bull Publishing.

Shepherd, R. (1989). Factors influencing food preferences and choice. *Handbook of the psychophysiology of human eating.* New York: Wiley.

Simons-Morton, B. G., Parcel, G. S., Baranowski, T., Forthofer, R., & O'Hara, N. M. (1991). Promoting physical activity and a healthful diet among children: Results of a school-based intervention study. *American Journal of Public Health, 81,* 986–991.

Singleton, J. C., Achterberg, C. L., & Shannon, B. M. (1992). Role of food and nutrition in the health perceptions of young children. *Journal of the American Dietetic Association, 92,* 67–70.

Spiro, M. E. (1984). Some reflections on cultural determinism and relativism with special reference to emotion and reason. In R. A. Shweder & R. A. LeVine (Eds.), *Culture theory: Essays on mind, self and emotion* (pp. 323–346). Cambridge: Cambridge University Press.

Stark, L., Collins, F. L., Jr., Ocnes, P. G., & Stokes, T. F. (1986). Using reinforcement and cueing to increase healthy snack food choices in preschoolers. *Journal of Applied Behavior Analysis, 19,* 367–379.

Steinmetz, K. A., & Potter, J. D. (1991). Vegetables, fruit and cancer. I. Epidemiology. *Cancer Causes and Control, 2,* 325–357.

Story, M., & Brown, J. E. (1987). Do young children instinctively know what to eat? The studies of Clara Davis revisited. *The New England Journal of Medicine, 316,* 103–106.

Story, M., & Faulkner, P. (1990). The prime time diet: A content analysis of eating behavior messages in television program content and commercials. *American Journal of Public Health, 80,* 737–740.

Story, M., & Resnick, M. D. (1986). Adolescents' views on food and nutrition. *Journal of Nutrition Education, 18,* 188–192.

Strong, J. P. (1986). Coronary atherosclerosis in soldiers: A clue to the natural history of atherosclerosis in the young. *Journal of the American Medical Association, 256,* 2863–2866.

Taras, H. L., Sallis, J. F., Patterson, G. L., Nader, P. R., & Nelson, J. A. (1989). Television's influence on children's diet and physical activity. *Journal of Developmental and Behavioral Pediatrics, 10,* 176–180.

Troccoli, K. B. (1993). *Eat to learn, learn to eat: the link between nutrition and learning in children.* Washington, DC: National Health/Education consortium.

Turner, R. E., & Evers, W. D. (1987). Development and testing of a microcomputer nutrition lesson for preschoolers. *Journal of Nutrition Education, 19,* 104–108.

U.S. Department of Agriculture, U.S. Department of Health and Human Services. (1995). *Nutrition and your health: Dietary guidelines for Americans* (4th ed.). Home and Garden Bulletin no. 232. Washington, DC: U.S. Government Printing Office.

U.S. Department of Agriculture. (1992). *The food guide pyramid.* Home and Garden Bulletin No. 252. Washington, DC: U.S. Government Printing Office.

U.S. Department of Agriculture. (1994). *Dietary status of school children.* Alexandria, VA: U.S. Department of Agriculture, Food and Nutrition Service.

U.S. Department of Health and Human Services. (1986). *1985 President's Council on physical fitness and sports youth fitness survey.* Washington, DC: U.S. Government Printing Office.

Wachs, T. D. (1995). Relation of mild-to-moderate malnutrition to human development: Correlational studies. *Journal of Nutrition, 125* (Supplement), 2245S–2254S.

Wadden, T. A., & Stunkard, A. J. (1985). Social and psychological consequences of obesity. *Annals of Internal Medicine, 103,* 1062–1067.

Walter, H. J. (1989). Primary prevention of chronic disease among children: The school-based "Know Your Body" intervention trials. *Health Education Quarterly, 16,* 201–214.

Wardle, J., & Beales, S. (1986). Restraint, body image and food attitudes in children from 12 to 18 years. *Appetite, 7,* 209–217.

Wardle, J., & Marsland, L. (1990). Adolescent concerns about weight and eating: A social-developmental perspective. *Journal of Psychosomatic Research, 34,* 377–391.

White, A. A., & Skinner, J. D. (1988). Can goal setting as a component of nutrition education effect behavior change among adolescents? *Journal of Nutrition Education, 29,* 327–335.

Witschi, J. C., Capper, A. L., & Ellison, R. C. (1990). Sources of fat, fatty acids, and cholesterol in the diets of adolescents. *Journal of the American Dietetic Association, 40,* 1429–1431.

Yip, R., Binkin, N. J., Fleshood, L., & Trowbridge, F. L. (1987). Declining prevalence of anemia among low-income children in the United States. *Journal of the American Medical Association, 258,* 1619–1623.

Yperman, A. M., & Vermeersch, J. A. (1979). Factors associated with children's food habits. *Journal of Nutrition Education, 11,* 72–76.

CHAPTER 17

THE EFFECTS OF EXERCISE ON CHILDREN AND ADOLESCENTS

Bruce W. Tuckman, FLORIDA STATE UNIVERSITY

The purpose of this chapter is to (1) examine the amount of exercise typically engaged in by children and adolescents, (2) see what effects exercise has on physical fitness and various other characteristics of persons within these age groups, and (3) consider what can be done to increase the participation of today's youth in exercise programs. Exercise can take a variety of forms, such as running around as a part of play, participation in competitive sports, formal strengthening and stretching activities (e.g., body building, dance, calisthenics, yoga), and aerobic activities undertaken for fitness or fun (e.g., jogging, walking, swimming, biking, "aerobics"). The focus in this chapter will be particularly on the last category, aerobic exercise, or exercise that involves maintenance of an elevated heart rate over periods of time, because of its presumed relationship to fitness (Cooper, 1977).

The possible outcomes of exercise to be considered include the following:

1. *Aerobic fitness,* generally measured as the time taken to run either 800 meters (about a half-mile) or a mile
2. *"Fatness"* or body adiposity, which is an important component of fitness (Bar-Or, 1987), measured by skinfold thickness

3. *Cardiovascular health,* measured through pulse rate, blood pressure, or analysis of fat in the blood
4. *Cognitive ability,* including intelligence and various specific mental abilities, measured by paper-and-pencil tests
5. *Creativity,* measured by the number of divergent response alternatives generated on a verbal or figural test
6. *Self-esteem,* based on scores on various published, self-report tests
7. *Mood,* also based on self-report
8. *Behavioral self-control,* generally measured by observations and judgments of teachers

Outcomes 1, 2, and 3 are all regarded as indicators of *physical fitness.*

The chapter will proceed by considering a number of propositions about children's fitness, health, and exercise in the light of available research, and will conclude by considering the issue of how, if desirable, children's participation in exercise can be increased.

• **Proposition 1. Children and adolescents are (1) relatively inactive and (2) relatively unfit.**

The National Children Youth and Fitness Study (NCYFS; Ross & Gilbert, 1985) reported that although 82 percent of fifth- through twelfth-graders in the United States participated in physical activity, only 41 percent were exerting themselves enough to enhance cardiorespiratory functioning. Even though children in this age group reported engaging in over 12 hours of physical activity a week (Ross, Dotson, Gilbert, & Katz, 1985), such activity is not typically of the variety that contributes directly to fitness because it is not sustained and continuous. Although it may not be strictly true that older children and adolescents are inactive, the nature of their activity, when it occurs, is not of the type that contributes greatly to cardiovascular health.

Another way to view 12 hours of physical activity per week is to compare it to the amount of time spent watching television. Raithel (1988), reporting on the results of the second National Children's Youth and Fitness Study (NCYFS II), indicates that children in grades 1 to 4 watch an average of 17 hours of television a week. Also, physical education classes have been cut back in schools so that opportunities for physical activity during school time are reduced (Werner & Durham, 1988).

Simons-Morton, O'Hara, Simons-Morton, and Parcel (1987) present data on the activity patterns of children as documented by heart rate recordings and direct observation that contradict the presumption that children are physically active. Their evidence leads them to conclude that children receive limited amounts of physical activity, thus detracting from (1) their current physical health and (2) their establishment of a healthy life-style pattern that might carry over into adulthood. They see schools as the place where such activity should logically take place. However, Parcel and colleagues (1987) report that in elementary school physical education classes, students spend only about 6 percent of class time (less than 2 minutes per 30-minute class) in vigorous, fitness-inducing activity. Armstrong and Koenig-McIntyre (1992) review studies that indicate that not only in the United States but also in the United Kingdom, children lead life-styles that can be regarded as "sedentary."

Inactivity is as common in preschool children as in older children and adolescents. Sallis, Patterson, McKenzie, and Nader (1988) report that among a sample of low-income, multiethnic 4-year-olds, 58 percent of free-play time was spent in sedentary activities, such as sitting, and only 11 percent of that time was spent in vigorous activity. There is certainly reason to conclude that activity levels of young and older children and adolescents are less than optimal.

Given that children today are not especially active in a way that contributes to cardiovascular fitness, the next question is whether or not they are indeed unfit. Ross and Pate (1987), reporting on the results of NCYFS II on a sample of 4,678 elementary school students (grades 1 to 4), indicate scores on triceps and subscapular skinfold thicknesses being 2 to 4 mm greater, on average, than they were for children 20 years ago. This represents a substantial increase in this measure of "fatness." For a sample of 8,800 upper-grade students (grades 5 through 12), an average increase of 2 to 3 mm of skinfold thickness was reported in NCYFS I (Raithel, 1988). Research estimates suggest that 15 to 25 percent of school children in the United States are obese (Raithel, 1988).

That reduced activity may be the explanation for this increase in obesity in children and adolescents is supported by the work of Moffatt and Gilliam (1979), who found that decreased levels of aerobic activity were associated with increased fat weight, triglycerides, resting heart rate and decreased maximum oxygen consumption, high-density lipoprotein, and efficiency of heart function. Moreover, a sedentary lifestyle in childhood and adolescence is associated with an increase in the risk factors of blood pressure, lipid levels, and body mass associated with cardiovascular disease in adulthood (Sallis, 1987; Sallis, Patterson, Buono, & Nader, 1988). More physically fit and physically active individuals have more favorable risk profiles.

This last point, that children tend to maintain their relative ranking on variables such as blood pressure and serum cholesterol over time, called *tracking*, is what makes the inactivity of children and adolescents so worrisome. Since such inactivity leads to lower cardiorespiratory fitness and its associated characteristics (high blood pressure, etc.), and that these characteristics persist into adulthood (Woynarowska, Mukherjee, Roche, & Siervogel, 1985; Orchard, Donahue, Kuller, Hodge, & Drash, 1983), it can be expected that relatively inactive children and adolescents will face a higher risk of cardiovascular disease in adulthood than their more active counterparts.

Much of the evidence on the association between activity levels and levels of fitness cited here is based on correlational studies. Reports of activity levels of specific children are related to indices of their fitness, such as performance on a one-mile run, with greater reported activity being associated with better performance (Ross & Pate, 1987). However, it is difficult to establish cause-and-effect linkages in such research since certain types of children may be predisposed toward both higher activity and superior performance. For that reason, it is worthwhile to consider experimental evidence linking activity, specifically in the form of exercise, with physical fitness in children and adolescents.

• **Proposition 2. Children and adolescents who participate in a systematic program of exercise will become more physically fit than those who do not participate.**

The validity of this proposition has been well documented. Duncan, Boyce, Itami, and Puffenbarger (1983) compared fitness levels of two groups of 17 fifth-graders each, one that completed a nine-month (i.e., school year) physical fitness program based on aerobic conditioning techniques, and one that participated in customary physical education class activities over the same period. The aerobic conditioning program included calisthenics (e.g., pull-ups, sit-ups), rope jumping, ball handling, walking, jogging, and running. The physical education class activities involved mostly game playing (e.g., softball, kickball). At the end of nine months, children in the aerobic conditioning program exceeded those in the physical education class activity in endurance, strength, and flexibility (using the battery of tests described in the guidelines developed by the American Alliance for Health, Physical Education, and Recreation; Hunsicker & Reiff, 1976). These differences tended to persist for the three months immediately following cessation of the study.

Tuckman and Hinkle (1986) studied 154 fourth-, fifth-, and sixth-graders, half of whom were randomly assigned to a running group, the other half to regular physical education class activities over a 12-week period. The running program consisted of three 30-minute sessions per week, undertaken in lieu of attendance in the regular physical education classes. Fitness was measured by performance on an 800-meter run, skinfold thickness, and pulse rate. Children in the running group significantly outperformed children in the regular physical education classes in the 800-meter run immediately following treatment, and the difference persisted five months later for boys but not for girls. Children in the running group also had significantly lower pulse rates than those in the comparison group. On skinfold thickness, boys in the running group had significantly lower values than boys in the comparison group, but differences for girls were not significant.

Interestingly, after completing treatments, the groups in this study did not differ on a measure of an aerobic performance (time to complete a 50-meter dash). This indicates that aerobic training, which involves maintaining an elevated heart rate, does not affect an aerobic "fitness," which is reflected in the capacity for energy "bursts." However, results of this well-controlled, true design experiment showed that aerobic exercise improved aerobic function and fitness in children, although somewhat more so in boys than in girls.

Werner and Durham (1988) studied 130 fourth- and sixth-grade students in four intact classes. Two classes, one from each grade, received an hour of extra physical education a week (20 minutes a day, three days a week). During the extra time, students engaged in exercises related to flexibility, strength, and cardiorespiratory endurance. The remaining two classes only received regular physical education class activities. The South Carolina Physical Fitness Test was administered before and after the nine-week treatments. Children receiving special fitness training reduced their skinfold measurements by an average of 3.3 mm, whereas children in the control group showed increases of 0.9 mm, on average. On the mile run, children in the fitness training group improved their times by an average of 83 seconds compared to 22 seconds for controls. Again, aerobic exercise was found to yield improved fitness in children.

Lungo (1991) studied adolescent female volunteers, 86 of whom had completed a physical education class six months prior to the study, and 79 of whom participated in a 12-week aerobic exercise program during physical education classes. The aerobic exercise program was found to produce a significant reduction in total cholesterol, apolipoprotein B, and body fat levels (all risk factors for cardiovascular disease), whereas high-density lipoprotein (HDL) and apolipoprotein A-1 levels remained the same. Only total cholesterol and HDL levels decreased for members of the control group, the latter being an undesirable outcome. It was concluded that risk reduction for cardiovascular disease is possible during adolescent years through participation in aerobic exercise.

Hinkle, Tuckman, and Sampson (1993) carried out a replication and extension of the Tuckman and Hinkle (1986) study with eighth-graders. A total of 85 students were randomly assigned to either a running exercise group or regular physical education class group. After eight weeks, students receiving the daily 30-minute, running exercise treatment showed significantly greater improvement than students receiving regular physical education on aerobic capacity (i.e., time to complete an 800-meter run), greater reductions in systolic blood pressure, and greater reductions in subcutaneous adipose tissue (body fat) measured at the tricep. This is further evidence of the positive effect of aerobic exercise on cardiorespiratory fitness and "fatness." Unfortunately, eight weeks after completion of the experiment, no differences were found between groups in an 800-meter follow-up run, indicating that cardiorespiratory effects of exercise are not guaranteed to persist if exercise itself does not persist.

Results of the preceding experiments, all of which compared aerobic exercise to regular physical education class-type activities, clearly indicate that the proposition that aerobic exercise enhances physical fitness is valid for children and adolescents. Aerobic exercise is the type in which participants maintain steady levels of heart rate beyond a normal resting level and below a maximal level over a period of 20 to 30 minutes, two to three times a week. As a result, there is a tendency for improvement in the following indicators of fitness:

1. Aerobic performance (such as running endurance) as reflected by a reduction in the time required to complete either a half-mile or mile course
2. Pulse rate and blood pressure (both being reduced)
3. Skinfold thickness or body fat (being lessened)

4. Content of unhealthy fats in the bloodstream (being decreased)

In all, the result is a reduction in the risk factors associated with cardiovascular disease during the period in which aerobic exercise is maintained. Those fitness gains can be lost, however, when aerobic exercise ceases.

- **Proposition 3. Children and adolescents who participate in a systematic program of exercise will, for the most part, not manifest greater cognitive ability than those who do not participate, but will show greater creativity.**

Results of research shows that exercise has only limited effects on cognitive ability. In other words, exercise does not necessarily make people "smarter." Tomporowski and Ellis (1986) reviewed studies of the relationship between exercise and cognitive functioning and discovered conflicting findings: Some report a facilitative effect, some report cognitive impairment, and some report no difference. They hypothesize that exercise may simultaneously arouse the central nervous system and fatigue the skeletal-motor system, making the result of exercise a function of its duration and intensity, and the fitness state of the exerciser. Few, if any, of the studies they cite were done with either children or adolescents.

Thomas, Landers, Salazar, and Etnier (1993) report on results of meta-analyses of studies that related exercise to a variety of cognitive measures. Most of the studies were carried out with college students and, as in the review just cited, most of the studies were of an ex-post facto nature rather than experimental. Effect sizes are reported for eight cognitive measures, with only three attaining significance (but not of great magnitude). Significant effect sizes were attained for math (es = 0.48), acuity (es = 0.36), and reaction time (es = 0.15). Nonsignificant effect sizes were attained for short-term memory, fluid intelligence, crystallized intelligence, WAIS digit span, and learning.

There are a few studies of children that bear on the question of the impact of exercise on cognitive ability. Molloy (1989) compared two groups of elementary school children after one of the groups had engaged in a "dose" of aerobic exercise. No differences were found between groups on either problem solving or attention span, but differences were found in arithmetic in favor of the exercise group. (Recall that Thomas et al., 1993 found in their meta-analyses that exercise had its greatest effect on math test performance.)

Tuckman and Hinkle (1986), in their controlled comparison of the effects of exercise and nonexercise treatments on fourth-, fifth-, and sixth-graders, included two measures of perceptual coordination generally regarded as reflecting cognitive processing. One was the *Bender-Gestalt Test* (Bender, 1938), the other the *Maze Tracing Speed Test* from the ETS Cognitive Test Kit (French, Ekstrom, & Price, 1963). No significant differences were found between exercise and nonexercise groups. Finally, Ewing, Scott, Mendez, and McBride (1984) compared responses to Rorschach and Holtzman inkblots by exercise and nonexercise groups and found no differences in cognitive process.

In sum, the impact of exercising on cognition seems minimal, other than perhaps some small but consistent effect on math performance. Yet all of the cognitive processes described here have a certain similarity—they are regarded as left-brained. In other words, they are analytical, reductive, and convergent, focusing on obtaining the correct solution to a problem. But there are also right-brained cognitive functions that are more divergent and expansive, often subsumed under the name "creativity." Subjectively, aerobic exercisers—long-distance runners, in particular—report instances of euphoria accompanied by highly fanciful thinking, a phenomenon referred to as the "runner's high" (Sachs, 1984). Perhaps creativity is a by-product of aerobic exercise, brought on by right-brain stimulation.

Using college students, Tuckman and Gondola (1984) compared an aerobic exercise treatment group to a control group on two test measures of creativity. Both tests required subjects to invent numbers of creative solutions—in one case unusual uses for familiar objects, and in the other remote consequences of strange happenings. On both measures, subjects in the exercise group showed greater gains than subjects in the control group.

Tuckman and Hinkle (1986) replicated the effect of exercise on creativity, but this time for fourth-, fifth-, and sixth-graders, in a study that featured random assignment of subjects to exercise and nonexercise groups. They used one of the two creativity tests used by Tuckman and Gondola (1984), *Alternate Uses* (Christensen, Guilford, Merrifield, & Wilson, 1960), a test on which respondents are given the names of familiar objects (e.g., a shoe) and are asked to list as many uses for them as they can. The creativity score is the number of acceptable uses given other than the common one. Tuckman and Hinkle (1986) found a substantial advantage to the those in the exercise group: They produced almost 40 percent more of the creative responses following 12 weeks of running (after adjusting for pretest scores) than did children who attended regular physical education classes.

Hinkle, Tuckman, and Sampson (1993) replicated the relationship between exercise and creativity yet again, this time on a sample of eighth-graders, using different tests than those used in the two preceding studies. They used the lengthy and detailed Torrance Tests of Creative Thinking (Torrance, 1966, 1974), one of which was verbal (and included Ask-and-Guess, Product Improvement, Unusual Uses, Unusual Questions, and Just Suppose) and one figural (and included Picture Construction, Incomplete Figures, and Repeated Figures) These tests measure the ability to make mental leaps in order to avoid the commonplace, and to use elaboration, originality, and fluency. (The preceding studies had used only verbal tests of creativity, and not the same one used in this study.) Results again showed a substantial advantage in creativity accruing as a result of the exercise experience (gains by running treatment subjects ranged from 3 to 10 times greater than gains by controls). This advantage was primarily on the figural measures, and applied to the creativity dimensions of fluency, flexibility, and originality.

The impact of exercise on creativity was also found by Curnow and Turner (1992) in a study of 46 college students. Exercise alone and exercise with music were found to increase scores on a measure of creative fluency, but not on either originality or elaboration.

Explanation for the physical benefits resulting from exercise is quite straightforward and obvious, but explanation for the effect of exercise on creativity is much more speculative. There is little inclination to question a physical activity having physical benefits, since this is expected. But when a physical activity has a mental benefit, an explanation must be sought. One can only hypothesize at this time about possible biochemical changes resulting from aerobic exercise that affect brain function in such a way to produce creativity. (The details of such an explanation are beyond the scope and purpose of this chapter.) There is much anecdotally, primarily in the literature of the running culture, that supports a connection between exercise and creativity.

• **Proposition 4. Children and adolescents who participate in a systematic program of exercise will not, for the most part, attain higher levels of self-esteem, nor more positive moods, than those who do not participate.**

Scherman (1989) reviewed 22 studies that examined the influence of physical fitness activities on the self-esteem and mood of children and adolescents. The great majority of these studies, especially the ones that were done in the school setting, showed no differences in either self-esteem or mood as a result of participation or nonparticipation in physical activity programs. Exercise as an intervention strategy was not found to be particularly effective in enhancing either self-esteem or mood.

However, when used in a camp setting, especially for students with special needs, exercise interventions did tend to show more influence on self-esteem. In a pair of classic studies, Collingwood and Willett (1971) and Collingwood (1972) did find that fitness training improved self-concept and body image among a group of obese adolescents. Also, exercise improved self-esteem for a group of students with special needs (Culhane, 1979).

Among other, more well-controlled experimental studies, the evidence is almost uniformly strong that both self-esteem and mood are unaffected by exercise in children and adolescents. Bruya (1977) compared fourth-graders who did and did not experience eight half-hour physical activity treatments on the Piers-Harris Children's Self-Concept Scale (Piers & Harris, 1969) and found no difference. Tuckman and Hinkle (1986) used the same instrument to evaluate the effect of exercise on fourth-, fifth-, and sixth-graders and found no difference, as well, between exercise

and nonexercise groups. Hinkle, Tuckman, and Sampson (1993) used the Coopersmith Self-Esteem Inventory and found no difference between eighth-graders in the exercise and nonexercise groups. Mauser and Reynolds (1977) found no difference for elementary school students in exercise and nonexercise groups on the Martinek-Zaichkowsky Self-Concept Scale (Martinek & Zaichkowsky, 1975), a correlate of both the Piers-Harris and Coopersmith instruments. An exception was a study by Percy, Dziuban, and Martin (1981), where sixth-graders who ran a mile three times a week showed significantly greater mean gain scores on the Coopersmith test than their nonrunning counterparts.

It is not entirely surprising to find a minimal influence of exercise on self-esteem. Self-esteem is a highly central psychological concept, and one that is based on a wide variety of life experiences. It is likely to be relatively stable, and hence not something that would be expected to change easily, particularly in the short term. It is also not likely to be influenced by one's biochemistry or cardiovascular state, the areas in which exercise has its greatest influence.

Mood, on the other hand, is much more likely to be affected by biochemistry, and thus should be susceptible to the influence of exercise. Several studies (e.g., Morgan & Pollack, 1977; Morgan, 1978; Joesting, 1981; Gondola & Tuckman, 1982, 1983a) have found runners to have more positive mood states than nonrunners, as measured by the Profile of Mood States (McNair, Lorr, & Droppleman, 1981). But these tend to be ex post facto studies of adults, and since adults self-select themselves for running, it is hard to account for cause and effect or to generalize the findings to people of other ages and other circumstances. Even those more recent experimental studies that found a connection between exercise and mood enhancement (e.g., Ewing, Scott, Mendez, & McBride, 1984) were done with college-age students.

Given the expectation of a relationship, Hinkle, Tuckman, and Sampson (1993) included the Profile of Mood States (McNair, Lorr, & Droppleman, 1981), the State Anxiety Scale of the State-Trait Anxiety Inventory (Spielberger, Goruch, Lushene, Vagg, & Jacobs, 1983), and the Discomfort Scale of the Psychological Screening Inventory (Lanyon, 1973) in their experimental study of exercise among eighth-graders. The Discomfort Scale was included because Gondola and Tuckman (1983b) had found a negative correlation between amount of reported exercise and psychological discomfort among college students. For eighth-graders, no differences were found between exercise and nonexercise groups on any of the mood measures, although girl exercisers tended to report fewer symptoms of discomfort than nonexercisers following the treatment, whereas for boys it was just the reverse.

In fact, in a more in-depth study of the moods of eighth-graders associated with exercise and nonexercise programs, Tuckman (1988) found that daily running as a required alternative to regular physical education class activities greatly worsened student's moods, with mood improvement coming only when the running requirement had ended. Rather than experiencing some kind of biochemical euphoria as a result of running, students reported an enormous sense of relief that they would no longer be forced to run. Perhaps this same sense of relief at no longer having to run was true of the girls in the Hinkle, Tuckman, and Sampson (1993) study, thus accounting for their reduction in discomfort as cited above.

The fact that programs of systematic exercise, such as those that use running, may not be expected to produce the same sense of mood elevation in children and adolescents who participate in them involuntarily as they do in adults who participate in them voluntarily has strong motivational implications regarding the incorporation of exercise as a life-style. Perhaps mood enhancement cannot be counted on to motivate young people to engage in vigorous exercise. This is an issue that will be returned to later.

• **Proposition 5. Children and adolescents who participate in a systematic program of exercise will show essentially no greater behavioral self-control than those who do not participate.**

It is possible that exercise, with its physical demands, might provide children and adolescents with a means of using up their "nervous energy," the result being a heightened manifestation of behavioral self-control at home and in the classroom. To test this hypothesis, Tuckman and Hinkle (1986), in their experimental study of exercising and nonexercising fourth-, fifth-, and sixth-graders, had teachers complete the Devereaux Elementary School Behavior Rating Scale

(Swift, 1982) for children in the two groups. This instrument measures the following behaviors: work organization, creative initiative/involvement, positive behavior toward teacher, need for direction, social withdrawal, failure anxiety, impatience, irrelevant thinking/talking, blaming others, and negative/aggressive behavior. No differences were found between exercise and nonexercise groups on any of these measured behaviors.

Hinkle, Tuckman, and Sampson (1993) compared exercise and nonexercise groups of eighth-graders on impulsive behavior as measured by participant and parent responses to the Behavior Rating Profile (Brown & Hammill, 1983). No differences were found on parent ratings, but differences that approached significance were found on the self-ratings, with eighth-graders in the exercise group rating themselves more favorably than nonexercisers.

In contrast to these results are those of one study carried out with a special population—namely, elementary school students with learning disabilities (Bass, 1985). Six subjects served as their own controls, running on alternate days. On running days, five of the six children demonstrated greater attention span in classroom tasks, and three of the six demonstrated more impulse control in classroom behavior. This study was, of course, limited in both scope and sample, and used a group of children for whom behavioral self-control was a serious problem.

It would appear that exercise cannot be counted on to help most children (particularly so-called normal ones) behave themselves, but it may have some potential in this regard for children with special behavioral problems. Overall, the hypothesis that exercise uses up "excess energy" is without support.

• **Proposition 6. Overall, exercise improves cardiovascular fitness and enhances creativity among children and adolescents, but has little, if any, predictable effect on cognitive ability, self-esteem, mood, or behavioral self-control.**

One can now see the extent and dimensions of the exercise effect in children and adolescents. Exercise as a physical activity has primarily physical effects. Training aerobically for between one and two hours a week, for five to eight weeks, has the direct effect of enhancing aerobic capacity as long as the training continues. (Actually there may be some residual effect, but it is definitely limited.) Training aerobically also produces related cardiovascular benefits in pulse rate, blood pressure, and blood chemistry—particularly as related to the digestion of fats. Finally, a reduction in skinfold thickness, an indicator of body fat content (American Alliance for Health, Physical Education, Recreation, and Dance 1980), may also be expected.

A secondary benefit, apparently related to the aerobic enhancement process, is an increase in creativity, demonstrated for children, adolescents, and college students (and even for the elderly; see Palmer & Tuckman, 1994). The effect of such increase in creativity will not necessarily be evident in school performance since most schoolwork requires convergent rather than divergent thinking. However, the legitimacy of the phenomenon of improved creativity as an exercise outcome is difficult to challenge after repeated findings.

Other possible cognitive, psychological, emotional, and behavioral outcomes seem largely unrelated to exercise despite an occasional positive finding under special circumstances. Although exercise advocates may argue for the benefits of exercising on all areas of functioning, evidence strongly suggests that exercise can be expected to directly contribute little, if anything, to the intelligence, cognitive skills, self-esteem, behavioral self-control, or even mood of most children and adolescents under most circumstances. This does not devalue exercise as a recommended part of life for young people, since the physical benefits alone are so reliable and substantial. Moreover, since both life-style patterns and cardiovascular risk factors tend to persist from childhood into adulthood (Charney, Goodman, McBride, Lyon, & Pratt, 1976; Sallis, 1987), exercising in childhood and adolescence would be highly recommended.

• **Proposition 7. To ensure that children and adolescents exercise on a continuing basis in order to maintain cardiovascular health, physical exercise should become a regular part of the program in the public schools.**

Given the data on the low level of cardiovascular health in children and adolescents with high body fat content, it is clear that during this period of life, human beings do not engage in a systematic program of aerobic exercise. Children and adolescents spend most of their school time in sedentary social and intellectual endeavors, while out-of-school activities mostly constitute play. Aerobic exercises such as sustained running, vigorous walking, bicycling, swimming, or aerobic "dancing," all of which involve maintaining a continuously elevated heart rate, represent effort expenditure rather than fun. Although, as George Sheehan (1978) contends, an aerobic activity such as running can constitute "play" for some adults, it is less likely to fulfill this role for young people. And yet, because of the carry-over effect of life-style (Sallis, 1987), the likelihood of cardiovascular health and long life would seem to depend on some continuing involvement in systematic exercise during one's youth.

Given the apparent lack of intrinsic motivation among children and adolescents to engage in vigorous exercise, how then is their involvement in exercise to be accomplished? If children and adolescents are left to their own motivational devices, evidence already presented indicates that aerobic exercising will not occur to any significant degree. Moreover, how is society to get its youth to exercise, when many of its adults do not? In many ways, children appear to learn their sedentary, unmotivated pattern of behavior from their parents, since Sallis, Patterson, McKenzie, and Nader (1988) report a significant correlation between parental physical activity habits and the observed activity of 4-year-olds. Therefore, to increase healthful, physical activity in young people, we must turn to other, more externally based strategies.

One such possible strategy to get today's youth to exercise is to make exercising a compulsory part of schooling, as has essentially been proposed by Simons-Morton and colleagues (1987). Making exercise a part of school will not guarantee that all students will cooperate; indeed, all students do not apply themselves to the intellectual requirements of school. However, imposing such a requirement can be expected to increase children's participation in exercise. Seefeldt (1984) recommends focusing on the tasks of which locomotion and skilled performance are comprised, particularly for young children. However, he himself reports that preschoolers, when given time for "free play," spend most of it sitting in small groups engaged in social play, rather than engaging in vigorous physical activity. Since young children show little initiative practicing fundamental motor skills, they must be directed into it as part of the instructional process.

Sallis (1987) recommends an alteration in school physical education programs in order to provide children with training in health-related physical activity skills. Change is needed, he contends, because "the current generation of school physical education programs are not serving the public health needs of children" (p. 329). It is noteworthy that in so many of the experimental studies of the effect of exercise on children (e.g., Tuckman & Hinkle, 1986; Hinkle, Tuckman, & Sampson, 1993), the "nonexercising" control group activity is represented by regular physical education classes. Clearly, physical education in the schools as currently constituted, and physical exercise, are not synonymous. However, in fairness, it must be pointed out that even physical education classes in school are not the daily requirement they once were. Raithel (1988) reported that even in grades 1 to 4, only about one-third of the students take physical education on a daily basis.

Sallis (1987) also contends that "school physical education programs can be effective in increasing exercise if children are *required* to do vigorous physical activity" (p. 328, italics his). Data collected by Ross, Dotson, Gilbert, and Katz (1985) show that the only potentially aerobic activities popular among children between the ages of 5 and 12 are bicycling and swimming, and these are undoubtedly often done in a manner that is more social than aerobic. Effective aerobic activities that would lend themselves to the format of physical education classes—such as jogging, walking quickly, or aerobic dance—are either unpopular or not done at all (Ross et al., 1985).

Greene and Adeyanju (1991) cite exercise guidelines provided by the American College of Sports Medicine that include exercising three to five days a week for 15 to 60 minutes each time at a continuous rate of 50 to 85 percent of maximal oxygen uptake. As examples of acceptable aerobic activities, they cite running/jogging, walking/hiking, swimming/skating, bicycling, rowing, cross-country skiing, rope skipping, and various endurance games and activities. (These authors also cite a specific and detailed list of guidelines for the development of an exercise program for children that are consistent with the Sports

Medicine guidelines cited earlier.) Kobberling, Jankowski, and Leger (1991) found that adolescents require a minimum of 30 minutes of daily activity at a minimal oxygen consumption rate of 28 milliliters of oxygen per kilogram of body weight per minute to attain and maintain their age-predicted normal aerobic capacity. This represents a fairly vigorous activity level such as would be true of running or walking at a rate of five miles per hour, swimming at a rate of 40 yards per minute, or jumping rope.

What form should this exercise take, particularly if it is to be carried out in school? Cooper, Purdy, Friedman, Bohannon, Harris, and Arends (1975) demonstrated that a running program in school can improve the fitness of elementary and high school students, while Hinkle and Tuckman (1987) describe the details of such a model for using running as part of the physical education program. Greene (1989) recommends what he calls sport-specific aerobics, a combination of sport-specific skills such as making different basketball passes choreographed to music. The intensity of such routines is high, and they are easy to learn. Walking would be a third possibility. Stalnaker (1988) and Fletcher (1989) both showed that the aerobic benefits to elementary school children of walking were equal to those of running. Aerobic dance would seem to be another good possibility for an in-school exercise routine, given its popularity among adults, its use of music, and its many and various forms and focuses. Although mostly popular with women, aerobic dance might gain in its appeal to men if it were practiced in school.

SUMMARY AND CONCLUSIONS

In conclusion, one cannot expect the vast majority of children and adolescents to voluntarily engage in physical exercise, despite its obvious, healthful benefits. They are not so motivated. Since starting an exercise program early and realizing its healthful benefits may be expected to carry over into adulthood, it becomes society's responsibility to make exercising a part of the requirements of school, probably as a major component of physical education. To make physical education serve this purpose, it must

1. Be a regular requirement of a student's program of studies throughout the years of schooling

2. Include physical exercising
3. Be of the type of exercising that yields cardiovascular benefits (i.e., it requires maintenance of a continuous elevated heart rate at a submaximal level for 20 to 30 minutes)

To accomplish this, changes in the program of the schools and of physical education curricula will be required. The cost of not making these changes will be the continuation of poor cardiovascular health in a large segment of the population.

Short of such changes in the programming of the schools, parents are encouraged to enroll their children in after-school and summer sport programs and camps that involve children in physical activity. Such out-of-school programs have been shown to have some benefits (Anshel, Muller, & Owens, 1986; Bowlsby & Iso-Ahola, 1980), although the nature and degree of these benefits will depend on the quantity and quality of activity engaged in. The primary emphasis should be on participation in vigorous physical activity rather than on organized, competitive sports, although the latter can be used to motivate the former, given the proper circumstances (e.g., universal participation, deemphasis on winning and losing). In other words, activity should be carried out in the way that Nicholls (1984) calls *task-involving* or focused on mastery, rather than *ego-involving* or focused on performance. The potential benefit of enrollment in such programs can be particularly great for children who exhibit little self-motivation to exercise. Also, parents should encourage and prompt their children to spend time outdoors and to be physically active, since both have been found to be associated with increased physical activity among children (Sallis, Nader, Broyles, Berry, Elder, McKenzie, & Nelson, 1993).

Although exercise may not deliver the enormous variety of benefits its devotees claim for it, the issue of whether or not exercising is healthful seems quite well resolved. What remains to be found are ways to motivate children and adolescents to engage in it. This can be partially accomplished by enhancing its "fun" aspects. Largely, however, the responsibility for ensuring that young children and teens exercise will remain with adults, a population whose own exercise habits are far short of ideal.

NOTE

The author is indebted to Michele Mason for her assistance in reviewing the literature.

REFERENCES

American Alliance for Health, Physical Education, Recreation, and Dance. (1980). *Health related physical fitness test manual.* Reston, VA: Author.

Anshel, M., Muller, D. I., & Owens, V. (1986). Effect of a sports camp experience on the multidimensional self-concepts of boys. *Perceptual and Motor Skills, 63,* 363–366.

Armstrong, N., & Koenig-McIntyre, C. (1992). Are American children and youth fit?: Some international perspectives. *Research Quarterly for Exercise and Sport, 63,* 449–452.

Bar-Or, O. (1987). A commentary to children and fitness: A public health perspective. *Research Quarterly for Exercise and Sport, 58,* 304–307.

Bass, C. K. (1985). Running can modify classroom behavior. *Journal of Learning Disabilities, 1,* 160–161.

Bender, L. (1938). *A visual motor gestalt test and its clinical use* (Research Monograph No. 3). Albany, NY: American Orthopsychiatric Association.

Bowlsby, R., & Iso-Ahola, S. (1980). Self-concepts of children in summer baseball programs. *Perceptual and Motor Skills, 51,* 1202.

Brown, R. S., & Hammill, D. D. (1983). *Behavior rating profile: An ecological approach to behavioral assessment.* Austin, TX: ProEd.

Bruya, L. D. (1977). Effect of selected movement skills on positive self-concept. *Perceptual and Motor Skills, 45,* 252–254.

Charney, E., Goodman, H. C., McBride, M., Lyon, B., & Pratt, R. (1976). Childhood antecedents of adult obesity: Do chubby infants become obese adults? *New England Journal of Medicine, 295,* 6–9.

Christensen, P. R., Guilford, J. P., Merrifield, P. R., & Wilson, R. C. (1960). *Alternate uses: Manual of administration, scoring, and interpretation.* Beverly Hills, CA: Sheridan Supply.

Collingwood, T. R. (1972). The effects of physical training on behavior and self attitudes. *Journal of Clinical Psychology, 28,* 583–585.

Collingwood, T. R., & Willett, L. (1971). The effects of physical training upon self-concept and body attitude. *Journal of Clinical Psychology, 27,* 411–412.

Cooper, K. H. (1977). *The aerobics way.* New York: M. Evans.

Cooper, K. H., Purdy, J. G., Friedman, A., Bohannon, R. L., Harris, R. A., & Arends, J. A. (1975). An aerobics conditioning program for the Fort Worth, Texas School District. *Research Quarterly for Exercise and Sport, 4,* 345–350.

Coopersmith, S. (1981). *Self-esteem inventories*. Palo Alto, CA: Consulting Psychologists Press.

Culhane, J. C. (1979). Physical fitness and self-concept: An investigation of self-concept modification by aerobic conditioning. *Dissertation Abstracts International*, 40-B, 1985.

Curnow, K. E., & Turner, E. T. (1992). The effects of exercise and music on the creativity of college students. *Journal of Creative Behavior, 26,* 50–52.

Duncan, B., Boyce, W. T., Itami, R., & Puffenbarger, N. (1983). A controlled trial of a physical fitness program for fifth grade students. *Journal of School Health, 53,* 467–471.

Ewing, J. A., Scott, D. G., Mendez, A. A., & McBride, T. J. (1984). Effects of aerobic exercise upon affect and cognition. *Perceptual and Motor Skills, 59,* 407–414.

Fletcher, C. E. (1989). Comparative analysis of cardiovascular endurance in fifth-grade children participating in a walking and a running fitness program. Unpublished master's thesis, University of Kansas, Lawrence.

French, J. W., Ekstrom, R. B., & Price, L. A. (1963). *Manual for kit of reference tests for cognitive factors*. Princeton, NJ: Educational Testing Service.

Gondola, J. C., & Tuckman, B. W. (1982). Psychological mood state in "average" marathon runners. *Perceptual and Motor Skills, 55,* 1295–1300.

Gondola, J. C., & Tuckman, B. W. (1983a). Diet, exercise, and physical discomfort in college students. *Perceptual & Motor Skills, 57,* 559–565.

Gondola, J. C., & Tuckman, B. W. (1983b). Extent of training and mood enhancement in woman runners. *Perceptual & Motor Skills, 57,* 333–334.

Greene, L. (1989). *Sport specific aerobic routines*. Dubuque, IA: Eddie Bowers.

Greene, L., & Adeyanju, M. (1991). Exercise and fitness guidelines for elementary and middle school children. *The Elementary School Journal, 91,* 138–144.

Hinkle, J. S., & Tuckman, B. W. (1987). Children's fitness: Managing a running program. *Journal of Physical Education, Recreation and Dance, 58,* 58–61.

Hinkle, J. S., Tuckman, B. W., & Sampson, J. P. (1993). The psychology, physiology, and creativity of middle school aerobic exercisers. *Elementary School Guidance & Counseling, 28,* 133–145.

Hunsicker, P., & Reiff, G. G. (1976). *Youth fitness test manual*. Washington, DC: American Alliance for Health, Physical Education, Recreation and Dance.

Joesting, J. (1981). Comparison of personalities of athletes who sail with those who run. *Perceptual and Motor Skills, 52,* 514.

Kobberling, G., Jankowski, L. W., & Leger, L. (1991). The relationship between aerobic capacity and physical activity in blind and sighted adolescents. *Journal of Visual Impairment and Blindness, 34,* 382–384.

Lanyon, R. I. (1973). *Psychological Screening Inventory*. Goshen, NY: Research Psychologists Press.

Lungo, D. (1991). The effect of aerobic exercise on total cholesterol, high density lipoprotein, apolipoprotein B, apolipoprotein A-1 and percent body fat in adolescent females. ERIC Document No. 335326.

Martinek, T. J., & Zaichkowsky, L. D. (1975). *The development and validation of the Martinek-Zaichkowsky Self-Concept Scale for Children*. Boston: Department of Movement, Health and Leisure, School of Education, Boston University.

Mauser, H. J., & Reynolds, R. P. (1977). Effects of a developmental physical activity program on children's body coordination and self-concept. *Perceptual and Motor Skills, 44,* 1057–1058.

McNair, D. M., Lorr, M., & Droppleman, L. F. (1981). *Profile of Mood States*. San Diego: Educational and Industrial Testing Service.

Moffatt, R., & Gilliam, T. (1979). Serum lipids and lipoproteins as affected by exercise: A review. *Artery, 6,* 1–19.

Molloy, G. N. (1989). Chemicals, exercise and hyperactivity: A short report. *International Journal of Disability, Development and Education, 36,* 57–61.

Morgan, W. P. (1978). The mind of the marathoner. *Psychology Today, 11* (4), 38–49.

Morgan, W. P., & Pollack, M. L. (1977). Psychologic characterization of the elite distance runner. *Annals of the New York Academy of Sciences, 301,* 382–403.

Nicholls, J. G. (1984). Achievement motivation: Conceptions of ability, subjective experience, task choice, and performance. *Psychological Review, 91,* 328–346.

Orchard, T. J., Donahue, R. P., Kuller, L. H., Hodge, P. N., & Drash, A. L. (1983). Cholesterol screening in childhood: Does it predict adult hypercholesterolemia? The Beaver County experience. *Journal of Pediatrics, 103,* 687–691.

Palmer, A., & Tuckman, B. W. (1994). Exercise, optimism, and age as predictors of cognitive ability and creativity in the elderly. *Journal of Aging and Physical Activity*. (Submitted)

Parcel, G. S., Simons-Morton, B. G., O'Hara, N. M., Baranowski, T., Kolbe, L. J., & Bee, D. E. (1987). School promotion of healthful diet and exercise behavior: An integration of organizational change and social learning theory interventions. *Journal of School Health, 57,* 150–156.

Percy, L. E., Dziuban, C. D., & Martin, J. B. (1981). Analysis of effects of distance running on self-concepts of elementary students. *Perceptual and Motor Skills, 52,* 42.

Piers, E. V., & Harris, D. B. (1969). *The Piers-Harris Children's Self-Concept Scale: The way I feel about myself*. Los Angeles: Western Psychological Services.

Raithel, K. S. (1988). Are American children really unfit? (Part 1 of 2). *The Physician and Sportsmedicine, 16,* 146–154.

Ross, J. G., Dotson, C. O., Gilbert, G. G., & Katz, S. J. (1985). The national children and youth fitness study:

Physical activity outside of physical education programs. *Journal of Physical Education, Recreation & Dance, 56,* 35–39.

Ross, J. G., & Gilbert, G. G. (1985). The national children and youth fitness study: A summary of findings. *Journal of Physical Education, Recreation & Dance, 56,* 45–50.

Ross, J. G., & Pate, R. R. (1987). The national children and youth fitness study II: A summary of findings. *Journal of Physical Education, Recreation & Dance, 58,* 51–56.

Sachs, M. L. (1984). The runner's high. In M. L. Sachs & G. W. Buffone (Eds.), *Running as therapy: An integrated approach* (p. 273–287). Lincoln: University of Nebraska Press.

Sallis, J. F. (1987). A commentary on children and fitness: A public health perspective. *Research Quarterly for Exercise and Sport, 58,* 326–330.

Sallis, J. F., Nader, P. R., Broyles, S. L., Berry, C. C., Elder, J. P., McKenzie, T. L., & Nelson, J. A. (1993). Correlates of physical activity at home in Mexican-American and Anglo-American preschool children. *Health Psychology, 12,* 390–398.

Sallis, J. F., Patterson, T. L., Buono, M. J., & Nader, P. R. (1988). Relation of cardiovascular fitness and physical activity to cardiovascular disease risk factors in children and adults. *American Journal of Epidemiology, 127,* 933–941.

Sallis, J. F., Patterson, T. L., McKenzie, T. L., & Nader, P. R. (1988). Family variables and physical activity in preschool children. *Developmental and Behavioral Pediatrics, 9,* 57–61.

Scherman, A. (1989). Physical fitness as a mode for intervention with children. *The School Counselor, 36,* 328–332.

Seefeldt, V. (1984). Physical fitness in preschool and elementary school-aged children. *Journal of Physical Education, Recreation & Dance, 55,* 33–37.

Sheehan, G. A. (1978). *Running and being.* New York: Simon and Schuster.

Simons-Morton, B., O'Hara, N. M., Simons-Morton, D., & Parcel, G. S. (1987). Children and fitness: A public health perspective. *Research Quarterly for Exercise and Sport, 58,* 295–302.

Spielberger, C. D., Goruch, R. L., Lushene, R., Vagg, P. R., & Jacobs, G. A. (1983). *Manual for the state-trait anxiety inventory (Form Y).* Palo Alto, CA: Consulting Psychologists Press.

Stalnaker, M. L. (1988). Differences in aerobic fitness of seven and eight year old children after participation in a walking or jogging program. Unpublished master's thesis, University of Kansas, Lawrence.

Swift, M. (1982). *Devereaux Elementary School Behavior Rating Scale II manual.* Devon, PA: Devereaux Foundation.

Thomas, J. R., Landers, D. M., Salazar, W., & Etnier, J. (1993). *Exercise and cognitive function.* Paper given at Consensus Symposium on Physical Activity, Fitness and Health, Toronto, CA.

Tomporowski, P. D., & Ellis, N. R. (1986). Effects of exercise on cognitive processes: A review. *Psychological Bulletin, 99,* 338–346.

Torrance, E. P. (1966). *Torrance Tests of Creative Thinking: Directions manual and scoring guide: Figural test booklet A.* Bensenville, IL: Scholastic Testing Service.

Torrance, E. P. (1974). *Torrance Tests of Creative Thinking: Directions manual and scoring guide: Verbal test booklet A.* Bensenville, IL: Scholastic Testing Service.

Tuckman, B. W. (1988). The scaling of mood. *Educational and Psychological Measurement, 48,* 419–427.

Tuckman, B. W., & Gondola, J. C. (1984). *The effects of exercise on creativity in college students.* Paper presented at the Olympic Scientific Congress, Eugene, OR.

Tuckman, B. W., & Hinkle, J. S. (1986). An experimental study of the physical and psychological effects of aerobic exercise on schoolchildren. *Health Psychology, 5,* 197–207.

Werner, P., & Durham, R. (1988). Health related fitness benefits in upper elementary school children in a daily physical education program. *Physical Educator, 45,* 89–93.

Woynarowska, B., Mukherjee, D., Roche, A. F., & Siervogel, R. M. (1985). Blood pressure changes during adolescence and subsequent adult blood pressure level. *Hypertension, 7,* 695–701.

CHAPTER 18

ENHANCING DENTAL ADHERENCE

Michele A. Keffer, STATE UNIVERSITY OF NEW YORK AT BUFFALO

During the last half of the twentieth century, researchers and clinicians learned a great deal about oral health. With this gain in knowledge and technique, the science of dentistry has focused a large portion of its energy on the prevention of oral disease, particularly caries and, more recently, periodontal disease. Caries are progressive lesions in the teeth caused by breakdown of enamel through acids produced by bacteria. Periodontal disease involves bacterial infection of the gingivae, or tissues that support the teeth. Gingivitis, an early stage of periodontal disease, is an inflammation of the gingivae and may be indicated by sensitive and bleeding gums during brushing, flossing, or probing. If periodontal disease progresses, bone loss may occur, and pockets may form so that there is loss of attachment between teeth and surrounding tissue. Eventual tooth loss can follow (Nikias, 1976).

Children are not exempt from oral disease. Some research suggests that as many as 55 to 65 percent of children have gingivitis or more advanced periodontal disease (Sinkford, 1981). Preventive dental recommendations should be followed from the time children get their first teeth (Schneider, 1993). Preventive oral care necessitates removal or prevention of plaque formation—that soft, adhesive bacterial deposit that allows for oral disease to take hold. Several dental health care practices focus on preventing or removing plaque. Fluoride, whether present in the water system or applied directly to the teeth, helps protect them

from plaque. Sealants placed by a dentist can also armor teeth against plaque formation. Regularly scheduled dental prophylaxes remove plaque and its calcified form from the teeth and gingivae, and dental check-ups allow for the early treatment of incipient disease.

Daily oral home care (brushing and flossing) is an important adjunct to these methods of prevention. Brushing thoroughly removes plaque on the surface of the teeth and gingivae, and flossing removes plaque from the interproximal surfaces, or areas between the teeth and between the teeth and gingivae. A combination of these preventive efforts is the key to preventing tooth loss (American Academy of Pediatric Dentistry Clinical Affairs Committee, 1987; Frazier, 1980; Horowitz, 1979).

Given that optimal oral health may depend on these methods of fighting plaque, what can be done to improve pediatric and adolescent oral health? This chapter will focus on two sets of behaviors affecting the removal of plaque: oral home care (brushing and flossing) and professional care. Adherence to brushing and flossing behavior is the first topic, and studies that focus on increasing these two behaviors will be reviewed. The ability of children to receive professional care (including prophylaxis, restorative treatment, and the application of topical fluoride or sealants) can be affected by dental fear (leading to canceled appointments) and behavioral management problems (which prevent successful treatment and perpetuate anxiety). Research that examines these factors affecting professional care will be discussed.

ENHANCING BRUSHING AND FLOSSING BEHAVIOR

Education, Attitudes, and Beliefs

The first organized attempt to prevent oral disease in children on a widespread scale involves education in the dental office and in schools. The assumption is that if children understand how to take care of their teeth, and why it's beneficial, they will do so. The amount and type of education judged to be necessary varies greatly, and the following programs range from one-shot educational programs to highly intensive programs with repetition of components.

Podshadley and Shannon (1970) tested the effect of an educational program including a lecture, a film-strip, and a demonstration in which fifth- and sixth-grade children used disclosing solution to view plaque in their own mouths, and then were taught to brush and floss properly to remove the stained plaque. The group who received the intervention showed greater improvement (indicated by decreased plaque scores) than the no-treatment control group two weeks after intervention, but the difference was not strong enough to be clinically significant (i.e., to be believed to make a difference in oral health). It is presumed that simply having several unannounced dental exams at school to take clinical plaque measures may have produced the general slight improvement in scores for both groups.

Walsh (1985) tested an intervention with similar components, but divided into four one-hour sessions, on a group of 12- to 14-year-olds from 10 different schools. Although tested knowledge improved for the group who received the education, no significant relationship was found between knowledge, attitude, and reported behavior. Unfortunately, no more objective measure (e.g., plaque or gingival indices) was assessed. The students had increased their knowledge, but this did not translate into behavioral improvement.

Boffa and Kugler (1970) prepared a similar educational program for junior high school students, but added a microbiological component: Students cultivated oral bacteria and viewed samples taken from

their own mouths. Once again, the group receiving this intervention learned more than the no-treatment control group did, but only a nonsignificant trend was found for improved plaque scores.

Bagley and Low (1992) provided an educational intervention for college freshmen, which included a pictorial diagram of periodontal disease progression and a discussion of the importance of flossing. Both experimental and control groups received dental exams, floss, a demonstration of how to floss correctly, a hygiene brochure, and daily record charts to assist in self-monitoring of flossing behavior. Both groups improved in plaque scores, interproximal plaque scores, and pocket depth scores (a measure of gingival health) over a period of 24 days. Unfortunately, no further follow-up was carried out. Although the authors' hypothesis focused on the educational program, their control conditions were apparently highly powerful as well. This may be because both experimental and control groups participated in self-monitoring of behavior, which can be a powerful behavioral intervention in its own right (Masters, Burish, Hollon, & Rimm, 1987). In addition, these subjects were older adolescents, as opposed to the young children and early adolescents used in most of these studies, and this factor may have influenced the results.

Ohler (1976) tested the effect of several highly intensive teaching programs involving 484 second-grade students. The children were divided into five groups, one that emphasized behavioral skills, one didactic, one combined group, one yoked control group (who received dental aids without instruction), and one no-treatment control group. The skill and didactic groups received 28 teaching sessions over the course of a 22-week period, which provided for repetition of instructions and feedback on progress. Despite the extent of such education, by the end of this study the initial improvement in plaque scores in the intervention group was dwindling.

Clearly, education alone, even when extensive, is not powerful enough to increase dental health behaviors. Several researchers attempted to augment the effects of education by appealing to emotions or by trying to affect changes in attitudes and beliefs about dental care.

Evans and colleagues conducted two large-scale studies with early adolescents that compared fear arousal and positive affect arousal. Evans, Rozelle,

Lasater, Dembroski, and Allen (1970) tested groups who were presented with high and low fear appeals, a positive appeal (correlating good health and popularity), oral health recommendations, or elaborated recommendations. Initially, all groups reported increased behavior and showed decreased plaque scores, with the greatest improvement in the elaborated recommendations and the positive appeal groups. However, by a six-week follow-up, all groups had returned to baseline behavior. Once again, knowledge was not related to behavior. Initial cleanliness of teeth was related to final oral health (i.e., adolescents who entered the study in the best oral health left it the same way). The analyses used unfortunately did not directly compare this past behavior effect with the effect of the intervention.

Evans, Rozelle, Noblitt, and Williams (1975) compared fear and positive appeals again, but added intervention groups who also experienced a visual display and verbal statement about the individuals' plaque scores. Interventions were repeated five times over a period of 10 weeks, at intervals of increased length. At the end of the study, all groups, including the control group, had improved, suggesting that the fear and positive appeals were no more effective than simply having subjects' teeth examined with disclosing solution on a frequent basis. What is notable is that decrease in plaque scores did not attenuate over time, as in most other studies, although the clinical significance of this decrease is unknown. Perhaps repetition of the exams and the decrease in frequency, or fading, over time, had the effect of maintaining this behavior.

Albino (1978) designed an intervention to induce change by creating cognitive dissonance with a group of 171 seventh-grade students. Subjects ranked personal characteristics and were asked to compare good oral hygiene to some of the characteristics valued highly by themselves and their peers (i.e., good oral hygiene might be associated with popularity, taking care of oneself, or cleanliness). Dissatisfaction was aroused by having the student rate his or her satisfaction in relation to the valued characteristics and his or her dental behaviors. Other groups received no intervention, traditional instruction, or a behavioral rehearsal approach (which involved guided visualization of the behavioral steps needed to incorporate dental health care habits into their daily lives). The belief consistency approach was most effective (mainte-

nance of reduced plaque levels at a 12-week follow-up), but again, improvements were small.

Albino, Juliano, and Slakter (1977) examined the belief consistency approach again in a large-scale, three-year study. Three groups were compared: (1) traditional prophylaxis, (2) intensive dental care (including topical fluoride and sealant application), and (3) an intervention group that included the belief consistency approach and, for some children, a parent-administered behavioral modification program and intergroup competition. Over the course of the study, the intervention group again had a significantly lower plaque score compared with the other groups; clinical significance is unknown. A treatment effect was not found for gingival index scores; however, these were low to begin with, and so there may not have been enough room for measured improvement in periodontal health.

Kegeles, Lund, and colleagues (Kegeles & Lund, 1982, 1984; Kegeles, Lund, & Weisenberg, 1978; Weisenberg, Kegeles, & Lund, 1980) tested the application of the Health Belief Model to seventh-graders' dental health behaviors. The Health Belief Model as originally proposed states that people will perform health-related behaviors if they feel they are susceptible to a health problem, they believe the problem is serious, they know of methods that will be beneficial to the problem, and the behavior would not be perceived as worse than the health problem itself. This model has undergone several modifications and has been predictive (retrospectively) of a number of health behaviors performed by adults (e.g., obtaining a Pap smear) (Kegeles, 1969), and complying with a prophylactic regimen following rheumatic fever (Heinzelmann, 1962). Fewer studies have been carried out with the model prospectively, and fewer still have applied the model to adolescents.

Kegeles and colleagues conducted two studies, one that required compliance with receiving several topical fluoride treatments over a period of time and one that required daily use of a mouth rinse at home. The behavioral intervention (contingency management) appeared to produce positive oral hygiene behavior during the study, in contrast to information or group discussion groups. However, the Health Belief Model did not fare well. Measures were taken of health beliefs, both specifically for dental behaviors and more generally for health behaviors, but neither were consistently related to adherence in the study. In particular, susceptibility sometimes was found to be related to behavior in a manner opposite to that predicted by the model; that is, those children who perceived themselves as less susceptible were actually more compliant. The authors suggest that this result is an effect of past behavior as a strong predictor for future behavior (as in Evans et al., 1970). That is, children who have been compliant in the past continue to be compliant in the present, and they feel less susceptible to oral disease because they have taken care of their teeth in the past (Kegeles & Lund, 1984).

This review of interventions focusing on increasing or changing knowledge, beliefs, or attitudes towards dental health indicates that knowledge is not necessarily associated with the behaviors needed for good oral health in either children or adolescents. It also becomes clear that maintaining brushing and flossing behavior after completion of an intervention is difficult and often unsuccessful. Evans and colleagues (1975) did have success in maintenance after low fear and positive appeals at a brief follow-up, however, improvements were small. Albino (1978) and Albino and her colleagues (1977) achieved similar results with a belief consistency approach, but some of these subjects were also involved in a behavioral intervention involving tangible rewards.

Bagley and Low (1992) found significant results for flossing, a more difficult behavior than brushing. This study also included a behavioral component (self-monitoring), as did the Kegeles study, which found at least temporary success with contingency management. However, there was no follow-up in this study. Unfortunately, many of these studies had several possibly active components (e.g., instruction, feedback through use of disclosing solution, repeated exams) and it is often impossible to know which components had effects on subjects' behavior.

Behavioral Interventions

Given that knowledge and positive attitudes are not sufficient to induce brushing and flossing by young people, how do programs based on behavior modification fare? Although some of the preceding studies on education and attitudes reviewed had some behavioral components, the following studies were designed to test specific behavioral techniques.

Several programs have focused on relatively simple strategies to motivate young children to brush and floss. Lee, Friedman, McTigue, Carlin, Cline, and Flintom (1981) tested the use of a chart that required self-monitoring on a group of 8- and 9-year-old children. The control group experienced only exams with disclosing solution, oral hygiene instruction, and feedback. There were no differences in plaque and gingival indices between groups, but there were differences for both groups over time, suggesting that simply participating in the exam and feedback baseline had a significant effect on behavior. Unfortunately, there was no long-term follow-up.

Blount and Stokes (1984) used a multiple baseline design with first- and second-graders, testing the effects of feedback, praise, encouragement, and public reinforcement, which consisted of posted photographs of the children contingent on low levels of plaque in the classroom. Trends in reduction of plaque occurred in both classrooms when photograph posting was added to the previous feedback and reinforcement conditions.

Swain, Allard, and Holborn (1982) designed the Good Toothbrushing Game (based on the Good Behavior Game, see Barrish, Saunders, & Wolf, 1969) for use in first- and second-grade classrooms. Children are randomly divided into teams, and each day four children from each team are randomly selected for dental examination. Children received feedback on areas that were not well brushed. The team whose evaluated members have the lower plaque scores wins. Winning team members receive stickers and have their names posted in front of the class. Plaque scores decreased greatly during the program, and were maintained at a 9-month follow-up—a finding that is in stark contrast to those of the educational programs discussed earlier.

Pinkham and Stacey (1975) attempted to use modeling to initiate and maintain toothbrushing behavior in 35 third-grade classrooms. Sociometrically defined "leaders" and "nonleaders" were taught to be models for the rest of the class. Children were given time to brush during school, or could use this time for rest and relaxation. Brushing behavior was 100 percent in 20 of the schools tested, regardless of whether the models were "leaders" or "nonleaders." However, there were some indications that by the end of the 10-day program, the number of children brushing in some schools was already beginning to decline. Certainly, the novelty of the idea likely had an effect on the children's behavior in the beginning, and it is possible that brushing was simply a more desirable choice than resting for these children. However, it is also possible that the modeling did indeed have the desired effect, but that the characteristics of the model were not important in demonstrating this behavior.

Martens, Frazier, Hirt, Mesking, and Proshek (1973) designed a more elaborate program at school for second-grade children. Experimental group members were given the opportunity to earn plastic chips by brushing effectively (judged by exam) and trade these in for prizes. When the children requested help, they were given individualized instruction in brushing, which varied according to the child's dexterity, loss of deciduous teeth, and eruption of secondary teeth. After two months, children could also contract to earn chips by participating in learning activities related to dental health knowledge. Parents were given the opportunity to come to the school to learn about the program and how to reinforce their children at home.

The control group only participated in the periodic examinations to assess plaque level. The experimental groups reduced plaque levels by 30 percent and maintained them 6 months after the program had ended (which included summer vacation). The control group maintained a plaque reduction of 15 percent (possibly a result of feedback with exams and general improvement in motor skills and dexterity over time). There is some indication that students in the experimental group improved their brushing skills, and this may have been as important as frequency of brushing in producing the lower plaque scores. No differences were found between children whose parents participated in the program and those whose parents did not participate. Interestingly, one classroom in the study lost its regular teacher during the year and did not do well throughout the rest of the study, suggesting the importance of teacher involvement in this intervention.

Stacey, Abbott, and Jordan (1972) conducted a behavioral study with 17 children, aged 5 to 17, at an eight-week summer camp for speech disorders. The program included individualized instructions in oral hygiene, verbal feedback and reinforcement, supervision of use of disclosing solution and brushing at

night, cuing using a poster, modeling of brushing behavior by camp counselors, and tangible reinforcement for individually adjusted goals. The children showed modest but continued improvement on plaque indices at the final posttest. Follow-up (two months after the program was discontinued) was available for only 3 children; although they showed some regression in hygiene, scores were still improved from pretest. Unfortunately, there was no control group in this study, and it is impossible to know which elements involved in the study resulted in decrease of plaque.

Several programs were school based, but involved the parents more directly. Greenberg (1977) studied a 16-week behavior modification program with 344 eighth-grade children. All subjects were part of a larger study that already provided the students with annual dental prophylaxes, application of topical fluoride and sealant, and dental health education. Some of the intervention group subjects were chosen from the group of students with the poorest oral health. Other intervention group subjects were sociometrically determined "leaders" of their classes. (The investigator was hoping for a modeling effect with the latter condition, but this nonrandom choice of subjects makes interpretation of the results inherently difficult.) Parents of children in the intervention group rewarded their children weekly for brushing and flossing every day of the week; rewards were negotiated between parents and children.

Project staff conducted four surprise examinations at school and rewarded students for moderately low plaque scores. Staff also visited the students' homes to check progress and guide parents in administering rewards. The intervention group had lower plaque scores at the end of the study than did the control group; however, the clinical significance of this difference is unknown. These results were not replicated for gingival indices, but it should be noted that initial gingival scores were low, leaving little room for improvement. The investigators also noted that all subjects had already experienced a good deal of oral care intervention as part of the larger study, and this may have weakened the results in comparison to using the program with individuals who had not experienced such intervention.

Blount, Baer, and Stokes (1987) evaluated an intensive program with Head Start children whose ages ranged from 3.3 to 5 years, using their parents as rein-forcing agents. Two girls and four boys served as the experimental group and five boys served as the control. Treatment consisted of two phases. The first, Intensive Training, was a multiple component intervention, including repeated home training of the parents and children, and in-school examination and feedback. Plaque levels were checked daily at school. Parents received feedback sheets from the school regarding the child's progress, and confirmed this with the experimenters. Intensive Training was discontinued when plaque scores reached a low level at home visits without brushing instructions from the trainer.

The next phase in treatment was called Thinning, and during this phase, feedback was sent to the home on random days, but less and less often if plaque scores continued to drop or were maintained at a low level. The study design involved both reversals and multiple baseline procedures in order to test the effectiveness of the two phases of treatment. The control group simply received plaque assessment at the beginning and end of treatment conditions for the experimental group. Results showed that preschool children are able to achieve and maintain very low levels of plaque given intensive intervention involving feedback and reinforcement from the parents (a presumed step in the involvement of the parents, supported by anecdotal reports from parents and children, see Stokes, Fowler, & Baer, 1978). Children in the experimental group achieved significantly lower plaque levels and had a trend toward fewer caries. Maintenance of low plaque levels was found 3 to 12 months following completion of the study, but only when Thinning followed Intensive Training.

Thinning procedures used alone did not work as well as Thinning following Intensive Training. The researchers noted that Thinning provides a decreasing, intermittent schedule of feedback, which is likely to result in greater maintenance than continuous reinforcement (Kazdin & Polster, 1973). (Evans and associates, 1975, also showed positive results with a similar procedure, discussed earlier.) In addition, the criterion for feedback during thinning was individualized and determined by the child's previous achievement level, so that feedback was given as needed, not according to a standard, less meaningful criterion.

Claerhout and Lutzker (1981) developed individualized programs for four children, aged 7 to 9,

whose dentists had recommended them as especially noncompliant to brushing and flossing behaviors. All children had received prior dental health education from their dentists. Procedures differed for each child, ranging from reinforcement using stars on a calendar to a token economy and feedback system. The children were instructed to ask their parents to monitor the occurrence of brushing and flossing. Parents were instructed not to remind the children about responsibilities and never to scold them for nonadherence. Multiple baseline designs were used, with reversal as needed to demonstrate effect of the intervention. Four dependent measures were recorded: parents and children's self-report of behavior, plaque indices, and Snyder's test, which tests saliva for bacteria related to oral health. Reported brushing and flossing increased, plaque scores decreased, and bacteria level found in saliva improved, even though baseline levels were moderately low already. Unfortunately, follow-up 6 to 12 months later did not include any objective measures. Parents reported high maintenance effects, and one child's parents kept the contingencies in effect for one year without decline in adherence.

Dahlquist, Gil, Hodges, Kalfus, Ginsberg, and Holburn (1985) designed a home-based behavioral program to increase the flossing behavior of three 9-year-old children. In the first phase of treatment, the children were taught proper flossing technique and demonstrated their ability to floss correctly. In the second phase, cues were supplied, such as prompt cards and a bag to collect used floss. The child was instructed to record the time of day she flossed. The experimenter visited the home to conduct plaque checks and collect used floss, and the child was allowed to select a prize if flossing had occurred daily. During the third phase, the child was given feedback on the location and extent of her plaque scores, and flossed while the experimenter provided corrective feedback. During this phase, prizes were contingent on an individualized criterion level of plaque rather than just the behavior of flossing. Criteria were lowered as performance improved.

Two of the three subjects showed some improvement in plaque scores by the second phase of treatment, but striking and clinically significant improvements were evident for all three children during phase three. Self-monitoring, then, was not enough to achieve good oral health (in contrast to the results of Bagley and Low, 1992, with a group of older adolescents), although it did increase frequency of flossing. It may be that children of this age need repeated corrective feedback in order to acquire the skill required to remove plaque. A finding of particular importance was that plaque scores also decreased on the facial/lingual surfaces of the teeth, which are not affected by flossing. Brushing apparently improved during this intervention although it was not targeted at all. Unfortunately, no long-term follow-up of the children was conducted, and so the resiliency of the treatment effects are not known.

Dahlquist and Gil (1986) conducted another study using a condensed version of the preceding design with three 9-year-old children who had never flossed. Parents were taught a simplified version of scoring plaque on their children's teeth and were taught to give corrective feedback, thus taking over the experimenters' role toward the end of the study. Low levels of plaque were maintained over a period of three to four months, with the parent providing all feedback and reinforcement. Once again, plaque scores indicated that brushing had improved as well, although not the focus of treatment. While this intervention design involves less time on the part of an experimenter or a professional, it does require highly motivated parents in order to be successfully implemented, and this may not be feasible on a large scale.

Summary of Studies on Brushing and Flossing Behavior

The preceding review suggests strongly that educational programs alone are not effective in promoting long-term health care in children and adolescents. This is found to be true whether the educational effort is brief or intensive and repetitive. Some short-term effects have been found, particularly with interventions that simply highlight the salience of oral health (e.g., with repeated dental examinations). However, improvements are small, and the clinical significance of these improvements is unclear, as will be discussed shortly.

The Health Belief Model, widely used to predict various health behaviors, does not explain oral health care behavior in young people. Neither knowledge, beliefs, nor attitudes are necessarily predictive of oral

health behavior with this population. Interventions that attempt to appeal to emotions or induce cognitive dissonance have had some success; again, however, effects tend to be small. In addition, studies that were successful sometimes included a behavioral component such as self-monitoring (Bagley & Low, 1992), or tangible positive reinforcement (Albino et al., 1977). These studies were often not able to define what aspects of the intervention were effective, as many contained several possibly effective factors (e.g., combinations of education, repeated measurements, feedback, and reinforcement).

Behavioral interventions have had more success in improving the brushing and flossing of both children (as young as 3 years of age) and adolescents. (This is consistent with the conclusions of an earlier review by Blount, Santilli, and Stokes, 1989.) Interventions used modeling, self-monitoring, and positive reinforcement in terms of praise, public recognition, or tangible reward. Many of these studies suffered from no follow-up or a too brief follow-up. Studies that did find positive results at an adequate follow-up utilized group norms or competition with young children (Swain et al., 1982), provided token economies (Martens et al., 1973), and/or provided for variable reinforcement in a direct attempt at maintenance of behavior (Blount et al., 1987). These studies were conducted with youth from a wide range of socioeconomic backgrounds, and results did not appear to vary substantially along these lines. (For specifics and some exceptions, see Cipes, Kegeles, Lund, & Otradovec, 1983; Lund & Kegeles, 1982.)

Few age differences in effectiveness could be found in these studies of behavioral interventions. However, researchers who study adolescent medical adherence in general have several observations that might apply. Jay, Litt, and Durant (1984) focused largely on adolescent adherence to medication regimens. The authors emphasize that long-term compliance (which is necessary for good oral health) with this population is particularly difficult, and note that working toward a long-term goal of good health is too abstract for most adolescents (and admittedly, younger children). They suggest continued interventions with proximal consequences as solutions. Friedman and Litt (1986) point out that preventive programs are particularly difficult to maintain with a population that sees itself as invulnerable.

On the other hand, adolescents tend to be highly conscious of their peers' evaluations, and might take an appeal to appearances and attractiveness more to heart. Evans and associates (1970, 1975) took advantage of this in their "positive affect" condition. Friedman and Litt (1986) also emphasize the reactance of adolescents and their issues around emancipation. They suggest that because of these factors, goal setting by the adolescent is more beneficial than contracting with parents or a dentist. Placing responsibility with the adolescent will help avoid rebellion, and self-monitoring is one effective way of accomplishing this (see Bagley & Low, 1992). Habits are difficult to break, and one way to deal with the problem of adolescent adherence is to instill good oral health habits in early childhood so that they may be a matter of course in adolescence.

One problem previously noted in the studies of educational programs is also true with some of the behavioral studies. Some employed designs that specifically tested various components of treatment (e.g., Blount & Stokes, 1984), but others used a number of behavioral techniques (e.g., Stacey and colleagues, 1972, using modeling, reinforcement, cuing, or even experimental demand), and the effects of each of these aspects of the intervention were not teased out.

A major drawback to these studies is the effort and energy required to put them in place and maintain them. Some of the most effective (e.g., Blount et al., 1987) require considerable professional attention. Short-term effects are not likely to offset the cost in energy and time of instituting a behavioral program, particularly those tailored to suit individual needs. Of course, motivated parents may be trained to cut professional costs of managing behavioral modification (Blount et al., 1989), but getting some parents to participate might require another separate intervention!

Another difficulty with these studies that is often not discussed is the imperfect correlation between plaque indices and caries or periodontal disease. It is not known exactly how much plaque is necessary, or how long the plaque must remain on the teeth before disease sets in (Blount et al., 1987), and this is likely to vary with individuals in relation to genetic factors, immune system changes, and so on. Because of this uncertainty, it is difficult to evaluate studies with small changes in oral health. How much of a change is really clinically significant? Fortunately, several of the behavioral studies provided improvements that were large and more likely to be clinically significant.

Some researchers, however, emphasize that oral home care is not enough—professional care is necessary as well. (Orthodontal treatment is a specialty within professional dental care. Much has been written on adherence with orthodontic treatment; for example, see Albino, Lawrence, Lopes, Nash, & Tedesco, 1991; Gross, Sanders, Smith, & Samson, 1990. However, this field of research was viewed by the author as out of the scope of this brief review.) Good professional care requires that dental fear and anxiety not be so high as to engender avoidance behavior or to cause behavioral management problems that affect provision of care. Research on these factors will be reviewed in the next section of this chapter.

DENTAL FEAR AND ANXIETY

Fear of or anxiety about dental procedures is a worldwide problem that often begins in childhood (Bedi, Sutcliffe, Donnan, & McConnachie, 1993; Weinstein et al., 1992). Milgrom, Fiset, Melnick, and Weinstein (1988) found that 66 percent of fearful adults in their survey of Seattle residents reported their fear of the dentist was acquired by or during elementary school, with another 17.9 percent becoming fearful in early adolescence. Dental anxiety tends to decrease as the child ages, but during adolescence this trend often appears to stop or can even be reversed (Winer, 1982). There is some debate about the etiology of dental fear. Dental anxiety has been connected to painful treatment and lack of control in the office (Milgrom, Vignehsa, & Weinstein, 1992).

Weinstein (1990) suggests that dental treatment in developing countries and emergency-based treatment in the United States creates a cycle of fear: Treatment is avoided until there is a serious problem, requiring invasive and perhaps painful treatment. This unpleasant experience leads to anxiety about dental procedures, which leads to further avoidance, and results in poor oral health and more invasive treatment. Weinstein suggests that a strong focus on prevention can break this cycle by reducing the need for invasive procedures that breed fear. Davey (1989) suggests that those who do not experience pain early in treatment experience latent inhibition (i.e., later painful experience is less likely to cause fear unless it is excessive, because earlier positive experience serves as a buffer). On the other hand, Berggren and Meynert (1984) found that adults who reported early acquisition of dental fear believed the dentist's behavior, not pain, to be the most important factor in the etiology of their fear.

Several other factors have been associated with children who exhibit dental anxiety. Alwin, Murray, and Britton (1991) found that children who have higher expectations of pain, lower pain tolerance, and poor attention span had higher dental anxiety. Several studies found that females report more fear (Bedi, Sutcliffe, Donnan, Barrett, & McConnachie, 1992; Weinstein et al., 1992), although it is unclear whether they are experiencing more fear or are less uncomfortable reporting it. Some studies argue that more general psychological attributes play a role in dental anxiety. For example, Brown, Wright, and McMurray (1986) found that the factor most predictive of dental fear was level of general anxiety; and Williams, Murray, Lund, Harkiss, and deFranco (1985) found that children with dental fear were generally more fearful in novel situations of any kind. Venham, Murray, and Gaulin-Kremer (1979) found that children who came from homes that were less structured, who had less responsive and less self-assured mothers, and who had parents who did not provide adequate rewards and punishments experienced more fear than children who did not experience these conditions, again suggesting the impact of a more general coping variable.

Whatever the etiology, children's dental anxiety is believed to have potential negative consequences on oral health. Several studies support the belief that fearful children will avoid dental care (Bedi et al., 1992, 1993; Milgrom et al., 1988; Weinstein et al., 1992), and have more missing teeth and fewer teeth protected by sealants (Bedi et al., 1992). While some studies indicate that very young fearful children have oral health equivalent to nonfearful children (Vignehsa, Chellappah, Milgrom, Going, & Teo, 1990), oral disease sometimes develops gradually, and effects on dental health may take time to become evident (Bedi et al., 1993). In addition, sometimes children are taken to the dentist by parents despite their fear, while fearful parents are more likely to avoid their own treatment (Kleiman, 1982). Fear that begins in childhood and is not arrested may lead to a lifetime of treat-ment avoidance and subsequent poor oral health (Milgrom et al., 1988).

Anxiety is also a major cause of behavioral management problems in young children, whose distress is acted out in behaviors such as kicking, flailing arms, and refusing to comply with directions. These actions make dental treatment difficult or impossible, and in fact can cause injury to the child if unintended contact is made with dental equipment (Stokes & Kennedy, 1980). The next section will focus on strategies designed to decrease fear and increase behavioral adherence so that professional treatment can be performed.

Behavioral Management

The following fear reduction and behavioral management strategies will be discussed: communication (including verbal reinforcement, punishment, and shaping), desensitization, modeling, distraction, escape (negative reinforcement), and teaching coping strategies. Although it is recognized that pharmacological methods are widely employed, they will not be discussed in this chapter. This is not meant to decry their use as adjuncts to behavioral strategies (see Veerkamp, Gruythuysen, Hoogstraten, & van Aermongen, 1993) or as methods of last resort, but rather, to investigate other methods that do not have the same potential dangers or side effects as do pharmacological treatments. There is no evidence at this time to conclude that pharmacological treatment is any more cost effective than the behavioral management techniques discussed in this chapter (Allen, Stanley, & McPherson, 1990). Invasive techniques, such as hand-over-mouth and restraint, will not be discussed in this chapter, as they can be seen as aggressive, are in disfavor among many parents (Weinstein & Nathan, 1988), and are viewed as ethically questionable in some cases (Griffin & Schneiderman, 1992).

Communication Strategies

Communication from the dentist to the child or adolescent has been shown to have significant effects on the behavior of some children. Weinstein, Getz, Ratener, and Domoto (1982) studied communication strategies with children aged 3 to 5. They found that of all communication strategies, immediate direction and specific reinforcement (stating which behavior was targeted) were most consistently associated with a reduction in fear-related behaviors (uninstructed movement, crying, screaming, whimpering, protest, hurt, and discomfort). Physical patting and stroking were also followed by a reduction in fear behaviors. Questioning for feelings had a positive effect, while ignoring feelings, denying feelings, giving reassurance, and simple explanations were not helpful. As might be expected, coercion, coaxing, and put-downs ("you're acting like a baby") were often followed by an increase in fearful behavior. Weinstein also suggests that dental communication should occur while treatment is being performed, as stopping treatment to talk to the child reinforces their fearful behavior.

Melamed and colleagues (Melamed et al., 1982) studied the effect of verbal positive reinforcement (e.g., "Great, you did that very well"), punishment ("Not good. I need you to hold still while I put this in your mouth"), combined use of reinforcement and punishment, and neutral messages. Their subjects were children ranging in age from 4 to 12 years old who received varying amounts of restorative treatment. Children who underwent repeated treatment showed a reduction in anxiety and improved behavior when given specific instructions, regardless of the type of feedback. Children who were initially fearful, were disruptive, or had previous experience with dental treatment did better when the combined strategy of positive reinforcement and punishment was used, as indicated by decreased arousal, increased reported pleasure, and greater behavioral cooperation. Punishment alone was found to have a detrimental effect, particularly for children who were older than 7.5 years, who had previous dental experience, or who were initially reported as less fearful. Boys in the study showed increased arousal in the neutral condition, emphasizing again (as in Weinstein et al., 1982) the importance of feedback, positive and negative, so that the child's behavior is directed.

Greenbaum, Lumley, Turner, and Melamed (1993) studied the effect of touch combined with simultaneous verbal reassurance versus verbal reassurance without touch on children from 3.5 to 10 years of age who had previously experienced dental treatment. Touch consisted of a pat on the upper arm or shoulder two times during treatment. The older children (7 to 10 years) displayed less fidgeting, which was assumed to be related to fear or anxiety, when touch was

used. Children who were touched also reported more subjective pleasure about being at the dentist. Subjective arousal and nonadherence (as measured by inappropriate mouth closing) were not affected. It is unclear whether touch alone would be effective without verbal reassurance. The authors note that type of and amount of touch used was rather arbitrary, and much more research could focus on varying these factors. They also point out that treatment (an examination) used in the study was minimally stressful, and wonder about the effects of touch for first-time patients, or during more frightening procedures, such as restorations.

Desensitization

Desensitization, in the form of acquainting children with dental equipment and procedures in a nonthreatening manner before treatment is initiated, has a long history in dentistry. Weinstein and Nathan (1988) have reviewed a number of these studies, and conclude that use of separate "previsits" to the dental office before invasive treatment is begun can be quite helpful. Unfortunately, this method is not currently in common use because of the extra unbillable time required by dental personnel.

Machen and Johnson (1974) studied a desensitization treatment more closely modeled on systematic desensitization with preschoolers. Children in the experimental group were seen for a therapy visit before their first appointment. A hierarchy of dental fears was constructed for the children based on previous research (e.g., Howitt & Stricker, 1965) as the children had no prior dental experience. Children were exposed to the hierarchy in a nondental room in groups of three for a 30-minute session; then the children were introduced to the operatory. Results at later restorative appointments showed improved behavior following this treatment when compared with no-treatment controls. The difficulty with this procedure, as in desensitization treatment, is the extra cost in terms of time needed, as well as training for the person leading the treatment.

Modeling

Greenbaum and Melamed (1988) reviewed a number of studies that used modeling to reduce children's fear of dentistry. Modeling in this case involves watching a filmed or live model, usually another child, experiencing a visit to the dentist. Coping models show children who are initially anxious but cope with the situation, whereas mastery models show children who are comfortable with the procedures from the start. These investigators found that modeling has been shown to improve behavior in the operatory, improve self-report of emotions, and reduce physiological signs of anxiety. They note that modeling can be used with children of varying ages, both sexes, and varying levels of fear. No difference has been shown between mastery and coping models, but studies on this distinction were few. They believe the determinants of modeling effects involve the information given and the viewers vicariously experiencing rewards. Both filmed and live models have worked, but modeling is most effective with children who have had no previous experience with the dentist, suggesting that some of the effect may be due to desensitization.

Several other studies of modeling are notable. Klingman, Melamed, Cuthbert, and Hermecz (1984) tested a modeling videotape that showed children practicing relaxation skills, controlled respiration, and imagery techniques with fearful children aged 8 to 13. The group in the symbolic modeling condition saw the videotape and were told that it might help them with their own treatment. The active participant group was told to practice relaxation strategies along with the children in the tape. Children in the active participant group reported more reduction in anxiety and had slower respiration during the videotape, and disruption was less in their dental treatment following the videotape. The authors note that this finding is consistent with Bandura's theory of participant observation, and stress the importance of increased attention and coding of the coping strategies due to the instructions to participate along with the models.

Stokes and Kennedy (1980) and Williams, Hurst, and Stokes (1983) conducted two studies that used live modeling. The first involved eight 7-year-old children whose behavior was initially too disruptive for successful dental treatment. During baseline, these children all received instructions about appropriate behavior, a description of the procedures they would experience along with accompanying physical sensations, praise for good behavior, and a colorful stamp. The experimental procedure involved each child coming early for his or her appointment, and ob-

serving the child before he or she received treatment in the dental chair and received rewards if behavior was good. (Reinforcement was a small trinket that was a by-product of the procedure, and the chance to raise the seat for the next patient). Their behavior was also observed by the child following them.

Children's behavior in the visits following observation was greatly improved, whereas the baseline conditions before observation had had no effect, suggesting that children were probably not simply becoming desensitized to treatment. The second study involved four boys aged 4 to 9, three of whom observed and were observed as above, and two who were only observed by a peer. This study eliminated the two reinforcers for good behavior used in the previous study. Despite this modification, all the boys showed substantially improved cooperation during treatment, even though some treatments were more aversive than in the earlier study. Heart rate and ratings of anxiety also decreased or remained at low baseline levels. Two factors particular to this study are noteworthy. Behavior was improved in all cases, regardless of whether the model being observed exhibited cooperative or moderately uncooperative behavior (none were extremely uncooperative). This suggests that a coping model is effective for young children experiencing dental treatment. Also important is the ease with which this intervention can be implemented—essentially no additional cost, professional time, or equipment was necessary.

Distraction

Distraction has been effective in reducing anxiety with adult patients in dental treatment (Corah, Gale, & Illig, 1979). However, methods used to decrease anxiety in adults generally focus on emotional response, whereas those with children focus on behavioral response. Several studies examined the effect of distraction on anxiety and/or behavior with children. Weinstein and colleagues (1982) found that distraction was useful with very young children if used early in treatment, but warn that after an injection, children become wary of attempted distraction. Venham, Goldstein, Gaulin-Kremer, Peteros, Cohan, and Fairbanks (1981) used children's television programs to distract children aged 2 to 6 over a period of four visits. Distraction was not effective; in fact, the children were observed to attend only sporadically to the television, no doubt being more concerned about what was going on in their mouths.

Stark, Allen, Hurst, Nash, Rigney, and Stokes (1989) utilized a more intensive distraction procedure, involving a poster with accompanying story on headphones. Children (aged 4.5 to 7 years) then had to correctly answer a certain number of questions about the poster and stories in order to get a prize. Initially this procedure reduced disruptive behavior, but cooperation was not maintained over the following visits. The children apparently discovered that they could attend part of the time, be disruptive part of the time, and still answer questions correctly and receive the prize. In addition, the dentist's behavior in response to the child was not controlled, and so the child may have learned to be disruptive and thus delay treatment.

However, Ingersoll and colleagues (Ingersoll, Nash, Blount, & Gamber, 1984; Ingersoll, Nash, & Gamber, 1984) had more success with an intervention using contingent distraction. These studies worked with children aged 3.5 to 9, all of whom had had previous dental experience. In the first study, cartoons were viewed during treatment, with the condition that disruptive behavior would result in suspension of the viewing for a brief period of time. The second study was similar, but used audiotapes instead of television. Both studies found that disruptive behavior decreased greatly. The effects of audiotaped treatment were more robust, possibly because children who were listening and not viewing could close their eyes and screen out the visual stimuli of the operatory. Self-report of anxiety was not decreased using this procedure, but scores were initially low and offered little room for improvement. Unfortunately, no studies of which this author is aware have investigated the effects of similar distraction techniques with older children or adolescents.

Escape (Negative Reinforcement)

Two recent studies have used negative reinforcement, or the reinforcement of good behavior by the removal of an aversive stimulus, with children in dental treatment. Allen and Stokes (1987) utilized this method in a multiple baseline study of five children aged 3 to 6, whose behavior during dental treatment was rated as "excessively disruptive." Prior to treatment, each child experienced a reinforced practice procedure,

which involved presentation of the sights, sounds, and some sensations involved in dental treatment. Children were told that quiet and still behavior would result in a temporary "break" from the procedure. Children were not told how much time was required for the ensuing reward, but the length of time criterion was gradually increased as the child's behavior was shaped. Stickers and verbal praise were also used as reinforcers. When cooperation was not given, verbal and nonverbal (eye contact) feedback by the dentist was terminated. Following this practice session, children were allowed to choose a prize, and then told they could keep the prize if they remained cooperative during actual treatment. The escape contingency was used during treatment as well. This procedure was effective in reducing disruptive behaviors, even though some of the procedures were invasive. Children were also rated as more relaxed during treatment, and most exhibited a reduction in heart rate. The positive effects appear to be the result of the escape contingency, and not the prize or verbal reinforcement, as these latter two were not effective during baseline.

Allen, Loiben, Allen, and Stanley (1992) repeated this experiment. This time, the dentist was trained to initiate the contingency during treatment itself, without the prior practicing opportunity. When the dentist used the procedure at least 80 percent of the time, disruptive behavior was again reduced. The authors believe that the procedure interrupts disruptive behavior before it has the chance to escalate, and in fact, the longest time period before cooperation was gained was four minutes. Despite success, the dentist in this study tended to drift back toward traditional types of behavioral management, and additional training or perhaps more frequent use of the technique by peers (Allen, Stanley, & McPherson, 1990) might be useful in maintaining the dentist's behavior in this effective treatment.

Coping

Several studies examine the effects of coping skills on dental anxiety with children, following the suggestion of some studies (e.g., Venham et al., 1979) that coping skills may be deficient in dentally anxious children. The modeling procedure used by Klingman and colleagues (1984), discussed earlier, involved modeling of coping skills, and use of these was effective in reducing disruptive behavior in that study. Del Gaudio and Nevid (1991) studied dentally anxious children aged 9 to 13. Coping skills—including meditative relaxation, use of coping self-statements, and diaphragmatic breathing—were taught in four nondental sessions. Only the intensively taught coping skills with modeling videotape intervention was more effective in decreasing self-reported state anxiety than the control group. No differences were found among groups for pulse measures or disruptive behavior. These results are disappointing, as it is unlikely that such time-intensive pretreatment will be considered cost effective. However, the authors caution that behavior was initially not very disruptive, leaving little room for improvement, and the treatment given was noninvasive, perhaps not allowing for fear and disruptive behavior to build.

Siegel and Peterson (1980, 1981) created a coping skills intervention for use with 4- to 6-year-old children who had no previous dental treatment. The coping skills program involved body relaxation, deep and regular breathing, pairing of relaxing cue words with pleasant imagery, and calming self-talk. Another intervention group received detailed information about the typical physical sensations, sights, and sounds they would experience. A control group had a story read to them by research staff. Both experimental treatments were found to reduce disruptive behaviors, ratings of anxiety and discomfort, and pulse rate at both dental treatment following the intervention, and at a separate treatment one week later. These children were notably younger than in the two previous studies, suggesting that even very young children can learn effective behavioral and cognitive behavioral coping skills.

Summary of Dental Fear and Behavioral Management

It is clear from the preceding review that dental fear frequently develops in childhood and can influence a lifetime of dental health. Several strategies have been tested to decrease anxiety and improve behavior at the dental office, allowing for successful treatment of the child. Communication was found to be important, with an emphasis on feedback, positive reinforcement, questioning for feelings, and, in some cases, physical touch in the form of the dentist patting the child (Greenbaum et al., 1993; Melamed et al., 1983; Weinstein et al., 1982). Desensitization can be useful (Machen & Johnson, 1974; Weinstein & Nathan, 1988) and might be best paired with live modeling, which has been shown to be effective and cost and time efficient (Stokes & Kennedy, 1980, Williams et al., 1983). Distraction can be useful if applied contingently (Ingersoll et al., 1982, 1984). However, this technique requires some equipment, and is probably more difficult for the dentist to use than is escape, or negative reinforcement, in which the reinforcer is simply a short break from the dental procedure (Allen & Stokes, 1987; Allen et al., 1992).

Kuhn and Allen (1994) emphasize the promise and need for more research on the last three procedures mentioned (i.e., live modeling, contingent distraction, and escape). They focus on these as time and cost effective and easy to learn, although it is acknowledged that in one study (Allen, Loiben, Allen, & Stanley, 1992), the dentist did in fact have difficulty maintaining his use of escape with his young clients. Teaching coping skills, which in these studies consisted of behavioral and cognitive behavioral relaxation training and coping self-statements, is also effective, surprisingly, with children as young as 4 years old. Such teaching requires training and additional time of the dentist or other professional, but one might argue that these skills also have the benefit of being generalizable to other feared situations. In this way, dentists can be helpful social change agents (Weinstein & Nathan, 1988).

Outcome measures in the behavioral management studies varied. Some studies assessed measures of reported or rated anxiety, some assessed physiological response, and others assessed disruptive behavior or combinations of these. Anxiety and behavioral disruption are assumed to be closely linked (but not inseparable; see Pinkham, 1993) and measures often overlap. For example, behavioral disruption may include kicking, which could indicate fear and/or anger at lack of control, and crying, which could be an expression of fear and anger or a method of avoidance. The studies, grouped together under the behavioral technique used (e.g., distraction), each evidenced some measure of anxiety and behavior disruption, and further attempts at separating these behavioral responses are not likely to be useful for the purposes of this review.

Likewise, looking at age differences in effectiveness of techniques is not highly fruitful. Even the very young could participate in relaxation and cognitive behavioral coping exercises. Melamed and colleagues (1983) did find that verbal punishment had a more deleterious effect on the older children (older than 7.5 years) in their study. It has been suggested that modeling works best with children who have not had previous treatment (Greenbaum & Melamed, 1988), but Williams and associates (1983) found live modeling of peers to be effective with children who were already labeled as dental behavioral management problems. However, for the most part, the studies did not indicate specific age-related limits on behavioral management techniques. Guidelines specific to adolescents were discussed earlier in the section on brushing and flossing adherence.

SUMMARY

This chapter reviewed research studies focusing on the two basic ingredients of good oral health for children and adolescents: home care brushing and flossing, and professional care of the teeth and gums. A number of studies focused on interventions designed to increase brushing and flossing behaviors. These studies found that programs using behavior modification were generally more successful in improving adherence than were educational programs or programs focusing on attitudes and beliefs toward dental care. Unfortunately, many studies suffered from inadequate follow-up, and further research is necessary to discover just which aspects of these interventions were most effective. While time, cost, and energy are expended in implementing these programs, long-term gain in reduced oral health care costs might make these programs cost-beneficial in the long run for children who exhibit poor adherence. Prevention obviates the need for later expensive and sometimes painful professional treatment.

Professional care is also vitally important to good oral health. Dental fear/anxiety and behavioral management problems can interfere profoundly with the provision of professional treatment. Several studies were reviewed that focused on behavioral techniques to fight these barriers to care. Effective communication involved a combination of direction, positive reinforcement, punishment, and sometimes touch to al-

lay anxiety and shape the child's skills in adherence. Live modeling has been shown to be effective and cost efficient, as well. Contingent distraction works well with young children, but requires some special equipment. Negative reinforcement in the form of temporary escape appears to be highly effective, but further research should focus on ways to teach and maintain this technique. Teaching coping skills is somewhat time consuming, but can be done even with young children, and might be helpful if generalized to other fearful or anxiety-provoking situations.

A number of techniques, particularly those developed out of the field of behavioral modification, can be used both to improve young people's oral self-care and to provide for more effective professional treatment. Continued efforts on the part of dental health professionals to utilize these techniques in private practice, hospitals, clinics, educational, and research settings may further improve the health care of children and adolescents, and prevent extensive treatment and loss of teeth in adulthood.

REFERENCES

Albino, J. E. (1978). Evaluation of three approaches to changing dental hygiene behaviors. *Journal of Preventive Dentistry, 5,* 4–10.

Albino, J. E., Juliano, D. B., & Slakter, M. J. (1977). Effects of an instructional-motivational program on plaque and gingivitis in adolescents. *Journal of Public Health Dentistry, 37,* 281–289.

Albino, J. E. N., Lawrence, S. D., Lopes, C. E., Nash, L. B., & Tedesco, L. A. (1991). Cooperation of adolescents in orthodontic treatment. *Journal of Behavioral Medicine, 14,* 53–70.

Allen, K. D., Loiben, T., Allen, S. J., & Stanley, R. T. (1992). Dentist-implemented contingent escape for management of disruptive child behavior. *Journal of Applied Behavior Analysis, 25,* 629–636.

Allen, K. D., Stanley, R. T., & McPherson, K. (1990). Evaluation of behavior management technology dissemination in pediatric dentistry. *Pediatric Dentistry, 12,* 79–82.

Allen, K. D., & Stokes, T. F. (1987). Use of escape and reward in the management of young children during dental treatment. *Journal of Applied Behavior Analysis, 20,* 381–390.

Alwin, N. P., Murray, J. J., & Britton, P. G. (1991). An assessment of dental anxiety in children. *British Dental Journal, 171,* 201–207.

American Academy of Pediatric Dentistry Clinical Affairs Committee, 1985–1986 (1987). Guidelines for dental health of the adolescent—May 1986. *Pediatric Dentistry, 9,* 247–250.

Bagley, J. G., & Low, K. G. (1992). Enhancing flossing compliance in college freshmen. *Clinical Preventive Dentistry, 14,* 25–30.

Barrish, H. H., Saunders, M., & Wolf, M. M. (1969). Good behavior game: Effects of individual contingencies for group consequences on disruptive behavior in a classroom. *Journal of Applied Behavior Analysis, 2,* 119–124.

Bedi, R., Sutcliffe, P., Donnan, P. T., Barrett, N., & McConnachie, J. (1992). Dental caries experience and prevalence of children afraid of dental treatment. *Community Dentistry and Oral Epidemiology, 20,* 368–371.

Bedi, R., Sutcliffe, P., Donnan, P. T., & McConnachie, J. (1993). Oral cleanliness of dentally anxious schoolchildren and their need for periodontal treatment. *Journal of Dentistry for Children, 60,* 17–21.

Berggren, U., & Meynert, G. (1984). Dental fear and avoidance: causes, symptoms, and consequences. *Journal of the American Dental Association, 109,* 247–251.

Boffa, J., & Kugler, J. F. (1970). Development and testing of a junior high school oral hygiene education program. *The Journal of School Health, 40,* 557–560.

Blount, R. L., Baer, R. A., & Stokes, T. F. (1987). An analysis of long-term maintenance of effective toothbrushing by Head Start schoolchildren. *Journal of Pediatric Psychology, 12,* 363–377.

Blount, R. L., Santilli, L., & Stokes, T. F. (1989). Promoting oral hygiene in pediatric dentistry: A critical review. *Clinical Psychology Review, 9,* 737–746.

Blount, R. L., & Stokes, T. R. (1984). Contingent public posting of photographs to reinforce dental hygiene. *Behavior Modification, 8,* 79–92.

Brown, D. F., Wright, F. A. C., & McMurray, N. E. (1986). Psychological and behavioral factors associated with dental anxiety in children. *Journal of Behavioral Medicine, 9,* 213–217.

Cipes, M. H., Kegeles, S. S., Lund, A. K., & Otradovec, C. L. (1983). Differences in dental experiences, practices, and beliefs of inner-city and suburban adolescents. *American Journal of Public Health, 73,* 1305–1307.

Claerhout, S., & Lutzker, J. R. (1981). Increasing children's self-initiated compliance to dental regimens. *Behavior Therapy, 12,* 165–176.

Corah, N. L., Gale, E. N., & Illig, S. J. (1979). The use of relaxation and distraction to reduce psychological stress during dental procedures. *Journal of the American Dental Association, 98,* 390–394.

Dahlquist, L. M., & Gil, K. M. (1986). Using parents to maintain improved dental flossing skills in children. *Journal of Applied Behavior Analysis, 19,* 255–260.

Dahlquist, L. M., Gil, K. M., Hodges, J., Kalfus, G. R., Ginsberg, A., & Holburn, S. W. (1985). The effects of behavioral intervention on dental flossing skills in children. *Journal of Pediatric Psychology, 10,* 403–412.

Davey, G. C. L. (1989). Dental phobias and anxieties: Evidence for conditioning processes in the acquisition and modulation of a learned fear. *Behaviour Research and Therapy, 27,* 51–58.

Del Gaudio, D. J., & Nevid, J. S. (1991). Training dentally anxious children to cope. *Journal of Dentistry for Children, 58,* 31–37.

Evans, T. I., Rozelle, R. M., Lasater, T. M., Dembroski, T. M., & Allen, B. P. (1970). Fear arousal, persuasion, and actual versus implied behavioral change: New perspective utilizing a real-life dental hygiene program. *Journal of Personality and Social Psychology, 16,* 220–227.

Evans, R. I., Rozelle, R. M., Noblitt, R., & Williams, D. L. (1975). Explicit and implicit persuasive communications over time to initiate and maintain behavior change: New perspective utilizing a real-life dental hygiene situation. *Journal of Applied Social Psychology, 5,* 150–156.

Frazier, P. J. (1980). School-based instruction for improving oral health: Closing the knowledge gap. *International Dental Journal, 30,* 257–268.

Friedman, I. M., & Litt, I. F. (1986). Promoting adolescents' compliance with therapeutic regimens. *Pediatric Clinics of North America, 33,* 955–973.

Greenbaum, P. E., Lumley, M. A., Turner, C., & Melamed, B. G. (1993). Dentist's reassuring touch: Effects on children's behavior. *Pediatric Dentistry, 15,* 20–23.

Greenbaum, P. E., & Melamed, B. G. (1988). Pretreatment modeling: A technique for reducing children's fear in the dental operatory, *Dental Clinics of North America, 32,* 693–704.

Greenberg, J. S. (1977). A study of behavior modification applied to dental health. *The Journal of School Health, 47,* 594–596.

Griffin, A., & Schneiderman, L. J. (1992). Ethical issues in managing the noncompliant child. *Pediatric Dentistry, 14,* 178–183.

Gross, A. M., Sanders, S., Smith, C., & Samson, G. (1990). Increasing compliance with orthodontic treatment. *Child & Family Behavior Therapy, 12,* 13–23.

Heinzelmann, F. (1962). Factors in prophylaxis behavior in treating rheumatic fever: An exploratory study. *Journal of Health and Human Behavior, 3,* 73–87.

Horowitz, A. M. (1979). A comparison of available strategies to affect children's dental health: Primary preventive procedures for use in school-based dental programs. *Journal of Public Health Dentistry, 39,* 268–274.

Howitt, J. W., & Stricker, G. (1965). Sequential changes in response to dental procedures. *Journal of the American Dental Association, 70,* 70–74.

Ingersoll, B. D., Nash, D. A., Blount, R. L., & Gamber, C. (1984). Distraction and contingent reinforcement with pediatric dental patients. *Journal of Dentistry for Children, 51,* 203–207.

Ingersoll, B. D., Nash, D. A., & Gamber, C. (1984). The use of contingent audiotaped material with pediatric dental patients. *Journal of the American Dental Association, 109*, 717–719.

Jay, S., Litt, I. F., & Durant, R. H. (1984). Compliance with therapeutic regimens. *Journal of Adolescent Health Care, 5*, 124–136.

Kazdin, A. E., & Polster, R. (1973). Intermittent token reinforcement and response maintenance in extinction. *Behavior Therapy, 4*, 386–391.

Kegeles, S. S. (1969). A field experimental attempt to change beliefs and behavior of women in an urban ghetto. *Journal of Health and Social Behavior, 10*, 115–125.

Kegeles, S. S., & Lund, A. K. (1982). Adolescents' health beliefs and acceptance of a novel preventive dental activity: Replication and extension. *Health Education Quarterly, 9*, 96–112.

Kegeles, S. S., & Lund, A. K. (1984). Adolescents' health beliefs and acceptance of a novel preventive dental activity: A further note. *Social Science and Medicine, 19*, 979–982.

Kegeles, S. S., Lund, A. K., & Weisenberg, M. (1978). Acceptance by children of a daily home mouthrinse program. *Social Science and Medicine, 12*, 199–210.

Kleiman, M. B. (1982). Fear of dentists as an inhibiting factor in children's use of dental services. *Journal of Dentistry for Children, 49*, 209–213.

Klingman, A., Melamed, B. G., Cuthbert, M. I., & Hermecz, D. A. (1984). Effects of participant modeling on information acquisition and skill utilization. *Journal of Consulting and Clinical Psychology, 52*, 414–422.

Kuhn, B. R., & Allen, K. D. (1994). Expanding child behavior management technology in pediatric dentistry: A behavioral science perspective. *Pediatric Dentistry, 16*, 13–17.

Lee, M. M., Friedman, C. M., McTigue, D. J., Carlin, S. A., Cline, N. V., & Flintom, C. J. (1981). Affecting oral hygiene behaviors in children: Use of a chart as a motivational device. *Clinical Preventive Dentistry, 3*, 28–31.

Lund, A. K., & Kegeles, S. S. (1982). Increasing adolescents' acceptance of long-term personal health behavior. *Health Psychology, 1*, 27–43.

Machen, J. B., & Johnson, R. (1974). Desensitization, model learning, and the dental behavior of children. *Journal of Dental Research, 53*, 83–87.

Martens, L. V., Frazier, P. J., Hirt, K. J., Mesking, L. H., & Proshek, J. (1973). Developing brushing performance in second graders through behavior modification. *Health Service Reports, 88*, 818–823.

Masters, J. C., Burish, T. G., Hollon, S. D., & Rimm, D. C. (1987). *Behavior therapy: Techniques and empirical findings* (pp. 523–525). San Diego: Harcourt Brace Jovanovich.

Melamed, B. G., Bennett, C. G., Jerrell, G., Ross, S. L., Bush, J. P., Hill, C., Courts, F., & Ronk, S. (1983).

Dentist's behavior management as it affects compliance and fear in pediatric patients. *Journal of the American Dental Association, 106*, 324–330,

Milgrom, P., Fiset, L., Melnick, S., Weinstein, P. (1988). The prevalence and practice management consequences of dental fear in a major U.S. city. *Journal of the American Dental Association, 116*, 641–647.

Milgrom, P., Vignehsa, H., & Weinstein, P. (1992). Adolescent dental fear and control: Prevalence and theoretical implications. *Behavior Research and Therapy, 30*, 367–373.

Nikias, M. K. (1976). Prevention in oral health problems: Social behavioral aspects. *Preventive Medicine, 5*, 149–164.

Ohler, F. D. (1976). Oral health behavior: Acquisition and maintenance. *The Journal of School Health, 46*, 522–528.

Pinkham, J. R. (1993). The roles of requests and promises in child patient management. *Journal of Dentistry for Children, 60*, 169–174.

Pinkham, J. R., & Stacey, D. C. (1975). Using classroom leaders as models for teaching toothbrushing. *Journal of Public Health Dentistry, 35*, 91–94.

Podshadley, G., & Shannon, J. H. (1970). Oral hygiene performance of elementary school children following dental health education. *Journal of Dentistry for Children, 37*, 298–302.

Schneider, H. S. (1993). Parental education leads to preventive dental treatment for patients under the age of four. *Journal of Dentistry for Children, 60*, 33–36.

Siegel, L. J., & Peterson, L. (1980). Stress reduction in young dental patients through coping skills and sensory information. *Journal of Consulting and Clinical Psychology, 48*, 785–787.

Siegel, L. J., & Peterson, L. (1981). Maintenance effects of coping skills and sensory information on young children's response to repeated dental procedures. *Behavior Therapy, 12*, 530–535.

Sinkford, J. (1981). Dental health needs of children and adolescents. *Journal of the American Dental Association, 103*, 901–905.

Stacey, D. C., Abbott, D. M., & Jordan, R. D. (1972). Improvement in oral hygiene as a function of applied principles of behavior modification. *Journal of Public Health Dentistry, 32*, 234–242.

Stark, L. J., Allen, K. D., Hurst, M., Nash, D. A., Rigney, B., & Stokes, T. F. (1989). Distraction: Its utilization and efficacy with children undergoing dental treatment. *Journal of Applied Behavior Analysis, 22*, 297–307.

Stokes, T. F., Fowler, S., & Baer, D. M. (1978). Training preschool children to recruit natural communities of reinforcement. *Journal of Applied Behavior Analysis, 11*, 285–303.

Stokes, T. F., & Kennedy, S. H. (1980). Reducing child uncooperative behavior during dental treatment through modeling and reinforcement. *Journal of Applied Behavior Analysis, 13*, 41–49.

Swain, J. J., Allard, G. B., & Holborn, S. W. (1982). The Good Toothbrushing Game: A school-based dental hygiene program for increasing the toothbrushing effectiveness of children. *Journal of Applied Behavior Analysis, 15,* 171–176.

Veerkamp, J. S. J., Gruythuysen, R. J. M., Hoogstraten, J., & van Amerongen, W. E. (1993). Dental treatment of fearful children using nitrous oxide—Part 4: Anxiety after two years. *Journal of Dentistry for Children, 60,* 372–376.

Venham, L. L., Goldstein, M., Gaulin-Kremer, E., Peteros, K., Cohan, J., & Fairbanks, J. (1981). Effectiveness of a distraction technique in managing young dental patients. *Pediatric Dentistry, 3,* 7–11.

Venham, L. L., Murray, P., & Gaulin-Kremer, E. (1979). Child-rearing variables affecting the preschool child's response to dental stress. *Journal of Dental Research, 58,* 2042–2045.

Vignehsa, H., Chellappah, N. K., Milgrom, P., Going, R., & Teo, C. S. (1990). A clinical evaluation of high- and low-fear children in Singapore. *Journal of Dentistry for Children, 57,* 224–228.

Walsh, M. M. (1985). Effects of school-based dental health education on knowledge, attitudes and behavior of adolescents in San Francisco. *Community Dentistry and Oral Epidemiology, 13,* 143–147.

Weinstein, P. (1990). Breaking the worldwide cycle of pain, fear, and avoidance: Uncovering risk factors and promoting prevention in children. *Annals of Behavioral Medicine, 12,* 141–147.

Weinstein, P., Getz, T., Ratener, P., & Domoto, P. (1982). The effect of dentists' behaviors on fear-related behaviors in children. *Journal of the American Dental Association, 103,* 38–40.

Weinstein, P., & Nathan, J. E. (1988). The challenge of fearful and phobic children. *Dental Clinics of North America, 32,* 667–692.

Weinstein, P., Shimono, T., Domoto, P., Wohlers, K., Matsumura, S., Ohmura, M., Uchida, H., & Omachi, K. (1992). Dental fear in Japan: Okayama Prefecture school study of adolescents and adults. *Anesthesiology Progress, 39,* 215–220.

Weisenberg, M., Kegeles, S. S., & Lund, A. K. (1980). Children's health beliefs and acceptance of a dental preventive activity. *Journal of Health and Social Behavior, 21,* 59–74.

Williams, J. A., Hurst, M. K., & Stokes, T. F. (1983). Peer observation in decreasing uncooperative behavior in young dental patients. *Behavior Modification, 7,* 225–242.

Williams, J. M. G., Murray, J. J., Lund, C. A., Harkiss, B., & deFranco, A. (1985). Anxiety in the child dental clinic. *Journal of Child Psychology and Psychiatry, 26,* 305–310.

Winer, G. A. (1982). A review and analysis of children's fearful behavior in dental settings. *Child Development, 53,* 1111–1133.

CHAPTER 19

PREPARATION TO UNDERGO MEDICAL PROCEDURES

Ronald L. Blount, UNIVERSITY OF GEORGIA
Adina J. Smith, UNIVERSITY OF GEORGIA
Natalie C. Frank, GEORGE WASHINGTON UNIVERSITY

Hospitalization can be a very scary experience for children. Unknown hospital staff approach children and are often masked, unusual odors are abundant, a new environment is experienced, parents are sometimes absent, and the actual medical procedures can be frightening and painful. Relatively benign anesthesia inductions, for example, have been demonstrated to be intimidating and frightening.

Since the middle of this century, negative reactions by children to hospitalization have been noted by clinicians (e.g., Jensen, 1955). In 1975, Douglas identified lasting behavioral problems, learning difficulties, and delinquency present 20 years after hospitalization. In addition, other negative reactions—such as increased verbal and physical aggression, eating problems, sleep disturbances, enuresis, fear of death, increased anxiety, and regressive behavior—have been evidenced after hospitalization (Peterson & Mori, 1988). Furthermore, results of a recent meta-analysis (Thompson & Vernon, 1993) of studies examining effects of hospitalization indicated that children who received no psychosocial interventions during hospitalization tended to demonstrate poorer adjustment after hospitalization. Contrary to the findings in the earlier literature, these more recent studies indicated that adjustment problems appeared to remit after two weeks. Other studies have found greater variability in duration of problem behaviors, but most indicated that in the majority of posthospitalization adjustment difficulties subsided within six months of discharge (Carson, Council, & Gravely, 1991).

Therefore, the older literature indicates that hospitalization produced long-term detrimental effects, but more recent research suggests that ill effects are, in general, less severe and of shorter duration. However, while some children cope well before, during, and after such stressful situations (Mabe, Treiber, & Riley, 1991), other children do not, and many adjustment problems have been exhibited by some children after discharge (e.g., Lumley, Melamed, & Abeles, 1993). Determining those factors associated with variability in children's responses to hospitalization and specific medical procedures may prove heuristic in identifying high-risk individuals and in determining targets for intervention.

The following is a review of factors that have been studied as influencing children's distress during and after hospitalization. These include children's coping style, temperament parental factors, developmental factors, and previous medical experience. The intervention research on preparation for hospitalization will then be critiqued. Finally, research on children's coping and distress during the relatively discrete stressor of acute painful medical procedures will be presented.

FACTORS INFLUENCING CHILDREN'S DISTRESS DURING HOSPITALIZATION

Coping Style

A considerable amount of research has been conducted to determine whether an individual's coping style may be an important factor in his or her reactions to painful medical procedures. During medical procedures, one person may cope better by seeking and receiving information while another may cope better by using distraction techniques. Several researchers have categorized children as having either approaching or avoidant coping styles (e.g., Fanurik, Zeltzer, Roberts, & Blount, 1993). Those with approaching coping styles seek information about the procedure and direct their attention toward the threatening stimulus, whereas those with avoidant styles ignore or refuse to attend to the event, and use repression, denial, or distraction to avoid facing the stressful procedure.

Suls and Fletcher (1985) performed a meta-analysis to determine whether there was evidence for the efficacy of one coping style over the other. Overall, they did not find strong evidence favoring either strategy. However, supplementary analyses indicated that avoidance was correlated with more positive coping with a short-term stressor. In contrast, attention was associated with more positive outcomes when confronting long-term stressors. Therefore, temporal and other unique aspects of the stressor, as well as coping style, may influence coping outcomes.

The main question that has faced researchers in this area is whether children with different coping styles experience different amounts of distress during medical treatments. Siegel (1981) found that among children hospitalized for surgery, those who coped successfully requested more information about upcoming procedures. Peterson and Toler (1986) also found that information seeking was positively associated with the child's previous adjustment to medical

procedures. Similar results from other assessment studies (e.g., Burstein & Meichenbaum, 1979), as well as the conclusions drawn from recent literature reviews (e.g., Blount, Davis, Powers, & Roberts, 1991), have supported the utility of the information-seeking over the information-avoiding coping style with children. Treatment implications from these assessment studies are not readily clear, but the usual recommendation by researchers in this area is that children should be provided with information or distraction based interventions depending on their coping style.

Contrary to these recommendations, two treatment studies have found alternative intervention implications. A study by Fanurik and associates (1993) found that repressors showed greater tolerance when they were taught to use imagery (a matched intervention) when coping with cold pressor-induced pain. Pain ratings also tended to be lower for this matched group. Pain ratings were higher, however, for repressors who were in the sensory focusing group (a mismatched intervention). There were no differences for the sensitizer group across matched or mismatched interventions on the dependent variables.

Smith, Ackerson, and Blotcky (1989) also attempted to match coping styles (repressor, sensitizer) with behavioral interventions (verbal distraction, sensory information) for pediatric oncology patients undergoing bone marrow aspirations (BMAs) or lumbar punctures (LPs). Children who were matched with interventions to their coping style reported higher pain ratings than those with a seemingly inconsistent intervention. No significant main effects were found between sensitizers and repressors on self-reports of fear and anticipated pain.

More generally, however, the literature indicates that children who display a sensitizer or approach style of coping adjust better to prolonged stressors such as hospitalization. For this reason, perhaps all children should be given age-appropriate information about upcoming stressful events. Avoidance of such procedural information by children may be more indicative of current distress, and, according to the assessment literature in this area, predictive of distress during and after the medical stressor. As such, children's avoidance of age-appropriate information may be reconceptualized as a distress behavior and as a "lack of coping" strategy. Those children who are highly avoidant might, therefore, be considered at greater risk for adverse reactions to medical stressors and in need of additional treatment interventions. This view of coping styles differs greatly from others in the area, even though the authors believe that it has practical clinical utility and empirical support.

Temperament and Prehospital Adjustment

Additional factors, such as temperament, may also influence a patient's ability to cope. *Temperament* has been defined as "a collection of relatively consistent, basic dispositions which underlie and modulate the expression of activity, reactivity, emotionality, and sociability" (Goldsmith et al., 1987). During medical procedures, temperament may affect adjustment by influencing the type and range of coping behaviors that a person exhibits, as well as by influencing what is perceived as stressful (Carson et al., 1991).

McClowry (1990) performed an investigation with 75 8- to 12-year-old children who were seen during hospital admissions. She found that the temperament dimensions of predictability, approach or withdrawal, mood, threshold of responsiveness, and intensity of reaction were associated with children's prehospital behavior, behavior one week following hospitalization, and behavior one month after hospitalization. At all three measurement times, temperament explained more than 50 percent of the variance in their behavior. However, it is possible in this investigation that the association between behavior and temperament in the children would have been found even without the event of hospitalization.

Findings from a study on adjustment of children hospitalized for tonsillectomies indicated that adjustment before hospitalization and temperament were two of the strongest predictors of postsurgical adjustment (Carson et al., 1991). The better adjusted children were adaptable, positive in mood, generally predictable in behavior, approaching and approachable, distractible, less reactive to stimuli, and had less intense emotional reactions.

Lumley, Abeles, Melamed, Pistone, and Johnson (1990) investigated the combined effects of children's temperamental characteristics and maternal behavior during medical situations on children's reactions to those situations. Although no significant main

effects were present, an interaction effect was found showing that children who were rated by their mothers as "difficult" were more distressed if their mothers were not involved with them following the procedure. Difficult children with involved mothers demonstrated less distress. These relationships were not evidenced for children rated as highly adaptable. A second interaction was found between maternal behavior and child temperament. For children who withdrew from novel stimuli, maternal distraction was associated with better coping, whereas for approaching children, distraction was related to more distress. For withdrawing children, information provision was associated with increased distress, and for approachers, information provision was associated with decreased distress. This study indicates that a match between the temperament dimension of approach-withdrawal from novel stimuli and information provision may foster more adaptive outcomes.

In summary, the few studies that have been conducted on temperament indicate that an easy temperament is related to better coping and more positive adjustment to hospitalization (Carson et al., 1991). Children with a difficult temperament and a history of previous adjustment problems may be at greatest risk for adverse reactions to the stressor of hospitalization, and therefore most in need of therapeutic interventions. As Lumley and colleagues (1990) demonstrated, when approach/withdrawal temperament characteristics are matched with an intervention during a medical procedure, children appear to experience decreased distress. Such an exchange between environment and temperament may be a critical determinant of whether the child's needs are being recognized and met and should be considered when planning for hospital intervention. However, these conclusions must be seen as tentative due to the paucity of research investigating the association between temperament, therapeutic intervention, and coping in medical situations.

Parental Factors

Aspects of parent-child relationships have been shown to be related to the child's coping with surgery or hospital stays. For example, Carson and colleagues (1991) found that mothers who were more anxious before the child's surgery, as well as those who were more rejecting, overindulgent, and overprotective, had children who did not cope well with hospitalization. Wells and Schwebel (1987) also found that parents who were overly involved with their child had children at a greater risk for poor posthospitalization adjustment.

Zabin and Melamed (1980) assessed whether parenting styles would be strong predictors of children's adjustment to hospitalization. They found that parents who reported using positive reinforcement, modeling, and persuasion had children with lower anxiety and fear levels. In contrast, those parents who reported relying more on punishment, force, and reinforcement of dependency had children who displayed greater anxiety.

Separation from their parents continues to be a major factor associated with hospitalized children's distress. Children who have been allowed to have constant parental contact during their hospital stay have been rated as adjusting better during hospitalization and demonstrating fewer maladaptive behaviors at discharge and at a six-month follow-up than children whose mothers were not allowed to stay in the children's rooms (Brain & Maclay, 1968). Couture (1976) and Douglas (1975) later replicated these findings.

Shaw and Routh (1982) conducted a study in which mothers were either present or absent during their 18-month-old or 5-year-old children's injection. For both age groups, they found that the children whose mothers were present during the injections were more distressed. Similarly, in a study of 13-month- to 7¾-year-old children who were receiving injections, Gonzalez and associates (1989) also found that older children displayed more behavioral distress when the parent was present. However, despite these findings, the same children strongly preferred their parent to be present for future injections. Blount, Davis, and colleagues (1991) speculated that it was not the mothers' presence or absence, but what the parents did that increased or decreased the level of the children's distress.

Prugh, Staub, Sands, Kirschenbaum, and Lenihan (1953) noted that quality of the parent-child relationship was the salient factor influencing a child's adjustment to hospitalization. These investigators also found that parents who visited their children more frequently were more likely to have better relationships with their children than parents who visited less frequently. Furthermore, parents' attitudes and expectations (Jay, 1988; Peterson, 1989), their anxiety levels (e.g., Carson et al., 1991), and whether they are overly protective and reinforcing of dependence (Carson et al., 1991; Zabin & Melamed, 1980) are variables that appear to influence the parent-child relationship, and thus the child's ability to successfully cope. Also, some parents may inadvertently cue and reinforce their children's distress, while others may promote coping by the child (Blount, Davis et al., 1991). Due to the number of parental variables that may influence child coping, there is a need for continuing assessment in this area focusing on the particular characteristics of the parent, child, and parent-child interactions. Also, since a child's hospitalization is anxiety provoking for parents, and few parents have been trained to manage their own distress or effectively assist their child with coping, Blount, Davis, and associates (1991) recommend that parents receive training to promote their own and their children's coping both prior to and during hospitalization.

Developmental Issues

For years, it has been widely recognized that younger children appear to be more behaviorally distressed by medical procedures than older children (e.g., Azarnoff & Woody, 1981; Wolfer & Visitainer, 1975). According to Wells and Schwebel (1987), studies of 6-month- to 4-year-old children undergoing surgery have demonstrated that the younger children showed more anxiety and posthospitalization disturbances than the older children. It is possible that younger children are not capable of fully mastering concepts and that they have misconceptions about hospitalization or surgical procedures. As children grow, their language and reasoning skills and their ability to utilize abstract thinking all become more finely tuned so that they are better able to understand their illnesses. For example, Vernon and Thompson (1993) found that younger children were not as responsive to hospital interventions as older children. Their data suggested that this may be because most interventions to assist children during hospitalization are information based and thus may not be as easily grasped by such younger children.

Bibace and Walsh (1980) hypothesized that children's conception of illness follows a predictable course based on developmental changes. In their study, children were shown to move from prelogical explanations of illness characterized by spatial context (i.e., the sun gives you a cold) to formal operational explanations combining physiological and psychological causes (i.e., you worry too much, the tension affects your heart and gives you a heart attack). Simeonsson, Buckley, and Monson (1979) and Campbell (1975) presented similar findings demonstrating children's differential understanding of illness depending on developmental level.

It appears that there are important clinical implications derived from a consideration of children's cognitive abilities and developmental levels. Less-developed communication skills or lack of knowledge and understanding about the hospital environment may prevent the child from effectively expressing the pain he or she is experiencing or from understanding the information or help being offered (e.g., Thompson & Varni, 1986). Therefore, it is necessary to recognize and appreciate children's cognitive development and their understanding of medical procedures.

Previous Experience

Previous medical experiences may shape children's expectations, thereby influencing their tolerance of medical procedures. In a study examining the presurgical anxiety of 4- to 10-year-old children, quality of previous medical experiences, as indexed by maternal ratings of the child's past medical and dental treatments, were predictive of distress during an upcoming medical treatment. However, maternal prediction of child behavior was demonstrated to be an even better predictor, as it accounted for 22 percent of distress variance (Lumley et al., 1993). Parental predictions of their children's reactions to medical treatments probably take into consideration the child's previous experience in the specific procedure being examined, as well as a host of other factors such as experience with other procedures, temperament, maternal anxiety, mood, irritability, and physical condition (Pate & Blount, 1995).

Quinton and Rutter (1976) investigated the relationship between hospital admissions and behavioral disturbances in 10-year-old children. Psychiatric diagnoses (conduct disturbances and emotional disturbances) were assigned when deviant scores were evidenced on both teacher questionnaires and maternal interviews. Results indicated that multiple admissions, with at least one during preschool years, were more common in both the conduct and emotionally disturbed groups than in the normal group. Single hospitalizations of up to one week were not correlated with later emotional or behavioral disturbances. Therefore, repeated hospitalizations appeared to be related to disturbances in later childhood and adolescence. However, an alternative interpretation is that those children who displayed psychological difficulties may have been more likely to require repeated hospitalizations for a number of reasons, such as risk taking.

Other investigations of postsurgical disturbances have found mixed results. For example, Wells and Schwebel (1987), in their study of children with physical handicaps, found that fewer previous surgeries were associated with greater posthospital upset and slower recovery. Such results may indicate that those who have had previous surgeries have learned more adaptive coping responses and are therefore able to recover more rapidly than those who have had fewer hospital experiences (Wells & Schwebel, 1987).

In summary, although earlier investigations by Quinton and Rutter (1976) and Douglas (1975) suggest enduring disturbances from hospitalization, the more recent studies have yielded inconsistent findings. Based on these results, a child's reactions to previous medical experiences, rather than the presence or absence of previous medical experiences, should be assessed. Misconceptions could be addressed and other interventions could be developed, particularly for those who have had negative reactions in the past. Another factor that influences the amount of pain and distress a child experiences is the amount of analgesia administered during hospitalization. Effective postoperative analgesia is important since inadequate pain relief may be associated with a number of negative outcomes, including development of maladaptive behaviors and cognitions. Such negative outcomes could potentially contribute to a lack of future utilization of medical services (Bush, 1987), distrustful attitudes, and adverse emotional responses toward health care providers (e.g., Bush, 1990).

It must be realized that children may not always express their pain in ways that are recognized by adults (Craig, Grunau, & Branson, 1988). Thus, in the absence of clear signs of pain, nurses may assume that analgesics are not necessary. Therefore, it is crucial for nurses to understand children's pain expression at different developmental levels, be able to assess pain in children, and have solid knowledge concerning analgesics (Ross, Bush, & Crummette, 1991).

In summary, several factors have been identified that may influence the coping and adaptation of a child undergoing hospitalization. The literature indicates that a child's coping style, temperament, interaction with parents, developmental level, and previous experience all contribute to his or her ability to cope effectively with the stressor of hospitalization.

HOSPITAL PREPARATION PROGRAMS

It is estimated that 75 percent of pediatric hospitals utilize some sort of preparation with hospitalized children (Peterson & Ridley-Johnson, 1980). However, the design of these preparation programs is seldomly based on research evaluating the effectiveness of various alternatives for decreasing distress in hospitalized children. The most common types of preparation used in children's hospitals are group tours and group discussion (Azarnoff & Woody, 1981). Unfortunately, effectiveness of these easily administered, low-cost interventions is rarely evaluated (Blount, 1987). The types of preparation programs that have received the most research attention include providing information to the parent and/or child, modeling, and coping skills training. This section will describe and critique the general types of interventions utilized in preparation for medical procedures and hospitalization, as well as factors that influence the effectiveness of these interventions.

Information Provision

One of the earliest interventions for decreasing distress in pediatric populations was the provision of information. Giving information to the parent (Skipper & Leonard, 1968) and child (Haller, Talbert, & Dombro, 1967) regarding what to expect has been shown to be effective in decreasing distress in hospitalized children. More recent studies examine information provision in combination with other interventions. However, it should also be noted that many interventions have some component of information provision, whether it is specifically evaluated in the study or not. For example, both modeling of procedures and desensitization, through practice with play medical equipment, provide the patient with information.

In one of the earlier studies on this topic, Wolfer and Visintainer (1975) examined whether providing information to the parent and child, coupled with supportive care, influenced both child and parent distress and coping. Subjects were children ages 3 to 14 years (and their parents) admitted to a hospital for elective surgery. In the experimental group, children and parents were provided with stress point care, consisting of procedural and sensory information by nurses at several critical times during the hospitalization. Nurses also provided support and reassurance to the family and helped children rehearse responses that were expected of them during the procedures. Children and parents in the control group received standard nursing care. Results indicated that children who received information were less distressed and more cooperative at different points during the hospitalization than children in the control group. Parents who received information reported less anxiety, perceived the information provided as more adequate and were more satisfied with the care their child received than parents of the control group.

In a partial replication, Visintainer and Wolfer (1975) compared different interventions for hospitalized children and their parents. These families received either stress point care, information provision, a description of sensory expectations and rehearsal of responses at admission, supportive care without information provision, or standard nursing procedures. Results indicated that children in the stress point preparation group were significantly less distressed and more cooperative than those in the supportive care group or the control group and were less distressed during preoperative medication than children in the single session group. Children in the single session group were better adjusted after discharge compared to the control group. Parents in the stress point preparation group were less anxious, better informed, and more satisfied with care than all the other groups.

The next study by these researchers examined home preparation through reading material in an effort to decrease the cost and training time necessary for stress point nursing care (Wolfer & Visintainer, 1979). Preparatory materials included booklets explaining what to expect during the hospitalization, with pictures of children going through each procedure. Children were also provided with a medical bag with play equipment to be used along with the illustrations in the book. These materials were sent to the families three to four days prior to hospital admission. Home preparation was shown to be as effective in reducing child and parent distress during hospitalization as in-house preparation. Home preparation with either stress point nursing or with supportive care was more effective in reducing parent anxiety than home preparation or supportive care alone. Each of the experimental preparation groups was more effective in reducing child and parent distress than the standard control procedures.

Providing children and parents with information is effective in helping to decrease emotional and behavioral distress. Further, stress point care—consisting of providing information, support, and rehearsal of responses at several critical times during the hospitalization—appears to be more effective than providing information at a single point in time. Stress point care may help parents and children better remember information through prompting and the supportive nature in which the information is offered.

Modeling

Much of the research on hospital preparation has utilized modeling of upcoming procedures. Modeling provides the child with information through exposure to the situation via observation of another child. This is often accomplished through use of videotapes, illustrated materials, or puppets. The best recognized example of modeling is Melamed and Siegel's (1975) study comparing the film, "Ethan Has an Operation," with a control film. The experimental film, which followed a peer model through the steps and procedures involved in hospitalization for hernia repair surgery, was more effective than the control film in decreasing fear and distress in 4- to 12-year-old children.

Less expensive modeling preparations have also been demonstrated to be effective in decreasing dis-

tress. Peterson, Schultheis, Ridley-Johnson, Miller, and Tracy (1984) compared the professionally produced "Ethan Has an Operation" with a nonprofessional videotape of a child undergoing surgery in a local hospital, and a puppet modeling show. They found that all interventions were equally effective in decreasing anxiety and maladaptive responses in children prior to and after surgery. Schultz, Raschke, Dedrick, and Thompson (1981) and Peterson, Ridley-Johnson, Tracy, and Mullins (1984) also demonstrated utility of using an inexpensive puppet model to decrease anxiety and behavioral distress in children undergoing elective surgery.

Coping skills have also been included in modeling preparations to enhance the effects of the intervention. For example, Faust, Olson, and Rodriquez (1991) examined the utility of a modeling slide-audio show, which included information and modeling of a child undergoing medical procedures while utilizing relevant coping skills, such as deep breathing and imagery. This preparation was compared with a control condition, which consisted of information provision via a mock surgery exhibit and a 10-minute talk. The authors found the modeling intervention to be significantly more effective in reducing physiological and behavioral distress in same-day pediatric surgery patients than the mock surgery exhibit.

Pinto and Hollandsworth (1989) examined whether having the parent view the modeling film with the child added anything to the effects of the child viewing the film alone. Parents and children watched a video of a child undergoing the various steps leading up to and following surgery. Half of the children viewed a film narrated by a peer and half of the children viewed a film narrated by an adult. Results indicated that children who viewed the film alone responded best to the peer-narrated film, whereas children who viewed the film with their parents responded best to the adult-narrated film. Parents who viewed the film were better adjusted than parents who did not view the film. Overall, children who viewed the film with their parents were rated as less distressed on physiological measures than children who viewed the film alone, although the groups did not differ on behavioral or self-report measures.

Roberts, Wurtele, Boone, Ginther, and Elkins (1981) demonstrated effectiveness of a slide-audio peer modeling presentation made at a local hospital in reducing medical fears in a nonpatient population of third- and fifth-graders. Such preparation also modeled the children effectively coping with their hospital-related anxiety and fear through self-talk, relaxation, and modification of their cognitions. Elkins and Roberts (1985) compared this slide-audio preparation with the film "Ethan Has an Operation," the Mr. Rogers film "Let's Talk about Having an Operation," and a control film titled "The Case of the Elevator Duck," which models a child coping with a novel nonmedical situation. Results indicated that children who were rated as "high fear" prior to the intervention reported significant reductions in fear and anxiety levels following one of the medically related preparations, as compared to the control group. This effect was not found for children rated as having low fear prior to the intervention.

Previous Medical Experience and Modeling

Initial studies attempting to limit individual differences in prior medical experience have mostly included patients with no previous experience. However, this creates problems in generalization. For example, studies indicate that although modeling may decrease distress in children with no previous experience, this intervention is relatively ineffective with experienced children. These results have been demonstrated in dental patients (Klorman, Hilpert, Michael, LaGana, & Sveen, 1980) as well as in surgical patients (Melamed, Dearborn, & Hermecz, 1983). Melamed and colleagues (1983) indicated that young children with previous medical experience may actually be sensitized by a hospital modeling film, resulting in increased distress during the actual procedures. Thus, modeling interventions that provide redundant information or information that is conflicting with the child's experience may actually serve to increase anxiety and distress.

In summary, modeling procedures appear to be useful in preparing the child for what to expect during various medical treatments. Cost-effective modeling preparations, such as puppet shows and locally produced peer modeling slides or videotapes, have been effectively introduced into hospitals. Coping skills training can be added to these preparations to enhance their effects. However, these interventions may prove less effective with children who have previous medi-

cal experience, as modeling may increase anxiety. Alternative preparation programs may be more appropriate with these children.

Coping Skills Training

Coping skills training has been widely used, both singularly and in combination, with other interventions, to aid children in handling difficult medical situations. Three types of coping skills often taught are distraction, relaxation, and self-talk. Distraction consists of the use of imagery or focusing on external stimuli, such as watching movies. Relaxation can consist of simple procedures such as deep breathing or more elaborate techniques, such as visualization. Self-talk teaches the child to use coping statements such as: "I can handle this" or "Everything is alright" in attempting to block or counter anxiety-provoking statements such as "I can't stand this" (Melamed & Ridley-Johnson, 1988).

Peterson and Shigetomi (1981) compared the efficacy of information provision, coping skills training, and coping skills training plus filmed modeling in decreasing distress in children undergoing surgery and their parents. Coping skills consisted of a 15-minute presentation and practice of relaxation, self-talk, and distraction. Results indicated that children in the two coping skills conditions were less distressed than children in the information group, as demonstrated by greater food intake, nurses ratings of anxiety and cooperativeness, and child ratings of fear and anxiety. Parents in the coping skills condition also reported less anxiety, a greater sense of competence, and greater satisfaction.

Meng and Zastowny (1982) evaluated an intervention program that utilized several types of coping strategies. Children were trained in relaxation, distraction, strategies for coping with negative feelings, and the use of self-statements for dealing successfully with stress. Children receiving this intervention were rated as more cooperative and better adjusted following surgery than the other children. Further, parents of children in the prepared group reported less anxiety than parents of the unprepared children. Perhaps parents' knowledge that their child had participated in the intervention and/or children showing lower amounts of distress contributed to lower parental anxiety.

In an extension of this research, Zastowny, Kirschenbum, and Meng (1986) trained parents to direct their children in the use of relaxation and coping skills. Parents viewed a videotape one week prior to surgery, instructing them how to coach their children to utilize coping skills at various stress points during the hospitalization. Parents were also provided with a booklet with further instruction about coping skills and about how to inform their child regarding the upcoming surgery. Children were then coached by their parents to utilize the coping strategies throughout their hospital stay. Results indicated that children who were coached by their parents were rated as less distressed at six stress points during the hospitalizations as compared to children who were not coached. Parents in the coaching condition also rated their children as exhibiting less problematic behaviors in the week before and after hospitalization.

Summary and Future Directions

Coping skills training in distraction, relaxation, and self-talk has been demonstrated to be effective in reducing anxiety and distress in hospitalized children and their parents. Coping skills can be taught directly to the child, to the child and parent, or to the parent who then coaches the child. However, research examining whether these methods are differentially effective has not been conducted. Further, a more cost-effective method for teaching coping skills may be to train the nurses to coach the children. In this manner, nurses' prompts could augment the effects of filmed coping skills training.

Although it is useful to group interventions into discrete types for review and evaluation of their effectiveness, it should be noted that most studies include multiple intervention components. For example, Wolfer and Visintainer's (1975) stress point procedure included the child rehearsing various responses that could be conceived of as a type of coping skill. Meng and Zastowny (1982) taught coping skills training via a videotape, which could also be considered modeling. Finally, most modeling preparations provide some aspect of exposure to the potentially feared stimulus, thereby allowing for possible desensitization or habituation of the fear responses. Desensitization might also be accomplished through experience with play medical equipment, exposure to sensory in-

formation, or rehearsal of responses that are expected during the various procedures.

Although the previously cited literature clearly demonstrates effectiveness of various interventions in preparing children for hospitalization, much of the research has exclusively utilized elementary school children (Peterson & Brownlee-Duffeck, 1984). This is problematic because previous research suggests that children understand the illness concept differently depending on age (e.g., Bibace & Walsh, 1980). Therefore, generalizability of results from treatment outcome studies is suspect, particularly to preschool-aged children. Further, few studies have been conducted comparing the efficacy of different preparation programs in different age groups. One such study completed by Ferguson (1979) compared use of a preadmission visit with filmed modeling in 3- to 5-year-old and 6- to 7-year-old children. Results indicated that although the peer modeling film was effective in reducing distress behavior in both age groups, the preadmission visit was effective in reducing distress behavior only in the older group.

In a synthesis of the literature examining the effectiveness of intervention programs in decreasing children's distress conducted by Vernon and Thompson (1993), the meta-analysis indicated that children who received some sort of preparation for hospitalization exhibited less behavioral distress than children who did not receive an intervention. When divided into groups based on age, however, results indicated that children under 6 years benefited less from preparation than older children. Further analyses revealed that this may be due to the cognitive nature of many intervention programs.

Rasnake and Linscheid (1989) evaluated a preparation program that was based on developmental considerations. Children received either standard information, developmentally appropriate information, or developmentally advanced information. Developmentally appropriate information for preschool children consisted of sensory expectations and a simple description of what was to occur. Developmentally appropriate material for the concrete operational stage children consisted of more cognitively advanced descriptions. Results indicated that children given developmentally appropriate information demonstrated less distress than children in the other two groups.

The limited research available in this area suggests the importance of taking a child's developmental level into account when selecting a preparation program for them. Many researchers in the area believe that different preparation programs are needed for different age groups (e.g., Harbeck-Weber & McKee, in press). For younger children, it may be necessary to present ideas in a very concrete manner, whereas older children may be able to understand an explanation which includes more abstract concepts. It will be important to conduct further research examining the effectiveness of various preparation programs for different age groups in order to provide the most appropriate intervention for each child.

ACUTE PAINFUL MEDICAL PROCEDURES

Hospitalization can be thought of as a complex, multi-component series of stressors or demands. One of the many common stressors that children experience during hospitalization and in other medical environments is undergoing a painful medical procedure. Among the most frequently occurring acute painful medical procedures are finger sticks and intramuscular (IM), and intravenous (IV) injections. Further, children with cancer are exposed to other more invasive and recurrent events, including lumbar punctures (LP) and bone marrow aspirations (BMA). These painful procedures, while complex in their own right, are relatively discrete when contrasted to hospitalization. Although most children show moderate levels of distress to acute painful procedures, some experience severe to extreme distress while others appear to experience only mild distress or no apparent distress reactions. This suggests that not every child who undergoes a painful medical procedure is in need of coping skills training. For example, approximately 25 to 30 percent of pediatric oncology patients cope satisfactorily with LPs and BMAs (e.g., Blount et al., 1989; Zeltzer & LeBaron, 1982). Similar results occur with healthy preschool children undergoing immunizations (Blount et al., 1992).

Satisfactory coping does not mean an absence of distress during a medical procedure, although some children and parents seem to achieve this. Rather, satisfactory coping means that the event is seen as manageable, even though it is unpleasant. Learning what distinguishes those children and parents who cope more effectively from those who are highly distressed should be a goal of much of the assessment work in this area.

Assessment of Children's Reactions to Painful Medical Procedures

Assessment of pediatric pain and distress has been conducted using a variety of means, including self-reports of pain, ratings by medical staff and parents, physiological monitoring, and direct observation. Although each method has unique costs and benefits (for review, see Karoly, 1991), studies using direct observation methodology have yielded results that have greater heuristic implications for the development of effective coping skills training programs. For this reason, assessment studies using direct observation techniques will be the focus of this section.

Katz, Kellerman, and Siegel (1980) conducted the initial investigations using direct observation assessment measures for oncology patients undergoing BMAs and LPs. Using the Procedure Behavioral Rating Scale (PBRS), Katz and colleagues found differences in distress as a function of age and sex. About 6 to 7 years of age, children exhibited more self-control, fewer emotional outbursts, and fewer anxious behaviors than younger children. Also, girls generally appeared more anxious than boys and displayed a greater range of distress behaviors.

The Observation Scale of Behavioral Distress (OSBD; Jay, Ozolins, Elliott, & Caldwell, 1983) is a revised version of the PBRS. *Behavioral distress* is a term that encompasses both anxiety and pain because the two constructs are difficult to differentiate during acute medical procedures. Significant sex differences were not found using the OSBD. These results are inconsistent with the findings of Katz and colleagues (1980). Jay and associates speculate that this may be due to the small sample size in their study. The distress levels of children under 7 years old were five times that of older children. Jay and associates (1983) also found a positive association between parental anxiety and children's distress scores. Additionally, the OSBD is positively correlated with children's anxiety. Children displayed less distress after repeated BMAs, although two years were needed to show this effect for the younger children. Child's age, parental anticipation of child's pain, and the number of previous BMAs accounted for 86 percent of the variance in OSBD distress scores.

Expanding on previous research that focused exclusively on child distress, the Child-Adult Medical Procedure Interaction Scale (CAMPIS; Blount et al., 1989) was originally developed to code vocal interactions of all the people present in the pediatric treatment room. Behaviors of the staff, parent, and child were coded continuously throughout the procedure. Some 16 child codes encompassing distress, coping behaviors, and normal talk during a medical procedure and 19 adult behaviors including adult-adult and adult-child verbalizations were utilized on the CAMPIS. The 35 CAMPIS codes were combined into the 6 category CAMPIS-R, which includes child coping (making coping statements, deep breathing, humor, and nonprocedural talk), distress (crying, screaming, verbal resistance, request emotional support, verbal fear, verbal pain, verbal emotion, and information seeking), and neutral behaviors, and adult coping promoting (behaviors associated with child coping: humor to the child, nonprocedural talk to the child, and commands to engage in coping strategy), distress promoting (associated with child distress: criticism, reassuring comments, giving control to the child, apology, and empathy), and neutral behaviors that were not associated with child coping or distress (Blount, Sturges & Powers, 1990). These categorizations were based on the general literature on child coping and distress, as well as on the results from the earlier investigation (Blount et al., 1989). Transcripts made from audiotapes or videotapes have been used to code the vocal interactions.

In the initial study using the CAMPIS (Blount et al., 1989), data were analyzed across phases of the BMA or LP procedures for pediatric oncology patients who were not trained in the use of coping behaviors. Results of sequential analyses indicated that adults' nonprocedural talk and humor *to* the child was most often followed by nonprocedural talk and humor *by* the child. Adults' commands to the child to use coping strategies (typically saying "Breathe") most often resulted in the children using deep breathing, which rarely occurred without repeated coaching. Child coping seldomly occurred without frequent and sometimes repeated prompts by adults. Child distress was most often preceded by adults' reassuring comments, empathic comments, apologies, criticism, and giving control to the child (over the initiation or resumption of a painful procedure).

Also, adults typically attempted to reassure following child distress. Reassurance was the highest frequency adult behavior directed toward the children. Also important to note, adults often took their cues from other adults as to how to interact with each other and with the child. For 11 of the 19 adult behaviors, the most frequent behavior to follow was another adult behaving in the same manner. For example, if a parent observed a nurse distracting the child, the parent often joined in and also distracted the child.

To elaborate, adult behaviors of reassurance, empathic comments, and apologies to the child could be viewed as interacting with the child in an emotionally solicitous manner (also see Jay, 1988, p. 416). Although helpful in some situations, they may cue and reinforce child distress during painful medical procedures, particularly if adults do not prompt child coping behaviors. Bush, Melamed, Sheras, and Greenbaum (1986) found a similar association between parental reassurance and child distress. Gonzalez, Routh, and Armstrong (1993) experimentally manipulated reassurance in order to evaluate whether it has a causal, as opposed to a merely correlated, association with child distress. They found no significant differences between their control condition and the reassurance condition for children undergoing immunizations. However, parental reassurance was provided at least every 10 seconds for several minutes before, during, and several minutes after the immunizations. This time-driven schedule is very different from the way "naturally" occurring reassurance is provided. Research is currently underway evaluating the effects of experimentally manipulated reassurance that more closely approximates how it occurs in the natural environment (Manimala et al., 1995).

The second investigation (Blount et al., 1990; Sturges, Blount, James, Powers, & Prater, 1991) examined child and adult behavioral variations by phase of medical procedure. Children's distress increased at the beginning of the anesthetic and did not decrease significantly until after the final painful procedure. Early anticipatory phase distress was positively correlated with distress during the BMA. The types, but not the amount of coping, varied significantly during the anticipatory, painful, and recovery phases. During the anticipatory phase, children used relatively high levels of distraction (nonprocedural talk) and low levels of deep breathing. The reverse was true during the painful phases. Very high correlations were obtained within medical phases between children's use of distraction and breathing, and adults' attempts to distract the child or coach them to breathe.

Further, there was a negative association between adults' distracting or coaching the children to use a coping behavior, and the children's distress during the anticipatory and painful phases, respectively. Therefore, children's and adults' coping and coping promoting behaviors tended to be phase specific, at least for these children; distraction was used during the anticipatory phase and breathing during the painful phases.

In the final assessment study (Blount, Landolf-Fritsche, Powers, & Sturges, 1991), subjects were assigned to groups depending on whether the children engaged in high or low proportions of coping behaviors. Results indicated that (1) parents of high-coping children engaged in more distraction and coaching of their children than did the parents of low-coping children; (2) high-coping children were more likely to cope following adults' prompts than were the low-coping children; and (3) *both* high- and low-coping children were more likely to cope following adult distraction and coaching than following any other adult antecedents. Also, both groups were more likely to display distress following adult distress promoting behaviors than following any other adult statements. Children also were more likely to cope following either staff's or parent's distracting interactions or coaching than following any other staff or parent behaviors. These latter findings suggest some generalization of adult-child interactional probabilities across high- and low-coping children and across staff-child and parent-child interactions.

As with the OSBD and PBRS, the CAMPIS and CAMPIS-R have been modified according to the demands of the particular investigation. For example, the authors have used fewer phases, proportional or rate data, and the scale in treatment (Blount et al., 1992) and assessment (e.g., Frank, Blount, Smith, Manimala, & Martin, 1995) studies of healthy children undergoing immunizations. The reliability and validity of the CAMPIS-R adult and child categories were supported by the correlations between them and various observational, self-report, parental-report, and staff-report measures (Blount et al., 1997).

Further, Morrow, Armstrong, Routh, Gay, and Levy (1993) and Manne and colleagues (1992) have adopted several CAMPIS codes, rather than the entire scale, for use in their investigations. Morrow and associates (1993) also monitored the occurrence of the CAMPIS behaviors in a time sampling format. In addition, modifications of the CAMPIS have been used in an interval coding format (Cohen, Blount, Panopoulos, & Manimala, 1995; Manimala et al., 1995) and when coding only from videotapes (Cohen et al., 1995).

In several assessment studies, Manne, Jacobsen, Redd, and colleagues (Jacobsen et al., 1990; Manne et al., 1992) examined the dyadic interactions of parents and their children during their IV injections. Nurse behaviors during the medical procedures were not observed. Results of the first investigation (Jacobsen et al., 1990) indicated that the timing of parents giving procedural explanations (information) to the children may be important. Children who were distressed during the anticipatory phase who were given explanations did better during the injection phase than similarly distressed children who were not given explanations. However, children who were not distressed during the anticipatory phase and were not provided with explanations did better during the injection than similarly nondistressed children who were provided explanations. Explanations to distressed children during the injection did little good, and may have made the children more distressed.

In the second assessment study from this group, Manne and associates (1992) found that distraction was the only parent behavior that was both positively related to child coping and negatively related to distress. Also, parents' praise was unlikely to be followed by distress. Giving decisional control to the child, such as "Which hand do you want me to look at first?" (p. 248), was associated with less crying and screaming during the injection.

In summary, assessment of relevant variables during the BMAs, LPs, and IM and IV injections has become more complex and complete. In addition to monitoring child distress, child coping behaviors are also relevant, dependent variables that have recently been assessed with greater frequency by researchers. Also, the literature increasingly points to the influence of adult behaviors in the treatment room on child distress and coping. Interactions in the treatment room are triadic, at a minimum; there is at least one medical staff member, usually at least one parent, and the child present. There is compelling evidence that adults take many of their cues from other adults as to how to interact with one another and with the child (Blount et al., 1989) and there do not appear to be significant differences in how children react to the same behaviors produced by parents versus by staff (Blount, Landolf-Fritsche et al., 1991).

Further, parent and staff behaviors during the sessions account for at least 38 percent of the variance in child coping and 55 percent of the variance in child distress during immunizations (Frank et al., 1995). However, the amount of effort required for comprehensive assessments might prove prohibitive for some investigations. Therefore, the authors recommend focusing on those parent and medical staff behaviors that have been shown to be associated with child distress and coping, as well as on child coping and distress behaviors, as the minimum requirements for a sufficiently comprehensive instrument.

A primary goal of assessment research should be to aid in the development of better interventions to reduce child distress. Such treatment intervention research would also experimentally validate the assessment findings. Assessment research that does not eventually assist in either the identification of children in need of training or in the design of therapeutic interventions is of limited clinical value (also see Roberts, 1992, p. 798). From the studies reviewed, parent and child anxiety (Jay et al., 1983); reassurance, apologies, empathic statements, and criticism (Blount et al., 1989); giving the child different types of control (Blount et al., 1989; Manne et al., 1992; Ross & Ross, 1988); distraction and coaching the child to use coping behaviors (Blount et al., 1989; Blount et al., 1990; Manne et al., 1992), and explanations (Jacobsen et al., 1990) are potential variables influencing child distress which should be manipulated experimentally.

Cognitive-Behavioral Treatment of Acute Procedural Pain

The best-known cognitive behavioral program for reducing children's distress was developed by Susan

Jay and colleagues (e.g., Jay & Elliott, 1990; Jay, Elliott, Katz, & Siegel, 1987; Jay, Elliott, Woody, & Siegel, 1991). This treatment package combines filmed modeling using a commercially available videotape developed by the authors, breathing exercises, imagery/distraction, incentives, behavioral rehearsal, and coaching of the child by the therapist during the medical treatment. Jay and associates (1987) compared effectiveness of the coping skills intervention to 0.3 mg/kg of oral Valium administered 30 minutes prior to the BMA, and to an attention control condition during which the children watched cartoons for 30 minutes prior to the BMA. The order of each child's exposure to the three treatment conditions was counterbalanced for the 56 3½- to 13-year-old children with leukemia.

For the medical procedure considered as a whole, the behavioral intervention was superior to the control condition on behavioral distress, self-report, and heart rate measures. The Valium treatment only resulted in lower systolic blood pressure scores taken just prior to cleansing for the BMA, than the control condition. Later research (Jay et al., 1991) indicated that combination of the cognitive behavioral program plus 0.15 mg/kg of oral Valium provided no measurable benefit beyond that obtained from the cognitive behavioral program alone for reducing distress during BMAs and LPs.

Jay and Elliott (1990) examined the effectiveness of child-focused compared to parent-focused interventions as a means of lowering parental distress during their child's BMA or LP. In the child-focused intervention, the children received either the cognitive behavior therapy alone or in combination with oral Valium. In the parent-focused intervention, the child was trained with or without the addition of Valium while the parent was provided with a stress inoculation program consisting of viewing a videotape about BMAs and LPs, and direct training in making coping statements and in relaxation.

There were no significant differences between the conditions on either parents' distress behaviors or on parents' physiological measures. Parents in the stress inoculation group reported lower anxiety and higher positive self-statement scores. Parents in both groups engaged in more coaching and interaction with the child after the interventions than they did during a baseline observation. From the authors' own research, it is possible that such change in parental behavior was due to parental imitation of the therapist's coaching of the child to use the coping behaviors (Blount et al., 1989).

In the most recent study by Jay and colleagues (Jay, Elliott, Fitzgibbons, Woody, & Siegel, in press), cognitive behavior therapy was compared to halothane-induced anesthesia for 18 3- to 12-year-old pediatric oncology patients undergoing BMAs. Each child was exposed to both conditions in a counterbalanced, repeated measures design. Results were equivocal and indicated that children in the halothane condition displayed less distress from when they first entered the treatment room until they were on the table. No differences were found on children's self-report of pain. No data were reported on child distress during and after the BMAs.

There were a number of side effects for children in the halothane condition, including displaying a variety of behavioral adjustment symptoms within the 24-hour period following the BMA when compared to children in the cognitive-behavior therapy condition. Transient elevations in the liver enzymes SGOT and SGPT postanesthesia and other low frequency side effects—including nausea and vomiting, dizziness, and headaches—were found. The average time the children were in the treatment room in the anesthesia condition was 30 minutes and in the cognitive-behavior therapy condition, 11 minutes. Nurses reported more stress during the anesthesia condition. However, parents expected the anesthesia condition to be most effective, and there was a slight preference by parents for that intervention after completion of the study.

There have been attempts to incorporate nurses as coaches of children during acute painful medical procedures. However, these efforts to gain control over nurse behavior have proven difficult, in that there have been either fairly small differences (Smith, Ackerson, & Blotcky, 1989) or no differences in nurse behavior between experimental conditions (Manne, Bakeman, Jacobsen, Gorfinkle, & Redd, 1994). Using stimulus control techniques, Cohen and associates (1995) gained control over nurse prompting of child coping behavior during immunizations. In two treatment conditions, nurses were instructed to prompt children to attend to a cartoon distraction before, during, and after immunizations. Nurse training

consisted of instructions, practice, feedback, and praise. In the control condition, the video monitor was off, obviating the possibility of nurse prompting. Nurse coaching, when used singularly, was found to be as effective and less costly than nurse coaching plus training the parents and children. Both treatment conditions resulted in lower distress than the standard medical treatment control condition.

Manne and associates (1990) used a behavioral intervention to reduce distress for 23 3- to 9-year-old children undergoing IV injections for chemotherapy. The treatment consisted of having the child blow a party blower while the parent counted to pace the rate of blowing, and giving stickers to the child for holding still and blowing during the IV. During the IV, the experimenter prompted the parent to coach the child during the injection. The therapist reviewed training procedures before two subsequent IVs and accompanied the parent and child during the IV procedure, but did not prompt during the final injection. This procedure was compared to a control condition. Results indicated that observational distress and parent rated distress were lower during three intervention sessions only for the behavior therapy group. Parents in the behavior therapy condition also showed a significant decrease in their own anxiety.

It should be noted that the intervention by Manne and colleagues (1990) represents a different approach to decreasing parental anxiety than was included in the stress inoculation program by Jay and Elliott (1990). In this case, the assumption seems to be that parental anxiety will be lower when parents are taught how to help their children and when their children are less distressed. Blount and colleagues (1992) also found that parents who had been trained to coach their healthy preschool children during immunizations reported that their own distress was lower than usual when their child received injections. In contrast, untrained parents reported that their distress was the same or worse than usual. Without training, many parents do not seem to know what to do to help their child during painful medical procedures. Training parents to coach the children and training the children to be responsive to that coaching may go far in alleviating parental, as well as child, distress.

In treatment research with healthy and ill children undergoing painful medical procedures (Blount et al., 1992; Blount, Powers, Cotter, Swan, & Free,

1994; Cohen et al., 1995; Manimala et al., 1995; Powers, Blount, Bachanas, Cotter, & Swan, 1993) the authors used an empirically guided, matching-to-sample type of approach to aid in the selection of therapeutic interventions. The coping skills intervention was, therefore, an attempt to teach the children who were having difficulty coping to use the behaviors, which were found to be incompatible with distress in the authors' assessment studies (Blount et al., 1989; 1990; Blount, Landolf-Fritsche et al., 1991; Sturges et al., 1991).

In a multiple baseline design with pediatric oncology patients, three 4½- to 7-year-old children undergoing BMA or LP procedures (Blount et al., 1994) were trained initially to use nonprocedural talk and deep breathing. However, nonprocedural talk proved difficult to train, with long silences ensuing even after a list of conversational topics had been prepared with parents' input. Toys, books, coloring books, and so on, were used to prompt distracting interactions between the parent and child during the occasional long periods of time between when the child went into the treatment room and when procedures began.

Also, these young children had a difficult time using deep breathing. Therefore, the party blower was adopted to replace deep breathing. Training consisted of providing a rationale to the parents about the effects of distraction on distress, modeling use of toy play and parental distraction during the anticipatory phases, modeling blowing and coaching to blow during the medical treatment, and behavioral rehearsal of coping and coping promoting behaviors during a BMA/LP role-play. Repeated role-plays, feedback, and praise were provided until the child and parent(s) were proficient and until the child ceased to flinch when touched on the back with pretend medical equipment during the role-play.

Unlike the previous cognitive-behavioral or behavioral treatment packages described, the components of this package were designed to be used in a phase-specific manner, with distracting interaction prescribed for the phase prior to the procedure and blowing for the phase just before and during the painful aspects of the procedure. The therapist accompanied the families to the medical treatment room, providing minimal prompts to the parent to coach the child on a progressively decreasing schedule across sessions. Dependent variables included parent's coping promoting behaviors, children's coping behaviors, and child distress. Results indicated that all children and parents changed in the therapeutic direction on all variables. This change was short-lived for one child, whose distress returned to baseline levels despite his father's continued coaching. Also, there was an increase in family stressors outside the medical environment between the first and subsequent intervention sessions for this family, and the child never became proficient in the use of the blower. The other two children and their parents continued to make and maintain their treatment gains, with the therapist ceasing to train or to accompany them during the last few sessions.

Powers and colleagues (1993) used a variation of the training package described above to teach four 3- to 5-year-old oncology patients and their parents to use an active distraction procedure prior to, and blowing or counting during, IM or IV injections. A multiple baseline design was used. The trainers did not accompany the families during the medical treatment during any phase. Results indicated that parents' coaching and children's coping increased, and children's distress decreased. Also, nurses rated the children as more cooperative across intervention sessions. Maintenance of children's coping, parents' coping promoting behaviors, and lower child distress was found.

Although the treatments were successful, Powers and associates point out that not all trained children at all times maintained their behavior change following, or even during, training. They note that there are multiple sources of variability inherent in the display of children's procedural distress. For a description of the potential sources of variability, see reviews by Varni, Blount, Waldron, and Smith (1995) and Varni, Blount, and Quiggins (in press).

Summary and Future Directions for the Assessment and Treatment of Acute Pediatric Pain

Cognitive behavioral techniques have proven useful for reducing the distress that children experience during medical treatments. Training programs varied from a multicomponent intervention package (e.g., Jay & Elliott, 1990), from which the child and therapist selected different components for use; to the child using only a blower throughout IV procedures (Manne et al., 1990); to phase-specific training programs with particular coping behaviors being performed at particular times (e.g., Blount et al., 1992, 1994).

Some evidence for maintenance of treatment gains was found in the studies by Dahlquist, Gil, Armstrong, Ginsberg, and Jones (1985), Manne and associates (1990), Blount and associates (1994), and Powers and associates (1993). However, the number of sessions during which maintenance was evaluated ranged only from one to three. Long-term maintenance has not been assessed. The range of dependent variables was broadened in some of the studies reviewed in this section to include child coping (e.g., Blount et al., 1992, 1994; Cohen et al., 1995; Manimala et al., 1995), parental distress, as well as other parent behaviors (e.g., Blount et al., 1992; Jay & Elliott, 1990; Manne et al., 1990) during the medical treatment. Parents' coaching of their children to cope was taught and monitored by Blount and colleagues (1994) and Powers and colleagues (1993). Nurse behaviors were also monitored in investigations of children undergoing immunizations (Blount et al., 1992; Cohen et al., 1995) and injections for chemotherapy (Manne et al., 1994). Some evidence of generalization of coping-promoting behavior from the therapist/coach to the untrained parents was found by Jay and Elliott (1990) and Cohen and colleagues (1995). Similarly, some evidence of generalization of coping-promoting behavior from trained parents to untrained nurses was found by Blount and colleagues (1992).

Treatment comparison studies were conducted (Jay et al., 1991; Jay & Elliott, 1990; Smith et al., 1989; Gonzalez et al., 1993; Cohen et al., 1995; Manimala et al., 1995). The other investigations critiqued were of treatment as compared to baseline or no-treatment conditions. As effectiveness of the interventions becomes established, research should move from demonstrating that a treatment works to comparing the relative effectiveness of different interventions. Research by Jay and colleagues, which evaluates the incremental effectiveness of adding Valium or anesthesia to their coping skills training program, might serve as a model for future investigations of other frequently used pharmacological interventions for helping children endure painful procedures. Such investigations would be timely and clinically useful.

There also is a need for further investigation of the effects of the social environment in the treatment room. Assessment research with pediatric oncology patients conducted in the authors' laboratory and by Manne, Jacobsen, Redd, and colleagues has emphasized and helped clarify the role of adults' behavior on children's coping and distress. However, in the two settings in which this research was conducted, there were differences in the types of control that adults offered children. Also, reassurance, the most frequent adult behavior in the sample, was not included in the studies by Manne and colleagues. Further, in the original sample, adults engaged in high rates of coaching of children to breathe.

The authors have not observed those same high rates in other settings in which they have worked. Such differences suggest two things. First, there is a need for replication studies. Second, researchers and clinicians should be good observers of the behaviors of adults and children in their own clinics. The authors believe that results of their studies are generalizable, but they also believe that different behaviors are displayed in different proportions in different settings. Therefore, for any particular child, assessment of the effects of the social environment should necessarily be idiographic, while still guided in large part by the literature.

Assessment research also indicates that some adult behaviors may lead to increases in child distress. Thus far, the authors have worked on the assumption that increasing parents' coping promoting behaviors would lead to decreases in other possibly undesirable parent behaviors. However, it is also important to conduct experimental research manipulating those adult behaviors, which were positively associated with child distress (e.g., Gonzalez et al., 1993; Manimala et al., 1995). If the validity of these particular findings from the assessment studies is also upheld, it may be desirable to train some adults what *not* to do, as well as what to do, when interacting with children during acute painful medical treatments.

There are a number of additional directions for future treatment research in the area of acute pain experienced by pediatric oncology patients and by other pediatric populations. The most obvious is to develop more effective interventions. Distraction, or cognitive refocusing (Varni, Blount, & Quiggins, in press), is a common component of the treatments reviewed.

Developing treatments that help assure greater distraction seems to be a promising approach. Second, efforts to incorporate medical staff as coaches for the child or parent should be continued (Blount, 1987; Cohen et al., 1995).

Third, evaluating the effects of additional commonly used medications for children undergoing painful treatments seems to be a valuable direction for future research. Effects of medication might be evaluated either in conjunction with, or when compared to, the effects of powerful coping skills programs. These types of investigations could also result in the development of criteria for matching particular pharmacological and/or psychological treatment to the unique characteristics of the child and family. EMLA, a topical anesthetic, and midazolam, used for conscious sedation, are two such medications (for a review, see Varni, Blount, & Quiggins, in press). It will be especially important in investigations using pharmacological interventions for child distress to be assessed for longer periods of time to determine possible side effects from pharmacological interventions (Jay et al., in press).

Fourth, promoting long-term maintenance of adults' coping promoting and children's coping behaviors should be a goal of much of the treatment research on acute distress. Similarly, there are other dimensions of generalization, such as children and parents using their coping and coping promoting skills during other painful medical treatments. Generalization of coping skills across medical treatments should be promoted and assessed.

SUMMARY AND CONCEPTUALIZATION

Assessment of the effects of complex, relatively long-term medical stressors, such as hospitalization, indicates that for many children there are ill effects that last for several weeks or more. Some of the psychological variables that have been associated with more problematic adjustment to hospitalization include difficult temperament, prehospital adjustment problems, a history of painful and unpleasant medical care, and a younger age. Interventions that have been developed to help children cope with stresses they encounter during hospitalization are based on information provision, modeling, support by medical staff, and cop-

ing skills training. Although there is evidence for effectiveness of these approaches, they have been developed largely without regard to the findings from the assessment literature in this area. Restated, the assessment literature has done little to influence development of clinical interventions to assist children coping with hospitalization.

In observational studies of the assessment of children's reactions to acute painful medical procedures, several parental, staff, and child variables have been identified that were related to children's coping and distress. Researchers in this area have utilized these findings to develop more effective therapeutic interventions to assist children, their parents, and medical staff during injections, LPs, and BMAs. One promising direction for future research in this area is to evaluate the effects of various pharmacological interventions when compared to, and when used in conjunction with, powerful psychosocial treatments.

It is clear that there are differences in the ways that children have been prepared for longer-term, more complex, and multifaceted stressors, such as hospitalization, versus more discrete, time-limited stressors, such as injections. For hospitalization, the general approach has been to provide the child with information, while also possibly teaching various coping strategies, some of which may include aspects of distraction. In contrast, for time-limited discrete stressors, such as injections, the general approach is to teach and prompt high levels of distraction or cognitive refocusing strategies, while, as a matter of course, also providing some information about the upcoming painful procedure.

Information is included in both cases, but the proportion is generally greater for the stressor of hospitalization than for acute painful procedures. Children have been prepared in ways consistent with this description, without regard to their usual coping styles, and the efficacy of these treatment approaches generally has been supported. A recent meta-analysis of studies of the effectiveness of approach or avoidant coping styles (Suls & Fletcher, 1985) support this interpretation of the literature. For short-term stressors, Suls and Fletcher (1985) found that attention to the sensory aspects of the stressful situation was superior to avoidance. However, avoidance was the superior strategy for short-term stressors if attention was focused on the emotional aspects of the situation, such as fear and anxiety. For long-term stressors, attention was associated with better outcomes.

What is needed is a coping strategy x stressful situation model for conceptualizing children's coping with stressful medical treatments, as well as for developing coping skills programs. Those children who must undergo acute stressors, such as injections, should be provided with some procedural information in the service of teaching and prompting high levels of distraction, or cognitive refocusing, away from their emotional reactions and the threatening aspects of the situation, particularly during the actual painful phases of the procedure. Such information is usually provided in coping skills programs during practice prior to the painful procedure and, perhaps to some extent, information may be provided during the painful procedures as well.

It should also be noted here that distraction is not necessarily the same as avoidance. Distraction is an active and focused cognitively oriented coping behavior over which the person exerts conscious control. Also, in the case of children undergoing acute painful medical treatments, distraction is very much facilitated by external cues, such as adult prompts to attend to something else or highly engaging cartoons. Avoidance, however, may simply reflect an attempt to escape from the threatening situation, a low level of control over the threatening situation, and a generally ineffective approach to coping with medical stressors. Thus, while distraction can be viewed as an active coping technique, avoidance may actually be a distress behavior.

In contrast to how best to cope with acute stressors, when confronted with complex and long-term stressors, it is important to provide the child with as much information as he or she needs, given that child's developmental level, while simultaneously teaching coping behaviors, which may include distraction or other techniques that involve aspects of cognitive refocusing, such as making coping statements or deep breathing. The prescription for the desired mix of information and distraction approaches for preparing children, given the nature of the stressful medical situation, is illustrated in Figure 19.1.

This model avoids the pitfalls of thinking only in terms of distraction versus information provision

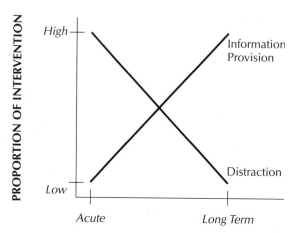

Figure 19.1 Prescription for the Relative Proportion of Information Provision- and Distraction-Based Interventions for Children Undergoing Acute or Long-Term Medical Stressors

types of treatments to be selected dependent on the coping style of the child. In fact, most treatments include varying degrees of information and distraction. Further, from the authors' clinical experience, it is common for individuals to shift from distraction to information gathering, and visa versa, during stressful situations. For example, some individuals who use distraction well during acute painful procedures switch to attending when the medical procedure moves to another phase or if a problem is encountered while performing the procedure. As this new information is incorporated and a routine is again attained, distraction is employed. What seems to be important is relative mix of information seeking/provision and distraction, given the characteristics of the stressor. Children's preferred coping styles in this context may be seen as more or less adaptive, depending on whether the style facilitates or hinders use of effective coping strategies in that situation. The clinician's task of preparing children might be made easier when the desired coping strategy for a particular stressor is consistent with the person's style, or usual coping pattern, and more difficult when it is at variance with that usual pattern.

REFERENCES

Azarnoff, P., & Woody, P. D. (1981). Preparation of children for hospitalization in acute care hospitals in the United States. *Pediatrics, 68,* 361–368.

Bibace, R., & Walsh, M. E. (1980). Development of children's concepts of illness. *Pediatrics, 66,* 912–917.

Blount, R. L. (1987). The dissemination of cost-effective psychosocial programs for children in health care settings. *Children's Health Care, 15,* 206–213.

Blount, R. L., Bachanas, P. J., Powers, S. W., Cotter, M. C., Franklin, A., Chaplin, W., Mayfield, J., Henderson, M., & Blount, S. D. (1992). Training children to cope and parents to coach them during routine immunizations: Effects on child, parent and staff behaviors. *Behavior Therapy, 23,* 689–705.

Blount, R. L., Cohen, L. L., Frank, N. C., Bachanas, P. J., Smith, A. J., Manimala, R. M., & Pate, J. T. (1997). The Child-Adult Medical Procedure Interaction Scale-Revised: An assessment of validity. *Journal of Pediatric Psychology, 22,* 73–88.

Blount, R. L., Corbin, S. M., Sturges, J. W., Wolfe, V. V., Prater, J. M., & James, L. D. (1989). The relationship between adults' behavior and child coping and distress during BMA/LP procedures: A sequential analysis. *Behavior Therapy, 20,* 585–601.

Blount, R. L., Davis, N., Powers, S., & Roberts, M. C. (1991). The influence of environmental factors and coping style on children's coping and distress. *Clinical Psychology Review, 11,* 93–116.

Blount, R. L., Landolf-Fritsche, B., Powers, S. W., & Sturges, J. W. (1991). Differences between high and low coping children and between parent and staff behaviors during painful medical procedures. *Journal of Pediatric Psychology, 16,* 795–809.

Blount, R. L., Powers, S. W., Cotter, M. W., Swan S. C., & Free, K. (1994). Making the system work: Training pediatric oncology patients to cope and their parents to coach them during BMA/LP procedures. *Behavior Modification, 18,* 6–31.

Blount, R. L., Sturges, J. W., & Powers, S. W. (1990). Analysis of child and adult behavioral variations by phase of medical procedure. *Behavior Therapy, 21,* 33–48.

Brain, D. J., & Maclay, I. (1968). Controlled study of mothers and children in hospital. *British Medical Journal, 1,* 278–280.

Burstein, S., & Meichenbaum, D. (1979). The work of worrying in children undergoing surgery. *Journal of Abnormal Child Psychology, 7,* 121–132.

Bush, J. P. (1987). Pain in children: A review of the literature from a developmental perspective. *Psychology and Health, 1,* 215–235.

Bush, J. P. (1990). Understanding pediatric pain: A developmental perspective. In T. W. Miller (Ed.), *Chronic pain: Clinical issues in health care management* (Vol. 2, pp. 757–786). Madison, CT: International Universities Press.

Bush, J. P., Melamed, B. G., Sheras, P. L., & Greenbaum, P. E. (1986). Mother-child patterns of coping with anticipatory medical stress. *Health Psychology, 5* (2), 137–157.

Campbell, J. D. (1975). Illness is a point of view: The development of children's concepts of illness. *Child Development, 46,* 92–100.

Carson, D. K., Council, J. R., & Gravley, J. E. (1991). Temperament and family characteristics as predictors of children's reactions to hospitalization. *Developmental and Behavioral Pediatrics, 12* (3), 141–147.

Cohen, L., Blount, R. L., Panopoulos, G., & Manimala, M. R. (1995). *Training nurses to administer coping skills program to parents and children undergoing immunizations.* Manuscript in preparation.

Couture, C. J. (1976). The psychological responses of young children to brief hospitalization and surgery: The role of parent-child contact and age. *Dissertation Abstracts International, 37*(B), 1427B.

Craig, K. D., Grunau, R. V., & Branson, S. M. (1988). Age-related aspects of pain: Pain in children. In R. Dubner, G. F. Gebhart, & M. R. Bond (Eds.), *Pain research and clinical management: Vol. 3. Proceedings of the Fifth World Congress on Pain* (pp. 317–328). Amsterdam: Elsevier.

Dahlquist, L., Gil, K., Armstrong, F., Ginsberg, A., & Jones, B. (1985). Behavioral management of children's distress during chemotherapy. *Journal of Behavior Therapy and Experimental Psychiatry, 16,* 325–329.

Douglas, J. W. B. (1975). Early hospital admission and later disturbances of behavior and learning. *Developmental Medicine and Child Neurology, 17,* 456–480.

Elkins, P. D., & Roberts, M. C. (1985). Reducing medical fears in a general population of children: A comparison of three audiovisual modeling procedures. *Journal of Pediatric Psychology, 10,* 65–75.

Fanurik, D., Zeltzer, L. K., Roberts, M. C., & Blount, R. L. (1993). The relationship between children's coping styles and psychological interventions for cold pressor pain. *Pain, 53,* 213–222.

Faust, J., Olson, R., & Rodriguez, H. (1991). Same-day surgery preparation: Reduction of pediatric patient arousal and distress through participant modeling. *Journal of Consulting and Clinical Psychology, 59,* 475–478.

Ferguson, B. F. (1979). Preparing young children for hospitalization: A comparison of two methods. *Pediatrics, 64,* 656–664.

Frank, N. C., Blount, R. L., Smith, A. J., Manimala, M. R., & Martin, J. K. (1995). Parent and staff behavior, previous child medical experience, and maternal anxiety as they relate to child distress and coping. *Journal of Pediatric Psychology, 20,* 277–289.

Goldsmith, H. H., Buss, A. H., Plomin, R., Rothbart, M. K., Thomas, A., Chess, S., Hinde, R. A., & McCall, R. B. (1987). Roundtable: What is temperament? Four approaches. *Child Development, 58,* 505–529.

Gonzalez, J. C., Routh, D. K., & Armstrong, F. D. (1993). Effects of maternal distraction versus reassurance on children's reactions to injections. *Journal of Pediatric Psychology, 18* (5), 593–604.

Gonzalez, J. C., Routh, D. K., Saab, P. G., Armstrong, F. D., Shifman, L., Guerra, E., & Fawcett, N. (1989). Effects of parent presence on children's reactions to injections: Behavioral, physiological, and subjective aspects. *Journal of Pediatric Psychology, 14* (3), 449–462.

Haller, J., Talbert, J. L., & Dombro, R. H. (Eds.). (1967). *The hospitalized child and his family.* Baltimore: Johns Hopkins University Press.

Harbeck-Weber, C., & McKee, D. H. (in press). Prevention of emotional and behavioral distress in children experiencing hospitalization and chronic illness. In M.C. Roberts (Ed.), *Handbook of pediatric psychology* (2nd ed.). New York: Guilford.

Jacobsen, P., Manne, S., Gorfinkle, K., Schorr, O., Rapkin, B., & Redd, W. H. (1990). Analysis of child and parent activity during painful medical procedures. *Health Psychology, 9,* 559–576.

Jay, S. M. (1988). Invasive medical procedures: Psychological intervention and assessment. In D. K. Routh (Ed.), *Handbook of pediatric psychology* (pp. 401–425). New York: Guilford.

Jay, S. M., & Elliott, C. H. (1990). A stress inoculation program for parents whose children are undergoing painful medical procedures. *Journal of Consulting and Clinical Psychology, 58,* 799–804.

Jay, S. M., Elliott, C. H., Fitzgibbons, I., Woody, P., & Siegel, S. (in press). A comparative study of cognitive behavior therapy versus general anesthesia for painful medical procedures for children. *Pain.*

Jay, S. M., Elliott, C., Katz, E., & Siegel, S. (1987). Cognitive-behavioral and pharmacologic interventions for children's distress during painful medical procedures. *Journal of Consulting and Clinical Psychology, 55,* 860–865.

Jay, S. M., Elliott, C. H., Woody, P. D., & Siegel, S. (1991). An investigation of cognitive-behavior therapy combined with oral valium for children undergoing painful medical procedures. *Health Psychology, 10,* 317–322.

Jay, S. M., Ozolins, M., Elliott, C. H., & Caldwell, S. (1983). Assessment of children's distress during painful medical procedures. *Health Psychology, 2* (2), 133–147.

Jensen, R. A. (1955). The hospitalized child: Round table. *American Journal of Orthopsychiatry, 25,* 293–318.

Karoly, P. (1991). Assessment of pediatric pain. In J. P. Bush & S. W. Harkins (Eds.), *Children in pain: Clini-* cal and research issues from a developmental perspective. New York: Springer-Verlag.

Katz, E. R., Kellerman, J., & Siegel, S. E. (1980). Distress behavior in children with cancer undergoing medical procedures: Developmental considerations. *Journal of Consulting and Clinical Psychology, 48,* 356–365.

Klorman, R., Hilpert, P. L., Michael, R., LaGana, C., & Sveen, O. B. (1980) Effects of coping and mastery modeling on experienced and inexperienced pedodontic patients' disruptiveness, *Behavior Therapy, 11,* 156–168.

Lumley, M. A., Abeles, L. A., Melamed, B. G., Pistone, L. M., & Johnson, J. H. (1990). Coping outcomes in children undergoing stressful medical procedures: The role of child-environment variables. *Behavioral Assessment, 12,* 223–238.

Lumley, M. A, Melamed, B. G., & Abeles, L. A. (1993). Predicting children's presurgical anxiety and subsequent behavior changes. *Journal of Pediatric Psychology, 18* (4), 481–497.

Mabe, P. A., Treiber, F. A., & Riley, W. T. (1991). Examining emotional distress during pediatric hospitalization for school-aged children. *Children's Health Care, 20* (3), 162–169.

Manimala, M. R., Blount, R. L., Panopoulos, G., Cohen, L., Pate, J., & Smith, A. (1995). *The effects of distraction and reassurance on the coping and distress of children undergoing immunizations.* Manuscript in submission.

Manne, S. L., Bakeman, R., Jacobsen, P. B., Gorfinkle, K., Bernstein, D., & Redd, W. H. (1992). Adult-child interaction during medical procedures. *Health Psychology, 11* (4), 241–249.

Manne, S. L., Bakeman, R., Jacobsen, P. P., Gorfinkle, K., & Redd, W. H. (1994). An analysis of a behavioral intervention for children undergoing venipuncture. *Health Psychology, 13,* 556–566.

Manne, S., Redd, W. H., Jacobsen, P., Gorfinkle, K., Schorr, O., & Rapkin, B. (1990). Behavioral intervention to reduce child and parent distress during venipuncture. *Journal of Consulting and Clinical Psychology, 58,* 565–572.

McClowry, S. G. (1990). The relationship of temperament to the pre and post behavioral responses of hospitalized school-age children. *Nursing Research, 39* (1), 30–35.

Melamed, B. G., Dearborn, M., & Hermecz, D. A. (1983). Necessary conditions for surgery preparation: Age and previous experience. *Psychosomatic Medicine, 45,* 517–525.

Melamed, B. G., & Ridley-Johnson, R. (1988). Psychological preparation of families for hospitalization. *Journal of Developmental and Behavioral Pediatrics, 9,* 96–102.

Melamed, B. G., & Siegel, L. J. (1975). Reduction of anxiety in children facing hospitalization and surgery by use of filmed modeling. *Journal of Consulting and Clinical Psychology, 43,* 511–521.

Meng, A., & Zastowny, T. (1982). Preparation for hospitalization: A stress inoculation training program for parents and children. *Maternal-Child Nursing Journal, 11,* 87–94.

Morrow, C. E., Armstrong, F. D., Routh, D. K., Gay, C., & Levy, J. (1993, April). *Correlates of child distress during lumbar punctures: Parent behavior and parenting characteristics.* Paper presented at the Florida Conference on Child Health Psychology, Gainesville, FL.

Pate, J. T., & Blount, R. L. (1995). *The effects of medical experience on future medical care: A review and critique.* Manuscript in submission.

Peterson, L. (1989). Coping by children undergoing stressful medical procedures: Some conceptual, methodological, and therapeutic issues. *Journal of Consulting and Clinical Psychology, 57* (3), 380–387.

Peterson, L., & Brownlee-Duffeck, M. (1984). Prevention of anxiety and pain due to medical and dental procedures. In M. C. Roberts & L. Peterson (Eds.), *Prevention of problems in childhood: Psychological research and applications* (pp. 266–308). New York: Wiley-Interscience.

Peterson, L., & Mori, L. (1988). Preparation for hospitalization. In D. K. Routh (Ed.), *Handbook of pediatric psychology* (pp. 460–491). New York: Guilford.

Peterson, L., & Ridley-Johnson, R. (1980). Pediatric hospital response to survey on prehospital preparation for children. *Journal of Pediatric Psychology, 5,* 1–7.

Peterson, L., Ridley-Johnson, R., Tracy, K., & Mullins, L. L. (1984). Developing cost-effective presurgical preparation: A comparative analysis. *Journal of Pediatric Psychology, 9,* 439–455.

Peterson, L., Schultheis, K., Ridley-Johnson, R., Miller, D. J., & Tracy, K. (1984). Comparison of three modeling procedures on the presurgical and postsurgical reactions of children. *Behavior Therapy, 15,* 197–203.

Peterson, L., & Shigetomi, C. (1981). The use of coping techniques to minimize anxiety in hospitalized children. *Behavior Therapy, 12,* 1–14.

Peterson, L. J., & Toler, S. M. (1986). An information seeking disposition in child surgery patients. *Health Psychology, 5,* 343–358.

Pinto, R. P., & Hollandsworth, J. G. (1989). Using videotape modeling to prepare children psychologically for surgery: Influence of parents and costs versus benefits of providing preparation services. *Health Psychology, 8,* 79–95.

Powers, S. W., Blount, R. L., Bachanas, P. J., Cotter, M. C, & Swan, S. C. (1993). Helping preschool leukemia patients and their parents cope during injections. *Journal of Pediatric Psychology, 18,* 681–695.

Prugh, D. G., Staub, E. M., Sands, H. H., Kirschenbaum, R. M., & Lenihan, E. A. (1953). A study of the emotional reactions of children and families to hospitalization and illness. *American Journal of Orthopsychiatry, 23,* 70–106.

Quinton, D., & Rutter, M. (1976). Early hospital admissions and later disturbances of behavior: An attempted replication of Douglas' findings. *Developmental Medicine & Child Neurology, 18,* 447–459.

Rasnake, L. K., & Linscheid, T. R. (1989). Anxiety reduction in children receiving medical care: Developmental considerations. *Journal of Developmental and Behavioral Pediatrics, 10,* 169–175.

Roberts, M. C. (1992). Vale dictum: An editor's view of the field of pediatric psychology. *Journal of Pediatric Psychology, 17,* 785–805.

Roberts, M. C., Wurtele, S. K., Boone, R. R., Ginther, L. J., & Elkins, P. D. (1981). Reduction of medical fears by use of modeling: A preventive application in a general population of children. *Journal of Pediatric Psychology, 6,* 293–300.

Ross, D. M., & Ross, S. A. (1988). *Childhood pain: Current issues, research, and management.* Baltimore: Urban & Schwarzenberg.

Ross, R. S., Bush, J. P., & Crummette, B. D. (1991). Factors affecting nurses' decisions to administer PRN analgesic medication to children after surgery: An analog investigation. *Journal of Pediatric Psychology, 16* (2), 151–167.

Schultz, J. B., Raschke, D., Dedrick, C., & Thompson, M. (1981). The effects of a preoperational puppet show on anxiety levels of hospitalized children. *Journal of the Association for the Care of Children's Health, 9,* 118–120.

Shaw, E. G., & Routh, D. K. (1982). Effect of mother presence on children's reaction to aversive procedures. *Journal of Pediatric Psychology, 7* (1), 33–42.

Siegel, L. J. (1981, April). *Naturalistic study of coping strategies in children facing medical procedures.* Paper presented at the meeting of the Southwestern Psychological Association, Atlanta.

Simeonsson, R. J., Buckley, L., & Monson, L. (1979). Conceptions of illness causality in hospitalized children. *Journal of Pediatric Psychology, 4,* 77–84.

Skipper, J. K., & Leonard, R. C. (1968) Children, stress and hospitalization: A field experiment. *Journal of Health and Social Behavior, 9,* 275–280.

Smith, K., Ackerson, J., & Blotcky, A. (1989). Reducing distress during invasive medical procedures: Relating behavioral interventions to preferred coping style in pediatric cancer patients. *Journal of Pediatric Psychology, 14,* 405–419.

Sturges, J. W., Blount, R. L., James, L. D., Powers, S. W., & Prater, J. M. (1991). Analysis of child distress by phase of medical procedure. In J. H. Johnson & S. B. Johnson (Eds.), *Advances in child health psychology* (pp. 63–76). Gainesville: University of Florida Press.

Suls, J., & Fletcher, B. (1985). The relative efficacy of avoidant and nonavoidant coping strategies: A meta-analysis. *Health Psychology, 4* (3), 249–288.

Thompson, K. L., & Varni, J. (1986). A developmental cognitive-behavioral approach to pediatric pain management. *Pain, 25,* 283–296.

Thompson, R. H., & Vernon, D. T. A. (1993). Research on children's behavior after hospitalization: A review and synthesis. *Developmental and Behavioral Pediatrics, 14* (1), 28–35.

Varni, J. W., Blount, R. L., & Quiggins, D. J. L. (in press). Oncologic disorders. In R. T. Ammerman & J. V. Campo (Eds.), *Handbook of pediatric psychology and psychiatry.* Boston: Allyn and Bacon.

Varni, J. W., Blount, R. L., Waldron, S. A., Smith, A. J. (1995). Management of pain and distress. In M. C. Roberts (Ed.), *Handbook of pediatric psychology* (2nd ed. pp. 105–123). New York: Guilford.

Vernon, D. T., & Thompson, R. H. (1993). Research on the effect of experimental interventions on children's behavior after hospitalization: A review and synthesis. *Journal of Developmental & Behavioral Pediatrics, 14,* 36–44.

Visintainer, M. A., & Wolfer, J. A. (1975). Psychological preparation for surgical pediatric patients: The effect on children's and parents' stress responses and adjustment, *Pediatrics, 56,* 187–202.

Wells, R. D., & Schwebel, A. I. (1987). Chronically ill children and their mothers: Predictors of resilience and vulnerability to hospitalization and surgical stress. *Developmental and Behavioral Pediatrics, 8* (2), 83–89.

Wolfer, J. A., & Visitainer, M. A., (1975). Pediatric surgical patients' and parents' stress responses and adjustment. *Nursing Research, 24,* 244–255.

Wolfer, J., & Visitainer, M. (1979). Prehospital psychological preparation for tonsillectomy patients: Effects on children and parents' adjustment, *Pediatrics, 64,* 646–655.

Zabin, M. A., & Melamed, B. G. (1980). Relationship between parental discipline and children's ability to cope with stress. *Journal of Behavior Assessment, 2* (1), 17–38.

Zastowny, T. R., Kirschenbaum, D. S., & Meng, A. L. (1986). Coping skills training for children: Effects on distress before, during and after hospitalization for surgery. *Health Psychology, 5,* 231–247.

Zeltzer, L. K. & LeBaron, S. (1982). Hypnosis and nonhypnotic techniques for reduction of pain and anxiety during painful procedures in children and adolescents with cancer. *Journal of Pediatrics, 101,* 1032–1035.

PART V

SPECIAL ISSUES

Relative to adults, research on children's health issues has lagged behind. However, this emerging arena offers many exciting opportunities. The chapters in this section address some of the topics in the evolving fields of child and adolescent health psychology. The first chapters of this section deal with a variety of issues, most of which have only begun to receive any significant attention. Chapter 20 deals with posttraumatic stress disorder (PTSD) and Chapter 21 discusses daily stress. The former introduces the two-factor model and discusses diagnostic considerations; the latter addresses the difficulties inherent in measuring stress and goes on to identify common childhood stressors. The authors also discuss measurement of and coping with these common stressors.

Chapter 22 highlights the continued need for prevention programs that target sexually transmitted diseases (STDs). Chapter 23 presents information on classification and assessment issues confronting clinicians and researchers who work with children complaining of sleep disorders. How parental chronic illness affects children is dealt with in Chapter 24, which reviews theoretical models and recent data-based studies. Chapter 25 focuses on the physical health of children with mental retardation. Chapter 26 addresses suicide risk factors and prevention as well as how to work effectively with suicidal adolescents and children. A comprehensive review of the abuse and violence literature is presented in Chapter 27. In addition to reviewing literature regarding characteristics of children and parents in abusive environments, the authors discuss the effects of abuse and violence on children, including the effects of spousal abuse and community violence. The final chapter (Chapter 28) discusses many ethical issues that confront practicing pediatric health psychologists, including confidentiality issues with minors and cultural sensitivity. The authors also review a variety of legal areas.

CHAPTER 20

POSTTRAUMATIC STRESS DISORDER

Judith A. Lyons, JACKSON VETERANS AFFAIRS AND UNIVERSITY OF MISSISSIPPI MEDICAL CENTERS
Christina Adams, JACKSON VETERANS AFFAIRS AND UNIVERSITY OF MISSISSIPPI MEDICAL CENTERS

The clinical and scientific study of posttraumatic stress disorder (PTSD) is evolving rapidly (see Lyons, 1987). This makes the field both an exciting one that offers many opportunities for ground-breaking work and, simultaneously, a frustrating one in which diagnostic criteria have undergone frequent revisions and few standardized measures or treatment protocols have been available. This chapter will briefly review the historical development of theories of PTSD and diagnostic criteria. A practical review of assessment and treatment strategies from the perspective of the two-factor model of PTSD is also presented.

HISTORY AND THEORETICAL MODELS

Throughout history, scholars have recognized that extreme events, such as war, can lead to the constellation of symptoms identified as posttraumatic stress disorder. Although debate continues regarding the precise difference between a traumatic event and a highly stressful but nontraumatic event, mental health professionals generally accept that an element of physical threat and a subjective experience of distress regarding the event must both be present for PTSD to develop (American Psychiatric Association, 1994). War, family/neighborhood violence, sexual abuse, natural disasters, and transportation disasters are among the traumatic events commonly reported for both adults and children.

Over the past century, researchers have proposed various models to explain the distress and dysfunction some individuals display following a traumatic event. Early models of trauma assumed a biological basis for the symptoms, (e.g., soldier's heart, battle fatigue, shell shock), thereby assuming physical recuperation was sufficient treatment. Even when professionals acknowledged trauma-related psychopathology as a "gross stress reaction" (American Psychiatric Association, 1952), therapy remained largely supportive.

By the time the label *posttraumatic stress disorder* was coined, emphasis had shifted to dynamic models of phasic shifts between intrusive and avoidant symptoms (e.g., Horowitz, 1976). Phasic models tend to emphasize the dissociative aspects of PTSD (March, 1990). The belief that repression or avoidance of traumatic memories often suppress intrusive reexperiencing of the trauma was evident in the fact that the original diagnostic criteria for PTSD (American Psychiatric Association, 1980) included a separate subcategory for chronic/delayed PTSD. This classification has since been abolished (American Psychiatric Association, 1987, 1994) due to the recognition that delays in diagnosis are often caused by delays in reporting of symptoms, rather than delays in onset of psychopathology.

Although the phasic cycles proposed by these models have not received consistent support in the literature (March, 1990), data do indicate that dissociative reactions at the time of the traumatic event mark an increased risk for developing the disorder (e.g., Koopman, Classen, & Spiegel, 1994; Marmar et al., 1994). In addition to their impact on the original diagnostic criteria for PTSD, the influence of models such as Horowitz's is also evident in one of the major assessment tools in use today, the Impact of Events Scale (Horowitz, Wilner, & Alvarez, 1979; Zilberg, Weiss, & Horowitz, 1982). Renewed attention to phasic models may also emerge in response to the ongoing false/recovered memory debate (e.g., Loftus, 1994, and related letters in the *American Psychologist;* September–December 1994 issue of *Consciousness and Cognition).*

Behavioral (Keane, Zimering, & Caddell, 1985) and cognitive (Foa & Kozak, 1986) models of PTSD developed during the 1980s continue to be examined and refined. These models focus on the anxiety-related aspects of PTSD. They emphasize cues associated with perceptions of threat/arousal and the coping strategies individuals use to reduce their distress. Many of the components of these models are empirically testable. The evidence to date supports these models over the phasic models (March, 1990; Pitman, 1993) and, although there has been much debate, PTSD remains classified as an anxiety disorder rather than a dissociative disorder. The behavioral and psychophysiological assessment paradigms for PTSD and most of the treatment strategies that employ some form of therapeutic exposure to trauma cues have their roots in behavioral and cognitive theoretical models.

Recently, researchers have proposed intriguing new biological models (e.g., Burges Watson, Hoffman, & Wilson, 1988; Kolb, 1987; van der Kolk, 1994; see review by ver Ellen & van Kammen, 1990). Far more complex than the old biological models, which posited a single cause, such as fatigue or artillery reverberations, recent models incorporate psychological as well as physical factors. Paradigms for biological/physiological assessments are becoming more commonplace, and pharmacotherapy regimens based on these models are undergoing clinical trials (see reviews by Friedman, 1991; Pitman, 1993). The authors anticipate that future model building will combine features of biological, behavioral, and cognitive models of PTSD to enhance understanding of this complex disorder.

The Two-Factor Model of PTSD

Of the models presently available, the authors of this chapter find the behavioral two-factor model to be the most helpful and parsimonious in conceptualizing the development, assessment, and treatment of PTSD. Originally developed by Mowrer (1947), this model incorporates both classical and instrumental conditioning to explain anxiety disorders, such as PTSD. *Classical conditioning* is the learning process by which previously unrelated stimuli become associated with an involuntary response and gain the capacity to elicit that response. In the case of PTSD, classical conditioning begins at the time of the trauma. By *DSM-IV* definition, the traumatic event elicits intense fear, helplessness, or horror. Thus, the trauma serves as an unconditioned stimulus (UCS) eliciting physiological arousal and psychological distress (the unconditioned response, UCR). Other internal and external cues present at the time of the trauma (conditioned stimuli, CS) become paired with these responses. Thus, when trauma survivors later encounter these conditioned stimuli, they reexperience psychophysiological distress (conditioned response, CR). Such CRs constitute one of the main diagnostic criteria for PTSD (Criterion B), as detailed in the section on *DSM-IV* later.

Instrumental conditioning is the process by which an organism learns to behave in ways that yield desired outcomes. According to the two-factor model, it is through instrumental conditioning that trauma survivors learn to avoid or escape trauma-related cues. Such behavior becomes reinforced because it allows survivors to escape from or avoid psychophysiological reexperiencing and thus reduces acute distress. Over time, such avoidance can lead to marked restrictions in activities and emotional responding (as detailed in discussion of *DSM-IV* Criterion C later).

Most trauma-related cues (CSs) are inherently innocuous. Repeated encounters with such cues during which nothing disastrous occurs would, according to classical conditioning theory, serve as extinction trials that would eventually extinguish the conditioned distress. However, the combination of classically conditioned distress and instrumentally conditioned avoidance makes symptoms self-perpetuating in many cases. Successful avoidance behavior can preclude exposure to trauma-related cues and thus limit the number of extinction trials that survivors experience. The range of trauma-associated cues can then expand over time through stimulus generalization. Furthermore, many CSs consist of complex stimuli and involve serially ordered cues; these complications contribute to the persistence of reexperiencing symptoms and avoidance because all major components of the cue complex must become deconditioned in order for survivors to obtain lasting symptom relief (Levis, 1981, 1985).

DSM-IV DIAGNOSTIC CRITERIA

When the original *DSM-III* diagnostic criteria for PTSD were developed, the literature on children's responses to trauma was minimal. Subsequently, Lenore Terr's clinical research on trauma reactions in children, even though it did not follow a structured protocol, was pivotal in ensuring inclusion of numerous characteristics of children's responses in *DSM-III-R* criteria (see review, Terr, 1985). The new *DSM-IV* criteria continue to specify variations of symptoms specific to children, including some of the behavior patterns first identified by Terr. However, the co-chairs of the committee that developed the *DSM-IV* criteria for PTSD, John Davidson and Edna Foa (1991), admit that there is only limited research on the factor structure and internal consistency of the diagnostic criteria as they apply to children.

The Traumatic Event

The first element required for the diagnosis of PTSD (Criterion A) is *identification of a specific traumatic experience*. Based on empirical data, the definition of the stressor in *DSM-IV* no longer requires that the event must be outside the range of usual human experience (March, 1993). By the *DSM-IV* definition, an event must both (A1) encompass a degree of physical threat to the patient directly or to someone else and (A2) evoke a subjective reaction of intense fear, helplessness, or horror. Two variants of these guidelines apply in the case of children. First, sexual experiences that exceed the appropriate developmental level of a

child qualify as a traumatic stressor, even in the absence of threats, violence, or injury. Second, observance of agitated or disorganized behavior can serve as a substitute for subjective reports of distress.

In reviewing existing literature, McNally (1993) concluded that broadening the stressor criterion to include nonrare events is unlikely to increase greatly the number of cases of PTSD detected. The events most likely to lead to PTSD symptomatology in children involve acts of violence, such as shootings and warfare, that would qualify under either *DSM-III-R* or *DSM-IV* criteria.

It is important to note that occurrence of a traumatic event is a necessary but not sufficient condition for development of PTSD. Reported incidence of PTSD secondary to disasters and child abuse varies widely across studies, perhaps due to variability in discrete components of the trauma experience (McNally, 1991, 1993) as well as differences in diagnostic procedures used. The probability/severity of PTSD symptomatology increases in both children and adults as a function of intensity of the stressor, physical proximity to the actual event, and degree to which the trauma results from deliberate actions of another person rather than the result of an accident or natural causes (Davidson & Fairbank, 1993; Lonigan, Shannon, Taylor, Finch, & Sallee, 1994; Nader, Pynoos, Fairbanks, Al-Ajeel, & Al-Asfour, 1993; Nader, Pynoos, Fairbanks, & Frederick, 1990; Pynoos, Frederick, et al., 1987; Pynoos, Nader, Frederick, Gonda, & Stuber, 1987). Those who have experienced multiple events are at increased risk (Burton, Foy, Bwanausi, Johnson, & Moore, 1994). However, chronic states of stress tend to produce effects other than PTSD (McNally, 1993; Terr, 1991).

Reexperiencing

The second diagnostic criterion (Criterion B) stipulates that, to qualify for the diagnosis, *survivors must persistently reexperience the traumatic event in one of several ways*. This criterion is essentially the key to differential diagnosis of PTSD because it is the one set of symptoms unique to PTSD (Davidson & Foa, 1991). In adults, such reexperiencing most commonly takes the form of intrusive thoughts or nightmares in which survivors relive the event. In children, repetitive play that expresses themes or components of the event and/or general frightening dreams are common, and are sufficient to meet Criterion B. Intense psychological distress or physiological reactivity in response to internal or external trauma-related cues is also sufficient evidence of reexperiencing. Dissociative flashbacks may occur, but these are rare in adults and appear to be even rarer in children (Terr, 1985).

Avoidance and Numbing

Numbing of responsiveness and/or persistent avoidance of cues associated with the trauma (Criterion C) must be present to diagnose PTSD. These can include symptoms such as avoidance of thoughts, feelings, situations, or activities related to the trauma; psychogenic amnesia regarding important aspects of the event; diminished interest in activities; emotional detachment from others; restricted range of affect; and sense of a foreshortened future. Three of these symptoms must be present to make a diagnosis of PTSD. Research indicates that these symptoms may be infrequent and difficult to assess following a single-event trauma (Terr, 1991).

Hyperarousal

Persistent increased arousal (Criterion D) must also be present, as evidenced by problems such as insomnia, irritability/anger, trouble concentrating, hypervigilance, and exaggerated startle response. This criterion will be somewhat more difficult to meet under *DSM-IV* than it was under *DSM-III-R* due to the fact that physiological reactivity, in *DSM-IV*, now falls under Criterion B. Thus, individuals must now show two of five hyperarousal symptoms rather than two of a list of six. This difference may be particularly important in light of the fact that both Schwarz and Kowalski's (1991) work with survivors of a school shooting and Realmuto and colleagues' (1992) work with Cambodian adolescent refugees found Criterion D symptoms to be the limiting factor in how many of their subjects met full diagnostic criteria for PTSD.

Duration of Symptoms

Symptoms must persist for longer than one month in order to meet criteria for the diagnosis of PTSD (Cri-

terion E). However, a new *DSM-IV* diagnosis, "acute stress disorder," describes briefer/immediate reactions. This new category may prove sensitive in PTSD case finding because most cases of PTSD include acute reactions to the event. However, specificity as a marker for PTSD may be low because most cases of acute reaction do not develop into PTSD (see reviews by Blank, 1993; Rothbaum & Foa, 1993).

Level of Functioning

DSM-IV Criterion F is new. It stipulates that *symptoms must be sufficiently severe as to cause clinically significant distress or impairment in functioning.* Studies have found that children can score within the normal range on measures of general functioning even though they may meet other criteria for PTSD (e.g., Belter, Dunn, & Jeney, 1991; Lonigan et al., 1994), and children can often maintain satisfactory school functioning in spite of meeting PTSD Criteria A–E (e.g., Terr, 1985).

Other Symptoms

Additional symptoms frequently associated with PTSD in children, but neither necessary nor sufficient for diagnosis, include omen formation and somatic complaints (American Psychiatric Association, 1994). Terr (1985) reported finding regressive behavior (e.g., incontinence), perceptual distortions (time, auditory, visual), limited life philosophy, and death dreams among traumatized children. Other researchers also reported dependent behavior and separation difficulties in children following a trauma (Vogel & Vernberg, 1993).

Use of *DSM* Criteria

Not all researchers and clinicians urge strict adherence to *DSM* diagnostic criteria. Some have focused on the existence of a life-threatening stressor and advocate diagnosis of PTSD even in the absence of clear signs of reexperiencing or hyperarousal (e.g., Stuber, Nader, Yasuda, Pynoos, & Cohen, 1991). Others have argued that a history of chronic neglect or "toxic" surroundings produces PTSD even without a specifiable "traumatic event" (Earl, 1991). It is the authors' view, however, that PTSD is a very specific syndrome that is one of many possible responses to extreme stress. (Vogel and Vernberg's [1993] American Psychological Task Force report on children's responses to disasters provides an excellent outline of alternative outcomes.) Furthermore, it is important to differentiate PTSD from other Axis I and Axis II alternatives. By doing so, mental health professionals enhance their ability to predict, diagnose, and successfully treat the disorder.

AGE DIFFERENCES IN SYMPTOM PRESENTATION

Some studies have found more PTSD symptoms in younger children than older children (e.g., Lonigan et al., 1994; Pynoos & Nader, 1988a), whereas others found the opposite (e.g., Green et al., 1991). Some studies have obtained no significant differences in symptoms as a function of age (e.g., Pynoos, Frederick et al., 1987), although in some cases this may be a function of the limited age range in the sample (Yule, 1992). The literature is more consistent regarding reports of qualitative differences in symptom presentation across age levels than it is with quantitative aspects. For example, younger children's verbal reports of intrusive thoughts and avoidance/denial symptoms may be less common than those of older children, yet younger children still display distress behaviorally (Greene et al., 1991; Stuber et al., 1991; Terr, 1989; Vogel & Vernberg, 1993). Vogel and Vernberg (1993) suggested that several potential mediating factors (e.g., event appraisal, coping strategies, locus of control) may differ with age. Similarly, the effect of parental distress may vary according to the age of a child. There tends to be more similarity between distress levels of parents and children when the children are young as compared to when they are older, whereas older children's reactions may more directly relate to the degree of trauma exposure than do younger children's reactions (e.g., Green et al., 1991).

ASSESSMENT

For clinicians using the two-factor model of PTSD, the goal of assessment is to identify the unconditioned stimulus (traumatic event), conditioned stimuli (internal and external cues related to the traumatic event), extent and content of conditioned responses (severity and pattern of symptoms), and any avoidance responses that have precluded natural exposure to the conditioned stimuli. A thorough assessment based on *DSM* criteria, therefore, provides clinicians with not only a diagnostic label but also with baseline data and a blueprint for intervention. Assessment of traumatized children must also investigate potential comorbid disorders, particularly depression (Kinzie, Sack, Angell, Clarke, & Ben, 1989).

Symptom reports differ across assessment tools (e.g., Jones, Ribbe, & Cunningham, 1994) and also appear influenced by choice of informant (e.g., Belter et al., 1991; Famularo, Kinscherff, & Fenton, 1992). Although there have been exceptions (e.g., Breton, Valla, & Lambert, 1993; Martini, Ryan, Nakayama, & Ramenofsky, 1990), most studies indicate that parents and teachers report fewer symptoms when describing children's functioning than children report when describing themselves (e.g., Belter et al., 1991; Stallard & Law, 1993). This may be particularly true regarding subjective or covert symptoms, such as intrusive thoughts, rather than objective symptoms or overt behavior. Yule and Williams (1990) also found that children tend to report fewer symptoms in the presence of their parents. In light of such findings, multimethod and multiinformant assessment protocols are essential. Some of the commonly used assessment tools are described next.

Structured Interviews

PTSD Reaction Index (PTSD-RI)

The PTSD-RI is the most widely used structured interview for childhood PTSD (e.g., Belter et al., 1991; Lonigan, Shannon, Finch, Daugherty, & Taylor, 1991; Lonigan et al., 1994; Martini et al., 1990; Stuber et al., 1991). It is an adaptation of the adult PTSD-RI (Frederick, 1985), a self-report questionnaire (Pynoos, Frederick, et al., 1987). Reliability and validity of the 20-item interview/questionnaire have been satisfactory, and there are cut-off scores for various categories of symptom severity using a five-point scale for each item, as summarized by Nader and associates (1990, 1993). Other investigators, however, have used a four-point scale (Bradburn, 1991). Difficulties thus arise in comparing PTSD-RI results across studies. Realmuto and colleagues (1992) suggested the need for further content revision of the PTSD-RI and recommended the addition of frequency and duration indices.

Children's Posttraumatic Stress Disorder Inventory (CPTSDI)

Saigh (1989) constructed the CPTSDI based on *DSM-III* and clinical observations. The interview contains four subtests: mode of trauma induction (experienced directly, observed), intrusive ideation, general affect, and miscellaneous symptoms. Like the PTSD-RI, the CPTSDI is specific to PTSD symptomatology and does not assess comorbid difficulties.

Diagnostic Interview for Children and Adolescents (DICA)

The DICA, developed to assess a range of *DSM-III* disorders in children and adolescents (Welner, Reich, Herjanic, Jung, & Amado, 1987), underwent revision (DICA-R) for *DSM-III-R* and is now available in parent, adolescent, and child versions (Reich & Welner, 1990). Numerous studies have used the DICA or DICA-R to diagnose children with PTSD (e.g., Famularo, Kinscherff, & Fenton, 1991; Jones et al., 1994). For example, in a large prospective study of psychiatric admissions, Adam, Everett, and O'Neal (1992) found that 29 percent of abused children met criteria for PTSD according to the DICA-R. In light of the relatively poor performance of the adult Diagnostic Interview Schedule in identifying PTSD, however, further evaluation of the DICA's sensitivity and specificity for PTSD diagnosis appears warranted (McNally, 1991; Saigh, 1992).

Questionnaires

Impact of Events Scale (IES)

The IES (Horowitz et al., 1979), a 15-item questionnaire comprised of Intrusion and Avoidance subscales, is perhaps the most widely used of all assessment instruments in the study of both adult and child PTSD (e.g., Jones et al., 1994; Joseph, Brewin, Yule, & Williams, 1993). However, utility of the IES as a standard remains limited because of inconsistency across scoring systems and lack of normative data

(Vogel & Vernberg, 1993). High scores may reflect either grief reactions or PTSD (Pynoos, Nader, et al., 1987), a finding that is not surprising given that the original research sample consisted largely of bereaved adults (Horowitz et al., 1979).

Revised Children's Manifest Anxiety Scale (RCMAS)

The RCMAS (Reynolds & Richard, 1978) is a measure of general anxiety that numerous investigators have used in studies of PTSD. Following Hurricane Hugo, Lonigan and colleagues (1994) found that children who scored above the median on the RCMAS were nine times more likely to meet criteria for PTSD than those who scored below the median, even though their RCMAS scores remained within the normal range. Several studies (Joseph et al., 1993; Stallard & Law, 1993; Yule & Williams, 1990) have used the RCMAS in conjunction with the IES and the Birleson Depression Inventory (Birleson, 1981) to assess traumatized children. Despite differences in traumatic events (e.g., schoolbus accident versus cruise ship sinking), scores on this battery were similar across studies.

Behavioral Observation and Self-Monitoring

Behavioral observation of anxiety symptoms can be documented via formal counts and ratings or informal commentary, and can be a useful tool in diagnosis and measurement of treatment gains. One formal approach used in a series of studies by Saigh (1992) is the behavioral avoidance test (BAT) to measure avoidance of trauma cues. In a BAT, children are asked to approach the conditioned stimuli they fear. It is then possible to quantify their avoidance responses by measuring proximity attained, duration of stimulus tolerance, and so on. The primary drawback of the BAT is the lack of standardization, which limits efforts to examine reliability, validity, and generalizability (Caddell & Drabman, 1992).

Self-monitoring of intrusive thoughts, nightmares, avoidance, and the like, is often an option. For example, Saigh (1987a, 1987b) trained youths to self-monitor trauma-related ideation through different phases of flooding treatment with the use of pocket frequency counters. Parents and teachers may also monitor behaviors they observe. Report bias and reactivity to the monitoring process, however, may affect reliability and validity of self-monitoring data (Caddell & Drabman, 1992).

Physiological Recording

Physiological techniques, common in the adult PTSD literature, are rare in the assessment of childhood PTSD (McNally, 1991; Saigh, 1992). The need for funding and technical expertise to purchase and operate psychophysiological assessment equipment and the strain that complex laboratory procedures may place on patients might have discouraged the use of psychophysiological procedures in the past (Caddell & Drabman, 1992). However, the availability of inexpensive and easily operated devices for measuring heart rate, blood pressure, and so on, has reduced such concerns (Lyons, Alexander, Smith, Veltum, & Vogeltanz, 1993).

In the only available study of physiological reactivity in children with PTSD, Ornitz and Pynoos (1989) evaluated the exaggerated startle response in children traumatized by a sniper attack. Normally, it is possible to modulate a person's startle response by presenting a brief nonstartling warning tone prior to exposure to the louder, more abrupt test stimulus. Not only was this typical pattern of inhibitory startle modulation not present among the children with PTSD but these children also evidenced an increased startle response when the warning tone was of longer duration. Pitman and Orr (1990) challenged Ornitz and Pynoos's statistical analyses and interpretations. However, if future studies can replicate Ornitz and Pynoos's results, examination of startle modulation may prove useful in the assessment of PTSD in children. Pitman, Orr and colleagues' (Pitman, Orr, et al., 1990) protocol for presenting trauma cues via verbal scripts may also prove effective with youths.

TREATMENT

In comparison to the number of publications on assessment, there has been relatively little research on treatment of PTSD in children. The quality of research has also been quite variable, with few well-controlled empirical studies.

Crisis Intervention
Secondary Prevention

It is becoming increasingly common to hold post-trauma debriefings following an event that affects a large sector of the community or a defined group of individuals. Most posttrauma debriefings are based on, or are consonant with, the procedure developed by Jeffrey Mitchell, in which trauma survivors are encouraged to gather as a group and express their thoughts and feelings about the event. Restated in terms of the two-factor model, the goal is to provide group exposure to the internal (physiological, cognitive, emotional) and external (situational) cues associated with the trauma. Theoretically, the debriefing procedure's emphasis on immediacy (usually within 48 hours of the trauma) promotes therapeutic exposure before stimulus cues can generalize further and before complex avoidance patterns develop.

There really is little evidence by which to evaluate the impact of such interventions, either in the child literature or the adult literature. Robinson and Mitchell (1993) reported retrospective self-report data indicating that adults perceive such interventions help normalize reactions, reduce stress, and enhance coping. Follow-up studies of children are few and usually do not include control groups of exposed but not treated children (e.g., Milgram, Toubiana, Klingman, Raviv, & Goldstein, 1988; Stallard & Law, 1993; Yule & Udwin, 1991). When using control groups, it is important to conduct assessments of each group within similar time frames (compare methodologies and conclusions of Yule & Udwin, 1991, versus Yule, 1992). Overall, confounds between symptomatology and attrition are problematic, and outcomes are often inconsistent across measures/time.

Readers who are designing a crisis intervention for children may refer to Crabbs (1981), Pynoos and Nader (1988b) and Toubiana, Milgram, Strich, and Edelstein (1988) for guidelines on the topic. These references detail specific strategies, including projective/art techniques and use of guest speakers who stimulate discussion, to promote children's self-expression regarding the trauma and their losses. In the absence of stronger empirical support than is currently available regarding the efficacy of debriefings with children or adults, mental health professionals and administrators must rely on their professional judgment in recommending or prioritizing resources for such interventions.

Treatment Once PTSD Has Developed

Within the two-factor model of PTSD, the therapist's role is straightforward. Therapists must first provide a sufficiently supportive environment and convincing rationale so that patients are willing and able to tolerate exposure to trauma-related cues. Second, therapists guide patients through paced therapeutic exposure to the trauma cues. Third, therapists quickly identify any avoidance behaviors that are obstructing therapeutic exposure and intervene to minimize such avoidance. Although it is possible to identify each of these tasks and make them sound easy to perform, actual implementation is much more complex.

Rapport and Rationale

The authors strongly agree with Saigh (1992) that education regarding treatment rationale and the treatment procedures being used is a critical initial step in treatment. Therapists must inform both children and caregivers that the children will be focusing on distressing details of their trauma and that this process will be stressful. Therapists must also clearly inform children and caregivers that a transient increase in symptomatology may occur as therapists begin to prevent the children's avoidant coping strategies and begin to expose the children to trauma cues.

During assessment as well as during treatment, clinical rapport is crucial. As interviews with patients proceed to elicit detailed information about the trauma and related reexperiencing, the line between assessment and treatment often blurs because information gathering borders on therapeutic exposure to the trauma memories. It is important to be supportive and encouraging and to let clinical judgment guide the pace of such sessions. Clinician must be aware that there are marked individual differences in children's abilities to tolerate trauma cues without outbursts/ withdrawal (avoidant behavior) or dissociation (reexperiencing).

Therapeutic Exposure and Avoidance Response Prevention

Therapeutic exposure to trauma-related cues is the central component of all PTSD treatment, regardless of theoretical model (Fairbank & Nicholson, 1987). Trauma-focused groups, play therapy, art therapy, and expressive writing (Terr, 1989) are interventions used by therapists from various theoretical schools. Other techniques for therapeutic exposure—such as implosive therapy, imaginal and in vivo flooding, and systematic desensitization (Lyons & Keane, 1989; Saigh, 1992)—are specific to behaviorally oriented therapists. More important than the selection of a specific technique is the underlying emphasis on providing patients with an opportunity to voluntarily reexperience elements of the traumatic experience in a safe and supportive environment, with the goal of extinguishing the patients' conditioned responses to trauma-related cues.

Given that avoidance of trauma cues is a central feature of PTSD, the tasks of exposure and response prevention go hand in hand. As patients learn that they are able to reexperience internal and external cues associated with the trauma, they will be increasingly willing and able to reduce their avoidance behavior. Unfortunately, many clinicians not trained in the treatment of PTSD often allow or even encourage patients to engage in avoidance of trauma cues because it does produce a temporary reduction in acute distress. As March (1990, p. 77) noted, however, avoidance behaviors maintain PTSD symptoms and avoidance prevention "may be one key to successful therapy."

Saigh's work with war-related trauma in Lebanon is the only known series of programmatic studies regarding individual therapy for PTSD in children. Saigh studied exposure-based therapy (flooding) using multiple-baseline across traumatic scenes designs (reviewed in Saigh, 1992). His well-conducted work includes children of various ages. The children engaged in relaxation exercises followed by several hour-long imaginal flooding sessions. During each individual flooding session, children imaged various aspects of their trauma experience until their distress abated. Another brief relaxation exercise followed each flooding session. Across studies, Saigh has consistently found flooding to be efficacious in treating child and adolescent PTSD, with improvement documented on behavioral avoidance tests, subjective ratings, self-monitored intrusive thoughts, academic GPA, and a variety of standard tests and questionnaires.

Cocco and Sharpe (1993) reported a case study using an auditory variant of eye movement desensitization to treat a 4-year-old boy one year after a violent robbery. The therapist alternatingly clicked his fingers to each side of the child's head while the boy focused on a drawing of the crime. The therapist also integrated a drawing of the boy's favorite movie hero into the procedure, and the boy received prompts to describe what his superhero would do to the robbers. The boy stabbed the drawing of the attackers, acting out the conquering of the robbers. Additional forms of therapy were necessary to address recurring post-trauma behavioral problems, but the traumatic reexperiencing resolved after a single session using this procedure. Cocco and Sharpe's findings are consistent with reports in the adult literature, which demonstrates that procedures similar to those in Shapiro's (1989) eye-movement desensitization/reprocessing technique do offer effective protocols for conducting exposure therapy for PTSD; however, these studies also suggest that basic exposure/extinction, not the eye movement paradigm, is the active ingredient (see discussions by Acierno, Hersen, Van Hasselt & Tremont, 1994, and Dyck, 1993).

The Emotional Toll of Treating Trauma

Those who work with trauma survivors know that such work can extract an emotional toll. During therapy, clinicians must often deal with many of the same questions with which their patients are struggling. Why do terrible things happen? How can people be so cruel? In a similar crisis, how would I react? Coming to terms with these issues often forces therapists to alter their own world views (Eldridge, 1991; McCann & Pearlman, 1990). The details of a trauma may become nearly as vivid for therapists as for patients, and therapists may occasionally experience intrusive images of the event a patient has depicted. Although this phenomenon, known as *vicarious traumatization,* has received attention when working with adult patients also, the strain may be even greater when survivors are children (Dyregrov & Mitchell, 1992). Just as it is important for trauma survivors to know that their initial distress is normal and that support is available, clinicians should be aware that occasional bouts of vicarious traumatization are normal and that clinicians seek the support of peers familiar with trauma work.

FUTURE DIRECTIONS

In working with trauma survivors, it is vital to remember that the majority of those who experience a trauma never develop PTSD. Some experience intrusive and avoidant symptoms soon after an event but suffer no future distress; some develop symptoms of other disorders (Green et al., 1994; McFarlane, 1992). Many may endorse symptoms if surveyed, yet they continue to function well without seeking treatment. Some exhibit remarkable resilience following trauma and seem to suffer no ill effects (Lyons, 1991).

In an essay on the debate over mental health versus illness in war veterans, Smith, Parson, and Haley (1983) concluded that such apparently conflicting findings suggest that stress recovery is a normal process through which survivors can expect to evolve. The challenge for mental health professionals is to identify and assist the subgroup of survivors whose recovery seems to have derailed. Studies need to specifically diagnose for PTSD rather than merely reporting a list of symptoms. Efforts to standardize test batteries, cut-off scores, and symptom thresholds for the diagnosis of PTSD in children would greatly enhance the ability to compare findings across studies (Schwartz & Kowalski, 1991; Udwin, 1993). Researchers also need to include broadband instruments in assessment packages to allow for normative comparisons and examination of alternative (non-PTSD) responses to trauma.

Papers on child abuse and incest constitute 14 percent of all references on the effects of psychological trauma published during the 1970s and 1980s (Blake, Albano, & Keane, 1992). Additionally, there have been numerous studies of the effects of war, disaster, and other events on children. In spite of the number of studies on children and adolescents, virtually all the theoretical and clinical advances regarding PTSD have come from the adult literature and subsequently been adapted to work with younger populations. The extent to which theoretical models apply to children must be carefully examined. Developmental differences in symptom expression also deserve further investigation. For example, some researchers have not been able to replicate the finding of some of Terr's child-specific symptoms (e.g., Kiser et al., 1988), and the parameters of these features remain vague. For example, what level of inference is acceptable in defining posttraumatic play? When does a missequencing of events relate to a child's developmental level rather than to "time skew"?

Several areas of research that have shown promise in the adult PTSD literature have not received extensive study in children and adolescents. Research on psychophysiological reactivity is a major area that remains underinvestigated among youths (McNally, 1991; Saigh, 1992). Ornitz and Pynoos's (1989) study of eye blink startle responses and Yule, Udwin, and Murdoch's (1990) finding that scores on the physiological factor of the RCMAS differentiate traumatized children from others suggest that psychophysiological assessment could prove to be as valuable with children as it has with adults. Similarly, pharmacological interventions and the tendency of some survivors to self-medicate with nonprescribed substances are areas that have yet to undergo as thorough evaluation in children as has occurred with adults.

Self-mutilation, eating disorders (especially subsequent to sexual abuse), and sex differences in trauma response remain underexplored in both the adult and child literatures. Similarly, further study is necessary to compare the effects of cumulative, ongoing, repeated trauma versus "single-blow" events (Terr, 1985, 1991). Perhaps the most striking need in both the child and adult literatures is for well-controlled and theoretically grounded intervention studies.

The understanding of PTSD, both in children and adults, has advanced at a phenomenal pace over the past two decades. As the field continues to evolve, many questions remain. The challenge will be to define clinical and research efforts carefully to advance and test new models that integrate this rapidly expanding knowledge base.

SUMMARY

Researchers have made considerable progress in the study of PTSD in recent years. There is now substantial documentation that PTSD does occur in children, although symptoms may take different forms at different ages and some risk factors may vary with age. Mental health experts continue to refine diagnostic criteria and theoretical models, and numerous assessment tools are now available. There has been less systematic research on treatment issues than on diagnostic and epidemiological questions. However, one widely accepted premise is that treatment for PTSD, whether in adults or children, must focus on therapeutic exposure to trauma-related cues rather than on secondary symptoms. The two-factor model provides a useful framework for conceptualizing diagnostic and treatment issues with this population.

NOTE

The authors would like to thank Drs. Bonnie Green and Joseph Scotti for their extremely helpful feedback on an earlier draft of this chapter.

REFERENCES

Acierno, R., Hersen, M., Van Hasselt, V. B., & Tremont, G. (1994). Review of the validation and dissemination of eye-movement desensitization and reprocessing: A scientific and ethical dilemma. *Clinical Psychology Review, 14,* 287–299.

Adam, B. S., Everett, B. L., & O'Neal, E. (1992). PTSD in physically and sexually abused psychiatrically hospitalized children. *Child Psychiatry & Human Development, 23,* 3–8.

American Psychiatric Association. (1952). *Diagnostic and statistical manual of mental disorders.* Washington, DC: American Psychiatric Association.

American Psychiatric Association. (1980). *Diagnostic and statistical manual of mental disorders* (3rd ed.). Washington, DC: American Psychiatric Association.

American Psychiatric Association. (1987). *Diagnostic and statistical manual of mental disorders* (3rd ed. rev). Washington, DC: American Psychiatric Association.

American Psychiatric Association. (1994). *Diagnostic and statistical manual of mental disorders* (4th ed.). Washington, DC: American Psychiatric Association.

Belter, R. W., Dunn, S. E., & Jeney, P. (1991). The psychological impact of Hurricane Hugo on children: A needs assessment. *Advances in Behavior Research and Therapy, 13,* 155–161.

Birleson, P. (1981). The validity of depressive disorder in childhood and the development of a rating scale: A research report. *Journal of Child Psychology and Psychiatry, 22,* 73–78.

Blake, D. D., Albano, A. M., & Keane, T. M. (1992). Twenty years of trauma: Psychological Abstracts 1970 through 1989. *Journal of Traumatic Stress, 5,* 477–484.

Blank, A. S. (1993). The longitudinal course of posttraumatic stress disorder. In J. R. T. Davidson & E. B. Foa (Eds.), *Posttraumatic stress disorder: DSM-IV and beyond* (pp. 3–22). Washington, DC: American Psychiatric Press.

Bradburn, I. S. (1991). After the earth shook: Children's stress symptoms 6–8 months after a disaster. *Advances in Behavior Research and Therapy, 13,* 173–179.

Breton, J., Valla, J., & Lambert, J. (1993). Industrial disaster and mental health of children and their parents. *Journal of the American Academy of Child and Adolescent Psychiatry, 32,* 438–445.

Burges Watson, I. P., Hoffman, L., & Wilson, G. V. (1988). The neuropsychiatry of posttraumatic stress disorder. *British Journal of Psychiatry, 152,* 164–173.

Burton, D., Foy, D., Bwanausi, C., Johnson, J., & Moore, L. (1994). The relationship between traumatic exposure, family dysfunction, and post-traumatic stress symptoms in male juvenile offenders. *Journal of Traumatic Stress, 7,* 83–93.

Caddell, J. M., & Drabman, R. S. (1992). Post-traumatic stress disorder in children. In R. T. Ammerman & M. Hersen (Eds.), *Handbook of behavioral therapy with children and adults: A longitudinal perspective.* Boston: Allyn and Bacon.

Cocco, N., & Sharpe, L. (1993). An auditory variant of eye movement desensitization in a case of childhood posttraumatic stress disorder. *Journal of Behavior Therapy and Experimental Psychiatry, 24,* 373–377.

Crabbs, M. A. (1981). School mental health services following an environmental disaster. *The Journal of School Health, 51,* 165–167.

Davidson, J. R. T., & Fairbank, J. A. (1993). The epidemiology of posttraumatic stress disorder. In J. R. T. Davidson & E. B. Foa (Eds.), *Posttraumatic stress disorder: DSM-IV and beyond* (pp. 147–169). Washington, DC: American Psychiatric Press.

Davidson, J. R. T., & Foa, E. B. (1991). Diagnostic issues in posttraumatic stress disorder: Considerations for the DSM-IV. *Journal of Abnormal Psychology, 100,* 346–355.

Dyck, M. J. (1993). A proposal for a conditioning model of eye movement desensitization treatment for posttraumatic stress disorder. *Journal of Behavior Therapy and Experimental Psychiatry, 24,* 201–210.

Dyregrov, A., & Mitchell, J. T. (1992). Work with traumatized children—Psychological effects and coping strategies. *Journal of Traumatic Stress, 5,* 5–17.

Earl, W. L. (1991). Perceived trauma: Its etiology and treatment. *Adolescence, 26,* 97–104.

Eldridge, G. D. (1991). Contextual issues in the assessment

of post-traumatic stress disorder. *Journal of Traumatic Stress, 4,* 7–23.

Fairbank, J. A., & Nicholson, R. A. (1987). Theoretical and empirical issues in the treatment of post-traumatic stress disorder in Vietnam veterans. *Journal of Clinical Psychology, 43,* 44–55.

Famularo, R., Kinscherff, R., & Fenton, T. (1991). Posttraumatic stress disorder among children clinically diagnosed as borderline personality disorder. *Journal of Nervous and Mental Disease, 179,* 428–431.

Famularo, R., Kinscherff, R., & Fenton, T. (1992). Psychiatric diagnoses of maltreated children: Preliminary findings. *Journal of the American Academy of Child and Adolescent Psychiatry, 31,* 863–867.

Foa, E. B., & Kozak, M. J. (1986). Emotional processing of fear: Exposure to corrective information. *Psychological Bulletin, 99,* 20–35.

Frederick, C. J. (1985). Selected foci in the spectrum of posttraumatic stress disorders. In J. Laube & A. Murphy (Eds.), *Perspectives on disaster recovery* (pp. 110–130). East Norwalk, CT: Appleton-Century-Crofts.

Friedman, M. J. (1991). Biological approaches to the diagnosis and treatment of posttraumatic stress disorder. *Journal of Traumatic Stress, 4,* 67–91.

Green, B. L., Grace, M. C., Vary, M. G., Kramer, T. L., Gleser, G. C., & Leonard, A. C. (1994). Children of disaster in the second decade: A 17-year follow-up of Buffalo Creek survivors. *Journal of the American Academy of Child and Adolescent Psychiatry, 33,* 71–79.

Green, B. L., Korol, M., Grace, M. C., Vary, M. G., Leonard, A. C., Gleser, G. C., & Smitson-Cohen, A. (1991). Children and disaster: Age, gender, and parental effects on PTSD symptoms. *Journal of the American Academy of Child and Adolescent Psychiatry, 30,* 945–951.

Horowitz, M. (1976). *Stress response syndromes.* New York: Jason Aronson.

Horowitz, M., Wilner, N., & Alvarez, W. (1979). Impact of Event Scale: A measure of subjective stress. *Psychosomatic Medicine, 41,* 209–218.

Jones, R. T., Ribbe, D. P., & Cunningham, P. (1994). Psychosocial correlates of fire disaster among children and adolescents. *Journal of Traumatic Stress, 7,* 117–122.

Joseph, S. A., Brewin, C. R., Yule, W., & Williams, R. (1993). Causal attributions and posttraumatic stress in adolescents. *Journal of Child Psychology and Psychiatry and Allied Disciplines, 34,* 247–253.

Keane, T. M., Zimering, R. T., & Caddell, J. M. (1985). A behavioral formulation of posttraumatic stress disorder in Vietnam veterans. *The Behavior Therapist, 8,* 9–12.

Kinzie, J. D., Sack, W., Angell, R., Clarke, G., & Ben, R. (1989). A three-year follow-up of Cambodian young people traumatized as children. *Journal of the Ameri-*

can Academy of Child and Adolescent Psychiatry, 28,
501–504.

Kiser, L. J., Ackerman, B. J., Brown, E., Edwards, N. B.,
McColgan, E., Pugh, R., & Pruitt, D. B. (1988). Posttraumatic stress disorder in young children: A reaction
to purported sexual abuse. *Journal of the American
Academy of Child and Adolescent Psychiatry, 27,*
645–649.

Kolb, L. C. (1987). A neuropsychological hypothesis explaining posttraumatic stress disorders. *American
Journal of Psychiatry, 144,* 989–995.

Koopman, C., Classen, C., & Spiegel, D. (1994). Predictors
of posttraumatic stress symptoms among survivors of
the Oakland/Berkeley, Calif., firestorm. *American
Journal of Psychiatry, 151,* 888–894.

Levis, D. J. (1981). Extrapolation of two-factor learning
theory of infrahuman avoidance behavior to psychopathology. *Neuroscience and Biobehavioral Reviews, 5,*
355–370.

Levis, D. J. (1985). Implosive theory: A comprehensive extension of conditioning theory of fear/anxiety to psychopathology. In S. Reiss & R. R. Bootzin (Eds.), *Theoretical issues in behavior therapy* (pp. 49–82).
Orlando: Academic Press.

Loftus, E. F. (1994). The repressed memory controversy.
American Psychologist, 49, 439–445.

Lonigan, C. J., Shannon, M. P., Finch, A. J., Daugherty, T.
K., & Taylor, C. M. (1991). Children's reactions to a
natural disaster: Symptom severity and degree of exposure. *Advances in Behaviour Research and Therapy, 13,* 135–154.

Lonigan, C. J., Shannon, M. P., Taylor, C. M., Finch, A. J.,
& Sallee, F.R. (1994). Children exposed to disaster: II.
Risk factors for the development of post-traumatic
symptomatology. *Journal of the American Academy of
Child and Adolescent Psychiatry, 33,* 94–105.

Lyons, J. A. (1987). Posttraumatic stress disorder in children and adolescents: A review of the literature. *Developmental and Behavioral Pediatrics, 8,* 349–356.

Lyons, J. A. (1991). Strategies for assessing the potential for
positive adjustment following trauma. *Journal of
Traumatic Stress, 4,* 93–111.

Lyons, J. A., Alexander, J., Smith, P. O., Veltum, L., &
Vogeltanz, N. (1993, October). Physiological assessment of hyperarousal during treatment. Paper presented at the annual meeting of the International Society for Traumatic Stress Studies, San Antonio, TX.

Lyons, J. A., & Keane, T. M. (1989). Implosive therapy for
the treatment of combat-related PTSD. *Journal of
Traumatic Stress, 2,* 137–152.

March, J. S. (1990). The nosology of posttraumatic stress
disorder. *Journal of Anxiety Disorders, 4,* 61–82.

March, J. S. (1993). What constitutes a stressor? The "Criterion A" issue. In J. R. T. Davidson & E. B. Foa (Eds.),
Posttraumatic stress disorder: DSM-IV and beyond
(pp. 37–54). Washington, DC: American Psychiatric
Press.

Marmar, C. R., Weiss, D. S., Schlenger, W. E., Fairbank, J.
A., Jordan, B. K., Kulka, R. A., & Hough, R. L. (1994).
Peritraumatic dissociation and posttraumatic stress in
male Vietnam theater veterans. American *Journal of
Psychiatry, 151,* 902–907.

Martini, D. R., Ryan, C., Nakayama, D., & Ramenofsky, M.
(1990). Psychiatric sequelae after traumatic injury:
The Pittsburgh Regatta accident. *Journal of the American Academy of Child and Adolescent Psychiatry, 29,*
70–75.

McCann, I. L., & Pearlman, L. A. (1990). Vicarious traumatization: A framework for understanding the psychological effects of working with victims. *Journal of
Traumatic Stress, 3,* 131–168.

McFarlane, A. C. (1992). Commentary. Posttraumatic
stress disorder among injured survivors of a terrorist
attack: Predictive value of early intrusion and avoidance symptoms. *The Journal of Nervous and Mental
Disease, 180,* 599–600.

McNally, R. J. (1991). Assessment of posttraumatic stress
disorder in children. *Psychological Assessment: A
Journal of Consulting and Clinical Psychology, 3,*
531–537.

McNally, R. J. (1993). Stressors that produce posttraumatic
stress disorder in children. In J. R. T. Davidson & E. B.
Foa (Eds.), *Posttraumatic stress disorder: DSM-IV
and beyond* (pp. 57–74). Washington, DC: American
Psychiatric Press.

Milgram, N. A., Toubiana, Y. H., Klingman, A., Raviv, A.,
& Goldstein, I. (1988). Situational exposure and personal loss in children's acute and chronic stress reactions to a school bus disaster. *Journal of Traumatic
Stress, 1,* 339–352.

Mowrer, O. H. (1947). On the dual nature of learning: A re-
interpretation of conditioning and problem solving.
Harvard Educational Review, 17, 102–148.

Nader, K. O., Pynoos, R. S., Fairbanks, L. A., Al-Ajeel, M.,
& Al-Asfour, A. (1993). A preliminary study of PTSD
and grief among the children of Kuwait following the
Gulf crisis. *British Journal of Clinical Psychology, 32,*
407–416.

Nader, K., Pynoos, R., Fairbanks, L., & Frederick, C.
(1990). Children's PTSD reactions one year after a
sniper attack at their school. *American Journal of Psychiatry, 147,* 1526–1530.

Ornitz, E. M., & Pynoos, R. S. (1989). Startle modulation in
children with posttraumatic stress disorder. *American
Journal of Psychiatry, 146,* 866–870.

Pitman, R. K. (1993). Biological findings in posttraumatic
stress disorder: Implications for DSM-IV classifications. In J. R. T. Davidson & E. B. Foa (Eds.), *Posttraumatic stress disorder: DSM-IV and beyond* (pp.
173–189). Washington, DC: American Psychiatric
Press.

Pitman, R. K., & Orr, S. P. (1990). Modulation of the startle
response in children with PTSD. *American Journal of
Psychiatry, 147,* 815–816.

Pitman, R. K., Orr, S. P., Forgue, D. F., Altman, B., de Jong, J. B., & Herz, L. R. (1990). Psychophysiologic responses to combat imagery of Vietnam veterans with posttraumatic stress disorder versus other anxiety disorders. *Journal of Abnormal Psychology, 99,* 49–54.

Pynoos, R. S., Frederick, C., Nader, K., Arroyo, W., Steinberg, A., Eth, S., Nunez, F., & Fairbanks, L. (1987). Life threat and posttraumatic stress in school-age children. *Archives of General Psychiatry, 44,* 1057–1062.

Pynoos, R. S., & Nader, K. (1988a). Children who witness the sexual assaults of their mothers. *Journal of the American Academy of Child and Adolescent Psychiatry, 27,* 567–572.

Pynoos, R. S., & Nader, K. (1988b). Psychological first aid and treatment approach to children exposed to community violence: Research implications. *Journal of Traumatic Stress, 1,* 445–473.

Pynoos, R. S., Nader, K., Frederick, C., Gonda, L., & Stuber, M. (1987). Grief reactions in school age children following a sniper attack at school. *Israel Journal of Psychiatry and Related Sciences, 24,* 53–63.

Realmuto, G. M., Masten, A., Carole, L. F., Hubbard, J., Groteluschen, A., & Chhun, B. (1992). Adolescent survivors of massive childhood trauma in Cambodia: Life events and current symptoms. *Journal of Traumatic Stress, 5,* 589–599.

Reich, W., & Welner, Z. (1990). *Diagnostic Interview for Children and Adolescents-Revised.* St. Louis: Washington University.

Reynolds, C. R., & Richard, B. O. (1978). What I Think and Feel: A revised measure of children's manifest anxiety. *Journal of Abnormal Child Psychology, 6,* 271–280.

Robinson, R. C., & Mitchell, J. T. (1993). Evaluation of psychological debriefings. *Journal of Traumatic Stress, 6,* 367–382.

Rothbaum, B. O., & Foa, E. B. (1993). Subtypes of posttraumatic stress disorder and duration of symptoms. In J. R. T. Davidson & E. B. Foa (Eds.), *Posttraumatic stress disorder: DSM-IV and beyond* (pp. 23–35). Washington, DC: American Psychiatric Press.

Saigh, P. A. (1987a). In vitro flooding of an adolescent's posttraumatic stress disorder. *Journal of Clinical Child Psychology, 16,* 147–150.

Saigh, P. A. (1987b). In vitro flooding of childhood posttraumatic stress disorders: A systematic replication. *Professional School Psychology, 2,* 133–145.

Saigh, P. A. (1989). The development and validation of the Children's Posttraumatic Stress Disorder Inventory. *International Journal of Special Education, 4,* 75–84.

Saigh, P. A. (1992). The behavioral treatment of child and adolescent posttraumatic stress disorder. *Advances in Behavior Research and Therapy, 14,* 247–275.

Schwarz, E. D., & Kowalski, J. M. (1991). Posttraumatic stress disorder after a school shooting: Effects of symptom threshold selection and diagnosis by DSM-III, DSM-III-R, or proposed DSM-IV. *American Journal of Psychiatry, 148,* 592–597.

Shapiro, F. (1989). Efficacy of eye movement desensitization procedure in the treatment of traumatic memories. *Journal of Traumatic Stress, 2,* 199–223.

Smith, J. R., Parson, E. R., & Haley, S. H. (1983). On health and disorder in Vietnam veterans: An invited commentary. *American Journal of Orthopsychiatry, 53,* 27–33.

Stallard, P., & Law, F. (1993). Screening and psychological debriefing of adolescent survivors of life-threatening events. *British Journal of Psychiatry, 163,* 660–665.

Stuber, M. L., Nader, K., Yasuda, P., Pynoos, R. S., & Cohen, S. (1991). Stress responses after pediatric bone marrow transplantation: Preliminary results of a prospective longitudinal study. *Journal of the American Academy of Child and Adolescent Psychiatry, 30,* 952–957.

Terr, L. C. (1985). Psychic trauma in children and adolescents. *Psychiatric Clinics of North America, 8,* 815–835.

Terr, L. C. (1989). Treating psychic trauma in children: A preliminary discussion. *Journal of Traumatic Stress, 2,* 3–20.

Terr, L. C. (1991). Childhood traumas: An outline and overview. *American Journal of Psychiatry, 148,* 10–20.

Toubiana, Y. H., Milgram, N. A., Strich, Y., & Edelstein, A. (1988). Crisis intervention in a school community disaster: Principles and practices. *Journal of Community Psychology, 16,* 91–99.

Udwin, O. (1993). Children's reactions to traumatic events. *Journal of Child Psychology and Psychiatry and Allied Disciplines, 34,* 115–127.

van der Kolk, B. A. (1994). The body keeps the score: Memory and the evolving psychobiology of posttraumatic stress. *Harvard Review of Psychiatry, 1,* 253–265.

ver Ellen, P., & van Kammen, D. P. (1990). The biological findings in post-traumatic stress disorder: A review. *Journal of Applied Social Psychology, 20,* 1789–1821.

Vogel, J. M., & Vernberg, E. M. (1993). Task Force Report, Part I: Children's psychological responses to disasters. *Journal of Clinical Child Psychology, 22,* 464–484.

Welner, Z., Reich, W., Herjanic, B., Jung, K. G., & Amado, H. (1987). Reliability, validity, and parent-child agreement studies of the Diagnostic Interview for Children and Adolescents. *Journal of the American Academy of Child and Adolescent Psychiatry, 26,* 649–653.

Yule, W. (1992). Post-traumatic stress disorder in child survivors of shipping disasters: The sinking of the 'Jupiter.' *Psychotherapy & Psychosomatics, 57,* 200–205.

Yule, W., & Udwin, O. (1991). Screening child survivors for post-traumatic stress disorders: Experiences from the 'Jupiter' sinking. *British Journal of Clinical Psychology, 30,* 131–138.

Yule, W., Udwin, O., & Murdoch, K. (1990). The 'Jupiter' sinking: Effects on children's fears, depression, and anxiety. *Journal of Child Psychology and Psychiatry and Allied Disciplines, 31,* 1051–1061.

Yule, W., & Williams, R. M. (1990). Post-traumatic stress reactions in children. *Journal of Traumatic Stress, 3,* 279–295.

Zilberg, N. J., Weiss, D. S., & Horowitz, M. J. (1982). Impact of Event Scale: A cross-validation study and some empirical evidence supporting a conceptual model of stress response syndromes. *Journal of Consulting and Clinical Psychology, 50* (3), 407–414.

CHAPTER 21

DAILY STRESS AND COPING IN CHILDHOOD AND ADOLESCENCE

Rena L. Repetti, UNIVERSITY OF CALIFORNIA, LOS ANGELES
Emily P. McGrath, UNIVERSITY OF CALIFORNIA, LOS ANGELES
Sharon S. Ishikawa, UNIVERSITY OF CALIFORNIA, LOS ANGELES

This chapter summarizes research on how children respond to common negative experiences, such as feeling rejected by peers or overhearing an argument between parents. It does not focus on major traumatic events in a child's life, such as the loss of a parent, nor does it include growing up in high-risk environments, such as those characterized by poverty and high levels of community violence. Instead, the focus is on the kinds of events that *all* children will be exposed to at some point in their lives, but that *some* children will experience almost every day. The research literature in this area is at an early stage of development, with limited substantive knowledge and few well-accepted conclusions. This chapter therefore focuses attention on the ways that questions are posed about responses to common stressful events in childhood and on the research methods that are used to address those questions. The chapter also summarizes the evidence that exists for effects of chronic stressors on the well-being of youth, in particular their psychological adjustment and development, and emerging information about the various ways that children react to and attempt to cope with these daily events. Several different research literatures are discussed. In addition to an overview of traditional child stress-and-coping research,

we look to other literatures for a possible foreshadowing of future directions in the field. In particular, our discussion centers on three bodies of research that health psychologists often seem to ignore: developmental psychologists' investigations of problems in peer relationships and academic failure, and the work of marital and developmental researchers on reactions to exposure to conflict and anger between parents.

DAILY STRESSORS IN CHILDHOOD AND ADOLESCENCE

The Conceptualization and Measurement of Daily Stressors

Like the research literature on adults, child stress-and-coping studies have focused primarily on the impact of major events on children's lives. This research tradition typically emphasizes unwanted and uncontrollable changes that confront some children, such as a move to a new neighborhood, a major illness in the family, parental divorce, or the death of a parent or sibling. There is no doubt that these events place an enormous strain on families and can cause emotional distress and significant adjustment problems in childhood and adolescence. In the late 1980s, researchers began to report that the impact of major events on children may be best understood by an analysis of the numerous, seemingly more minor, changes in a child's life that result from the initial event (Compas, Howell, Phares, Williams, & Ledoux, 1989; Tolan, Miller, & Thomas, 1988). For example, the effects of parental divorce, per se, may not be nearly as great as the quality of the child's subsequent family situation, such as the extent to which the child feels caught between the divorced parents or the level of organization and routine in the home provided by the custodial parent (Buchanan, Maccoby, & Dornbusch, 1991; Monahan, Buchanan, Maccoby, & Dornbusch, 1993). Similarly, the direct effects of having a seriously ill sibling may not be as strong as the indirect effects caused by changes in family relationships (Lobato, Faust, & Spirito, 1988). A move to a new neighborhood probably also requires an analysis of the immediate demands that the change imposes on a child, such as developing new friendships and adjusting to a new school.

Studies suggesting that daily stressors mediate the impact of major life events have spurred researchers' interest in the cumulative effects of more minor daily events. There is now a growing literature focusing on adolescents' reports of their exposure to common chronic stressors. Many of the measures used in this literature were developed on the basis of lists of daily hassles or minor negative events provided by adolescents. Interestingly, all of the adolescent-report scales include interpersonal problems, such as conflicts with parents, teachers, siblings, or friends; feeling lonely or left out of peer groups; boyfriend/girlfriend problems; or observations of parental arguments. Some even focus exclusively on the interpersonal domain (Daniels & Moos, 1990; Timko, Moos, & Michelson, 1993). Most of these scales, however, assess a mixture of interpersonal difficulties and a wide variety of other stressors. A review of the items reveals the other kinds of daily problems, irritations, and difficulties that teens may experience, such as doing homework, getting a bad grade, skin problems, worries about health or the future, waiting in lines, racial tensions at school, peer pressures, fear of theft or violence, problems with a job, not doing well at sports, boredom, not being able to dress in a desired

manner, financial problems, and being overweight (Armacost, 1989; Bobo, Gilchrist, Elmer, Snow, & Schinke, 1986; Compas, Davis, Forsythe, & Wagner, 1987; DuBois, Felner, Brand, Adan, & Evans, 1992; Ham & Larson, 1990; Siegel & Brown, 1988). Some of the daily hassles scales have been used with children in younger age groups as well (Banez & Compas, 1990).

In addition to great heterogeneity in the substantive content of the daily events that are studied, some measures combine chronic ongoing problems with major life events (e.g., Cowen et al., 1991; Compas, Davis, Forsythe, & Wagner, 1987) to obtain an omnibus rating of the child's overall level of exposure to stressors. Although measures of chronic or daily stressors in childhood and adolescence include quite disparate kinds of experiences, attempts are sometimes made to categorize the stressors in meaningful ways. For example, some studies distinguish between expected and unexpected events (Ham & Larson, 1990) or controllable and uncontrollable situations (DuBois et al., 1992).

Effects of Daily Stressors on Child and Adolescent Development

Does exposure to a wide variety of common daily stressors increase a child's or an adolescent's risk for developing emotional or behavioral problems? Several cross-sectional correlational studies suggest that the answer is yes. Investigations of children, ranging from fourth grade through high school, indicate that self-reported mood, illness symptoms, and behavior problems correlate with child reports of daily hassles (Siegal & Brown, 1988; Tolan, 1988). The significant association between experiences with daily hassles and psychological adjustment persists even when researchers control for the effects of other important factors, such as the occurrence of major negative life events or positive daily events in the child's life (Daniels & Moos, 1990; Kanner et al., 1987), or exposure to parents' daily hassles and psychological symptoms (Banez & Compas, 1990). Some studies have found that perceived exposure to many minor daily stressors also predicts increases, over a one- to two-year period, in children's and adolescents' reports of their psychological adjustment (Compas, Howell, Phares, Williams, & Giunta, 1989; DuBois et al., 1992). However, in one study of girls, a prospective association between common negative events and two outcomes, depressed mood and illness symptoms, was found only for some of the girls, specifically those who felt that there had been few concurrent positive changes in their lives (Siegel & Brown, 1988).

The literature on daily hassles presents several challenges for researchers trying to understand how stressors influence children's health and development. A strong reliance on child self-reports raises a question about the role of respondent biases in these data. For example, it is interesting that results of studies like those just cited are not as strong when parents' ratings of child outcomes are used instead of child self-reported well-being (Banez & Compas, 1990; Compas, Howell, Phares, Williams, & Giunta, 1989). Even more important than the possibility of respondent biases inflating correlations is the complex problem of determining causal priority in this literature. Many of the stressful events assessed in measures of daily hassles are the kinds of experiences that may be evoked by the child. For example, interpersonal problems with peers, parents, or teachers are determined, in part, by certain aspects of a child's psychological functioning, such as his or her general mood and level of aggressive behavior. It is therefore not surprising that some prospective analyses suggest a reciprocal association between child maladjustment and daily stress. Just as stress predicts future adjustment, emotional or behavioral problems in children can predict subsequent increases in their reports of daily stressors (Compas, Howell, Phares, Williams, & Giunta, 1989; DuBois et al., 1992). However, this type of reciprocal effect is not always found (Siegel & Brown, 1988).

The problems associated with disentangling complex reciprocal linkages among correlated variables are compounded by the fact that the large majority of studies do not distinguish between different categories of daily hassles. Therefore, it is impossible to determine which types of daily experiences might play a more important role in accounting for developmental outcomes. In one exception, Daniels and Moos (1990) found that the best correlates of adolescent psychological adjustment were school stressors (such as problems with fellow students) and parent stressors (such as problems in the parents' marriage or their parenting style).

Researchers are in a much stronger position to address the possible causal relations between daily hassles and child adjustment when they attempt to identify effects associated with specific types of stressful experiences. This point is illustrated next by a discussion of three different stressful situations in childhood: *problems with peers*, *academic failure*, and *conflict between parents*. We focus on these particular situations for three reasons. First, they are common. Almost all children and adolescents will be exposed to these stressors at some point. Second, they often recur on a daily basis. Indeed, they appear on most or all measures of daily hassles. Third, growing evidence suggests that these environmental conditions are associated with important childhood outcomes. The discussion that follows emphasizes the assessment techniques and other research methods being developed in the literatures that focus on these three common stressors.

The Stress of Peer Problems

It is generally recognized that good relationships with peers are an important component of a child's healthy social and psychological adjustment. Research has shown that positive peer relationships contribute to the acquisition of social skills and the development of a positive self-concept (Asher & Coie, 1990). Poor peer relationships, on the other hand, act as chronic stressors that are associated with feelings of loneliness (Parker & Asher, 1993), and poor peer relationships may lead to serious adjustment problems in childhood and later in life (Parker & Asher, 1987).

Child development researchers distinguish between two aspects of children's experiences with peers: friendship and popularity. *Friendship* refers to children's experiences in close, one-to-one relationships with other children. *Popularity* refers to the extent to which children are more generally liked or accepted by their peer group. A child who is popular among peers might not have many close friends. Conversely, a generally unpopular child may be in a few close, one-to-one relationships with other children. Although the child development literature has focused primarily on children's popularity in peer groups, close friendships are also believed to be an important component of children's experiences with peers (Bukowski & Hoza, 1989; Parker & Asher, 1993).

Developmental psychologists often use sociometric scales to assess classmates' reports of a child's level of social acceptance in the classroom. The rationale behind this approach is that peers are the best informants about a child's peer-group status. Data from peers may also be less biased by social desirability concerns. Two types of sociometric scales are commonly used: likability rating scales and positive and negative peer nominations. *Likability rating scales* ask children to rate the degree to which they like each of their classmates. When ratings are averaged across all children in a classroom, these scales indicate social preference, or how much any given child is liked by his or her peers. *Positive peer nomination scales* ask all of the children in a classroom to name the classmates who they consider to be their best friends. *Negative peer nomination scales* ask the children to name the classmates with whom they do not like to play. Positive and negative peer nominations assess a child's social impact, or the degree to which he or she is noticed by peers.

Based on both sociometric ratings and nominations, children are classified into five sociometric categories: popular, rejected, neglected, controversial, and average (Newcomb, Bukowski, & Pattee, 1993). A *popular* child is one who receives very high likability ratings as well as many positive peer nominations from his or her peers. A *rejected* child is one who receives very low likability ratings and many negative nominations from his or her peers. A *neglected* child is not positively or negatively nominated by his or her peers and is neither liked nor disliked. A *controversial* child is nominated by many peers and is liked by some peers and disliked by others. An *average* child is one who scores about the mean on likability and nominations scales.

Informants other than peers are also used to assess a child's level of peer-group acceptance. Children are sometimes asked to describe their own level of social acceptance in their peer group. However, children's self-reports are not always accurate. For example, research suggests that some rejected children overrate their level of social acceptance (Hymel, Bowker, & Woody, 1993; Patterson, Kupersmidt, & Griesler, 1990). Teachers are also sometimes asked to rate the extent to which children are accepted by their peer group. Although teachers are able to identify most children who are not accepted by their peers, they are sometimes biased in their ratings. For example, teachers tend to rate children who are experiencing academic difficulties as low in peer-group acceptance (French & Waas, 1985). In order to minimize response bias, sociometric procedures are generally the preferred method in the child development literature for identifying children who are not accepted by their peers.

The use of sociometric procedures in longitudinal studies has enabled child development researchers to identify important outcomes associated with different types of sociometric categories. For example, Hymel, Rubin, Rowden, and LeMare (1990) found that children who were rejected by their peers in the second grade were more likely to exhibit externalizing problems, such as aggression, in the fifth grade. Kupersmidt and Patterson (1991) found that second- through fourth-grade girls who were neglected by their peers were at an increased risk for depression two years later. Thus, when examining long-term outcomes for children in different sociometric categories, distinctions between different types of unpopular children, such as rejected versus neglected, have proven to be important.

Rejected children may be more likely than neglected and controversial children to experience serious adjustment problems in childhood and later in life. For example, rejected children report more loneliness than do other unpopular children, such as neglected children (Asher & Wheeler, 1985). In addition, rejected children are at an increased risk for dropping out of high school, for becoming engaged in juvenile and adult crime, and for adult psychopathology (Parker & Asher, 1987).

Because rejected children appear to be at heightened risk for adjustment problems, psychologists are particularly interested in the factors that may lead children to be rejected by their peers. Many studies have been conducted examining the behavioral correlates of peer rejection. Newcomb and associates (1993) concluded, on the basis of a meta-analysis of numerous studies, that rejected children are more aggressive and withdrawn and less sociable than other children. However, the extent to which these behaviors *cause* children to be rejected by their peers, rather than develop as a result of peer rejection, is still unclear.

Coie and Kupersmidt (1983) employed a novel methodology to examine this question. They took unacquainted fourth-grade boys who had been classified as popular, average, neglected, or rejected according to classroom sociometrics and placed them in a free-play group for six weeks. Experimenters observed the behaviors of the children in the group setting. Social status rankings for the boys in the new setting were obtained by asking each child with whom he preferred to play in the group. Evidence of stability in the boys' social acceptance was found in the high correlation between the boys' social status rankings in the new setting and their classroom social status rankings. More important, boys who were rejected by peers in the free-play group were observed making more hostile and aversive comments and engaging in physical aggression more often than the other children. In a similar study conducted by Dodge (1983), second-grade boys who came to be rejected in experimental play groups made more hostile comments and were observed to hit other boys more than did the nonrejected boys in the group. These studies suggest that display of certain problematic behaviors, in particular verbal and physical aggression, may *cause* children to be rejected by their peers.

There is additional evidence suggesting that behavior problems may cause children to be rejected by their peers. Patterson, DeBaryshe, and Ramsey (1989) proposed a model suggesting that ineffective parenting practices result in child behavior problems, which, in turn, lead to peer rejection. Consistent with this model, Bierman and Smoot (1991) found that punitive and ineffective parental discipline was related to 6- to 10-year-old children's conduct problems at home and at school. Children's conduct problems, in turn, predicted poor peer relations at school. Dishion (1990) found that poor parenting techniques, such as the use of inconsistent and punitive behaviors, were associated with 9- and 10-year-old children's maladaptive, antisocial behaviors. Children's antisocial behaviors, in turn, were associated with rejection by peers. These studies suggest that children's behavior problems may mediate the link between poor parenting practices and peer-related difficulties.

Developmental psychologists have made important advances in the study of peer problems. The use of sociometric scales has enabled researchers to minimize problems associated with response bias as well

as identify important outcomes associated with different types of sociometric categories. For example, rejected children are more likely than neglected children to experience serious adjustment problems in childhood and later in life. As a result of these findings, child development researchers have utilized novel methodologies in order to examine the processes that may lead children to be rejected by their peers.

The Stress of Academic Failure

Academic failure, another common chronic stressor in childhood, can refer to children's actual experiences with school failure, children's perceptions of scholastic failure, or both. Children's *actual experiences* with academic failure are indicated by poor school grades or low standardized test scores. Children's *perceptions of scholastic failure* refer to children's beliefs that they are doing poorly in school. These beliefs are often measured by the cognitive competence subscale of the Perceived Competence Scale (Harter, 1982). The seven items that comprise this subscale assess how well children feel they are doing in class, how smart they think they are, how well they understand their classwork, how easy it is for them to figure out assignments, and how quickly they are able to perform academic tasks. Children's beliefs may or may not be associated with actual school failure. For example, some children earn very high grades on their report cards, yet believe they are not doing well in school (Phillips, 1987). Thus, exposure to academic failure in childhood may, for some children, refer to actual experiences with school failure. For others, it may consist entirely of a perception of scholastic failure.

Actual academic failure is associated with a variety of psychological disorders, such as attention-deficit hyperactivity disorder (ADHD), conduct disorder (Frick, Kamphaus, Lahey, Loeber, Christ, Hart, & Tannenbaum, 1991; Hinshaw, 1992), and depression (Blechman, McEnroe, Carella, & Audette, 1986). Because these findings are based on cross-sectional data, the extent to which exposure to actual academic failure actually *causes* child adjustment problems is unclear. It is certainly the case that adjustment problems in childhood can cause academic difficulties. For example, distractibility, difficulty concentrating, and lack of self-control cause many ADHD children to perform poorly in school. It is also possible that antecedent variables, such as low socioeconomic status or family adversity, cause both adjustment problems and academic failure (Hinshaw, 1992). Longitudinal investigations would help to clarify the reciprocal causal relations between actual academic failure and different child adjustment problems.

Children's perceptions of scholastic failure are also associated with psychological disorders, such as depression (Weisz, Weiss, Wasserman, & Rintoul, 1987). In addition, children's perceptions of school failure are associated with a wide range of academic difficulties, such as low expectancies for future success (Eccles, 1983; Phillips & Zimmerman, 1990), low achievement motivation (Harter, 1992), and lack of persistence in the face of challenge (Bempechat, London, & Dweck, 1991). Many investigators believe that children's perceptions of academic failure may be more powerful predictors of negative outcomes than are children's actual experiences with school failure. For example, students' interpretations of their academic performance are more powerful predictors of negative affective reactions to achievement than are objective indicators of school performance (Meece, Wigfield, & Eccles, 1990). Thus, although actual experiences with school failure are believed to be important, the focus here will be on *perceptions* of scholastic failure as a common chronic stressor in childhood.

Child development researchers have begun to use prospective longitudinal designs in order to examine causal relationships between perceptions of academic inability and negative achievement outcomes. For example, Meece, Wigfield, and Eccles (1990) found that seventh- through ninth-grade children who held negative perceptions of their abilities in the first year of the study had lower expectancies for success in math, believed that being good in math was not important, and were more anxious about math one year later. These findings suggest that children's perceptions of scholastic inability may lead to a set of attitudes that could impede future achievement.

Factors That Influence Children's Perceptions of Academic Failure

Because children's perceptions of academic inability appear to be powerful predictors of important child outcomes, child development researchers have investigated the factors that cause some children to perceive academic failure in their lives. Not surprisingly, parents seem to play a central role in shaping their children's perceptions of their scholastic competence. For example, Parsons, Adler, and Kaczala (1982) found that parents' perceptions of and expectations for their fifth- through eleventh-grade children were related to the children's self-perceptions of ability. The investigators assessed parents' beliefs about their children's math abilities and parents' perceptions of how difficult math is for their children. Parents' beliefs and perceptions were more directly related to children's self-perceptions of math ability than were the children's actual grades in math. Parents who thought math was hard for their children and who thought their children were not good at math had children who saw themselves as less academically competent, who believed math was difficult, and who had low expectations for future success in math.

Phillips (1987) also believes that parents contribute to children's perceptions of their academic competence. Among highly competent third-grade children, Phillips (1987) found that parents' perceptions of their children's academic competence were more predictive of children's self-perceptions than were actual indicators of performance such as grades and test scores. According to Phillips, parents use their interpretations of objective information, such as grades or test scores, to provide feedback to their children about their performance. Children, in turn, use this information to construct their self-perceptions. Consistent with this hypothesis, McGrath and Repetti (1995) found that parents' satisfaction with their fourth-grade children's school performance, independent of their children's actual school performance, correlated positively with children's self-perceptions of academic competence.

Teachers and peers may also exert a substantial influence on children's self-perceptions of ability. For example, teachers' use of both praise and criticism in the classroom has been found to be associated with fifth- through ninth-grade boys' perceptions of their academic abilities (Parsons, Kaczala, & Meece, 1982). Phillips (1984) similarly reported that fifth-grade children who believed they were less competent had teachers who expected lower levels of performance from them. In a separate analysis it was found that these children accurately perceived their teachers' low expectations. In another study, fourth-graders whose teachers and peers evaluated their scholastic competence negatively near the start of the year saw themselves as less academically able at the end of the school year than at the beginning of the school year (Cole, 1991). Interestingly, although both teachers' and peers' evaluations were important, Cole found that peers' evaluations were even more predictive of changes in children's self-perceptions than were teachers' evaluations.

Although it is still unclear whether exposure to *actual* academic failure causes child adjustment problems, through use of prospective longitudinal designs child development researchers have been able to demonstrate that children's *perceptions* of scholastic failure lead to negative achievement outcomes. Parents, teachers, and peers may each play a role in shaping children's perceptions of their academic competence.

The Stress of Exposure to Interparental Conflict

In addition to the work done on peer rejection and perceived academic failure, a large body of research demonstrates that exposure to overt interparental conflict is associated with an increased risk for a wide variety of child emotional and behavioral problems. The problems range from aggression, conduct disorder, and delinquency or antisocial behavior to anxiety and depression (e.g., Emery, 1982, 1988; Grych & Fincham, 1990; Reid & Crisafulli, 1990). An understanding of the processes that account for the association of interparental conflict with child behavioral and emotional outcomes is beginning to emerge.

Most marital researchers working in this area ask parents to describe the level of conflict in their marriage and then link their descriptions to ratings of child mental health. A clear advantage to this method is that parents are obviously the best observers of their marriage. However, they may not always know the extent to which their child is aware of conflict between them (Grych, Seid, & Fincham, 1992). For example, parents may believe they are sparing their child by waiting to argue until he or she has gone outside to play or has gone to sleep for the night, not realizing that the child has come back inside the house or

has not yet fallen asleep. Thus, most researchers in this area believe that the child's own perception of marital conflict is critical to understanding how child outcomes are associated with marital conflict.

To address this issue, Grych and colleagues (1992) compared the Children's Perception of Interparental Conflict Inventory (CPIC) to the commonly used O'Leary-Porter Scale (OPS). The CPIC assesses children's awareness of and feelings about conflict between their parents; the OPS measures the parents' perceptions of how frequently marital conflict occurs in front of the children. Although ratings from the two conflict measures did not differ significantly from each other, children's perceptions of conflict consistently predicted child behavior problems as measured by parents, teachers, peers, and children better than did parents' perceptions of conflict.

In addition to interparental conflict, expressions of anger among other family members, such as between parents and children or between siblings, also appear to be related to child adjustment outcomes. For example, Jaycox and Repetti (1993) found that a child's well-being was more strongly related to the overall level of conflict within his or her family than to the degree of conflict in the parents' marriage. However, in another study, children reported greater sadness and anger after viewing a videotape of a verbal argument between two adults, compared to viewing an argument between an adult and a child (El-Sheikh & Cheskes, 1995).

Researchers have noted that, although conflict is generally equated with anger, conflicts may actually vary on several dimensions (Cummings & El-Sheikh, 1991). For example, in one family, a conflict may occur as a calm discussion between two parents in a private setting, whereas in another family, it may be a verbally hostile argument. In yet another family, the parents may engage in physical violence (Grych & Fincham, 1993). Some parents may communicate their anger nonverbally (e.g., giving the cold shoulder), verbally (e.g., yelling or insulting), or physically (e.g., pushing, slapping, or beating) (Cummings & El-Sheikh, 1991). Thus, anger within a marital relationship inherently involves some sort of conflict between the parents, whereas marital conflict does not necessarily involve anger. Marital researchers are currently investigating whether it is the anger underlying certain expressions of interparental conflict, and not the conflict per se, that leads to problems in adjustment for children.

Cummings (1987) and colleagues have provided evidence suggesting that children do experience background anger as a stressor. In this program of research, *background anger* was defined as anger between two adults that a child only observed, without any direct participation. In one study, mothers were trained to observe their toddlers' affect at home over a period of nine months. During times when the toddlers were exposed to naturally occurring background anger, they appeared more angry and distressed (Cummings, Zahn-Waxler, & Radke-Yarrow, 1981). In another study, ratings from 4- and 5-year-old children indicated that viewing live simulations of angry adult interactions elicited more negative emotions than did viewing affectionate adult interactions (Cummings, 1987). There is also evidence indicating that preschoolers respond physiologically through changes in heart rate and blood pressure when exposed to videotapes of angry adult interactions. Moreover, not only are these changes distinct from responses to friendly interactions, but changes in heart rate correlate with self-reported distress, as well as with observed behavioral and affective distress (El-Sheikh, Cummings, & Goetsch, 1989).

Cummings and colleagues have suggested that the *occurrence* of angry interparental conflict in itself is not as important as the *intensity* or *outcome* of the angry conflict (Cummings, Vogel, Cummings, & El-Sheikh, 1989). They found that as the intensity of anger between two adult actors increased (i.e., from nonverbal to verbal to physical), children reported more anger, sadness, and fear. Children in a more recent study also reported feeling more fearful while watching videotapes of physical conflicts between two adults than they did during tapes of verbal conflicts (El-Sheikh & Cheskes, 1995).

Interestingly, there was also an interaction between the child's age and the intensity of anger expressed between the conflicting adults in one of the studies, whereby older children were more sensitive to nonverbal adult anger than were younger children (Cummings et al., 1989). In addition, if the adults did not resolve the anger, then the children experienced more negative feelings. In a follow-up study, not only were 4- to 9-year-old children upset by unresolved anger, but older children (the 6- to 9-year-olds in the sample) could distinguish among different degrees of conflict resolution (Cummings et al., 1989). Recent findings also suggest that children prefer complete resolutions over incomplete resolutions of adult conflicts (El-Sheikh & Cheskes, 1995).

Expanding on this research, Grych and Fincham (1993) investigated the *content* of parent arguments. Children listened to an audiotape of two adult actors arguing, and responded to questions as though they were "Chris," the couple's child. Children heard two types of arguments. In the first type of argument, the parents argued about a child-related topic, such as what time Chris was supposed to do homework or which one of the parents would take Chris to an activity. In the second type of argument, the parents argued about a nonchild-related topic, such as financial concerns or the husband's work schedule. When children listened to parents engaging in child-related conflict, they experienced greater shame, self-blame, and fear of becoming drawn into the conflict than when they listened to parents engaged in nonchild-related conflict.

In a follow-up study, Grych and Fincham (1993) demonstrated that if the parents in a child-related conflict absolved Chris from blame for the argument, the children later reported less shame, fear of involvement, and self-blame than did those who heard the parents blame Chris for the same argument. Children's different reactions to the content of interparental conflict implies that child-related conflict may play a greater role than does nonchild-related conflict in children's self-conscious emotions.

These studies illustrate some important methodological advances. First, through the use of multiple observers and experimental designs, these researchers have reduced the risk of artificially inflating correlations between ratings of conflict and child adjustment, thereby strengthening confidence in their findings. Second, because they focus specifically on interparental conflict, they have been able to identify critical dimensions of conflict, such as the intensity of expressed anger, the degree of conflict resolution, and the content of the conflict (i.e., whether it was about the child). These investigators have also begun to uncover developmental changes in children's sensitivity to angry adult conflict. Without the specific focus on interparental conflict, the discovery of such important differences would have been lost.

Conclusion

All three of the research literatures discussed here suggest some powerful alternatives to self-report techniques for assessing chronic daily stressors in childhood. Some examples are peer sociometric ratings to assess a child's level of social acceptance at school, simulated conflicts between adults, and naturalistic observations in the home. This is not to argue that child reports of stressors are not of unique value. In fact, a careful distinction between child perceptions and more objective indicators of one common stressor, academic failure, leads to the conclusion that perceptions may be more critical than reality. The point to be made here is that some of the assessment techniques developed in other fields can provide stress-and-coping researchers with rich information that would be impossible to obtain with self-report data alone. For example, many investigators seem to believe that it is difficult, or impossible, for children to accurately describe their exposure to daily stressors before they near their adolescent years. Therefore, another result of an almost exclusive reliance on self-report measures has been a focus on adolescents, with little attention paid to the daily experiences of younger children. Yet, the research reviewed shows that there is much that can be learned about the effects that common daily stressors have on the well-being of young children.

Although these approaches can be much more complex and expensive to use, they ultimately suggest more differentiated and informative stress-and-coping models. Two examples illustrate how, by concentrating on a single chronic stressor, researchers have been able to identify the significant dimensions of a stressor and link those dimensions in a much more precise way with child characteristics and outcomes. In the case of chronic problems with peers, distinctions between different types of unpopular children suggest that, whereas rejected children are more likely to exhibit aggressive behavior, neglected children may be at an increased risk for becoming depressed. Similarly, other research indicates that a child's exposure to interparental discord needs to be understood in terms of the content of parent arguments, the intensity of the anger that is expressed by the parents, and the manner in which the conflicts are resolved.

Perhaps most important, the preceding research strategies seem to bring one much closer to empirically validated process models. Findings from these literatures are beginning to disentangle the complex web of causal relations that connect chronic stressors to child adjustment outcomes. For example, evidence suggests that behavior problems, especially the display of hostile and aggressive behaviors, increase the likelihood that a child will be rejected by his or her peers. Another example is a line of research investigating factors that contribute to children's perceptions of their academic competence. Researchers now know that certain parental attitudes, beliefs, and expectations help to shape at least one common stressor in childhood, the perception that one is unsuccessful in school. The most informative strategies appear to be those that focus on a single type of stressor that is studied either within an experimental context or as part of a prospective longitudinal study that includes multiple measures (including nonchild-report techniques). However, even with sophisticated research designs, one's understanding of daily stressors and their effects is incomplete without a consideration of how individual children and adolescents differ from each other in their responses to the same stressful situation. Within the health psychology literature, these individual differences are usually studied in terms of coping style.

COPING WITH DAILY STRESSORS IN CHILDHOOD AND ADOLESCENCE

The Conceptualization and Measurement of Coping in the Child Stress-and-Coping Literature

Coping in childhood is typically conceived in the stress-and-coping field as a purposeful or effortful response to a stressful event (Compas, 1987). The different strategies that children use to cope with common stressful events are often discussed in terms of a theoretical model suggested by Lazarus and Folkman (1984). According to their model, *problem-focused coping* includes strategies that attempt to manage or change the source of the problem. These can include thinking about the problem and considering alternative solutions, as well as acting to change the situation, such as seeking the help of others or studying more in order to improve grades. *Emotion-focused coping* refers to efforts to regulate emotional responses to the stressor. For example, seeking emotional support from friends and ignoring or denying the problem are two emotion-focused strategies that a child may use to cope with a household in which parents are frequently angry and openly argue with one another. A similar theoretical system that distinguishes between primary and secondary control has been proposed by Band and Weisz (1988). Here the emphasis is on the goals that underlie a coping behavior. *Primary control coping* is aimed at changing or influencing objective conditions or events, such as by yelling at a friend who took something from you. *Secondary control coping* is aimed at maximizing one's goodness of fit with conditions as they are, such as trying to feel less upset about a problem with peers.

Given the almost universal definition of coping as a conscious, intentional reaction to a recognized stressor, it is not surprising that, with few exceptions, self-report measures of coping are the norm in the child stress-and-coping literature. In this tradition, children and adolescents are asked to describe the strategies that they have used or that they would use to deal with stressful situations. All of the studies described next focus on children's descriptions of how they cope with common, everyday situations.

Researchers interested in spontaneous descriptions of coping strategies can employ several means to elicit information about coping from children and adolescents. In some cases, children are presented with hypothetical scenarios, such as conflicts with peers (Dubow & Tisak, 1989) or waiting situations that entail frustration or fear (e.g., waiting for a candy bar or waiting at the doctor's office for a shot) (Altschuler & Ruble, 1989). Subjects then respond to open-ended questions about the things that one might do in that stressful situation. In other studies, the children are first asked to describe an actual stressful experience in their lives and then to describe all the ways that they could have handled that situation and/or the coping strategies that they actually used (Band & Weisz, 1988; Compas, Malcarne, & Fondacaro, 1988; Frydenberg & Lewis, 1991; Kliewer, 1991). Often, they are directed to recall specific types of stressful events, such as being in conflict with a friend or receiving a disappointing grade in school. A child may also be

asked to describe coping responses to stressful situations that have been reported by a parent (Hardy, Power, & Jaedicke, 1993).

Spontaneous descriptions of coping are typically categorized according to theoretically based dimensions, such as problem-focused and emotion-focused responses (Compas, Malcarne, & Fondacaro, 1988); approach and avoidance techniques (Altshuler & Ruble, 1989); assertive solutions and aggressive solutions (Dubow & Tisak, 1989); or primary, secondary, and relinquished control strategies (Band & Weisz, 1988). In some cases, researchers also use more fine-grained, content-based groupings (Band & Weisz, 1988; Kliewer, 1991), or code children's responses according to a combination of different theoretical dimensions (Hardy, Power, & Jaedicke, 1993).

Instead of spontaneous descriptions of coping generated by the subject, another approach to coping assessment involves the use of checklists (e.g., Hops, Lewinsohn, Andrews, & Roberts, 1990; Spirito et al., 1988). Here, the child or adolescent indicates how often he or she uses different types of coping responses, such as asking for advice, thinking of different ways to solve a problem, pretending nothing happened, going to a movie, crying, or getting angry. Some measures define stressful situations (e.g., poor grades, peer conflicts), for which the child describes his or her coping responses (Causey & Dubow, 1992). Others aim for a more global assessment of coping style by asking about how the child generally copes with "difficulties," "concerns," or "problems" (Frydenberg & Lewis, 1991; Kurdek, 1987; Patterson & McCubbin, 1987; Sandler, Tein, & West, 1994). Coping checklists are usually scored according to factor-based scales, which represent empirically generated categories of coping strategies, rather than the theoretically based systems commonly used to code responses to open-ended questions about coping.

Whether through use of checklists or open-ended questions, nearly all assessments of coping in the stress-and-coping literature rely on children's self-reports. This approach has provided researchers with rich information about how children construe stress in their environment, the kinds of responses to common stressors that they consider, and the reactions they observe in their own thoughts, emotions, and behavior. However, Repetti (1996) has pointed out that self-report techniques impose certain limitations on what one can learn about children's coping. First, it seems unlikely that children would be aware of all the different coping strategies that they use in difficult situations. This may be especially true of emotion-focused and secondary-control coping efforts, which often involve internal cognitive and emotional processes.

Difficulties involved in recognizing coping responses are compounded by the fact that the context in which coping occurs often changes over time. In particular, children may continue to cope with distress generated by even a minor event long after the incident has occurred and the situation has changed. For example, after school has ended and a child is home for the day, he or she may still deal with the hurt and anger of being left out of a group during a class recess period. Because emotion-focused coping efforts may take place in a situation that is different from the one that caused the distress, it should not be surprising that children sometimes fail to recognize the connection between their current coping responses and the original stressful situation.

A second problem with self-report techniques in this literature is that, when they are confronted with a questionnaire or interview, children may not recall or adequately describe even those coping strategies that they did originally recognize. The most obvious coping responses may be relatively easy to recall, such as trying to study more and keep up with homework in order to improve grades. However, a child may be less likely to remember other responses, such as teasing a classmate or sibling who is succeeding in school in an effort to cope with the frustration and distress of a disappointing report card. In general, less rational and intentional responses may be relatively difficult for a child to initially recognize as coping, to recall later, and to describe, even though they were part of an effort to manage emotional distress.

A reliance on self-report data has made it difficult for researchers to provide a comprehensive description of the different coping strategies that are actually used by children in any given stressful situation. Because it therefore seems premature to draw any conclusions about which strategies are most adaptive or maladaptive for a child to use, this chapter intentially avoids an analysis of coping along these lines. Instead, the discussion turns now to research on how children attempt to cope with the three particular situations that were discussed earlier: problems with peers, academic failure, and interparental conflict. Once again, the focus is on promising research designs and assessment techniques that suggest some alternatives to the use of children's own reports of their coping responses in questionnaires and interviews.

Coping with Peer Problems

The use of child self-reports to assess coping with peer problems is almost universal. One exception to this trend is work by Eisenberg and colleagues in which an emotion regulation paradigm is applied to children's coping with hostility (Eisenberg, Fabes, Nyman, Bernzweig, & Pinuelas, 1994; Fabes & Eisenberg, 1992). These developmental psychologists observe free-play periods at preschools and record children's reactions to overt anger provocations (e.g., responses to being teased or hit, or having a possession taken by another child). Reactions to the provocations are coded into descriptive categories, such as attempts to retaliate or seek revenge (e.g., hitting the provocateur), attempts to actively resist or object in a nonaggressive manner (e.g., telling someone to give a toy back), venting emotions (e.g., crying or throwing a tantrum), escape or avoidance (e.g., leaving the area), or adult seeking.

The obvious advantage to this approach is its ecological validity. Children's genuine reactions to hostility during natural social interactions are directly measured, without relying on the child's recall of the event and his or her reaction to it. Interestingly, Eisenberg and associates (1994) found that descriptions of child coping that were provided by teachers and mothers were consistent with observations of children's actual reactions to anger provocations. This finding suggests that teachers and parents may be able to provide accurate information about how a child tends to cope with certain types of common events.

A daily-report methodology can also be used to study coping during the course of normal day-to-day social interactions (Repetti, 1996). In this type of study, children keep records throughout the day of both their behavior and events that have occurred to them. Changes over time in perceptions of stressful situations are then associated with changes in the child's self-reported behavior. Thus, the child is not asked to describe his or her coping in response to the stressful event. Instead, the investigator notes the temporal connection between the report of a stressful event and a change in the child's behavior. Using this procedure, Repetti (1996) has found that perceptions of problems with peers at school are linked to a same-day increase in a child's self-reported demanding and difficult behavior at home, such as misbehaving and being loud and noisy.

These findings are consistent with Repetti's (1996) suggestion that a child's initial attempts to secure parental attention and support following a peer rejection at school can escalate into more aversive behaviors. There are several reasons why this type of escalation might take place. The child may not connect a current state of distress to a social problem that occurred earlier at school, which would make it difficult to adequately communicate his or her need for reassurance. Alternatively, the child may simply lack the language or social skills needed to directly communicate his or her need for support, and these skills may be especially deficient when the child is feeling distressed. As a result of either situation, the child may use immature or indirect bids for parental attention, such as clinging to a parent, or whining or nagging, and become frustrated if the parent fails to recognize and respond to his or her need for comfort and reassurance. Feelings of frustration and anger at home may also be fueled by lingering negative affect that was initially generated by events at school. The situation would be further inflamed by negative parent responses to the child's behavior, such as expressions of intolerance or anger and the use of discipline.

It is interesting to note that findings from the two research programs described here suggest that, whether it is hitting another child in immediate retaliation or behaving in a difficult and aversive manner with parents later on, expressions of anger and aggression may be a common child response to problems with peers. Consideration of self-report data alone would suggest that children only rarely resort to aggressive behavior as a coping strategy (Band & Weisz, 1988; Causey & Dubow, 1992).

Coping with Academic Failure

In contrast to the naturalistic approach represented in the preceding studies, some developmental psychologists use experimental research designs to observe children's responses to academic failure in the labora-

tory (Dweck & Licht, 1980). For example, in one study, children were trained to manipulate cans in order to match the configuration of an experimenter's cans. Once children learned the task, they were exposed to a failure condition in which they were given three unsolvable problems involving the cans (Bempechat, London, & Dweck, 1991). Observations of children's reactions to failure in this study and others like it suggest that children's beliefs about their academic abilities influence how they respond to failure situations.

Two types of responses have been identified. The first is exhibited by "helpless" children, who do not perceive themselves to be academically competent. When these children are exposed to difficult problems in a laboratory setting, they do not try to solve the problems. Dweck and colleagues hypothesize that children's negative beliefs about their competencies lead them to attribute failure experiences to a personal lack of ability, and that is why they simply give up when confronted with a difficult or challenging problem.

Mastery-oriented children, on the other hand, utilize problem-focused coping strategies in the face of failure. These children believe that they are academically competent and do not attribute failure to a personal lack of ability. In fact, they appear not to be concerned with the causes of their failures, and instead focus on strategies to solve difficult problems. Research has shown that such children try harder during challenging tasks. It is important to note that no differences have been found between helpless and mastery-oriented children's actual ability levels (Diener & Dweck, 1978; Dweck & Reppucci, 1973). It seems that their beliefs about their abilities, rather than their actual abilities, influence how they respond to failure.

Children who question their abilities may also attempt to cope with academic failure by avoiding situations in which failure might occur. For example, Harter (1992) found that a child's level of perceived cognitive competence predicted his or her choice of difficulty level in a laboratory setting. Children with lower perceptions of academic competence chose easier rather than more difficult anagrams in a problem-solving task. Harter suggests that perceptions of incompetence increase a child's level of worry or anxiety about challenging academic situations. One way to cope is by avoiding difficult problem-solving tasks in which failure might occur. Other research also indicates that self-reported perceptions of academic competence are related to preference for challenge in school activities (Boggiano, Main, & Katz, 1988). These studies, together with the work of Dweck and colleagues, suggest that children's perceptions of their academic competence may represent an important individual difference variable underlying the way that they attempt to cope with academic failure.

In the daily-report study described earlier, Repetti (1996) found that when children perceived more academic failure events at school (e.g., receiving a "bad" grade on a test or paper), they also reported both more aversive child behaviors and more aversive parent behaviors later in the evening. Moreover, the association between the children's perceptions of academic failure and negative parent responses (e.g., their reports of parental expressions of disapproval and anger) was independent of their own self-reported aversive behavior that evening. This finding suggests either that the parents were directly responding to the school failure event, or that the children were more apt to view their parents as disapproving when they believed that they had performed poorly at school. In either case, this study echoes the research pointing to the critical role that parents play in shaping children's responses to academic events. Not only do parents influence children's perceptions of their academic competence but they also may be intimately involved in their youngsters' attempts to cope with perceived failures at school.

Coping with Interparental Conflict

Marital researchers believe that, before age 5, children tend to cope with interparental conflict by managing their own emotional reaction and not attending to those around them. Around age 5, children appear to become more problem focused in their coping efforts and may try to mediate the dispute (Cummings & El-Sheikh, 1991). In the study mentioned earlier that used audiotapes of an adult couple arguing, Grych and Fincham (1993) asked children after each segment what they would do if the couple arguing was actually their own parents. Based on children's responses, the researchers identified four different ways that children cope with adult conflict.

Some children reported that they would engage in *direct intervention* by interrupting their parents while they were arguing. Other children responded that they would engage in *indirect intervention* and attempt to remove the perceived cause of conflict without becoming directly involved. For example, a child might clean up her room if she believes that is the cause of her parents' argument. In other cases, children indicated that they would cope with interparental conflict through *withdrawal* by either removing themselves from the situation or by seeking support from another family member or friend. As a fourth coping mechanism, children reported that they would *do nothing* and choose to ignore the conflict or distract themselves. This methodological approach, which elicits children's descriptions of coping in response to an immediate conflict situation, is also used in some of the studies described next. Although it relies on child self-report data, it does not require the child to recall past parental conflicts and his or her coping responses. Thus, by avoiding a retrospective design, investigators who use this strategy also avoid the problems of poor or selective recall.

Cummings (1987) supplemented child self-report data with observational data. He found that 4- and 5-year-old children responded to live simulations of anger between strangers in one of three ways. The *concerned emotional responders* were rated as more visibly distressed during the conflict and, in later reports, were most likely to indicate that they felt sad and had a desire to intervene while witnessing the dispute. The *ambivalent responders* were rated as showing both positive and negative affect during the conflict. These children reported behavioral and emotional arousal as indicated by their desire to cry and/or run away during the argument or to hit the arguing adults. They also showed increased physical and verbal aggression toward a friend in a playtime following the simulation.

Unresponsive children showed no overt behavioral or affective changes during the conflict, although they later reported that they had felt angry. When asked what they felt like doing during the conflict, these children reported a desire to use an avoidant coping strategy (i.e., they wanted to continue to play and ignore the actors). Results involving this last group of children are particularly interesting because they emphasize the importance of using multiple respondents. Had only the observers' ratings been used, the results would have indicated no change in the children's affect or behavior. Had only the children's responses been used, the results would have indicated an anger reaction. In either case alone, important information would have been lost.

In an interesting follow-up to this study, El-Sheikh and associates (1989) linked response style to physiological changes. Ambivalent responders showed the most variability in heart rate both to friendly and angry audiotaped adult interactions. Concerned emotional responders showed increased heart rate only to the angry interactions, and unresponsive children showed no significant heart rate changes either to the friendly or angry interactions.

In a recent study, children were shown segments of angry interactions between two adults and between an adult and a child (El-Sheikh & Cheskes, 1995). After each interaction, participants were asked to indicate how they had wanted to cope during the conflict by pointing to cards with either aggressive (i.e., hitting or yelling at people) or nonaggressive behavioral responses (i.e., crying, stopping the fight, leaving the room, ignoring the people, or doing nothing). The children tended to give more aggressive responses to adult-child conflicts than to adult-adult conflicts. However, their primary responses for both types of conflict were a desire to stop the fighting and a desire to leave the room.

Participants in this study were also asked how they might have lessened the actors' distress. Children endorsed two types of responses most frequently: *mediation*, in which the child attempts to stop the conflict through compromise, and *authority*, in which the child attempts to stop the conflict from a position of power (e.g., by using a directive such as "Stop that!"). Less frequently mentioned responses were *emotional support*, in which the child does not directly intervene but offers comfort by saying or doing something nice for both actors; *triangulation*, in which the child sides with or offers help to one person only; and *no involvement*, in which the child does not become involved in the conflict.

Researchers have also examined sex and age differences in children's emotional responses to adult conflicts. Young boys report more anger and aggression in response to interadult anger than do young girls. However, this sex difference appears to be less reliable among children over the age of 9 (Cummings, Ballard, & El-Sheikh, 1991; Cummings et al., 1989; El-Sheikh et al., 1989). Interestingly, there appears to be a general developmental progression in which there is a gradual reduction in children's self-reported emotional responses to angry adult interactions with increasing age (Cummings, Ballard, & El-Sheikh, 1991; Cummings, Ballard, El-Sheikh, & Lake, 1991; El-Sheikh et al., 1989; El-Sheikh & Cheskes, 1995).

Children's coping responses to interparental conflict appear to be determined by many factors, including the intensity of the conflict, the age and sex of the child, and individual differences among children in their emotional and physiological responses to adult anger. Researchers working in this field recognize the value of children's own perceptions and include child self-reports in their investigations. However, self-report measures and correlational studies are supplemented with observational techniques and analogue experimental designs. As a result, this literature presents a more complete picture of how children respond to signs of anger and conflict between parents.

Conclusion

The alternatives to self-report strategies discussed here contribute important information to the coping literature. In particular, children may use more emotion-focused coping than they are able to report. For example, the expression of anger and aggression appears to be a much more common way of responding to daily events than one would guess from children's descriptions of their own coping. In one study, increases in child aversive behavior at home appeared to be a delayed reaction to problems with peers and academic failure experiences that had occurred earlier at school (Repetti, 1995). In another study, Cummings (1987) observed increased aggression toward a friend in a playtime that followed a simulation of an adult conflict. These data also support the notion that coping responses unfold over time, even with a change in social context.

Another example of a possibly underreported emotion-focused coping response is a withdrawal from the challenge posed by the stressor. This type of strategy has been observed in Dweck's laboratory studies of failure situations, and has also been observed in Eisenberg's naturalistic studies of anger provocations. As suggested earlier, children may be unlikely to report responses like "giving up" because they do not recognize them as coping strategies or perhaps, when asked in an interview, they do not recall using them or are unable to describe them. Whatever the reason, the addition of new assessment techniques to the health literature should result in a more comprehensive description of the many different strategies that are used by children to cope with common daily stressors.

There also appear to be significant advantages to the study of child coping within a specified context. A focus on children's reactions to particular types of distressing situations (e.g., problems with peers at school, failure situations, or observations of conflicts between adults) makes it possible to learn much more about how children respond and attempt to cope within each context. So, for example, interrupting parents while they are arguing seems quite different from developing a strategy to solve a complex problem in a laboratory setting, even though both might be considered problem-focused coping responses. A more complete description of the process of coping within particular types of stressful situations will improve the inferences that researchers can make about what are adaptive and maladaptive coping responses within each context and about who are the most successful and unsuccessful copers. For example, distinguishing among children who are observed to be "concerned," "ambivalent," and "unresponsive" in the face of adult conflicts may ultimately reveal at least as much as do distinctions between children who generally report using more problem-focused or emotion-focused coping strategies.

FUTURE DIRECTIONS

Health psychologists and others who work within a stress-and-coping paradigm have recognized the importance of studying children's and adolescents' exposure to common psychosocial stressors and their responses to these seemingly minor events in daily life. In the long run, a youngster's experiences with events such as peer rejection, academic failure, or interparental conflict, and his or her way of reacting to them, contributes to the child's overall psychological development and adjustment. However, there remains much to be learned about stress-and-coping processes

and the role that they play in the mental and physical health of children and adolescents.

Our review suggests that the health psychology literature would be further advanced by some of the methods and approaches used in the other fields that were discussed here. In general, we recommend that global investigations of "daily stressors" be supplemented with studies that focus on specific types of stressful events or circumstances, that assessment techniques be broadened beyond the current reliance on the self-reports of children and adolescents, and that there be increased use of prospective longitudinal studies and experimental research designs in this literature.

NOTE

The preparation of this chapter was supported by a FIRST award (R29-48593) from the National Institute of Mental Health awarded to Rena Repetti. The authors would like to thank Jennifer Kelleher and the other members of the UCLA Family Development Study research group for their helpful comments on an earlier version of the paper.

REFERENCES

Altshuler, J. L., & Ruble, D. N. (1989). Developmental changes in children's awareness of strategies of coping with uncontrollable stress. *Child Development, 60,* 1337–1349.

Armacost, R. L. (1989). Perceptions of stressors by high school students. *Journal of Adolescent Research, 4,* 443–461.

Asher, S. R., & Coie, J. D. (1990). *Peer rejection in childhood.* New York: Cambridge University Press.

Asher, S. R., & Wheeler, V. A. (1985). Children's loneliness: A comparison of rejected and neglected peer status. *Journal of Consulting and Clinical Psychology, 53,* 500–505.

Band, E. B., & Weisz, J. R. (1988). How to feel better when it feels bad: Children's perspectives on coping with everyday stress. *Developmental Psychology, 24,* 247–253.

Banez, G. A., & Compas, B. E. (1990). Children's and parent's daily stressful events and psychological symptoms. *Journal of Abnormal Child Psychology, 18,* 491–605.

Bempechat, J., London, P., & Dweck, C. S. (1991). Children's conceptions of ability in major domains: An interview and experimental study. *Child Study Journal, 21,* 11–35.

Bierman, K. L., & Smoot, D. L. (1991). Linking family characteristics with poor peer relations: The mediating role of conduct problems. *Journal of Abnormal Child Psychology, 19,* 341–356.

Blechman, E. A., McEnroe, M. J., Carella, E. T., & Audette, D. P. (1986). Childhood competence and depression. *Journal of Abnormal Psychology, 95,* 223–227.

Bobo, J. K., Gilchrist, L. D., Elmer, J. F., Snow, W. H., & Schinke, S. P. (1986). Hassles, role strain, and peer relations in young adolescents. *Journal of Early Adolescents, 6,* 339–352.

Boggiano, A. K., Main, D. S., & Katz, P. A. (1988). Children's preference for challenge: The role of perceived competence and control. *Journal of Personality and Social Psychology, 54,* 134–141.

Buchanan, C. M., Maccoby, E. E., & Dornbusch, S. M. (1991). Caught between parents: Adolescents' experience in divorced homes. *Child Development, 62,* 1008–1029.

Bukowski, W. M., & Hoza, B. (1989). Popularity and friendships: Issues in theory, measurement, and outcome. In T. Berndt & G. Ladd (Eds.), *Peer relationships in child development* (pp. 15–45). New York: Wiley.

Causey, D. L., & Dubow, E. F. (1992). Development of a self-report coping measure for elementary school children. *Journal of Clinical Child Psychology, 21,* 47–59.

Coie, J. D., & Kupersmidt, J. B. (1983). A behavioral analysis of emerging social status in boys' groups. *Child Development, 54,* 1400–1416.

Cole, D. A. (1991). Change in self-perceived competence as a function of peer and teacher evaluation. *Developmental Psychology, 27,* 682–688.

Compas, B. E. (1987). Coping with stress during childhood and adolescence. *Psychological Bulletin, 101,* 393–403.

Compas, B. E., Davis, G. E., Forsythe, C. J., & Wagner, B. M. (1987). Assessment of major and daily stressful events during adolescence: The adolescent perceived events scale. *Journal of Consulting and Clinical Psychology, 55,* 534–541.

Compas, B. E., Howell, D. C., Phares, V., Williams, R. A., & Guinta, C. T. (1989). Risk factors for emotional/behavioral problems in young adolescents: A prospective analysis of adolescent and parental stress and symptoms. *Journal of Consulting and Clinical Psychology, 57,* 732–740.

Compas, B. E., Howell, D. C., Phares, V., Williams, R. A., & Ledoux, N. (1989). Parent and child stress and symptoms: An integrative analysis. *Developmental Psychology, 25,* 550–559.

Compas, B. E., Malcarne, V. L., & Fondacaro, K. M. (1988). Coping with stressful events in older children and young adolescents. *Journal of Consulting and Clinical Psychology, 56,* 405–411.

Cowen, E. L., Work, W. C., Hightower, A. D., Wyman, P. A., Parker, G. R., & Lotyczewski, B. S. (1991). Toward the development of a measure of perceived self-efficacy in children. *Journal of Clinical Child Psychology, 20,* 169–178.

Cummings, E. M. (1987). Coping with background anger in early childhood. *Child Development, 58,* 976–984.

Cummings, E. M., Ballard, M., & El-Sheikh, M. (1991). Responses of children and adolescents to interadult anger as a function of gender, age, and mode of expression. *Merrill-Palmer Quarterly, 37,* 543–560.

Cummings, E. M., Ballard, M., El-Sheikh, M., & Lake, M. (1991). Resolution and children's responses to interadult anger. *Developmental Psychology, 27,* 462–470.

Cummings, E. M., & El-Sheikh, M. (1991). Children's coping with angry environments: A process-oriented approach. In M. Cummings, A. Greene, & K. Karraker (Eds.), *Life-span developmental psychology: Perspective on stress and coping* (pp. 131–150). Hillsdale, NJ: Erlbaum.

Cummings, E. M., Vogel, D., Cummings, J. S., & El-Sheikh, M. (1989). Children's responses to different forms of expression of anger between adults. *Child Development, 60,* 1392–1404.

Cummings, E. M., Zahn-Waxler, C., & Radke-Yarrow, M. (1981). Young children's responses to expressions of anger and affection by others in the family. *Child Development, 52,* 1274–1282.

Daniels, D., & Moos, R. H. (1990). Assessing life stressors and social resources among adolescents: Applications to depressed youth. *Journal of Adolescent Research, 5,* 268–289.

Diener, C. I., & Dweck, C. S. (1978). An analysis of learned helplessness: Continuous changes in performance, strategy, and achievement cognitions following failure. *Journal of Personality and Social Psychology, 36,* 451–461.

Dishion, T. J. (1990). The family ecology of boys peer relations in middle childhood. *Child Development, 61,* 874–892.

Dodge, K. A. (1983). Behavioral antecedents of peer social status. *Child Development, 54,* 1386–1399.

DuBois, D. L., Felner, R. D., Brand, S., Adan, A. M., & Evans, E. G. (1992). A prospective study of life stress, social support, and adaptation in early adolescence. *Child Development, 63,* 542–557.

Dubow, E. F., & Tisak, J. (1989). The relation between stressful life events and adjustment in elementary school children: The role of social support and social problem-solving skills. *Child Development, 60,* 1412–1423.

Dweck, C. I., & Reppucci, N. D. (1973). Learned helplessness and reinforcement responsibility in children. *Journal of Personality and Social Psychology, 25,* 109–116.

Dweck, C. S., & Licht, B. G. (1980). Learned helplessness and intellectual achievement. In J. Garber & M. E. P. Seligman (Eds.), *Human helplessness: Theory and applications* (pp. 197–221). New York: Academic Press.

Eccles, J. P. (1983). Expectancies, values, and academic behaviors. In J. T. Spence (Ed.), *Achievement and achievement motives* (pp. 75–146). San Francisco: W. H. Freeman.

Eisenberg, N., Fabes, R. A., Nyman, M., Bernzweig, J., & Pinuelas, A. (1994). The relations of emotionality and regulation to children's anger-related reactions. *Child Development, 65,* 109–128.

El-Sheikh, M., & Cheskes, J. (1995). Background verbal and physical anger: A comparison of children's responses to adult-adult and adult-child arguments. *Child Development, 66,* 446–458.

El-Sheikh, M., Cummings, E. M., & Goetsch, V. L. (1989). Coping with adults' angry behavior: Behavioral, physiological, and self-reported responding in preschoolers. *Developmental Psychology, 25,* 490–498.

Emery, R. E. (1982). Interparental conflict and the children of discord and divorce. *Psychological Bulletin, 92,* 310–330.

Emery, R. E. (1988). *Marriage, divorce, and children's adjustment.* Newbury Park, CA: Sage.

Fabes, R. A., & Eisenberg, N. (1992). Young children's coping with interpersonal anger. *Child Development, 63,* 116–128.

French, D. C., & Waas, G. A. (1985). Teachers' ability to identify peer-rejected children: A comparison of sociometrics and teacher ratings. *Journal of School Psychology, 23,* 347–353.

Frick, P. J., Kamphaus, R. W., Lahey, B. B., Loeber, R., Christ, M. G., Hart, E. L., & Tannenbaum, L. E. (1991). Academic underachievement and the disruptive behavior disorders. *Journal of Consulting and Clinical Psychology, 59,* 289–294.

Frydenberg, E., & Lewis, R. (1991). Adolescent coping: The different ways in which boys and girls cope. *Journal of Adolescence, 14,* 119–133.

Grych, J. H., & Fincham, F. D. (1990). Marital conflict and children's adjustment: A cognitive-contextual framework. *Psychological Bulletin, 108,* 267–290.

Grych, J. H., & Fincham, F. D. (1993). Children's appraisals of marital conflict: Initial investigations of the cognitive-contextual framework. *Child Development, 64,* 215–230.

Grych, J. H., Seid, M., & Fincham, F. D. (1992). Assessing marital conflict from the child's perspective: The children's perception of interparental conflict scale. *Child Development, 63,* 558–572.

Ham, M., & Larson, R. (1990). The cognitive moderation of daily stress in early adolescence. *Journal of Community Psychology, 18,* 567–585.

Hardy, D. F., Power, T. G., & Jaedicke, S. (1993). Examining the relation of parenting to children's coping with everyday stress. *Child Development, 64,* 1829–1841.

Harter, S. (1982). The perceived competence scale for children. *Child Development, 53,* 87–97.

Harter, S. (1992). The relationship between perceived competence, affect, and motivational orientation within the classroom: Processes and patterns of change. In A. K. Boggiano & T. S. Pittman (Eds.), *Achievement and motivation: A social-developmental perspective* (pp. 77–114). New York: Cambridge University Press.

Hinshaw, S. P. (1992). Externalizing behavior problems and academic underachievement in childhood and adolescence: Causal relationships and underlying mechanisms. *Psychological Bulletin, 111,* 127–155.

Hops, H., Lewinsohn, P. M., Andrews, J. A., & Roberts, R. E. (1990). Psychosocial correlates of depressive symptomatology among high school students. *Journal of Clinical Child Psychology, 19,* 211–220.

Hymel, S., Bowker, A., & Woody, E. (1993). Aggressive versus withdrawn unpopular children: Variations in peer and self-perceptions in multiple domains. *Child Development, 64,* 879–896.

Hymel, S., Rubin, K. H., Rowden, L., & LeMare, L. (1990). Children's peer relationships: Longitudinal prediction of internalizing and externalizing problems from middle to late childhood. *Child Development, 61,* 2004–2021.

Jaycox, L. H., & Repetti, R. L. (1993). Conflict in families and the psychological adjustment of preadolescent children. *Journal of Family Psychology, 7,* 344–355.

Kanner, A. D., Weinberger, D. A., & Ford, M. E. (1987). Uplifts, hassles, and adaptational outcomes in early adolescents. *Journal of Early Adolescence, 7,* 371–394.

Kliewer, W. (1991). Coping in middle childhood: Relations to competence, type A behavior, monitoring, blunting, and locus of control. *Developmental Psychology, 27,* 689–697.

Kupersmidt, J. B., & Patterson, C. J. (1991). Childhood peer rejection, aggression, withdrawal, and perceived competence as predictors of self-reported behavior problems in preadolescence. *Journal of Abnormal Child Psychology, 19,* 427–449.

Kurdek, L. A. (1987). Gender differences in the psychological symptomatology and coping strategies of young adolescents. *Journal of Early Adolescence, 7,* 395–410.

Lazarus, R. S., & Folkman, S. (1984). *Stress, appraisal, and coping.* New York: Springer.

Lobato, D., Faust, D., & Spirito, A. (1988). Examining the effects of chronic disease and disability on children's sibling relationships. *Journal of Pediatric Psychology, 13,* 389–407.

McGrath, E. P., & Repetti, R. L. (1995). *Parents' attitudes toward their children's academic performance and children's perceptions of their academic competence.* Poster presented at the Biennial Meeting of the Society for Research in Child Development, Indianapolis, IN.

Meece, J. L., Wigfield, A., & Eccles, J. S. (1990). Predictors of math anxiety and its influence on young adolescents' course enrollment intentions and performance in mathematics. *Journal of Educational Psychology, 82,* 60–70.

Monahan, S. C., Buchanan, C. M., Maccoby, E. E., & Dornbusch, S. M. (1993). Sibling differences in divorced families. *Child Development, 64,* 152–168.

Newcomb, A. F., Bukowski, W. M., & Pattee, L. (1993). Children's peer relations: A meta-analytic review of popular, rejected, neglected, controversial, and average sociometric status. *Psychological Bulletin, 113,* 99–128.

Parker, J. G., & Asher, S. R. (1987). Peer relations and later personal adjustment: Are low-accepted children at risk? *Psychological Bulletin, 102,* 35–389.

Parker, J. G., & Asher, S. R. (1993). Friendship and friendship quality in middle childhood: Links with peer group acceptance and feelings of loneliness and social dissatisfaction. *Developmental Psychology, 29,* 1–11.

Parsons, J. E., Adler, T. G., & Kaczala, C. (1982). Socialization of achievement attitudes and beliefs: Parental influences. *Child Development, 53,* 310–321.

Parsons, J. E., Kaczala, C., & Meece, J. L. (1982). Socialization of achievement attitudes and beliefs: Classroom influences. *Child Development, 53,* 322–339.

Patterson, C. J., Kupersmidt, J. B., & Griesler, P. C. (1990). Children's perceptions of self and of relationships with others as a function of sociometric status. *Child Development, 61,* 1335–1349.

Patterson, G. R., DeBaryshe, B. D., & Ramsey, E. (1989). A developmental perspective on antisocial behavior. *American Psychologist, 44,* 329–335.

Patterson, J. M., & McCubbin, H. I. (1987). Adolescent coping style and behaviors: Conceptualization and measurement. *Journal of Adolescence, 10,* 163–186.

Phillips, D. A. (1984). The illusion of incompetence among academically competent children. *Child Development, 55,* 2000–2016.

Phillips, D. A. (1987). Socialization of perceived academic competence among highly competent children. *Child Development, 58,* 1308–1320.

Phillips, D. A., & Zimmerman, M. (1990). The developmental course of perceived competence and incompetence among competent children. In R. Sternberg & J. Kolligian (Eds.), *Competence considered* (pp. 41–66). New Haven, CT: Yale University Press.

Reid, R. J., & Crisafulli, A. (1990). Marital discord and child behavior problems: A meta-analysis. *Journal of Abnormal Child Psychology, 18,* 105–117.

Repetti, R. L. (1996). The effects of perceived daily social and academic failure experiences on school-age children's subsequent interactions with parents. *Child Development, 67,* 1467–1482.

Sandler, I. N., Tein, J., & West, S. G. (1994). Coping, stress, and the psychological symptoms of children of divorce: A cross-sectional and longitudinal study. *Child Development, 65,* 1744–1763.

Siegel, J. M., & Brown, J. D. (1988). A prospective study of stressful circumstances, illness symptoms, and depressed mood among adolescents. *Developmental Psychology, 24,* 715–721.

Spirito, A., Stark, L. J., & Williams, C. (1988). Development of a brief coping checklist for use with pediatric populations. *Journal of Pediatric Psychology, 13,* 555–574.

Timko, C., Moos, R. H., & Michelson, D. J. (1993). The contexts of adolescents' chronic life stressors. *American Journal of Community Psychology, 21,* 397–420.

Tolan, P. (1988). Socioeconomic, family, and social stress correlates of adolescent antisocial and delinquent behavior. *Journal of Abnormal Psychology, 16,* 317–331.

Tolan, P., Miller, L., & Thomas, P. (1988). Perception and experience of types of social stress and self-image among adolescents. *Journal of Youth and Adolescence, 17,* 147–163.

Weisz, J. R., Weiss, B., Wasserman, A. A., & Rintoul, B. (1987). Control-related beliefs and depression among clinic-referred children and adolescents. *Journal of Abnormal Psychology, 96,* 58–63.

CHAPTER 22

PREVENTION OF SEXUALLY TRANSMITTED DISEASES OTHER THAN HUMAN IMMUNODEFICIENCY VIRUS

Willard Cates, Jr., FAMILY HEALTH INTERNATIONAL, NORTH CAROLINA
Stuart M. Berman, CENTERS FOR DISEASE CONTROL AND PREVENTION

Sexually transmitted diseases (STDs) are a major health problem among adolescents and young adults in the United States (Cates, 1991). Although the human immunodeficiency virus (HIV) has commanded center stage both for the public's attention and for public health resources, the STDs other than HIV cause considerable morbidity (Cates, 1988). Not only do they increase the prevalence and incidence of HIV through "epidemiologic synergy," (Wasserheit, 1992) but also they lead to adverse reproductive sequelae such as tubal infertility (Cates et al., 1990), ectopic pregnancy (Chow et al., 1987), and genital neoplasms (Dalence, 1993). Thus, as we enter the twenty-first century, lowering the incidence of these STDs other than HIV has been designated as one of our nation's most important health objectives (DHHS, 1990).

This chapter addresses the epidemiology and prevention of STDs other than HIV in adolescents. Discussion will focus on the sexual behaviors that affect STD transmission in this group, the magnitude of the problem in the adolescent population, prevention approaches to reduce STDs in communities, and the

implications of STDs for future directions in adolescent health programs.

ADOLESCENT SEXUAL BEHAVIOR

Adolescence is a time of sexual curiosity and experimentation. During the last two decades, both the percentage of sexually active adolescents and the incidence of STDs in this group have grown to epidemic levels (Cates, 1991). During the 1980s, the proportion of adolescent women who reported having had premarital intercourse continued to increase. Furthermore, their first sexual experience occurred at progressively younger ages. Behaviorally, the increasing percentage of teenagers having sex at earlier ages has a cumulative impact on their number of sex partners (CDC, 1991; Kost & Forrest, 1992). The earlier sexual activity is begun, the longer a person is exposed to the risk of different sex partners. Moreover, unmarried females who have their first sexual experience at earlier ages have more partners per year than those who initiate later (CDC, 1991).

Thus, the teenage years appear to carry the highest risk for exposure to multiple sex partners, albeit usually in a pattern of serial monogamy. In 1988, over 25 percent of reproductive age women who began sexual activity by age 15 had 10 or more lifetime sex partners, compared with fewer than 6 percent of those beginning coitus at age 20 (Pratt & Eglash, 1990). In 1991, 24 percent of young urban heterosexuals had had more than one sex partner during the previous year (Binson et al., 1993).

Four measurable covariables are significantly associated with age of first premarital intercourse among young women: mother's education, religious affiliation, age at menarche, and family stability at age 14 (Hofferth et al., 1987; Hofferth, 1987). The lower the mother's education, the weaker the religious affiliation, the younger the age at menarche, and the less stable a family at age 14, the earlier the age at first intercourse.

Once adolescents have begun sexual activity, their use (or nonuse) of barrier contraception becomes important to preventing STDs. Condoms have received special attention because of fears regarding the spread of HIV and other STDs. Here, the recent data are hopeful but not ideal: from 27 percent to 66 percent of sexually active adolescents in different surveys reported using condoms at the last coital episode (Binson et al., 1993; DiClemente et al., 1992; Hingson et al., 1990). These percentages are two to three times higher than those reported in the 1970s. However, the level of condom use reported by adolescents may be elevated by what are perceived to be socially acceptable answers. Moreover, recency of condom use is not the same as consistency of use. In every survey in which the question was asked, fewer than half of the teenagers who recently used condoms reported doing so all the time (Pratt et al., 1990).

Factors associated with use of condoms by adolescents are related to both their underlying beliefs and the immediate availability of the prophylactic method (Kegeles et al., 1988). If adolescents are concerned about acquiring HIV, if they believe that condoms can prevent HIV transmission, if they are not embarrassed to ask a partner to use condoms, and if they have talked with a physician about condoms, they are more likely to use them. As expected, those who carry condoms with them are more likely to use

them consistently. In addition, use of drugs, especially cocaine and alcohol, is another behavioral determinant that increases high-risk sexual behaviors, including multiple partners and nonuse of condoms. Finally, inaccurate self-perceptions of STD risk among sexually active college students lead to inadequate planning for safer sex practices (MacDonald et al., 1990; Hernandez & Smith, 1990; Manning et al., 1989).

EXTENT OF THE PROBLEM

Gonorrhea

Because of the large numbers and the reporting stability, trends in gonorrhea provide the best estimates of STD patterns in adolescents (Mascola et al., 1983; Rice et al., 1987; Webster et al., 1993). From 1975 through 1993, the total number of gonorrhea cases reported to CDC decreased by 60 percent, from approximately 1 million to 400,000 (CDC, 1994b). This favorable trend was temporally associated with initiation in the early 1970s of a national gonorrhea control program to detect infected persons and interrupt transmission of the organism (Cates, 1987). To some extent, adolescents shared in this overall numerical decrease. In 1993, approximately 150,000 cases of gonorrhea were reported in teenagers, compared with over 200,000 in 1975.

However, while the *number* of gonorrhea *cases* declined among those aged 15 to 19 years, the *rates* of gonorrhea declined more slowly in adolescents than in older age groups (Webster & Rolfs, 1993). This apparent contradiction reflects both demographic and behavioral factors. First, the size of the teenage population, especially the white teenage population, began to shrink by the mid-1970s. Thus, the denominator was getting smaller. Conversely, the 25- to 44-year-olds, the tail end of the "baby boom" cohorts, constituted an increasing population base. Second, as described earlier, high-risk sexual behaviors continued to escalate among adolescents in the 1980s.

During the 1980s and into the 1990s, gonorrhea rates in both teenage males and females had the dubious distinction of increasing compared with rates in other age groups (see Figures 22.1 and 22.2). The incidence of gonorrhea in males aged 15 to 19 rose dur-

Figure 22.1 Gonorrhea Age-Specific Case Rates, Male (U.S. 1981–1992)

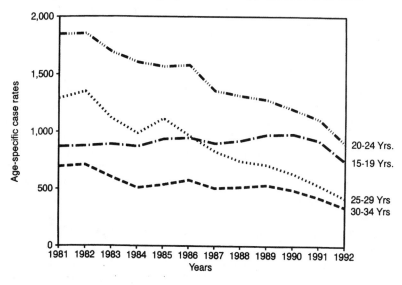

Figure 22.2 Gonorrhea Age-Specific Case Rates, Female (U.S. 1981–1992)

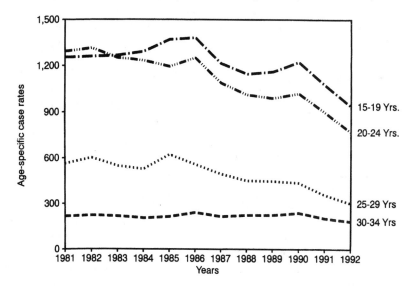

ing the decade, but declined for all other age groups. Only in 1992 was the gonorrhea rate in adolescent males lower than a decade earlier. Females aged 15 to19 had the highest age-specific gonorrhea rate in 1984, and the gap widened over the intervening years.

Although gonorrhea rates in adolescent females declined in the 1990s, they were still higher than in older women.

Racial differences are also apparent in gonorrhea trends among adolescents of both genders (Webster &

Rolfs, 1993; Gershman & Rolfs, 1991). Among white males, gonorrhea declined steadily in all age groups, yet those 15 to 19 years of age had the slowest decline. Similarly, rates among white adolescent women also had a slower decline than among older ages; their gonorrhea rate went from the second highest in 1981 to the highest by 1991. Unlike rates among white and Hispanic adolescents, gonorrhea rates for African American teenagers actually *increased* from 1981 through 1989. The incidence in African American males showed a pattern of gradual increase during the 1980s, whereas for African American females, the levels remained elevated throughout the decade (Webster & Rolfs, 1993). Because gonorrhea rates in older African American population have decreased, reasons for the increase in African American teenagers must be specific for this age group.

The effect of these temporal trends has further widened the gonorrhea racial gap between African American and white American adolescents. In 1981, the gonorrhea rates among African American male and female adolescents were twelvefold and ninefold, respectively, higher than among white adolescents. By 1991, these differences had risen to forty-fourfold and fifteenfold, respectively (Webster & Rolfs, 1993). Various hypotheses have been offered to account for the widening racial gap:

1. STD primary prevention messages, especially those aimed at HIV, have been more successful in white communities.
2. STD clinical care in public clinics has been overwhelmed by increasing responsibilities, which has a greater negative impact on the minority populations who disproportionately rely on these clinics.
3. STD interviewing and partner notification activities have been gradually shifted from gonorrhea to chlamydia and syphilis, again affecting gonorrhea control in minorities.
4. STD risk behaviors, fueled by illicit drugs, have created an increasing STD prevalence among low-income heterosexual minorities (Rolfs, Goldberg, & Sharrar, 1990; Fullilove et al., 1990; CDC, 1993a).

Because of marked geographic variation, each of these hypotheses probably played a role to a greater or lesser degree throughout the United States.

Syphilis

Syphilis is the other STD about which there is consistent data to measure trends. During the 1980s, syphilis rates decreased among white males, presumably because of safer sexual behaviors in response to HIV prevention messages (Rolfs & Nakashima, 1990). However, these gains have been more than offset by rapid increases since 1985 among minority heterosexuals, in part as a result of riskier sexual and health care seeking behaviors associated with illicit drugs. By 1990, syphilis in the United States was at its highest level since World War II; over the past few years, rates have declined (Webster & Rolfs, 1993).

Adolescents as a group apparently suffered less from the syphilis epidemic of the 1980s than older age groups (Webster & Rolfs, 1993), in part because the mean age of those with syphilis is older than those with gonorrhea (Webster et al., 1993). Nonetheless, the rate of syphilis in African American adolescent males and females increased from 1985 through 1990, and the racial gap widened. If teenagers with syphilis become pregnant, risks of congenital syphilis are heightened, especially if prenatal care is minimal. Congenital syphilis rose markedly in the United States beginning in 1989 (Dunn et al., 1993). Moreover, the genital ulcers of syphilis have been associated with increased risks of HIV infection (Wasserheit, 1992).

Chlamydia

Chlamydia trachomatis causes more lower genital tract infections among adolescents than gonorrhea (CDC, 1993b). Unlike gonorrhea, however, chlamydial infections are not reportable conditions in all 50 states, and national surveillance for chlamydia is based on pilot projects. Thus, consistent trends for this infection in adolescents are not available.

The prevalence of cervical chlamydia is from 8 to 40 percent of young women cultured during pelvic examinations (CDC, 1993b). Most investigations of adolescent females have found cervical chlamydia to be at least two times more common than gonorrhea

(CDC, 1993b). Similar ratios occur in urethral specimens from asymptomatic, sexually active adolescent males (Braverman et al., 1990). In virtually all studies, adolescent women appear to have an increased risk for chlamydial infections than do older age groups (CDC, 1993b). Both social/behavioral factors and/or an increased biologic susceptibility contribute to this higher percentage of chlamydia in adolescents (Ehrhardt & Wasserheit, 1991). High-risk sexual behavior interacts with increased cervical ectopy and presumed immunologic naivete to produce high levels of chlamydia prevalence (Arno et al., 1994).

Genital Herpes and Genital Warts

Trends in sexually transmitted viral infections among adolescents have followed the same course as that of bacterial infections (Becker et al., 1986; Becke et al., 1987). Based on consultations for genital herpes and genital wart infections in office-based fee-for-service practices, the number of visits for women aged 15 to 19 years increased for both these viral STDs during the past two decades. Cases of genital herpes increased from 15,000 yearly visits in 1966 to over 125,000 visits by 1992. Similarly, for genital warts, caused by the human papillomavirus (HPV), the number of visits for teenagers rose from approximately 50,000 in 1966 to nearly 300,000 in 1992. Student health authorities find genital warts to be the most prevalent symptomatic STD among their population (Budell, 1990).

For both these viral STDs, visits to private clinicians represent only the symptomatic tip of the iceberg. As physician awareness and availability of diagnostic methods have increased, subclinical herpes and HPV infections of the male and female genital tract are becoming increasingly recognized. Serologic examination of a representative sample of Americans using herpes simplex virus (HSV) type 2 antibody showed evidence of widespread asymptomatic infection (Johnson et al., 1989). By the end of their teenage years, approximately 4 percent of whites and 17 percent of African Americans have been infected with HSV-2. Most HSV transmission occurs from asymptomatic persons (Mertz et al., 1988; Brock et al., 1990). Similarly, for HPV, cervical cytologic evidence indicates at least threefold more women have

asymptomatic cervical HPV infection than report external genital warts (Stone, 1989). This ratio increases several times when more sensitive indicators (e.g., molecular probes, polymerase chain reaction) are used. Because adolescents with HPV are especially susceptible to future neoplasia (Koutsky et al., 1992), asymptomatic HPV infections in adolescents should be better documented so proper cancer screening services can be assured.

Hepatitis B Virus (HBV) Infections

Nationwide, the incidence of hepatitis B increased steadily during the 1980s in spite of both effective blood screening programs and the availability of a vaccine. By 1993, most HBV infections in the United States with known routes of transmission resulted from sexual and/or drug-related exposure. Adolescents are at special risk of heterosexual HBV, as with other STDs. Unfortunately, vaccination programs have not reached the risk groups that account for the most cases—injecting drug users, homosexual men, and persons acquiring the disease through heterosexual exposure.

The number of cases of hepatitis B caused by heterosexual exposure has increased over the past several years, primarily among inner-city minority heterosexuals (Alter et al., 1990). Approximately 30 percent of hepatitis B cases occur among student-age populations. Moreover, an estimated 5 percent of persons 24 years of age or younger have been infected with HBV. Clearly, young persons must be an increasing priority for vaccination programs addressing high-risk populations.

PREVENTION OF STDS

Primary Prevention

Primary prevention of STDs involves preventing persons from being exposed to infections and/or preventing acquisition of infection if exposure occurs. To prevent exposure to STDs, two behavioral approaches are possible: encouraging sexual abstinence and ensuring uninfected partners. Neither approach works well in the real world of teenage sexual decision making.

Sexual abstinence can be achieved either through postponing the initial sexual involvement or by encouraging periodic abstinence among sexually experienced persons. Despite the increasing awareness of the risks of HIV and AIDS, the 1980s saw an increasing percentage of adolescents having sex at early ages. By 1988, over one-quarter of African American and white 15-year-olds had experienced coitus; moreover, by age 19, over four-fifths of both races were sexually experienced (Aral & Cates, 1989). Some creative school education programs emphasizing peer-led discussion groups have had moderate success in encouraging high school students to postpone their sexual involvement (Howard & McCabe, 1990). The term *outercourse*—to connote sexual intimacy without intercourse, fellatio, or cunnilingus—has been derived to encourage a form of sexual expression that carries no STD risk.

Exposure can also be prevented by ensuring that coitus occurs with an uninfected partner. Mutual lifetime monogamy is one approach to this end. However, only a small minority of couples have each had only one sex partner their entire lives. Another approach is through asking potential sex partners about their sexual, drug, and STD history. Although some individuals will lie to have sex with others, most will not (Cochran & Mays, 1990). Thus, routinely asking will serve some protective function.

Once adolescents have chosen to be sexually active, preventing infection through use of barrier prophylaxis provides another tier of primary prevention. With adolescents and older students, current data on use of condoms by males show up to 66 percent of sexually active persons reported using condoms at last intercourse (DiClemente et al., 1992; Hingson et al., 1990; Sonenstein et al., 1989; Weisman et al., 1989). Female condoms, diaphragms, and spermicides also may help reduce some STDs other than HIV.

Finally, primary prevention can occur through vaccination. However, the only STD for which there is a vaccine—hepatitis B—has had a dismal vaccination record in the high-risk teenage populations. In the future, as additional vaccines become available, those concerned with providing adolescent health services will need to routinely screen and vaccinate susceptible persons for all vaccine-preventable conditions, including those transmitted sexually.

Secondary Prevention

Secondary prevention of STDs involves identifying infected persons and treating them before their infection either causes more costly complications or can be further transmitted within the community. In the latter sense, treating index cases also provides primary prevention to their partners. Achieving secondary STD prevention requires (1) screening asymptomatic persons, (2) diagnosing those with symptoms, (3) providing appropriate curative treatment for bacterial infections and suppressive treatment for viral infections, and (4) notifying partners who have been exposed to infected persons.

Screening persons for an STD can serve several purposes: early case detection and treatment, referral for clinical evaluation, changing high-risk behaviors, improved safety for health care providers, and documentation of STD prevalence. Most STD screening of adolescents occurs either in student health services or in public clinics (STD, family planning, maternal and child health, adolescent health). Screening tests in these settings should have high sensitivity to allow detection of as many infections as possible. Further testing can confirm false positives. For adolescents, noninvasive screening techniques may be most effective. For example, use of urine samples to detect evidence of genital inflammation or STD antigens would increase participation (Sadof et al., 1987; Getts, 1989; Shafer et al., 1993) and is cost beneficial (Genc et al., 1993). Recent experience with the ligase chain reaction and polymerase chain reaction tests for chlamydia has been encouraging (CDC, 1993b).

Diagnosing a particular STD usually occurs because of genital symptoms or notification of exposure to an STD. Presumptive diagnoses often form the basis for treatment, since most confirmatory diagnoses cannot be performed during a typical patient visit. Algorithms for approaching typical STD syndromes have been developed as a way of facilitating diagnosis (Stamm et al., 1988).

Early and adequate treatment of STDs is an effective way of preventing their spread within student populations (CDC, 1993c). Ideally, therapies should be inexpensive, simple, safe, and effective. Usually treatment is provided for specific infections or symptoms. In addition, based on epidemiologic indications, antibiotics can be administered to persons at high risk when infection is considered likely, in the interest of public health. This approach prevents complications that might occur between the time of testing and treatment, ensures treatment for infected persons with false-negative laboratory tests, and guarantees treatment for those who might not return when notified of positive tests.

Notification of the sex partners of infected persons is a traditional part of STD control programs in the United States (Bayer & Toomey, 1992). The privacy of patients and partners is rigorously protected. Two types of partner notification are possible: patient referral and provider referral (i.e., contact tracing). The latter service is more labor intensive, time consuming, and expensive. Therefore, provider referral is restricted to high-yield cases or to high-prevalence environments. As part of adolescent health services, partner notification can be arranged through collaboration with the local health department.

Implications for Adolescent Health

Preventing STDs among the adolescent population will require enlisting the entire spectrum of STD strategies, including behavioral, clinical, educational, and health promotional activities. First, we need renewed efforts both to learn more about and also to influence adolescent sexual behavior. For example, what modifiable determinants of teenagers' lives will help deter premature sexual activity? How can we influence peer values so that it is socially acceptable to postpone coital activity and socially unacceptable, if sexually active, to avoid using condoms? In this respect, many female adolescents apparently misinterpret the level of male reluctance to use condoms (Kegeles et al., 1988). We should emphasize to them that their male partners probably are willing to use condoms.

Second, we need better ways to detect and treat STD in adolescents. For example, using urine samples from males to screen for urethral chlamydia and gonorrhea has been encouraging (Sadof et al., 1987). Testing these specimens with leukocyte esterase, enzyme immunoassay, and ligase chain reaction for specific genetic material will have some future role (CDC, 1993b). Regarding treatment, single-dose oral antibiotics, such as cefixime and azithromycin, may promote better compliance than antibiotics (e.g., doxycycline) that require a week of therapy.

Third, we need continued efforts to reach health care providers, especially those concerned with adolescent health care. Clinicians providing health services for adolescents must first learn to deal with the sensitive area of teenage sexuality. Next, they should be up to date on the recommended approaches to diagnosing and treating the vast spectrum of STDs (Gilchrist & Rauh, 1985). Several opportunities for clinical training currently exist. The Centers for Disease Control and Prevention (CDC) sponsors 11 regional prevention/training centers that provide one- to two-week refresher courses at no cost to the participant. A simplified wall chart, also available from CDC, describes the symptoms, signs, laboratory approaches, therapy recommendations, and counseling message for each of the 15 most prevalent STDs (CDC, 1994a). The University of Washington has developed an up-to-date manual on a variety of STD syndromes, together with easily followed algorithms for clinical management (Stamm et al., 1988).

Fourth, we need increased STD/HIV school education programs, especially if offered within an environment of peer-led training and skills building, backed up by service availability. Most adolescents want to know more about STDs. Stimulated by recent concerns about AIDS, prototype school curriculum materials, using a self-instructional format and emphasizing behavioral messages, have been developed and field tested for both teachers and students in grades 6 through 12 (Yarber, 1989). Additionally, successful programs led by students themselves have helped adolescents both resist peer pressures to initiate sexual activity and use barrier methods if they become sexually active (Howard et al., 1990; Walter & Vaughan, 1993); we must build on this momentum.

Fifth, we need to go beyond school education programs by helping develop behavioral skills that reduce adolescents' sexual risks (St. Lawrence et al., 1994; St. Lawrence et al., in press). Understanding the social support structure, as well as influencing social norms, will be crucial to impacting both individual and aggregate sexual behaviors. Programs that have used cognitive-behavioral interventions have produced encouraging results, even in traditionally disenfranchised populations such as African American adolescents (St. Lawrence et al., in press).

Finally, we need to make better use of the mass media to convey effective health promotion messages to adolescents. Because they spend an average of 23 hours a week listening to radio or watching television, adolescents are a special audience for these electronic approaches (Strasburger, 1989). Messages should be aired to encourage condom use in high-risk settings or to publicize hotline numbers for further questions about STDs.

REFERENCES

Alter, M. J., Hadler, S. C., Margolis, H. S., & Alexander, W. J. (1990). The changing epidemiology of hepatitis B in the United States: Need for alternative vaccination strategies. *Journal of the American Medical Association, 263*, 1218–1222.

Aral, S. O., & Cates, W., Jr. (1989). The multiple dimensions of sexual behavior as a risk factor for STD: The sexually experienced are not necessarily sexually active. *Sexually Transmitted Diseases, 16*, 173–177.

Arno, J., Katz, B. P., McBride, R., Carty, G. A., Batteiger, B. E., Caine, V. A., & Jones, R. B. (1994). Age and clinical immunity to infections with *Chlamydia trachomatis. Sexually Transmitted Diseases, 21*, 47–52.

Bayer, R., & Toomey, K. E. (1992). HIV prevention and the two faces of partner notification. *American Journal of Public Health, 82*, 1158–1164.

Becker, T. M., Stone, K. M., & Alexander, E. R. (1987). Genital papillomavirus infection: A growing concern. *Obstetrics and Gynecology Clinics of North America, 14*, 389–396.

Becker, T. M., Stone, K. M., & Cates, W., Jr. (1986). Epidemiology of genital herpes infections in the United States: The current situation. *Journal of Reproductive Medicine, 31*, 359–364.

Binson, D., Dolcini, M. M., Pollack, L. M., & Catania, J. A. (1993). Multiple sexual partners among young adults in high-risk cities. *Family Planning Perspectives, 25*, 268–272.

Braverman, P. K., Biro, F. M., Brunner, R. L., Gilchrist, M. J., & Rauh, J. L. (1990). Screening asymptomatic adolescent males for chlamydia. *Journal of Adolescent Health Care, 11*, 141–144.

Brock, B. V., Selke, S., Benedetti, J., Douglas, J. M., Jr., & Corey, L. (1990). Frequency of asymptomatic shedding of herpes simplex virus in women with genital herpes. *Journal of the American Medical Association, 263*, 418–420.

Budell, J. W. (1990). Health problems in a university student health service. *Emory Journal of Medicine, 4*, 122–124.

Cates, W., Jr. (1987). Epidemiology and control of sexually transmitted diseases: strategic evolution. *Infectious Disease Clinics of North American, 1*, 1–23.

Cates, W., Jr. (1988). The "other STD"—Do they really matter? *Journal of the American Medical Association, 259*, 3606–3608.

Cates, W., Jr. (1991). Teenagers and sexual risk taking: The best of times and the worst of times. *Journal of Adolescent Health Care, 12*, 84–94.

Cates, W., Jr., Rolfs, R. T., Jr., & Aral, S. O. (1990). Sexually transmitted diseases, pelvic inflammatory disease and infertility: An epidemiologic update. *Epidemiologic Reviews, 12*, 199–220.

Centers for Disease Control and Prevention. (1991). Premarital sexual experience among adolescent women—United States, 1970–1988. *Morbidity and Mortality Weekly Report, 39*, 929–932.

Centers for Disease Control and Prevention. (1993a). Gang-related outbreak of penicillinase-producing *Neisseria gonorrhoea* and other sexually transmitted diseases—Colorado Springs, Colorado, 1989–1991. *Morbidity and Mortality Weekly Report, 42*, 25–28.

Centers for Disease Control and Prevention. (1993b). Recommendations for the prevention and management of *Chlamydia trachomatis* infections, 1993. *Morbidity and Mortality Weekly Report, 42*(RR-12), 1–3.

Centers for Disease Control and Prevention. (1993c). 1993 sexually transmitted diseases treatment guidelines. *Morbidity and Mortality Weekly Report, 42*(RR-14), 1–10.

Centers for Disease Control and Prevention.(1994a). *Sexually transmitted diseases summary, 1993*. Atlanta, GA: Centers for Disease Control and Prevention.

Centers for Disease Control and Prevention. (1994b). *Division of STD/HIV annual report 1993*. Atlanta, GA: Centers for Disease Control and Prevention.

Chow, W-H., Daling, J. R., Cates, W., Jr., & Greenberg, R. S. (1987). Epidemiology of ectopic pregnancy. *Epidemiologic Reviews, 9*, 70–94.

Cochran, S. D., & Mays, V. M. (1990). Sex, lies, and HIV (letter). *New England Journal of Medicine, 322*, 774–775.

Dalence, C. R. (1993). Human papillomavirus DNA testing in the management of cervical neoplasia. *Journal of the American Medical Association, 270*, 2975–2981.

Department of Health and Human Services (1990). Healthy people 2000. National Health Promotion and Disease Prevention Objectives. Washington, DC: Department of Health and Human Services.

DiClemente, R. J., Durbin, M., Siegel, D., Krasnovsky, F., Lazarus, N., & Comacho, T. (1992). Determinants of condom use among junior high students in a minority, inner-city school district. *Pediatrics, 89*, 197–202.

Dunn, R. A., Webster, L. A., Nakashima, A. K., & Sylvester, G. C. (1993). Surveillance for geographic and secular trends in congenital syphilis: United States, 1983–1991. *CDC Surveillance Summaries. Morbidity and Mortality Weekly Report, 42*(SS-6), 59–71.

Ehrhardt, A. A., & Wasserheit, J. N. (1991). Age, gender, and sexual risk behaviors for sexually transmitted diseases in the United States. In J. N. Wasserheit, S.O. Aral, & K. K. Holmes (Eds.), *Research issues in human behavior and sexually transmitted diseases in the AIDS era* (pp. 97–121). Washington, DC: American Society for Microbiology.

Fullilove, R. E., Fullilove, M. T., Bowser, B. P., & Gross, S. A. (1990). Risk of sexually transmitted disease among black adolescent crack users in Oakland and San Francisco, California. *Journal of the American Medical Association, 163,* 851–855.

Genc, M., Ruusuvaara, L., & Mardh, P-A. (1993). An economic evaluation for Chlamydia trachomatis in adolescent males. *Journal of the American Medical Association, 270,* 2057–2064.

Gershman, K. A., & Rolfs, R. T. (1991). Racial trends in gonorrhea in the United States, 1981–1988. Unpublished manuscript.

Getts, A. G. (1989). Diagnosing Chlamydia trachomatis urethritis by first-catch urine enzyme immunoassay in adolescent males. *Journal of Adolescent Health Care, 10,* 209–211.

Gilchrist, M. J. R., & Rauh, J. L. (1985). Office microscopic examination for sexually transmitted diseases: A tool to lower costs. *Journal of Adolescent Health Care, 6,* 311–320.

Hernandez, J. R., & Smith, F. J. (1990). Inconsistencies and misperceptions putting college students at risk of HIV infection. *Journal of Adolescent Health Care, 11,* 295–297.

Hingson, R. W., Strunin, L., Berlin, B., & Herren, T. (1990). Beliefs about AIDS, use of alcohol and drugs, and unprotected sex among Massachusetts adolescents. *American Journal of Public Health, 80,* 295–299.

Hofferth, S. L. (1987). Factors affecting initiation of sexual intercourse. In S. L. Hofferth & C. D. Hayes (Eds). *Risking the future: Adolescent sexuality, pregnancy, and childbearing* (Vol. 2, pp. 7–35). Washington, DC: National Academy Press.

Hofferth, S. L., Kahn, J. F., & Baldwin, W. (1987). Premarital sexual activity among U.S. teenage women over the past three decades. *Family Planning Perspectives, 19,* 46–53.

Howard, M., & McCabe, J. B. (1990). Helping teenagers postpone sexual involvement. *Family Planning Perspectives, 22,* 21–26.

Johnson, R. E., Nahmias, A., Madger, L. S., Lee, F. K., Brooks, C. A., & Snowden, C. B. (1989). A seroepidemiologic survey of the prevalence of herpes simplex virus type 2 infection in the United States. *New England Journal of Medicine, 321,* 7–12.

Kegeles, S. M., Adler, N. E., & Irwin, C. E. (1988). Sexually active adolescents and condoms. Changes over one year in knowledge, attitudes, and use. *American Journal of Public Health, 78,* 460–461.

Kost, K., & Forrest, J. D. (1992). American women's sexual behavior and exposure to risk of sexually transmitted diseases. *Family Planning Perspectives, 24,* 244–254.

Koutsky, L. A., Holmes, K. K., Critchlow, C. W., Stevens, C. E., Paavonen, J., Beckmann, A. M., DeRouen, T. A., Galloway, D. A., Vernon, D., & Kiviat, N. B. (1992). A cohort study of the risk of cervical intraepithelial neoplasia grade 2 or 3 in relation to papillomavirus infection. *New England Journal of Medicine, 327,* 1271–1278.

MacDonald, N. E., Wells, G. A., Fisher, W. A., Warren, W. K., King, M. A., Doherty, J. A., & Bowie, W. R. (1990). High-risk STD/HIV behavior among college students. *Journal of the American Medical Association, 263,* 3155–3159.

Manning, D., Balson, P. M., Barenberg, N., & Moore, T. M. (1989). Susceptibility to AIDS: What college students do and don't believe. *Journal of American College Health, 38,* 67–73.

Mascola, L., Cates, W., Jr., Reynolds, G. H., Blount, J. H., & Albritton, W. L. (1983). Gonorrhea and salpingitis among American teenagers, 1960–1981. CDC Surveillance Summaries. *Morbidity and Mortality Weekly Report, 32*(3SS), 25SS–30SS.

Mertz, G. J., Coombs, R. W., Ashley, R. L., Jourden, J., Remington, M., Winter, E. C., Fahnlander, A., Guinan, M., Ducey, H., & Corey, L. (1988). Transmission of genital herpes in couples with one symptomatic and one asymptomatic partner: a prospective study. *Journal of Infectious Diseases, 157,* 1169–1177.

Pratt, W. F., & Eglash, S. B. (1990). Premarital sexual behavior: Multiple partners and marital experience. Presented at the annual meeting of the Population Association of America, Toronto, Canada, May 4.

Rice, R. J., Aral, S. O., Blount, J. H., & Zaidi, A. A. (1987). Gonorrhea in the United States 1975–1984: Is the giant only sleeping? *Sexually Transmitted Diseases, 14,* 83–87.

Rolfs, R. T., Goldberg, M., & Sharrar, R. G. (1990). Risk factors for syphilis: cocaine and prostitution. *American Journal of Public Health, 80,* 853–857.

Rolfs, R. T., & Nakashima, A. K. (1990). Epidemiology of primary/secondary syphilis in the United States, 1981–1988. *Journal of the American Medical Association, 264,* 1432–1437.

Sadof, M. D., Woods, E. R., & Emans, S. J. (1987). Dipstick leukocyte esterase activity in first-catch urine specimens. *Journal of the American Medical Association, 258,* 1932–1934.

Shafer, M-A., Schachter, J., Moncada, J., Keogh, J., Pantell, R., Gourlay, L., Eyre, E. S., & Boyer, C. B. (1993). Evaluation of urine-based screening strategies to detect *Chlamydia trachomatis* among sexually active young males. *Journal of the American Medical Association, 270,* 2065–2070.

Sonenstein, F. L., Pleck, J. H., & Ku, L. C. (1989). Sexual activity, condom use and AIDS awareness among adolescent males. *Family Planning Perspectives, 21,* 152–160.

St. Lawrence, J. S., Brasfield, T. L., Jefferson, K. W., Alleyne, E., O'Bannon, R. E., & Shirley, A. (in press). Cognitive-behavioral intervention to reduce African-American adolescents' risk for HIV infection. *Journal of Consulting and Clinical Psychology.*

St. Lawrence, J. S., Brasfield, T. L., Jefferson, K. W., Alleyne, E., & Shirley, A. (1994). Social support as a factor in African-American adolescents sexual behavior. *Journal of Adolescent Research, 9,* 292–310.

Stamm, W. E., Kaetz, S. M., Beirne, M. B., et al. (1988). *The practitioner's handbook for the management of STDs.* Seattle: University of Washington.

Stone, K. M. (1989). Epidemiologic aspects of genital HPV infection. *Clinical Obstetrics and Gynecology, 32,* 112–116.

Strasburger, V. C. (1989). Adolescent sexuality and the media. *Pediatric Clinics of North America,* 747–773.

Walter, H. J., & Vaughan, R. D. (1993). AIDS risk reduction among a multiethnic sample of urban high school students. *Journal of the American Medical Association, 270,* 725–730.

Wasserheit, J. N. (1992). Epidemiological synergy: interrelationships between human immunodeficiency virus infection and other sexually transmitted diseases. *Sexually Transmitted Diseases, 19,* 61–77.

Webster, L. A., Berman, S. M., & Greenspan, J. R. (1993). Surveillance for gonorrhea and primary and secondary syphilis among adolescents, United States—1981–1991. *CDC surveillance summaries. Morbidity and Mortality Weekly Report, 42*(SS-3), 1–11.

Webster, L. A., & Rolfs, R. T. (1993). Surveillance for primary and secondary syphilis—United States, 1991. CDC surveillance summaries. *Morbidity and Mortality Weekly Report, 42*(SS-3), 13–19.

Weisman, C. S., Nathanson, C. A., Ensminger, M., Teitelbaum, M. A., Robinson, J. C., & Plichta, S. (1989). AIDS knowledge, perceived risk and prevention among adolescent clients of a family planning clinic. *Family Planning Perspectives, 21,* 213–217.

Yarber, W. L. (1989). *Curriculum for integrated STD/AIDS teaching.* Bloomington: University of Indiana.

CHAPTER 23

SLEEP DISORDERS

Jodi A. Mindell, ST. JOSEPH'S UNIVERSITY AND ALLEGHENY UNIVERSITY OF THE HEALTH SCIENCES

Sleep disorders are common in children and adolescents, and these sleep problems often get reported to those professionals working in the fields of medicine and health psychology. Unfortunately, however, most health professionals know little about sleep and sleep disorders (Mindell, Moline, Zendell, Brown, & Fry, in press). Therefore, the purpose of this chapter is to provide detailed information about the most common sleep disorders seen in children and adolescents.

CLASSIFICATION OF SLEEP DISORDERS

Before discussing any of the sleep disorders, it is important to mention the classification system of these disorders. Sleep disorders basically get classified into two major categories, the dyssomnias and the parasomnias, as delineated by the International Classification of Sleep Disorders (ICSD; Diagnostic Classification Steering Committee, 1990). The *dyssomnias* include those disorders that result in difficulty either initiating or maintaining sleep or involve excessive daytime sleepiness. The *parasomnias*, on the other hand, are disorders that disrupt sleep after initiation and are disorders of arousal, partial arousal, or sleep stage transitions. They are disorders that intrude into the sleep process but usually do not result in complaints of insomnia or excessive sleepiness.

Note that these terms, as defined by the ICSD, differ slightly from their use in the American Psychi-atric Association's *DSM-IV* (APA, 1994). *DSM-IV* defines *dyssomnias* as those sleep disorders in which the predominant disturbance is the amount, quality, or timing of sleep. The *parasomnias* are sleep disorders that involve abnormal behavioral or physiological events occurring in association with sleep, specific sleep stages, or sleep-wake transitions. Both methods of defining these terms, however, result in the same classification of specific sleep disorders into these two major categories. Note that coverage of the sleep disorders discussed in this chapter follows the ICSD classification system.

PREVALENCE AND PERSISTENCE

Survey studies have found that approximately 25 percent of children between the ages of 1 and 5 years experience some type of sleep disturbance (Bixler, Kales, Scharf, Kales, & Leo, 1976; Jenkins, Bax, & Hart, 1980; Lozoff, Wolf, & Davis, 1985; Richman, 1981; Richman, Stevenson, & Graham, 1975). Children's sleep disturbances come in many different forms. Salzarulo and Chevalier (1983) interviewed the families of 218 children, ages 2 to 15, referred for pediatric or child psychiatric consultation, and found that sleep talking was most common (32 percent), followed by nightmares (31 percent), waking at night (28 percent), trouble falling asleep (23 percent), enuresis (17 percent), bruxism (10 percent), sleep rocking (7 percent), and night terrors (7 percent).

Another survey (Dollinger, 1982), of mothers referring their children to a university clinic, found the most common sleep problems (among 3- to 15-year-olds) were sleep talking (53 percent), restless sleep and bedtime refusal (both 42 percent), and refusing to go to sleep without a nightlight (40 percent). Other sleep problems included bad dreams (35 percent), difficulty going to sleep (26 percent), crying out in sleep (16 percent), and nightmares (11 percent). An additional study of healthy preadolescents, ages 8 to 10 years, found that 43 percent of the children were experiencing a sleep problem that had lasted more than six months (Kahn et al., 1989). Looking at specific sleep disorders, parasomnias were present in 29 percent of the children, with enuresis (2 percent), sleep walking (5 percent), and night fears (15 percent) also frequently reported.

Sleep disturbances also tend to persist, especially from infancy throughout childhood. Kataria, Swanson, and Trevathan (1987) found that 84 percent of a sample of children had sleep disturbances that continued to persist after three years. Bixler and colleagues (1976) also reported that sleep problems in older children often relate to the presence of sleep-waking disorders in the first year of life. Furthermore, the children who had early disorders of the sleep-waking rhythm often had multiple sleep problems later.

In a third study, Abe, Ohta, Amatomi, and Oda (1982) found significant interyear associations, at five-year follow-up, for such sleep disorders as bruxism, sleepwalking, night terrors, and enuresis. Of all the behavior problems they assessed, sleep disturbances were the most persistent. However, sleep disturbances seen in early childhood are less likely to persist into adolescence and adulthood. For example, Klackenberg (1982a) reported that sleep disorders at 4 years of age predicted no more than 5 to 10 percent of sleep disturbances in later childhood and adolescence.

ASSESSMENT

A thorough assessment of sleep disorders in children and adolescents involves several steps. The first step is completion of a thorough sleep history. All aspects of the sleep-wake cycle need to be reviewed. Areas that need to be addressed include evening activities, such as television watching, medications, intake of caffeinated beverages, bedtime, and bedtime routines. Nighttime areas in need of evaluation include latency to sleep onset, behaviors during the night, and the number and duration of nighttime awakenings. Clinicians must also collect details about abnormal events during sleep, such as night terrors, confusional arousals, respiratory disturbances, seizures, and enuresis.

In the morning, wake time and sleepiness should be evaluated. Daytime variables in need of assessment include sleepiness, naps, meals, caffeine intake, medications, and feelings of anxiety and depression. Medication intake should also be reviewed because many medications can affect sleep. A review of psychological symptoms during the day is also important. Symptoms of anxiety and depression can be the result of lack of sleep. For example, feelings of fatigue, irritability, and sluggishness may simply be the result of sleep deprivation.

Other life events that may relate to acute sleep problems are significant life stressors and should also be assessed. Failure in school, death in the family, or a recent move can all contribute significantly to a sleep problem that resembles insomnia. A thorough evaluation must include questioning about school performance, social functioning, and family functioning. For example, a recent change in a family's financial status can result in sleep disturbances in children even when the parents do not believe that their children are aware of such problems. Often children, and especially adolescents, are much more aware of tensions in a family than parents are aware. Thus, it is important that clinicians conduct a thorough evaluation of all aspects of sleep and daytime functioning.

The second step in the evaluation of sleep problems is the keeping of sleep diaries. A typical sleep diary includes information on the time to bed, latency to sleep onset, number and duration of nighttime awakenings, time of arising in the morning, total sleep time, and duration and time of naps. For the most useful information, patients must keep at least two weeks of baseline sleep diaries. In this way, clinicians can clearly delineate sleep patterns.

In cases in which there is a concern about an underlying physiological problem, polysomnography (PSG) is an essential component of assessment. Even in some cases in which a client does not report any physiological symptoms, it may be important to conduct a PSG. For example, many children and parents are unaware of snore arousals or sleep apnea that may be interrupting sleep and resulting in complaints of insomnia and daytime sleepiness. Polysomnography typically consists of an overnight sleep study, which involves recordings of oxygen saturation, nasal and oral airflow, thoracic and abdominal respiratory movements, limb muscle activity, and electroencephalogram (EEG).

As an adjunct to a PSG, a multiple sleep latency test (MSLT) may serve a useful purpose. This test, performed in two-hour intervals throughout the day following the overnight study, evaluates a client's level of daytime sleepiness. The MSLT consists of four 20-minute nap opportunities given at two-hour intervals. Measures of sleep latency are taken. If sleep occurs, the nap gets terminated 15 minutes after sleep onset.

SPECIFIC SLEEP DISORDERS

Dyssomnias

Physiologically Based Dyssomnias

Two physiologically based dyssomnias are narcolepsy and obstructive sleep apnea. Although environmental circumstances may contribute to their presentation, these disorders have a primary physiological cause.

Narcolepsy. Children experience several sleep problems classified as dyssomnias. One such disorder is narcolepsy, which is a disorder characterized by excessive sleepiness often presenting itself as repeated episodes of naps or lapses into sleep of short duration throughout the day (Diagnostic Classification Steering Committee, 1990; Guilleminault, 1986, 1987; Mitler, Nelson, & Hajdukovic, 1987). Another common symptom unique to narcolepsy is cataplexy, which involves the sudden loss of bilateral muscle tone following the occurrence of a strong emotion, such as laughter, elation, or anger. This loss of muscle tone can be as minor as a mild sensation of weakness involving facial sagging or slurred speech, or it can be as severe as complete postural collapse. The duration of cataplexy typically lasts from a few seconds to several minutes, with complete and immediate recovery. Not all narcoleptics experience cataplexy, but for those who do, it is a pathognomonic symptom.

Narcolepsy occurs in approximately 0.03 to 0.16 percent of the population, with onset typically occurring in adolescence. This disorder rarely gets diagnosed in preteenaged children, although one study (Kotagal, Hartse, & Walsh, 1990) described the markers of narcolepsy in four children in this age group. Individuals with narcolepsy may also have associated psychosocial problems (Kavey, 1992). Children may get labeled as "apathetic" or "lazy" by parents or teachers. Often, difficulties in school arise prior to appropriate diagnosis and treatment. Especially in adolescence, social problems may occur, including social withdrawal and self-image problems.

There is no known cure for narcolepsy, so treatment focuses on management of this disorder. Treatment for narcolepsy often involves medications such as tricyclic antidepressants or stimulants (Wittig, Zorick, Roehrs, Sickelsteel, & Roth, 1983). Management of daytime sleepiness may require use of CNS stimulants, such as pemoline, methylphenidate, or dextroamphetamine. Cataplexy management may require use of tricyclics (e.g., desipramine, imipramine), which are REM suppressors (Reite, Nagel, & Ruddy, 1990). Unfortunately, most studies done on pharmacological treatments for narcolepsy involve adults; few studies include children.

Obstructive Sleep Apnea. A second dyssomnia often found in children is obstructive sleep apnea. This disorder involves repetitive episodes of upper airway obstruction during sleep, often causing a reduction in blood oxygen saturation (Diagnostic Classification Steering Committee, 1990; Guilleminault, Korobkin, & Winkle, 1981). The obstruction results from decreased muscle tone, during sleep, of the musculature maintaining the airway and the muscles involved in respiration. In children, the most common cause of sleep apnea is enlarged tonsils and adenoids, which usually do not interfere with respiration when awake. These apneic episodes cause frequent arousals and brief awakenings throughout the night. Most individuals with apnea are unaware of these occurrences.

In comparison with adults, in which apneic episodes often involve snoring and are easy to identify, diagnosis in children is more difficult (Brouillette, Fernback, & Hunt, 1982). Children with this disorder may be excessively sleepy during the day. They may exhibit daytime mouth breathing, difficulty swallowing, or poor speech articulation. During sleep, these children may snore, appear to be very restless sleepers, or sleep in unusual positions. One study found that evidence of breathing irregularities was a good indicator of sleep apnea in children, whereas snoring was not a good predictor (Croft, Brockbank, Wright, & Swanston, 1990). The mean age at diagnosis for children with sleep apnea is 7 years (Mauer, Staats, & Olson, 1983), and it is more common in boys than in girls (Guilleminault & Anders, 1976). Children who are morbidly obese (greater than 150 percent ideal body weight) are also at increased risk for sleep apnea (Mallory, Fiser, & Jackson, 1989).

The most common form of treatment for pediatric sleep apnea involves surgery to remove the airway obstructions (e.g., Croft et al., 1990; Guilleminault & Dement, 1988). Tonsillectomy or adenoidectomy relieves symptoms in about 70 percent of all child cases. Other treatments also recommended include weight loss and the use of pharmacological agents (Roth, Roehrs, & Zorick, 1988). Furthermore, nasal continuous positive airway pressure (CPAP), found to be extremely successful in the treatment of obstructive sleep apnea in adults (e.g., He, Kryger, Zorick, Conway, & Roth, 1988; Issa & Sullivan, 1986), may be an appropriate treatment for some children (Guilleminault, Riley, Powell, Simmons, & Nino-Murcia, 1985). Further systematic controlled studies are necessary to address the utility of CPAP for pediatric obstructive sleep apnea.

Environmentally Based Dyssomnias

Unlike narcolepsy or obstructive sleep apnea, each of which has a physiologically basis, other dyssomnias relate to environmentally circumstances. Four such disorders, adjustment sleep disorder, limit-setting sleep disorder, sleep-onset association disorder, and nocturnal eating (drinking) syndrome, are common among children. Other environmentally based dyssomnias include nighttime fears and delayed sleep phase disorder.

Adjustment Sleep Disorder. Adjustment sleep disorder is a form of insomnia related to emotional arousal caused by acute stress, conflict, or an environmental change (Diagnostic Classification Steering Committee, 1990). It is present among children following a move, after the death of a relative, or before the first day of school. The duration of such a sleep problem is often days, although in some cases, often associated with ongoing stressors, this form of sleep disturbance may last as long as several months.

One special population, hospitalized children, often experience an adjustment sleep disorder. Hospitals, and all that goes with a hospitalization, can be a major disrupter of sleep, and not surprisingly, hospitalized children often develop sleep problems (Beardslee, 1976; Prugh, Staub, Sands, Kirschbaum, & Lenihan, 1953; White, Powell, Alexander, Williams, & Conlon, 1988). Hospitalization also may exacerbate preexisting sleep difficulties (Anders & Weinstein, 1972). Hagemann (1981) found that hospitalized children, ages 3 to 8, lose up to 25 percent of their normal sleeptime because of difficulties falling asleep and delays in sleep onset.

Researchers have conducted some studies to explore means to reduce sleep difficulties in hospitalized children. Surprisingly, White and colleagues (1990) found that children felt more distressed and took longer to fall asleep when parents were present at bedtime or when children listened to a parent-recorded story compared to those children who listened to a stranger-recorded story at bedtime or had no intervention. They suggested that hospitalized children may have more difficulties falling asleep at night when reminders of home are present as opposed to when they are not present. These data are in contrast to popular opinion. A survey of 400 psychiatrists found that 44 percent believed that mothers should sleep in a hospitalized child's room whenever possible (Pietropinto, 1985).

Other suggestions to help hospitalized children sleep include instructing the nursing staff to institute structured bedtimes for the children and to modify the hospital environment (e.g., dimmed lights, reduced noise, television off) to reduce interferences with sleep. Mild sedatives may also be useful for hospitalized children experiencing sleep problems (Besana, Fiocchi, de Bartolomeis, Magno, & Donati, 1984).

Not only do hospitalized children have difficulties with sleep, but so may children with chronic illnesses or acute medical disturbances (Dinges et al., 1990; Mindell, Spirito, & Carskadon, 1990; Miser, McCalla, Dothage, Wesley, & Miser, 1987). For example, children with severe burns often experience nightmares (Noyes, Andreasen, & Hartford, 1971;

Tarnowski, Rasnake, & Drabman, 1987). One study (Roberts & Gordon, 1979) successfully treated a 5-year-old child who was having nightmares secondary to burns over 30 percent of her body. Treatment, consisting of response prevention and systematic desensitization, eliminated her nightmares within a two-week period. Unfortunately, few studies have targeted sleep problems related to other medical conditions, and much more research in this area is necessary.

In general, few studies have explored treatments for adjustment sleep disorders, other than those related to hospitalization, because these problems usually resolve naturally over time. If patients do seek treatment, primarily for longer-term sleep problems, psychological therapies typically focus on the disrupting events. With resolution of the precipitating event, the sleep problems typically dissipate, with sleep returning to normal.

Nighttime Fears. Bedtime problems can also relate to children's nighttime fears. These nighttime fears are the most common fears experienced by children and they are a normal, developmental occurrence in youngsters. They learn many of these fears through simple conditioning (Hewitt, 1981). For example, the bedroom may be a source of anxiety for some children, especially if the bedroom is the place where the child must go when punished. Also, in the middle of the night, when children have nightmares or awaken, distressed parents typically come into their children's room, turning on the lights. Thus, some children may associate light with comfort and associate darkness with distress or nightmares.

A variety of therapeutic techniques have been successful in treating nighttime fears. Connell, Persley, and Sturgess (1987) discussed the effective use of psychotherapy with six children (ages 10 to 12 years) who had phobic reactions to sleep after the death of a relative or friend. King, Cranstoun, and Josephs (1989) successfully utilized emotive imagery, a variant of systematic desensitization, with three children who had excessive fears at bedtime. Two large controlled studies have also been conducted in this area. Graziano and Mooney (1980) successfully treated bedtime fears with the use of relaxation training, self-instructions, guided imagery, and token reinforcement in a group of seventeen 6- to 12-year-olds. In

comparison with a waiting-list control group, the treated children had significantly fewer bedtime problems at posttreatment. Furthermore, at 2 1/2- to 3-year follow-up, 92 percent of the children demonstrated maintenance of improvement without additional treatment (Graziano & Mooney, 1982). This study, replicated by McMenamy and Katz (1989) with five 4- to 5-year-olds, also revealed that the use of relaxation training, self-instruction, imagery, and coping skills training was effective in reducing nighttime fears and inappropriate bedtime behavior.

In contrast, a recent study by Friedman and Ollendick (1989) involved a multiple-baseline design across subjects to examine the efficacy of a multicomponent treatment package for reducing nighttime fears in six children. Their results were positive in that disruptive bedtime behavior decreased in five of the six children. However, detailed analysis of the data showed that for those children with extended baseline, improvement preceded treatment. The authors argued that improvements may not have been a direct result of treatment but rather may have resulted from such variables as parent and child reactivity to home monitoring or maturation. Additionally, Ollendick, Hagopian, and Huntzinger (1991) found that reinforcement for engaging in appropriate nighttime behavior and self-control procedures were successful in reducing nighttime fears in two children. In their study, they found that the most important component of treatment was contingent reinforcement.

In summary, fear of the dark, which is common in young children, is often a result of associative learning. Although most children will outgrow their fears, in severe cases, cognitive-behavioral treatments can be effective.

Limit-Setting Sleep Disorder. The second environmentally related disorder, limit-setting sleep disorder, involves difficulty initiating sleep, typically characterized by stalling or refusing to go to bed (Diagnostic Classification Steering Committee, 1990; Ferber, 1987, 1989). Limit-setting sleep disorder incorporates a problem often called childhood insomnia. From 5 to 10 percent of the childhood population experience this sleep disorder, which is often as much a problem for caregivers as it is for children. For example, parents of children who have bedtime difficulties often experience increased depressive symptomatology, decreased marital satisfaction, and increased anxiety (Durand & Mindell, 1990). This disorder usually abates once caregivers set limits, and it is highly amenable to behavioral treatments, such as graduated extinction (Mindell, 1990; Mindell & Durand, 1993; Rickert & Johnson, 1988; Rolider & Van Houten, 1984) and the establishment of bedtime routines (Weissbluth, 1982).

Several case studies have focused on limit-setting sleep disorder. One early report by Williams (1959) described a single case study of a 4-year-old child who had temper tantrums at bedtime. His behavior rapidly extinguished after his parents stopped responding to his tantrums. Wright, Woodcock, and Scott (1970) successfully used a positive bedtime routine and extinction approach for a 3-year-old child who tantrummed at bedtime. Another case study of a 13-year-old boy demonstrated the efficacy of relaxation training and reduction of parental attention (Anderson, 1979). And, last, Weil and Goldfried (1973) demonstrated the effectiveness of self-relaxation for bedtime insomnia in an 11-year-old girl.

Researchers have also used larger-scale studies to evaluate the treatment of bedtime problems. Richman, Douglas, Hunt, Lansdown, and Levere (1985) found improvement in 77 percent of children, between the ages of 1 and 5 years, that they treated with behavioral methods. These researchers individualized their treatment for each child but typically included use of positive reinforcement for desired behaviors, elimination of parental attention to the child when awake following bedtime, shaping of an earlier bedtime, and a bedtime routine. There are some methodological concerns about this study, including lack of a control group and reliance on parental report and therapist ratings as outcome measures.

A study of six children between the ages of 24 months and 54 months had mixed results (three children improved, one child remained the same, and two children became worse) following a behavioral treatment that included establishment of a bedtime and bedtime routine, extinction of crying at bedtime, and mild punishment for being out of bed (Rapoff, Christophersen, & Rapoff, 1982). Adams and Rickert (1989), in a study of 36 toddlers and preschoolers, found both positive bedtime routines and graduated extinction to be equally effective in reducing bedtime

tantrum activity. Both treatments were significantly more effective than a control condition.

Additionally, a few studies have evaluated the efficacy of pharmacological treatments. Russo, Gururaj, and Allen (1976) treated fifty 2- to 12-year-olds with diphenhydramine. The medication was significantly better than placebo in improving the children's sleep. However, other studies have found drug treatments to be of limited value (e.g., Kales, Allen, Scharf, & Kales, 1970; Richman, 1985). And, as stated by Jackson and Rawlins (1977), "the problem of the sleepless toddler is not going to be solved by a three-minute consultation and a bottle of medicine."

Sleep-Onset Association Disorder. Sleep-onset association disorder, which is primarily a disorder found only in childhood, occurs when sleep onset becomes impaired due to the absence of a certain set of objects or circumstances, be it the presence of a bottle or pacifier or getting rocked to sleep (Diagnostic Classification Steering Committee, 1990; Ferber, 1987; Richman, 1981). When these objects or circumstances are present, sleep is normal. However, when these objects or circumstances are not present, sleep becomes disturbed and can result in sleep-onset difficulties and/or frequent night wakings.

To understand this disorder, it is important to realize that waking during the night is normal, and most children, called "self-soothers," are able to return to sleep easily. However, some children, known as "signallers," are unable to return to sleep until the conditions for sleep are reestablished. In children ages 6 months to 3 years, this disorder occurs in approximately 15 to 20 percent of the population. After age 3, the prevalence decreases, but some children continue to experienced it. Behavioral interventions have been successful in treating sleep-onset association disorder (Rickert & Johnson, 1988; Schaefer, 1990).

Studies have demonstrated that by implementing a behavioral program at bedtime, involving a positive bedtime routine and graduated extinction, generalization occurs to reduce frequent night wakings (Durand & Mindell, 1990; Mindell, 1990; Mindell & Durand, 1993). Other studies have found support for parent interventions (e.g., Jones & Verduyn, 1983; Milan, Mitchell, Berger, & Pierson, 1981; Richman et al., 1985; Seymour, Brock, During, & Poole, 1989).

However, one recent study did find that night waking problems in infancy are persistent and resistant to change (Scott & Richards, 1990). In this study, the investigators found no difference in the night waking behavior of 90 infants following written advice with therapist support or written advice only versus no intervention. The written advice included general background knowledge about sleep in infants, emphasized modifying parental expectations about sleep, and provided a listing of advantages and disadvantages of various behavior modification strategies to night waking problems.

Nocturnal Eating (Drinking) Syndrome. Another environmentally related sleep disorder is nocturnal eating (drinking) syndrome. This condition, which is similar to sleep-onset association disorder, "is characterized by recurrent awakenings, with the inability to return to sleep without eating or drinking" (Diagnostic Classification Steering Committee, 1990). This disorder is common in infancy and early childhood, when children require nursing or drinking a bottle to fall asleep. Bed-wetting may also be excessive and can cause increased night wakings. Treatment strategies for this disorder involve gradual removal of the eating or drinking behavior. For example, in one study (Mindell & Durand 1993), children received fewer and fewer ounces of milk per night at bedtime until they no longer drank any milk at the time of sleep onset. With removal of the drinking behavior, frequent night wakings ceased. This disorder occurs less often in children over the age of 3 than the other dyssomnias.

Delayed Sleep Phase Disorder. A common event that occurs especially with adolescents is staying up late at night. Some adolescents completely shift their sleep-wake schedule. The end result is that they may have symptoms of sleep-onset insomnia and extreme difficulty awakening at a desired time in the morning, otherwise known as delayed sleep phase disorder (Diagnostic Classification Steering Committee, 1990). Many adolescents do not go to sleep until the early morning hours and are unable to awaken on weekdays for school. On weekends, the adolescents have no problems sleeping but sleep on a delayed phase, often going to sleep at 2:00 A.M. and awakening anywhere

from 12:00 to 2:00 P.M. These individuals have little success trying to advance their timing of sleep onset to an appropriate schedule. Approximately 7 percent of adolescents experience delayed sleep phase syndrome (Thorpy, Korman, Spielman, & Glovinsky, 1988). The end result for many children and adolescents with this sleep disorder is difficulties in school, primarily because of chronic absenteeism and tardiness (Carskadon, Anders, & Hole, 1988).

The primary mode of treatment for this disorder is chronotherapy (Czeisler et al., 1981). The first step in this program is stabilizing sleep at the phase-delayed times, for example 3:00 A.M. to noon. For the next week to 10 days, patients receive instructions to delay the sleeping period by three hours every day until the desired sleeping times occur. For example, on night 1, sleep is to occur from 6:00 A.M. to 3:00 P.M., and on night 2, from 9:00 A.M. until 6:00 P.M. Patients must strictly follow the imposed scheduling of sleep for treatment to be effective. Once sleep is occurring at the appropriate times, patients must rigidly adhere to the new schedule, given that it is easy for these individuals to return to a delayed sleep phase pattern. Some adolescents will be resistant to treatment. In those cases, therapists will need to address psychological issues.

Parasomnias

Although many children do experience one of the preceding dyssomnias, the predominant sleep disorders found in children are parasomnias. These include confusional arousals, sleep terrors, sleepwalking, nightmares, sleep bruxism, rhythmic movement disorder, and sleep enuresis.

Confusional Arousals and Sleep Terrors. Confusional arousals occur almost universally in children before the age of 5 years (Ferber, 1985) and are much less common in older children. Confusional arousals, characterized by confusions following arousals from sleep mainly occurring in the first part of the night, are probably partial manifestations of sleep terror episodes and sleepwalking (Diagnostic Classification Steering Committee, 1990). Children with this disorder often become disoriented, have slowed speech, and are often slow to respond to commands or questions. This confusional behavior may last from several minutes to hours. There is relatively little research regarding treatment of this sleep disorder.

Sleep terrors occur in about 3 to 6 percent of all children and are more intense than confusional arousals (Broughton, 1968; DiMario & Emery, 1987; Soldatos & Lugaresi, 1987). Sleep terrors, also known as night terrors or pavor nocturnus, begin suddenly with a piercing scream or cry, and children experiencing night terrors appear intensely fearful during these events (Diagnostic Classification Steering Committee, 1990). Sleep terrors usually occur within 90 to 120 minutes of sleep onset and typically during the first period of slow wave sleep. When experiencing night terrors, children usually become extremely agitated, are often unresponsive to attempts at soothing, and may even become more agitated if held. If awakened, they may feel confused and disoriented.

Although sleep terrors and confusional arousals appear to be anxiety based, there is no evidence to confirm this and a fair amount to refute it. Parents often worry that their children are manifesting their daytime concerns or worries at night in the form of sleep terrors. This is not true. Sleep terrors are a developmental phenomenon, most common in children ages 4 to 12, and tend to resolve by adolescence (Kales, Kales, Soldatos, Caldwell, Charney, & Martin, 1980). In addition, sleep terrors have a genetic component in that there is usually a family history of such problems (Kales, Soldatos, & Kales, 1980), and are actually a disorder of impaired arousal (Broughton, 1968). One study that conducted a factor analysis on a multitude of sleep problems found that those items associated with night terrors did not in any way relate to items associated with anxiety (Fisher & McGuire, 1990). Unfortunately, many individuals unwittingly assume that night terrors are a form of child anxiety; this perpetuates the myth (e.g., Auchter, 1990; Taboada, 1975).

As with many sleep disorders, relatively little is known about treating these problems. The primary modes of treatment are reassurance to the family and an emphasis on safety (Clore & Hibel, 1993). Parents must erect gates across stairs and lock and bolt all windows and doors so that the child or adolescent is unable to leave the house. Two case studies successfully utilizing behavioral methods have appeared in the literature (Kellerman, 1979, 1980). Hypnosis also

has been useful as a treatment for night terrors (Koe, 1989; Kramer, 1989). Sometimes, pharmacological treatments have been successful. Studies have found diazepam (Valium) is effective (Fisher, Kahn, Edwards, & Davis, 1973; Glick, Schulman, & Turecki, 1971); however, relapse may occur after discontinuing use of the drug.

Other studies have reported successful treatment with a short-acting benzodiazepine, midazolam (Popoviciu & Corfariu, 1983), with alprazolam, a triazolobenzodiazepine (Cameron & Thayer, 1985), and even low doses of a tricyclic antidepressant (Reite et al., 1990). The use of medications to treat sleep terrors is controversial, with some individuals (e.g., Weissbluth, 1984) arguing strongly against their use. Some authors have implemented other treatments as well. Agrell and Axelsson (1972) significantly reduced sleep terrors following adenoidectomy in a group of 23 children. Unfortunately, researchers have conducted no further studies to replicate the benefits of adenoidectomy for children with sleep terrors.

Recently, studies have begun to look at the treatment of sleep terrors and confusional arousals with scheduled awakenings (Lask, 1988). Scheduled awakenings involve behavioral alteration of a child's sleep patterns. For example, in one case, seen at Allegheny University of the Health Sciences sleep center, a 7-year-old boy experienced, on average, three to four sleep terrors per week for approximately four years. Following a two-week regimen of scheduled awakenings, no future sleep terrors occurred. It is unclear what exactly is the mechanism of change. It may be that scheduled awakenings give an individual practice in changing sleep stages, as parasomnias occur during sleep stage transitions. Or it may be that scheduled awakenings simply interrupt sleep at the time of the night at which a parasomnia is likely to occur. However, no matter what the mechanism of change is, scheduled awakenings appear to be effective. This intervention is undergoing further study regarding its efficacy.

Sleepwalking. Another parasomnia common in children is sleepwalking, which often occurs in conjunction with sleep terrors and confusional arousals. Approximately 1 to 6 percent of children experience chronic sleepwalking, with as many as 15 percent of all children having at least one such episode (Anders,

1982; Broughton, 1968; Diagnostic Classification Steering Committee, 1990; Soldatos & Lugaresi, 1987). Sleepwalking is most prevalent in children between the ages of 4 and 8 years and usually spontaneously disappears after adolescence. The behavior may range from simply sitting up in bed to walking. These children are often difficult to awaken, and, upon awakening, they often appear confused. The frequency of the behavior can vary from infrequently to several times a week.

Sleepwalking can become exacerbated or induced by fever, sleep deprivation, and some medications, including lithium, prolixin, and desipramine (Klackenberg, 1982b). Other precipitating conditions are a distended bladder or external stimuli, such as noise. Little research has studied treatments for sleepwalking in children. Typically, parents receive instruction to safety-proof the house, as with sleep terrors and confusional arousals. Otherwise, parents receive reassurance about their child's sleepwalking and are informed that sleepwalking is usually a benign, self-limited maturational occurrence (Berlin & Qayyum, 1986).

The only study conducted in this area involved a 7-year-old boy referred for somnambulism accompanied by nightmares, crying, and talking in his sleep (Clement, 1970). Initial treatment with insight-oriented therapy proved to be ineffective. A behaviorally oriented conditioning procedure, instituted subsequent to the insight therapy, involved waking the child upon sleepwalking. The behavioral treatment led to a significant reduction in sleepwalking frequency. Unfortunately, this case study only presents preliminary data on the effectiveness of an awakening procedure for sleepwalking, and controlled experimental studies are necessary.

Nightmares. Nightmares occur in 10 to 50 percent of children between the ages of 3 and 6 years (Diagnostic Classification Steering Committee, 1990). Following a gradual onset, nightmares typically decrease in frequency over time. A small percentage of children will continue to have nightmares throughout adolescence and even possibly into adulthood (Diagnostic Classification Steering Committee, 1990). Nightmares occur during periods of rapid eye movement (REM) sleep; this is in contrast to sleep terrors, which happen during slow-wave sleep earlier in the night. They typically occur in the middle of the night or early morning hours, when REM is most likely to occur (Leung & Robson, 1993). Table 23.1 delineates unique characteristics of nightmares versus sleep terrors. Nightmares usually involve a specific danger, such as fears of attack, falling, or death (Kales, Soldatos, & Caldwell, 1980; Leung & Robson, 1993).

Stressful periods and traumatic events will exacerbate nightmares. Studies have found that distressing or frightening events, such as an automobile accident or death of a relative, occur in association with nightmares (Erman, 1987). Surprisingly, however, one study found that parents' most common causal attribution for nightmares was "overtiredness," with "stress" not highly rated as a factor (Fisher & Wilson,

Table 23.1 Characteristic Features of Sleep Terrors/Confusional Arousals and Nightmares

	SLEEP TERRORS/ CONFUSIONAL AROUSALS	NIGHTMARES
Time of night	First 1/3 of night	Mid to last 1/3
Behavior	Variable	Very little motor behavior
Level of consciousness	Unarousable or very confused if awakened	Fully awake
Memory of event	Amnesia	Vivid recall
Family history	Yes	No
Potential for injury	High	Low
Frequency	Common	Very common
Stage of sleep	Deep NREM	REM

1987). Some medications, including some beta blockers and antidepressants, may increase the likelihood of nightmares. Other medications—including alcohol, barbiturates, and benzodiazepines—produce nightmares as withdrawal symptoms. All in all, though, little is known about the causes of nightmares in children.

Infrequent nightmares typically only require reassurance. Frequent nightmares, however, are more likely to require some type of treatment. Treatment strategies for nightmares have focused on anxiety reduction techniques, such as relaxation and imagery, often combined with other behavioral strategies, such as systematic desensitization (Cavior & Deutsch, 1975) or response prevention (Roberts & Gordon, 1979). Kellerman (1980) successfully treated a 13-year-old girl for nightmares using reinforcement and anxiety management techniques. Others have used cognitive-behavioral treatments, including dream reorganization (Palace & Johnston, 1989), which involves both systematic desensitization with coping self-statements and guided rehearsal of mastery endings to dream content. A few case reports have also noted successful treatment of nightmares with hypnosis (Kingsbury, 1993) and eye-movement desensitization (Pellicer, 1993). However, as mentioned earlier, for most families, reassurance that nightmares are part of normal child development is beneficial and all the treatment that is necessary, especially to decrease the likelihood that parents will treat affected children as though they have psychological problems.

Sleep Bruxism.   Sleep bruxism, which involves grinding or clenching the teeth during sleep, occurs in over 50 percent of normal infants, with the average age of onset at 10 months (Diagnostic Classification Steering Committee, 1990; Kravitz & Boehm, 1971). Adult-related bruxism usually begins between the ages of 10 and 20 years. Bruxism may cause dental problems, such as abnormal wear of the teeth or periodontal tissue damage, and may also relate to headaches or jaw pain. To date, research on bruxism is primarily with adult populations. Studies have found bruxism amenable to EMG-activated biofeedback, as shown in naturalistic studies (e.g., Kardachi & Clarke, 1977), laboratory studies (e.g., Piccione, Coates, George, Rosenthal, & Karzmark, 1982; Wagner, 1981), and comparative studies of feedback alarms with other treatment approaches (e.g., Casas, Beemsterboer, & Clark, 1982; Kardachi, Bailey, & Ash, 1978).

Habit reversal has also been successful (Peterson & Schneider, 1991), as have stress management approaches (Casas et al., 1982). There are two thorough reviews of treatment for bruxism in adults, one focusing on biofeedback (Cassisi, McGlynn, & Belles, 1987) and the other on dental approaches (McGlynn, Cassisi, & Diamond, 1985). Unfortunately, few studies, if any, have researched the efficacy of treatment programs for bruxism in children.

Rhythmic Movement Disorder. Many children fall asleep while rocking their bodies, rolling back and forth, or banging their heads. Rhythmic movement disorder is a condition characterized by stereotyped movements that occur at sleep onset or when awakening from sleep (Diagnostic Classification Steering Committee, 1990). Body rocking, head rolling, or head banging are very common in infants, with 60 percent of 9-month-olds doing one of these behaviors. Until 2 years of age, 22 percent of children continue to engage in one of these behaviors. These behaviors continue to be present in 5 percent of children over age 2 and adolescents. Injuries are uncommon, and typically treatment is not necessary because this behavior is usually benign and self-limiting; thus, it usually dissipates on its own. These behaviors, again, are not a sign of anxiety or emotional disturbance; rather, they have a neurophysiological basis (Horne, 1992). The only major concern about this sleep disorder is that it can be disruptive to family members and can have psychosocial consequences in older children and adolescents.

Sleep Enuresis. The final parasomnia, and the most common, is sleep enuresis, or bed-wetting. A diagnosis of enuresis is appropriate when persistent bed-wetting occurs after age 5 (Diagnostic Classification Steering Committee, 1990; Schmitt, 1982). Estimates show that bed-wetting occurs in 30 percent of 4-year-olds, 10 percent of 6-year-olds, 5 percent of 10-year-olds, and 3 percent of 12-year-olds. The spontaneous rate of cure after age 6 is about 15 percent per year (DeJonge, 1973). Primary enuresis—that is, those who have had a continuous enuretic condition—comprises 70 to 90 percent of all cases of the disorder. Secondary enuresis, in which the child has had at least three to six months of dryness, comprises the remaining 10 to 30 percent of all cases. Males are more likely to experience this problem (up to age 10, about 50 percent likelier) than females.

Many studies have researched various aspects of enuresis, including diagnosis (see Butler, 1991, for an excellent review of the establishment of a working definition for nocturnal enuresis), assessment, and treatment. Enuresis is undoubtably the most well-studied sleep disorder of children. Several behavioral treatments have had proven high success rates (Azrin, Sneed, & Foxx, 1974; Doleys, 1977; Feldman, 1983; Weir, 1982). The most popular and effective technique is the bell-and-pad system, which sounds a bell when bedwetting occurs. Mowrer and Mowrer developed this method in 1938. Reported success rates for this technique have been as high as 75 percent (Forsythe & Redmond, 1974; Fraser, 1972), with the best results in children over 7 years of age (McClain, 1979). Other conditioning approaches have also been useful (e.g., Whelan & Houts, 1990).

Other treatment approaches for enuresis include bladder training (McClain, 1979; Troup & Hodgson, 1971), response prevention and contingency management (Luciano, Molina, Gomez, & Herruzo, 1993), hypnosis (Olness, 1975), and dietary control, such as a reduction in caffeine intake (Bond, Ware, & Hoelscher, 1990). Comprehensive treatment programs also exist for the treatment of enuresis. Scharf and Jennings (1988) instituted such a program incorporating five methods: bladder-stretching exercises, stream interruption, counseling for motivation and responsibility, visual sequencing, and conditioning therapy. Some 91 percent of children entering their multi-method treatment program showed significant improvements. Azrin and Thienes (1978) also developed a successful multimethod behavior modification program involving four basic procedures: a nightly waking schedule, positive practice, an alarm activated by wetness, and cleanliness training. This study, as well as others (e.g., Bollard & Nettelbeck, 1982), have included a nightly waking schedule as a component of their multimethod treatment program, and some investigators believe it is crucial for successful treatment.

Van Londen, Van Londen-Barentsen, Van Son, and Mulder (1993) found at a 2½ year follow-up of

their intervention that 92 percent of children whose treatment included arousal treatment remained continent; this compared to 77 percent of children who received the urine device with specific instructions and 72 percent of children who obtained the urine alarm alone. However, Whelan and Houts (1990) demonstrated that adding a waking schedule to full-spectrum home training (FSHT) did not produce increased benefits over FSHT alone.

In some cases of enuresis, tricyclic antidepressants may be helpful (Kales, Soldatos, & Kales, 1980). Studies show that imipramine can be successful in controlling enuresis in up to 70 percent of cases when taken regularly (Ambrosini, Bianchi, Rabinovich, & Elia, 1993; Bindeglas & Dee, 1978). However, upon withdrawal from the medication, few children stay dry. Because of imipramine's potential cardiotoxic effects and the high relapse rate following withdrawal, some authors have argued that is best not to use it for long periods of time (Scharf & Jennings, 1988).

Another drug that has been successful is desmopressin (DDAVP), an analogue of the antidiuretic hormone vasopressin (e.g., Miller, Goldberg, & Atkin, 1989; Warady, Alon, & Hellerstein, 1991). Desmopressin has success rates similar to imipramine, but like imipramine, it also almost always leads to relapse following discontinuation of the medication. Approximately 70 percent of cases, though, have persistent resolution of bed-wetting when maintained on desmopressin, with minimal side effects. Given that desmopressin is much more expensive and has higher relapse rates than other treatments, it may be the treatment of choice when used on a short-term, or as needed, basis (e.g., overnight camp, staying at a friend's house). Overall, results from the preceding studies indicate that enuresis is highly amenable to treatment.

DIFFERENTIAL DIAGNOSIS

Given the breadth and scope of the different sleep disorders just outlined, differential diagnosis is important. Often, the presenting complaints for many of the above sleep disorders are similar (e.g., "insomnia," excessive daytime sleepiness, or unusual behaviors during the night). It is important to conduct a thorough evaluation to fully assess which specific sleep disorder the child is experiencing. Thus, differential diagnosis in the area of sleep disorders is essential.

Differentiation between a sleep disorder and other medical or psychological problems is also important. A child with what looks like night terrors may actually be having seizures during sleep. In other cases, difficulties at bedtime may be symptomatic of a more general problem with noncompliance. Nighttime fears may be just one aspect of a child with extensive fears. In addition, it is important to assess for delayed sleep phase syndrome before making a diagnosis of school refusal. Given the similar characteristics of these two disorders, it appears likely that sleep phase disorder may sometimes present as school refusal, especially among adolescents who constitute the majority of individuals with delayed sleep phase syndrome.

Furthermore, it is important to keep in mind that some children may have more than one sleep disorder. For example, an adolescent may have narcolepsy and sleep apnea. Once a clinician has identified one sleep disorder, it is important for the clinician to continue to conduct a thorough evaluation for all other sleep disorders. If not, the clinician may miss vital information, and sleep problems may continue.

SUMMARY

Sleep disorders are a common problem experienced by children and adolescents. Many people believe that the primary contributing factors to sleep disturbances are psychological problems; however, in most cases, sleep problems are not the result of underlying psychopathology but have physiological, environmental, or behavioral bases. In addition, many sleep problems are highly amenable to treatment, but unfortunately they usually get underdiagnosed and undertreated.

In sum, given the prevalence of these problems in the child and adolescent population, it is important for all therapists to become knowledgeable about sleep and sleep disorders. This information is essential whether or not the therapist is going to treat the client directly or is going to refer for specialized services. People spend about one-third of their lives sleeping, or trying to sleep; thus, it is important to understand as much as we can about it.

REFERENCES

Abe, K., Ohta, M., Amatomi, M., & Oda, N. (1982). Persistence and predictive value of behaviors of 3-year-olds: A follow-up study at 8 years. *Acta Paedopsychiarica, 48,* 185–191.

Adams, L. A., & Rickert, V. I. (1989). Reducing bedtime tantrums: Comparison between positive routines and graduated extinction. *Pediatrics, 84,* 756–761.

Agrell, I. G., & Axelsson, A. (1972). The relationship between pavor nocturnus and adenoids. *Acta Paedopsychiatrica, 39,* 46–53.

Ambrosini, P. J., Bianchi, M. D., Rabinovich, H., & Elia, J. (1993). Antidepressant treatments in children and adolescents: II. Anxiety, physical and behavioral disorders. *Journal of the Academy of Child and Adolescent Psychiatry, 32,* 483–493.

American Psychiatric Association. (1994). *Diagnostic and statistical manual of mental disorders* (4th ed., rev.). Washington, DC: Author.

Anders, T. F. (1982). Neurophysiological studies of sleep in infants and children. *Journal of Child Psychology and Psychiatry and Allied Disciplines, 23,* 75–83.

Anders, T. F., & Weinstein, P. (1972). Sleep and its disorders in infants and children: A review. *Journal of Pediatrics, 22,* 137–150.

Anderson, D. R. (1979). Treatment of insomnia in a 13-year-old boy by relaxation training and reduction of parental attention. *Journal of Behavior Therapy and Experimental Psychiatry, 10,* 263–265.

Auchter, U. (1990). Anxiety in children: An investigation on various forms of anxiety. *Acta Paedopsychiatrica, 53,* 78–88.

Azrin, N. H., Sneed, T. J., & Foxx, R. M. (1974). Dry-bed training: Rapid elimination of childhood enuresis. *Behavior Research and Therapy, 12,* 147–156.

Azrin, N. H., & Thienes, P. M. (1978). Rapid elimination of enuresis by intensive learning without a condition apparatus. *Behavior Therapy, 9,* 342–354.

Beardslee, C. (1976). The sleep wakefulness pattern of young hospitalized children during nap time. *Maternal-Child Nursing Journal, 5,* 15–24.

Berlin, R. M., & Qayyum, U. (1986). Sleepwalking: Diagnosis and treatment through the life cycle. P*sychosomatics, 27,* 755–781.

Besana, R., Fiocchi, A., de Bartolomeis, L., Magno, F., & Donati, C. (1984). Comparison of niaprazine and placebo in pediatric behavior and sleep disorders: Double-blind clinical trial. *Current Therapeutic Research, 36,* 58–66.

Bindeglas, P. M., & Dee, G. (1978). Enuresis treatment with imipramine hydrochloride: A 10-year follow-up study. *American Journal of Psychiatry, 135,* 1549–1552.

Bixler, E. O., Kales, J. D., Scharf, M. B., Kales, A., & Leo, L. A. (1976). Incidence of sleep disorders in medical practice: A physician survey. *Sleep Research, 5,* 62.

Bollard, R. J., & Nettelbeck, T. (1982). A component analysis of dry-bed training for treatment for bedwetting. *Behavior Research and Therapy, 20,* 383–390.

Bond, T., Ware, J. C., & Hoelscher, T. J. (1990). Caffeine and enuresis: A case report. *Sleep Research, 19,* 195.

Broughton, R. J. (1968). Sleep disorders: Disorders of arousal? *Science, 159,* 1070–1078.

Brouillette, R. T., Fernback, S. K., & Hunt, C. E. (1982). Obstructive sleep apnea in infants and children. *Journal of Pediatrics, 100,* 31–40.

Butler, R. J. (1991). Establishment of working definitions in nocturnal enuresis. *Archives of Disease in Childhood, 66,* 267–271.

Cameron, O. G., & Thayer, B. A. (1985). Treatment of pavor nocturnus with alprazolam. *Journal of Clinical Psychiatry, 46,* 504.

Carskadon, M. A., Anders, T. F., & Hole, W. (1988). Sleep disturbances in childhood and adolescence. In H. E. Fitzgerald, B. M. Lester, and M. W. Yogman (Eds.), *Theory and research in behavioral pediatrics* (Vol. 4). New York: Plenum.

Casas, J. M., Beemsterboer, P., & Clark, G. T. (1982). A comparison of stress-reduction behavioral counseling and contingent EMG biofeedback with an arousal task. *Behaviour Research and Therapy, 20,* 9–15.

Cassisi, J. E., McGlynn, F. D., & Belles, D. R. (1987). EMG-activated feedback alarms for the treatment of nocturnal bruxism: Current status and future directions. *Biofeedback and Self-Regulation, 12,* 13–30.

Cavior, N., & Deutsch, A. (1975). Systematic desensitization to reduce dream induced anxiety. *Journal of Nervous and Mental Disease, 161,* 433–435.

Clement, P. W. (1970). Elimination of sleepwalking in a seven-year-old boy. *Journal of Consulting and Clinical Psychology, 34,* 22–26.

Clore, E. R., & Hibel, J. (1993). The parasomnias of childhood. *Journal of Pediatric Health Care, 7,* 12–16.

Connell, H. M., Persley, G. V., & Sturgess, J. L. (1987). Sleep phobia in middle childhood—A review of six cases. *Journal of the American Academy of Child and Adolescent Psychiatry, 26,* 449–452.

Croft, C. B., Brockbank, M. J., Wright, A., & Swanston, A. R. (1990). Obstructive sleep apnoea in children undergoing routine tonsillectomy and adenoidectomy. *Clinical Otolaryngology, 15,* 307–314.

Czeisler, C. A., Richardson, G. S., Coleman, R. M., Zimmerman, J. C., Moore-Ede, M. C., Dement, W. C., & Weitzman, E. D. (1981). Chronotherapy: Resetting the circadian clocks of patients with the delayed sleep phase syndrome. *Sleep, 4,* 1–21.

DeJonge, G. A. (1973). Epidemiology of enuresis: A survey of the literature: Bladder control and enuresis. *Clinical and Developmental Medicine, 48/49,* 39–46.

Diagnostic Classification Steering Committee. (1990). *The international classification of sleep disorders: Diagnostic and coding manual.* Rochester, MN: American Sleep Disorder Association.

DiMario, F. J., & Emery, E. S. (1987). The natural history of night terrors. *Clinical Pediatrics, 26,* 505–511.

Dinges, D. F., Shapiro, B. S., Reilly, L. B., Orne, E. C., Ohene-Frempong, L., & Orne, M. T. (1990). Sleep/wake dysfunction in children with sickle-cell crisis pain. *Sleep Research, 19,* 323.

Doleys, D. M. (1977). Dry-bed training and retention control training: A comparison. *Behavior Therapy, 8,* 541–548.

Dollinger, S. L. (1982). On the varieties of childhood sleep disturbance. *Journal of Clinical Child Psychology, 11,* 107–115.

Durand, V. M., & Mindell, J. A. (1990). Behavioral treatment of multiple childhood sleep disorders: Effects on child and family. *Behavior Modification, 14,* 37–49.

Erman, M. K. (1987). Dream anxiety attacks (nightmares). *Psychiatric Clinics of North America, 10,* 667–674.

Feldman, W. (1983). Nocturnal enuresis. *Canadian Medical Association Journal, 128,* 114–116.

Ferber, R. (1985). Sleep disorders in infants and children. In T. L. Riley (Eds.), *Clinical aspects of sleep and sleep disturbance.* Boston: Butterworth.

Ferber, R. (1987). The sleepless child. In C. Guilleminault (Ed.), *Sleep and its disorders in children.* New York: Raven Press.

Ferber, R. (1989). Sleeplessness in the child. In M. H. Kryger, T. Roth, & W. Dement (Eds.), *Principles and practice of sleep medicine.* Philadelphia: W. B. Saunders.

Fisher, B., & McGuire, K. (1990). Do diagnostic patterns exist in the sleep behaviors of normal children? *Journal of Abnormal Child Psychology, 18,* 179–186.

Fisher, B., & Wilson, A. (1987). Selected sleep disturbances in school children reported by parents: Prevalence, interrelationships, behavioral correlates, and parental attributions. *Perceptual and Motor Skills, 64,* 1147–1157.

Fisher, C., Kahn, E., Edwards, A., & Davis, D. M. (1973). A psychophysiological study of nightmares and night terrors: The suppression of stage 4 night terrors with diazepam. *Archives of General Psychiatry, 28,* 252–259.

Forsythe, W. I., & Redmond, A. (1974). Enuresis and spontaneous cure rate: Study of 1129 enuretics. *Archives of Disease in Childhood, 49,* 259–263.

Fraser, M. S. (1972). Nocturnal enuresis. *Practitioner, 208,* 203–211.

Friedman, A. G., & Ollendick, T. H. (1989). Treatment programs for severe night-time fears: A methodological note. *Journal of Behavior Research and Experimental Therapy, 20,* 171–178.

Glick, B. S., Schulman, D., & Turecki, S. (1971). Diazepam (Valium) treatment in childhood sleep disorders: A preliminary investigation. *Diseases of the Nervous System, 32,* 565–566.

Graziano, A., & Mooney, K. (1980). Family self-control instruction for children's nighttime fear reduction. *Jour-*

nal of Consulting and Clinical Psychology, 48, 206–213.

Graziano, A., & Mooney, K. (1982). Behavioral treatment of "nightfears" in children: Maintenance of improvement at 2½- to 3-year follow-up. *Journal of Consulting and Clinical Psychology, 50,* 598–599.

Guilleminault, C. (1986). Narcolepsy. *Sleep, 9,* 99–291.

Guilleminault, C. (1987). Narcolepsy and its differential diagnosis. In C. Guilleminault (Ed.), *Sleep and its disorders in children* (pp. 181–194). New York: Raven Press.

Guilleminault, C., & Anders, T. F. (1976). Sleep disorders in children. *Advances in Pediatrics, 22,* 151–174.

Guilleminault, C., & Dement, W. C. (1988). Sleep apnea syndromes and related sleep disorders. In R. L. Williams, I. Karacan, & C. A. Moore (Eds.), *Sleep disorders: Diagnosis and treatment* (pp. 47–72). New York: Wiley

Guilleminault, C., Korobkin, R., & Winkle, R. (1981). A review of 50 children with obstructive sleep apnea syndrome. *Lung, 159,* 275–287.

Guilleminault, C., Riley, R., Powell, N., Simmons, F. B., & Nino-Murcia, G. (1985). Obstructive sleep apnea syndrome in adolescents: Diagnosis and treatment [Abstract]. *Sleep Research, 14,* 159.

Hagemann, V. (1981). Night sleep of children in a hospital. Part I: Sleep duration. *Maternal-Child Nursing Journal, 10,* 113.

He, J., Kryger, M. H., Zorick, F. J., Conway, W., & Roth, T. (1988). Mortality and apnea index in obstructive sleep apnea: Experience in 385 male patients. *Chest, 94,* 9–14.

Hewitt, S. (1981). *The family and the handicapped child.* London: George Allan and Unwin.

Horne, J. (1992). Annotation: Sleep and its disorders in children. *Journal of Child Psychology and Psychiatry, 33,* 473–487.

Issa, F., & Sullivan, C. (1986). Reversal of central sleep apnea using nasal CPAP. *Chest, 90,* 165–171.

Jackson, H., & Rawlins, M. D. (1977). The sleepless child. *British Medical Journal, 2,* 509.

Jenkins, S., Bax, M., & Hart, H. (1980). Behavior problems in preschool children. *Journal of Child Psychology and Psychiatry, 21,* 5–17.

Jones, D. P. H., & Verduyn, C. M. (1983). Behavioral management of sleep problems. *Archives of Disease in Childhood, 58,* 442–444.

Kahn, A., Van de Merckt, C., Rebuffat, E., Mozin, M. J., Sottiaux, M., Blum, D., & Hennart, P. (1989). Sleep problems in healthy preadolescents. *Pediatrics, 84,* 542–546.

Kales, A., Allen, C., Scharf, M. B., & Kales, J. D. (1970). Hypnotic drugs and their effectiveness. *Archives of General Psychiatry, 23,* 226–232.

Kales, J. D., Kales, A., Soldatos, C. R., Caldwell, A. B., Charney, D. S., & Martin, E. D. (1980). Night terrors: Clinical characteristics and personality patterns. *Archives of General Psychiatry, 37,* 1406–1410.

Kales, J. D., Soldatos, C. R., & Caldwell, A. B. (1980). Nightmares: Clinical characteristics and personality patterns. *American Journal of Psychiatry, 137,* 1197–2001.

Kales, J. D., Soldatos, C. R., & Kales, A. (1980). Childhood sleep disorders. *Current Pediatric Therapy, 9,* 28–30.

Kardachi, B. J., Bailey, J. O., & Ash, M. M. (1978). A comparison of biofeedback and occlusal adjustment on bruxism. *Journal of Periodontology, 49,* 367–372.

Kardachi, B. J., & Clarke, N. G. (1977). The use of biofeedback to control bruxism. *Journal of Periodontology, 48,* 639–642.

Kataria, S., Swanson, M. S., & Trevathan, G. E. (1987). Persistence of sleep disturbances in preschool children. *Behavioral Pediatrics, 110,* 642–646.

Kavey, N. B. (1992). Psychosocial aspects of narcolepsy in children and adolescents. *Loss, Grief, and Care, 5,* 91–101.

Kellerman, J. (1979). Behavioral treatment of night terrors in a child with acute leukemia. *Journal of Nervous and Mental Disease, 167,* 182–185.

Kellerman, J. (1980). Rapid treatment of nocturnal anxiety in children. *Journal of Behavior Therapy and Experimental Psychiatry, 11,* 9–11.

King, N., Cranstoun, F., & Josephs, A. (1989). Emotive imagery and children's night-time fears: A multiple baseline design evaluation. *Journal of Behavior Therapy and Experimental Psychiatry, 20,* 125–135.

Kingsbury, S. J. (1993). Brief hypnotic treatment of repetitive nightmares. *American Journal of Clinical Hypnosis, 35,* 161–169.

Klackenberg, G. (1982a). Sleep behavior studied longitudinally: Data from 4-16 years on duration, night-awakening and bed sharing. *Acta Paediatrica Scandinavia, 71,* 501–506.

Klackenberg, G. (1982b). Somnambulism in childhood: Prevalence, course and behavioral correlations. *Acta Paediatrica Scandinavia, 71,* 495–499.

Koe, G. G. (1989). Hypnotic treatment of sleep terror disorder: A case report. *American Journal of Clinical Hypnosis, 32,* 36–40.

Kotagal, S., Hartse, K. M., & Walsh, J. K. (1990). Characteristics of narcolepsy in preteenaged children. *Pediatrics, 85,* 205–209.

Kramer, R. L. (1989). The treatment of childhood night terrors through the use of hypnosis—A case study: A brief communication. *The International Journal of Clinical Hypnosis, 4,* 283–284.

Kravitz, H., & Boehm, J. J. (1971). Rhythmic habit patterns in infancy: Their sequence, age of onset and frequency. *Child Development, 42,* 399–413.

Lask, B. (1988). Novel and non-toxic treatment for night terrors. British Medical Journal, 297, 592.

Leung, A. K., & Robson, W. L. (1993). Nightmares. *Jour-*

nal of the National Medical Association, 85, 233–235.

Lozoff, B., Wolf, A. W., & Davis, N. S. (1985). Sleep problems seen in pediatric practice. *Pediatrics, 75,* 477–483.

Luciano, M. C., Molina, F. J., Gomez, I., & Herruzo, J. (1993). Response prevention and contingency management in the treatment of nocturnal enuresis: A report of two cases. *Child and Family Behavior Therapy, 15,* 37–51.

Mallory, G. B., Fiser, D. H., & Jackson, R. (1989). Sleep-associated breathing disorders in morbidly obese children and adolescents. *Journal of Pediatrics, 115,* 892–897.

Mauer, K. W., Staats, B. A., & Olson, K. D. (1983). Upper airway obstruction and disordered nocturnal breathing in children. *Mayo Clinic Proceedings, 58,* 349–353.

McClain, L. G. (1979). Childhood enuresis. *Current Problems in Pediatrics, 9,* 1–36.

McGlynn, F. D., Cassisi, J. E., & Diamond, E. L. (1985). Diagnosis and treatment of bruxism: A behavioral dentistry perspective. In R. J. Daitzman (Ed.), *Diagnosis and intervention in behavior therapy and behavioral medicine* (Vol. 2, pp. 28–87). New York: Springer.

McMenamy, C., & Katz, R. C. (1989). Brief parent-assisted treatment for children's nighttime fears. *Developmental and Behavioral Pediatrics, 10,* 145–148.

Milan, M. A., Mitchell, Z. P., Berger, M. I., & Pierson, D. F. (1981). Positive routines: A rapid alternative to extinction for elimination of bedtime tantrum behavior. *Child Behavior Therapy, 3,* 13–25.

Miller, K., Goldberg, S., & Atkin, B. (1989). Nocturnal enuresis: Experience with long-term use of intranasally administered desmopressin. *Journal of Pediatrics, 114,* 723–726.

Mindell, J. A. (1990). Treatment of night wakings in early childhood through generalization effects. *Sleep Research, 19,* 121.

Mindell, J. A., & Durand, V. M. (1993). Treatment of childhood sleep disorders: Generalization across disorders and effects on family members. *Pediatric Psychology, 18,* 731–750.

Mindell, J. A., Moline, M. L., Zendell, S. M., Brown, L. B., & Fry, J. (in press). Pediatricians and sleep disorders: Training and practice. *Pediatrics.*

Mindell, J. A., Spirito, A., & Carskadon, M. A. (1990). Prevalence of sleep problems in chronically ill children. *Sleep Research, 19,* 337.

Miser, A. W., McCalla, J., Dothage, J. A., Wesley, M., & Miser, J. S. (1987). Pain as a presenting symptom in children and young adults with newly diagnosed malignancy. *Pain, 29,* 85–90.

Mitler, M. M., Nelson, S., & Hajdukovic, R. (1987). Narcolepsy: Diagnosis, treatment, and management. *Psychiatric Clinics of North America, 10,* 593–606.

Mowrer, O. H., & Mowrer, W. M. (1938). Enuresis—A method for its study and treatment. American *Journal of Orthopsychiatry, 8,* 436–459.

Noyes, R., Andreasen, N. O., & Hartford, C. (1971). The psychological reaction to severe burns. *Psychosomatics, 12,* 416–422.

Ollendick, T. H., Hagopian, L. P., & Huntzinger, R. M. (1991). Cognitive-behavior therapy with nighttime fearful children. *Journal of Behavior Therapy and Experimental Psychiatry, 22,* 113–121.

Olness, K. (1975). The use of self-hypnosis in the treatment of childhood nocturnal enuresis: A report on 40 patients. *Clinical Pediatrics, 14,* 273–279.

Palace, E. M., & Johnston, C. (1989). Treatment of recurrent nightmares by the dream reorganization approach. *Journal of Behavior Therapy and Experimental Psychiatry, 20,* 219–226.

Pellicer, X. (1993). Eye movement desensitization treatment of a child's nightmares: A case report. *Journal of Behavior Therapy and Experimental Psychiatry, 24,* 73–75.

Peterson, J. E., & Schneider, P. E. (1991). Oral habits: A behavioral approach. *Pediatric Clinics of North America, 38,* 1289–1305.

Piccione, A., Coates, T. J., George, J. M., Rosenthal, D., & Karzmark, P. (1982). Nocturnal biofeedback for nocturnal bruxism. *Biofeedback and Self-Regulation, 7,* 405–419.

Pietropinto, A. (1985). Children's reactions to illness and hospitalizations. *Medical Aspects of Human Sexuality, 19,* 129–136.

Popoviciu, L., & Corfariu, O. (1983). Efficacy and safety of midazolam in the treatment of night terrors in children. *British Journal of Clinical Pharmacology, 16,* 97–102.

Prugh, D., Staub, E., Sands, H., Kirschbaum, R., & Lenihan, E. (1953). A study of the emotional reactions of children and their families to hospitalization and illness. *American Journal of Orthopsychiatry, 23,* 70–106.

Rapoff, M. A., Christophersen, E. R., & Rapoff, K. E. (1982). The management of common childhood bedtime problems by pediatric nurse practitioners. *Journal of Pediatric Psychology, 7,* 179–196.

Reite, M. L., Nagel, K. E., & Ruddy, J. R. (1990). *Concise guide to evaluation and management of sleep disorders.* Washington, DC: American Psychiatric Press.

Richman, N. (1981). A community survey of characteristics of one to two year olds with sleep disruptions. *Journal of the American Academy of Child Psychiatry, 20,* 281–291.

Richman, N. (1985). A double-blind drug trial of treatment in young children with waking problems. *Journal of Child Psychology and Psychiatry, 4,* 591–598.

Richman, N., Douglas, J., Hunt, H., Lansdown, R., & Levere, R. (1985). Behavioral methods in the treatment of sleep disorders—A pilot study. *Journal of Child Psychology and Psychiatry, 26,* 581–590.

Richman, N., Stevenson, J. E., & Graham, P. J. (1975). Behavior problems in three-year-old children: An epidemiological study in a London borough. *Journal of Child Psychology and Psychiatry, 12,* 5–33.

Rickert, V. I., & Johnson, C. M. (1988). Reducing nocturnal awakening and crying episodes in infants and young children: A comparison between scheduled awakenings and systematic ignoring. *Pediatrics, 81,* 203–212.

Roberts, R. N., & Gordon, S. B. (1979). Reducing childhood nightmares subsequent to a burn trauma. *Child Behavior Therapy, 1,* 373–381.

Rolider, A., & Van Houten, R. (1984). Training parents to use extinction to eliminate nighttime crying by gradually increasing the criteria for ignoring crying. *Education and Treatment of Children, 7,* 119–124.

Roth, T., Roehrs, T., & Zorick, F. (1988). Pharmacological treatment of sleep disorders. In R. L. Williams, I. Karacan, & C. A. Moore (Eds.), *Sleep disorders: Diagnosis and treatment* (pp. 373–395). New York: Wiley

Russo, R., Gururaj, V., & Allen, J. (1976). The effectiveness of diphenhydramine HCL in pediatric sleep disorders. *Journal of Clinical Pharmacology, 16,* 284–288.

Salzarulo, P., & Chevalier, A. (1983). Sleep problems in children and their relationships with early disturbances of the waking-sleeping rhythms. *Sleep, 6,* 47–51.

Schaefer, C. E. (1990). Treatment of night wakings in early childhood: Maintenance of effects. *Perceptual and Motor Skills, 70,* 561–562.

Scharf, M. B., & Jennings, S. W. (1988). Childhood enuresis: Relationship to sleep, etiology, evaluation, and treatment. *Annals of Behavioral Medicine, 10,* 113–120.

Schmitt, B. D. (1982). Nocturnal enuresis: An update on treatment. *Pediatric Clinics of North America, 29,* 21–36.

Scott, G., & Richards, M. P. M. (1990). Night waking in infants: Effects of providing advice and support for parents. *Journal of Child Psychology and Psychiatry, 31,* 551–567.

Seymour, F. W., Brock, P., During, M., & Poole, G. (1989). Reducing sleep disruptions in young children: Evaluation of therapist-guided and written information approaches: A brief report. *Journal of Child Psychology and Psychiatry, 30,* 913–918.

Soldatos, C. R., & Lugaresi, E. (1987). Nosology and prevalence of sleep disorders. *Seminar in Neurology, 7,* 236–242.

Taboada, E. L. (1975). Night terrors in a child treated with hypnosis. *American Journal of Clinical Hypnosis, 17,* 270–271.

Tarnowski, K. J., Rasnake, L. K., & Drabman, R. S. (1987). Behavioral assessment and treatment of pediatric burn injuries: A review. *Behavior Therapy, 18,* 417–441.

Thorpy, M. M., Korman, E., Spielman, A. J., & Glovinsky, P. B. (1988). Delayed sleep phase syndrome in adolescents. *Journal of Adolescent Medicine, 9,* 22–27.

Troup, C., & Hodgson, N. (1971). Nocturnal functional bladder capacity in enuretic children. *Journal of Urology, 105,* 129–132.

Van Londen, A., Van Londen-Barentsen, M. W., Van Son, M. J., & Mulder, G. A. (1993). Arousal training for children suffering from nocturnal enuresis: A 2 1/2 year follow-up. *Behaviour Research and Therapy, 31,* 613–615.

Wagner, M. T. (1981). Controlling nocturnal bruxism through the use of aversive conditioning during sleep. *American Journal of Clinical Biofeedback, 4,* 87–92.

Warady, B. A., Alon, U., & Hellerstein, S. (1991). Primary nocturnal enuresis: Current concepts about an old problem. *Pediatric Annals, 20,* 246–255.

Weil, G., & Goldfried, M. R. (1973). Treatment of insomnia in an eleven-year-old child through self-relaxation. *Behavior Therapy, 4,* 282–294.

Weir, M. R. (1982). Things that go damp in the night: A review of childhood enuresis. *Military Medicine, 147,* 568–571.

Weissbluth, M. (1982). Modification of sleep schedule with reduction of night waking: A case report. *Sleep, 5,* 262–266.

Weissbluth, M. (1984). Is drug treatment of night terrors warranted? *American Journal of Diseases in Children, 138,* 1086.

Whelan, J. P., & Houts, A. C. (1990). Effects of a waking schedule on primary enuretic children treated with full-spectrum home training. *Health Psychology, 9,* 164–176.

White, M. A. (1990). Sleep onset latency and distress in hospitalized children. *Nursing Research, 39,* 134–139.

White, M., Powell, G., Alexander, D., Williams, P., & Conlon, M. (1988). Distress and self-soothing behaviors in hospitalized children at bedtime. *Maternal-Child Nursing Journal, 17,* 67–78.

White, M. A., Williams, P. D., Alexander, D. J., Powell-Cope, G. M., & Conlon, M. (1990). Sleep onset latency and distress in hospitalized children. *Nursing Research, 39,* 134–139.

Williams, C. D. (1959). The elimination of tantrum behavior by extinction procedures. *Journal of Abnormal Social Psychology, 59,* 269–273.

Wittig, R., Zorick, F., Roehrs, T., Sickelsteel, J., & Roth, T. (1983). Narcolepsy in a 7-year-old child. *Journal of Pediatrics, 102,* 725–727.

Wright, L., Woodcock, J., & Scott, R. (1970). Treatment of sleep disturbance in a young child by conditioning. *Southern Medical Journal, 63,* 174–176.

CHAPTER 24

ADAPTATION TO PARENTAL CHRONIC ILLNESS

Alice Kahle, TEXAS SCOTTISH RITE HOSPITAL FOR CHILDREN IN DALLAS, TEXAS
Glenn N. Jones, SCHOOL OF MEDICINE IN NEW ORLEANS, LOUISIANA STATE UNIVERSITY MEDICAL CENTER

Illness in a family member is an event encountered by everyone from time to time; but what are the consequences when a child must face the illness of a parent and the condition is chronic? Considerable speculation about the repercussions of this event exists.

The goal of this chapter is to integrate existing literature on the impact of parental chronic illness and to discuss children's adaptation to its presence. Possible outcomes predicted by various theoretical perspectives will be described. Many conventional assumptions about the effects of parental chronic illness will be challenged and factors that may relate to poor adaptation to parental chronic illness will be explored. Finally, the concluding portion of the chapter will be devoted to discussing possible directions for future research in this area.

IS CHRONIC ILLNESS IN PARENTS IMPORTANT?

There are several reasons why we should have an interest in discerning what, if any, impact parents' chronic illnesses might have on their children. First, there are reasons to believe that many children will have parents with chronic illnesses. Prevalence estimates differ according to one's definition of chronic

illness. Although a number of definitions are possible, one broad definition that will be used here is that *chronic illnesses* are biomedical conditions that persist over time (Koch-Hattern, Berolzheimer, & Thrower, 1988; Burish & Bradley, 1983) and are the result of nonreversible pathological alterations (Stuifbergen, 1990).

Current demographic, medical, and life-style trends suggest that a substantial number of parents have chronic illnesses and that the numbers will probably rise in the years ahead (Burish & Bradley, 1983). The coinfluence of these trends probably will increase the number of children who live with a chronically ill mother or father. For example, the authors of Healthy People 2000 (Department of Health and Human Services [DHHS], 1992) aptly describe the paradoxical consequences of the immense health care advances that have occurred during the last decade. They note that "unprecedented gains in life expectancy, combined with the increased ability of medical technology to avert death without always restoring health, add to the increasing prevalence of chronic conditions" (DHHS, 1992, p. 442).

Naturally, chronic conditions and disabilities are more prevalent among persons over 65 years of age than among those 65 years old and younger. However, if we loosely define parenting ages as 18 to 65, a surprising number of potential parents have chronic illnesses and disabilities. When one considers only the noninstitutionalized population, as many as 2 percent of the population have some disability interfering with activities of daily living to the extent that they need help with these activities (DHHS, 1992). The authors of Healthy People 2000 present another useful view on the problem. They describe data from the 1988 National Health Interview Survey (National Center for Health Statistics, 1989) concerning limitations in major activities (i.e., role as employee, student, homemaker, or independent older adult) due to chronic conditions. In 1988, over 9 percent of the U.S. population suffered a limitation in major activity due to a chronic condition. Among people aged 18 to 44, 5.9 percent experience limitations in major activities. In persons aged 45 to 64, the number rises to 16.9 percent (DHHS, 1992). Thus, a surprising number of people of parenting age are experiencing chronic illnesses and disabilities.

The increase in HIV incidence may also expose more children to parents with a chronic, life-threatening disease than has been the case in the past. In 1993, AIDS was the third largest cause of death among U.S. adults aged 25 to 44. The Centers for Disease Control and Prevention (CDC) estimates that 1 in 250 people have become infected with the HIV virus. Further, the CDC projects that AIDS will be one of the top five causes of death for women of childbearing age in the 1990s (CDC, 1993).

A growing health care practice may also affect children's exposure to chronic illness. A current trend is toward minimizing hospital stays by providing health care at home whenever feasible (Groce & Zola, 1993). The emphasis is on using family members, including children, to help chronically ill patients reach appropriate goals (Power, 1985; Burish & Bradley, 1983). These practices, supported by preliminary evidence that the family can play a crucial role in a patient's adjustment (Hough, Lewis, & Woods, 1991), may alter a child's experiences with an ill parent in several ways. First, the length of time a child and a sick parent are apart may decline. Also, increasing home health care and family involvement in caregiving may result in children having more extensive exposure to ill parents than they would have previously and encountering earlier illness stages that parents

previously would have experienced in the hospital. This trend in medical practice will apparently lead to more children getting raised by parents with chronic illnesses.

An additional reason that parental chronic illness is a potentially important area is that chronically ill parents express concerns about their own parenting ability. In separate studies (Allaire, 1988; Thorne, 1990), mothers with chronic illnesses were interviewed about parenting concerns related to their condition. In both, mothers expressed concern about physical limitations imposed by their illness that might interfere with parenting, as well as concerns about how their illness might affect their child's emotional adjustment and development. Thus, chronically ill parents themselves feel concerned about how their illness may interfere with their ability to parent.

In sum, multiple factors suggest that many children are (or will be) growing up in an environment that contains parents with chronic illnesses and disabilities. The combination of demographic trends, trends in prevalence of chronic illnesses, and trends in medical practice all support this contention. Further, changes in health care provision may alter the extent and nature of a child's exposure to a parent's condition. These trends, as well as the parenting concerns expressed by adults with chronic conditions, support the need for an understanding of children's adaptation to parental chronic illness.

THEORETICAL PERSPECTIVES

Hypotheses about the consequences of being the child of a chronically ill parent are available from several theoretical perspectives. In this section, possible outcomes predicted by the developmental, family systems, psychodynamic, and social learning perspectives will be presented. Empirical support drawn from these perspectives will be integrated into the following sections.

Developmental Model

The developmental model suggests that the presence of a chronically ill parent may interfere with a family's ability to achieve developmental goals in the normal progression. Transition from one developmental stage to the next is stressful under normal circumstances. When the strains of a chronically ill parent compound this process, the evolution of family development may become disrupted. For example, if an exacerbation of a chronic illness coincides with the developmental transition of a child, the presence of parental illness could interfere with this transition (Griffith & Griffith, 1987).

The developmental model also predicts that a child's response to parental illness may change as that child reaches typical developmental goals. For example, normal adolescent rebelliousness may play a part in a teenager's refusal to help with caregiving responsibilities (Allaire, 1988).

Family Systems

Family systems theory characterizes the family as a set of interacting, interrelating members functioning in relation to a broader sociocultural system and evolving over the life cycle (e.g., Jackson, 1957; Minuchin, 1974). A primary assumption is that the family strives to maintain stability in ongoing interactions. Family systems theory predicts that change in one part of the system will result in compensatory change in the other parts of the system (Jackson, 1957). With regard to an acute illness phase, family systems theory predicts that children may help compensate for system changes by filling roles that an impaired parent is unable to fulfill. Thus, family systems theory predicts adaptation to parental illness because such adaptation acts to preserve the system, but it may be an effective (e.g., Pratt, 1976) or ineffective (e.g., Minuchin, 1974) adaptation to the illness.

Working from a family systems perspective, Griffith and Griffith (1987) note three areas where chronic illness may disrupt family structure: boundaries, power hierarchies, and alliances and coalitions. As part of the family structure, children are as likely as other members to experience changes created by the disruption of chronic illness. For example, the authors suggest that chronic illness may allow a boundary between a child and afflicted parent to become so impermeable that effective parenting is impossible.

Psychodynamic Perspective

Traditional psychodynamic theory emphasizes that early developmental factors determine, to a large de-

gree, adult functioning long before people reach adulthood (Achenbach, 1992). Because chronic illness in a parent might produce intense anxiety within the family, it may have the potential to hinder smooth progression through the psychosexual developmental stages proposed by psychodynamic theorists.

Psychodynamic approaches to child development also stress that acquisition of personality characteristics, behavior, and values become most strongly influenced through identification with one's parents, with ultimate identification with one's same-sexed parent as particularly significant (e.g., Bandura, 1969; Bronfenbrenner, 1960; Lowrey, 1978). Consequently, one assumption is that if a chronic illness or disability influences the personality characteristics, values, and role functioning of a parent, the chronic illness will also influence children in the family as well. Much of the theoretical speculation about the effects of having a parent with a chronic illness has been in terms of maladjustment acquired through identification with a chronically ill parent (e.g., Beard, 1975; Heslinga, Schellen, & Verkuyl, 1974; Olgas, 1974). This prediction relies on the assumption that individuals with chronic illnesses or disabilities adopt poorly to the illness or disability. This assumption has only limited empirical and anecdotal basis (Buck & Hohmann, 1983), which will be more fully explored next.

Social Learning Perspective

Social learning theory is another theoretical perspective that makes predictions about the impact of exposure to parental chronic illness. Guided by the premise that early learning experiences affect future behavior, social learning theorists have argued that the sick role and how one functions when ill are learned behaviors (Mechanic, 1972). People identify with models who are prestigious and similar to oneself and are most likely to emulate these models. Thus, for most children, parents are very salient models. Parents' responses to their own illnesses and somatic sensations serve as a model for a child's future behavior (e.g., Turkat, 1982; Turkat & Noskin, 1983; Whitehead, Busch, Heller, & Costa, 1986; Whitehead, Winget, Fedoravicius, Wooley, & Blackwell, 1982).

Children learn how to interpret and respond to somatic sensations through observation and interactions with their parents. Beyond modeling, Whitehead and associates (1986) argue that parents also can shape future actions by reinforcing or punishing sick role or illness behavior. An intriguing hypothesis stemming from this area is that parents' experiences with chronic conditions affect not only their illness modeling but also their pattern of responding when their children are ill. This hypothesis deserves further investigation.

Nature of Research to Date

Although the potential impact of parental chronic illness is apparent, there is actually very little empirical evidence to guide one's understanding of the possible effects (Buck & Hohmann, 1983; Peters & Esses, 1985; Rustad, 1984). More than a decade ago, Buck and Hohmann (1983) extensively reviewed and summarized this material and emphasized that the majority of existing literature in the area consisted of unsystematic observations, anecdotal material, and mere opinionated speculation (Buck & Hohmann, 1983).

This chapter will attempt to focus on the methodologically advanced investigations and on evaluating literature that has emerged in the decade since Buck and Hohmann's review. Unfortunately, methodological problems (lack of control groups, unreliable measurement instruments of unknown validity, retrospective designs) have persisted and are a serious limitation of the few empirical investigations of parental chronic illness that have appeared recently (Peters & Esses, 1985; Stuifbergen, 1990).

Another critique of much of the existing literature is its tendency toward a negative bias. Crist (1993) makes the point that research on parental chronic illness often has worked from the perspective of stereotypical expectations about chronic illness in general or specific conditions in particular. Few researchers have attempted to examine whether presumed detrimental effects on parents' functioning or children's emotional state and adjustment truly occur. Crist notes that beginning with stereotypical negative expectations has led to a self-fulfilling prophecy of negative research outcomes rather than objective description. Most likely, the current, limited understanding of the implications of parental chronic illness has resulted from many researchers' failures to look for potential positive outcomes and the frequent use of subjective, bias-prone tools in their investigations.

The following sections describe the presentations and arguments of original authors accurately. However, it is important to communicate limitations of the existing literature explicitly. The limitations have had a significant influence on research outcomes, and only recently has the literature begun to address the questions effectively. With these limitations in mind, the text now examines various lines of research that appear to have bearing on the question of how parents' chronic illnesses may affect their children.

IMMEDIATE IMPACTS OF ACUTE PARENTAL ILLNESS ON CHILDREN

The scant nature of research on children's adaptation to parental chronic illness is unfortunate and leaves many unanswered questions. Support for the expectation that parental chronic illness indeed has an impact on children comes from research on children's responses to acute illnesses and their reactions at the onset of a chronic illness. If the acute illness phase has observable repercussions on children, these effects may have lasting implications for a child's adjustment. It seems well established that diagnosis of a serious illness has a stressful impact on the patient. For example, Cassileth and colleagues (1984) found that patients with recently diagnosed chronic illness (regardless of illness group) had poorer mental health scores than patients who had been diagnosed four months or longer. The initial impact of a chronic disease on the parents would seem likely to result in changes in children's behavior, as well.

Children's adjustment to their parent's cancer diagnosis is one acute illness phase that has received some attention in several empirical articles. Although the overall effect of parental cancer diagnosis on a child's emotional well-being remains poorly understood (Compass et al., 1994), some preliminary conclusions about its initial impact can be drawn from this literature. Lewis and colleagues have conducted a series of investigations of the impact of parental cancer diagnosis from both the parent's and child's perspectives (Lewis, Ellison, & Woods, 1985; Lewis, Woods, Hough, & Bensley, 1989). They found that, according to parental report, children in these families experienced few behavioral or emotional problems.

However, children's self-reports indicated some negative impact on their self-esteem and adjustment.

In another study, Compass and associates (1994) found that each family member's subjective appraisals of the seriousness and stressfulness of the cancer diagnosis (of the ill parent) moderately related to his or her own distress response. Importantly, the researchers found that both stress-response (e.g., intrusive thoughts and emotions, avoidant behavior) and anxiety/depression symptoms differed in children as a function of age, sex of the child, and sex of the patient. Distress was higher in children who were the same sex as the patient. Even after adjustment for normative sex differences, adolescent girls whose mothers had received a diagnosis of cancer reported far more distress than any other group. When comparing the responses of children and adolescents, these researchers noted that anxiety/depression symptoms were higher in adolescents than in children, but stress-response symptoms were more common in younger children than in adolescents. The younger children were also much higher on measures of social desirability than were the adolescents. The authors interpreted this as reflecting the children's use of denial as a coping mechanism.

In summary, the evidence suggests that diagnosis of a parent's catastrophic illness does have an impact on the immediate emotional state of other family members. The impact on children appears to vary as a function of age and sex. Adolescent girls appear most at risk, especially when their mother is the patient. However, the relations do not appear simple, and further empirical clarification certainly is necessary. Whether the immediate impact of a catastrophic illness has long-term effects on children and whether it serves as a good analogy for the possible effects of less dramatic, chronic illnesses remains in question. Other evidence regarding the long-term impact of parental chronic illness will be examined next.

THE IMPACTS OF PARENTAL CHRONIC ILLNESS ON CHILDREN'S ADJUSTMENT

The assumption that parental chronic illness relates to behavior problems in children is primarily because of retrospective, case control studies conducted in the 1950s and 1960s. These studies identified groups of disturbed (e.g., delinquent) and nondisturbed children and compared the incidence of parental illnesses for both groups. When comparing the parents of delinquent, institutionalized children to parents of nondelinquent children, a higher incidence of serious physical ailments was apparent in the parents of delinquents (Glueck & Glueck, 1950). Similarly, Rutter (1966) found higher incidences of chronic and recurrent illness among the parents of the psychiatrically disturbed children when compared to parents of controls matched on age and social class. Results such as these led Buck and Hohmann (1983) to state, "In general, parents of psychologically disturbed and delinquent children show a higher incidence of physical illness than parents in control groups" (p. 213).

The conclusiveness of these studies is questionable for a number of reasons. First, the case control design is subject to tremendous sampling biases. Also, researchers often poorly defined the methods they used of assessing child disturbance and parental illness, and in many cases, the only methods used were the subjective evaluations of unblinded observers. Further, the associations are only suggestive of a relation. Causality is virtually impossible to test with case-controlled designs. As Buck and Hohmann note in their critique of Rutter (1966), parental illness was confounded with the incidence of parental psychiatric disturbance, and there are alternative explanations of the association between parental illness and their children's psychological problems. In sum, the nature and direction of causality is undeterminable, and it is not easy to identify the strength of any association from studies of this type.

Recent work appears to contradict the conclusions and assumptions that children of chronically ill parents will exhibit problems. Crist (1993) examined the interactional patterns of mother-daughter dyads in standardized role-play tasks. Crist compared mothers with multiple sclerosis (MS) who were recruited from MS support groups and controls recruited through local Girl Scouts groups. Control mothers reported no physical disabilities or chronic illnesses. Daughters' ages ranged from 8 to 12 years, and Crist matched dyads on age of the daughter. Despite respectable sample sizes (MS group $n = 31$; Control group $n = 34$), Crist failed to identify a unique pattern of interacting between mothers with MS and their daughters. Both groups (i.e., MS group and control group) exhibited similar numbers of receptive, directive, and dissuasive interactions. Crist concluded that the data provided no evidence for a detrimental effect on children raised by a parent with a disability or chronic illness.

In another study, Dura and Beck (1988) also failed to find differences in communication patterns between children in families with a parent who had chronic pain ($n = 7$), diabetes ($n = 7$), and no illness ($n = 7$). They did find that children from families of a parent with chronic pain tended to have more days absent from school than children of mothers with no illness. However, a similar trend was not present among children from families with a diabetic parent. It is not clear if this difference was peculiar to chronic pain or was a chance occurrence. Replication is necessary to clarify their results.

Generalizability of the results of both studies remains limited due to their small sample sizes. Also, the study conducted by Crist (1993) may have been subject to a potential sampling bias because the authors recruited participants in the chronic illness group from an MS support group. Nevertheless, using better designs and more objective measures than their predecessors did, these studies yielded little evidence that children of chronically ill parents function differently than children with healthy parents.

IMPACTS OF PARENTAL CHRONIC ILLNESS ON THE FAMILY

Additional evidence of the impact of parental chronic illness comes from studies that examine the repercussions of chronic illness for the family as a whole. Typically, these studies have attempted to identify patterns or changes in family functioning or structure that might have an association with chronic illness. In addition, some have attempted to describe the impact of chronic illness on particular family dyads.

Family Environment

Stuifbergen (1990) examined Moos's Family Environment Scale ratings, a measure of perception of one's family environment, provided by 67 chronically ill parents and their spouses. The majority of participating families did not differ appreciably from families used to establish norms for the scale. Unfortunately, the author did not obtain a matched control group for comparison purposes. Nevertheless, descriptively, the researchers emphasized that the vast majority of participating families were within the normal range for the scales.

Peters and Esses (1985) also used the Family Environment Scale to explore differences between families with and without a chronically ill parent. The authors compared 33 children of a parent with multiple sclerosis (MS) to a sample of 33 control children whose parents did not have a chronic illness. The authors matched children in the index group with a control group participant on the basis of sex, age, number of siblings, and socioeconomic status. The children's ages ranged from 12 to 18. Children in the MS group, relative to children in the control group, reported higher scores on the Conflict subscale and lower scores on the Cohesion, Intellectual-Cultural Orientation, Moral-Religious Emphasis, and Organization subscales. The authors suggested that the lower Cohesion scores reported by children of MS parents may indicate that there is an overall lack of "feeling of togetherness" in families with a chronically ill parent. They interpreted the higher Conflict score as due to insufficient flexibility to accommodate changes in family roles produced by illness. The lower scores on Intellectual-Cultural Orientation and Moral-Religious Emphasis were possibly due to the extra consumption of the parents' time and energies by the additional instrumental needs created by the illness. Peters and Esses (1985) concluded that children of MS parents report perceptions of their family environment that are different from those reported by children of parents with no chronic disorders.

Peters and Esses's investigation represents one of the few studies to incorporate a control group of any sort. Unfortunately, imperfect matching may have yielded uninterpretable differences on the scales. Subjects in the chronic illness group were recruited from the membership roles of a national Multiple Sclerosis Society; control group children, on the other hand, were selected from a local, religiously affiliated parochial school. This sampling difference seems the most likely explanation for the dissimilarity on the Moral-Religious subscale and certainly confounds interpretation of the other differences.

Use of an objective scale represents an important advance in these research efforts. However, Peters and Esses (1985) note that the FES lacks a theoretical base, making its interpretation difficult. Thus, it is difficult to know what these results mean due to limited information about what each subscale measures. Although the scale has population-based norms, no empirical validation of the subscales is available.

Peter and Esses' results suggest intriguing differences in children's subjective perceptions of their family environment that may be due to a chronically ill parent's presence. However, these variations have no clear link to important differences in family adaptive functioning. Further, it is not clear whether these dimensions are important determinants of a child's later adult adjustment, illness attitudes, or future illness behavior. Finally, although groups differed on some subscales, it is impossible to determine if these differences were clinically meaningful.

Marital Discord

Further evidence that chronic illness may affect the family comes from its possible association with marital discord. In their series of case studies, Hough and colleagues (1991) noted that demands imposed by chronic illness in one member of a marital dyad associated with spousal depression and marital dissatisfaction in the other. A serious illness may increase marital distress (Klein, Dean, & Bogdonoff, 1967), and the spouses of patients have reported several marital complaints (see, e.g., Braham, Hauser, Cline, & Posner, 1975; Diamond, 1974).

Lewis and associates (1989) examined the effects of maternal chronic illness on marital satisfaction and child adjustment in a path analytic framework. They studied families whose mothers had a diagnosis of nonmetastatic breast cancer ($n = 19$), Type II Diabetes ($n = 13$) and, as a control, fibrocystic breast disease ($n = 16$). They examined the interrelations among several variables, including impact of the demands of the wife's illness on the father's level of depression, marital adjustment, and their children's psychosocial functioning. Lewis and associates found that the number of illness demands the father experienced was predictive of his level of depression. Although illness demands correlated with poorer marital

adjustment, in the path model this relationship appears mediated through the father's level of depression. Poorer child psychosocial adjustment correlated with higher illness demands, father's depression level, poorer marital adjustment, use of familial introspection as a coping mechanism, and the father's perception of the child-parent relationship. In the path model, better marital adjustment and quality of the father-child relation appeared to be the most important predictors of the child's higher psychosocial adjustment, mediating the impact of the other variables.

Lewis and colleagues (1989) concluded that the mother's illness has an impact on the spouse, leading to depression and reduced marital quality, poorer paternal relationships with children, and poorer child psychosocial adjustment. The conclusions seem overly strong, given the limits of the study. First, it was illness demands as perceived by the father that was the strongest predictor, not illness type. Illness type appears a misnomer because Lewis and co-workers combined the fibrocystic breast disease controls with the chronic illness group and contrasted them with the nonmetastatic breast cancer group. Illness demands did not particularly relate to this classification of illness type. It is unclear if the chronic illnesses were associated with higher illness demands, because Lewis and colleagues did not establish a link between illness groups and illness demands. Thus, it is difficult to conclude whether the effects are particular to the mother's chronic illness or whether the effects relate to illness behavior irrespective of diagnosis.

Second, Lewis and associates indicate that all of the variables involved the fathers' self-reports and perceptions. An obvious alternative hypothesis is that the fathers' levels of depression and/or marital dissatisfaction cause perceptions of poorer child psychosocial functioning. Certainly, collateral data from appropriate significant others would greatly strengthen the conclusions.

Lewis and associates (1989) findings do suggest that poorer marital adjustment is associated with poorer child adjustment. These results are consistent with current literature that suggests that marital discord is associated with distress in children and often undermines effective parenting (Maccoby & Mnookin, 1992; Goldberg, 1990).

In summary, marital discord may be more likely in families in which one parent is chronically ill than in families with no chronically ill parents, and marital discord relates to distress and problems in parenting. However, the probability that a chronic illness will affect marital adjustment and cause problems for the children remains uncertain. Further empirical evaluation of the linkages between parental chronic illness, marital distress, and adjustment problems of children is essential.

Life-Style Changes

Some literature documents the incidence of life-style changes that the entire family incorporates to enhance medical compliance of an ill parent. For example, family members of a cardiac patient may alter their diets to improve patient compliance (Sirles & Selleck, 1989). Many authors have speculated about the impact of chronic illness on a family's recreational pursuits (e.g., Anthony, 1970; Heslinga et al., 1974; Thomason & Clifford, 1972), but research on this topic has produced mixed results.

Some researchers have noted that active family recreation decreases after the onset of a chronic condition (McSweeny, Grant, Heaton, Adams, & Timms, 1982). Others, however, have failed to replicate this finding. For example, Peters and Esses (1985) found no differences between families with a parent with MS and control group families on the Active Recreational subscale of the Family Environment Scale. The authors interpret this result as indicating that the groups were similar in their recreational activities. Peters and Esses's data are consistent with Buck and Hohmann's (1981; see also Buck & Hohmann, 1982, 1983) findings. Buck and Hohmann matched children of fathers with spinal cord injuries and children of able-bodied fathers on several variables, including sex, race, father's age, and income. All of the fathers were veterans. Buck and Hohmann found that the two groups participated in similar patterns of recreational activities.

The findings of these separate investigations are surprising, given the physical limitations that often accompany MS and spinal cord injuries. Together, these results bring into question the common assumption that recreational activities will decrease for families of chronically ill or disabled parents.

Impacts on Adult Children of Chronically Ill Parents

Few researchers have attempted to examine how growing up in a family with an ill parent affects one's behavior as an adult. In a seminal work in the area, Buck and Hohmann (1981, 1982) examined the long-term effects of paternal disability. Participants were adult children whose fathers had spinal cord injuries (SCI). All fathers in both the index and control groups were veterans, and participants were matched on the variables of age, education, income, and sex of the adult child (SCI: $n = 45$, Control: $n = 36$). Using a variety of objective tests (e.g., MMPI, Sixteen Personality Factor Questionnaire) supplemented with survey-style questionnaires, Buck and Hohmann found no evidence of maladjustment in the adult children of disabled fathers. The adult children with SCI fathers appeared to be as well adjusted as the adult children of able-bodied fathers. Further, Buck and Hohmann found no differences in a variety of physical health patterns. They interpreted this result as a failure to confirm that children learned sick-role behaviors from their disabled parents. In an intriguing analysis, Buck and Hohmann found that the children's personality, behavior, and attitudes related more to their father's behavior (as assessed by the Parent-Child Relations Questionnaire II) than to his disability status. In general, Buck and Hohmann's results lent no credibility to the idea that growing up with a parent who has a disability is deleterious.

Limits to the work of Buck and Hohmann revolve around the self-report nature of the data, much of which was retrospective. The authors note the possibility of selection bias in the sampling, particularly a bias toward stable, intact families. The latter may limit the ability to generalize to the population. Although Buck and Hohmann conducted too many analyses of their data, this action would have operated to create more false differences rather than a consistent picture of similarity of the groups.

Another investigation conducted by Feeney and Ryan (1994), examined the relationship between, among other things, parental illness and attachment style. According to attachment theory, one can understand intimate relationships between adults in terms of attachment styles that develop from experiences with attachment figures during childhood. Secure attachment relates to trust, relationship satisfaction, and a constructive approach to conflict; avoidant attachment relates to low levels of commitment, intimacy, and care; anxious/ambivalent attachment correlates with dependency, relationship conflict, and low relationship satisfaction (Hazan & Shaver, 1987).

Feeney and Ryan's (1994) retrospective study used college students as participants. Reports of illness incidence in participants' parents were obtained and participants' current attachment styles. They found that frequent parental illness correlated with an avoidant attachment style. Paternal illness inversely related to a secure attachment style. Further, almost all of the students who reported frequent illness for both parents endorsed insecure forms of attachment. However, only paternal illness had an indirect effect on physical symptom reporting, mediated through attachment style and negative emotionality. Finally, participants' acknowledgment of a chronic illness in an immediate family member positively correlated with their reported number of visits to health care professionals during the previous ten weeks.

Unfortunately, the researchers did not require participants to designate which member of their family experienced a chronic illness, nor did participants indicate whether the parental illnesses were chronic or acute. Thus, none of the relations are clearly attributable to parental chronic illness. Finally, the retrospective nature of the study leaves many open questions about potential biases and recall problems. It may be that avoidant attachment styles lead to better recall of the illnesses of family members or the misperception of others as frequently ill. That is, though an association between the report of parental illnesses and avoidant attachment styles is apparent, the nature of the association deserves further exploration.

CHALLENGING ASSUMPTIONS ABOUT THE IMPACT OF PARENTAL CHRONIC ILLNESS

Buck and Hohmann (1983) criticized the assumption that chronic illness leads to maladjustment in children and their parents. Their point has received empirical support from various sources. For example, Cassileth and colleagues (1984) investigated psychosocial status in five groups of patients with chronic illness (arthritis, diabetes, cancer, renal disease, or dermato-

logic disorder) and compared them to groups of physically well individuals receiving treatment for depression and healthy adults not receiving mental health treatment. Cassileth and colleagues (1984) found few differences between groups of chronically ill persons on objective measures of distress and mental health and few differences between the chronically ill and healthy normals. Furthermore, all five chronic illness groups had significantly better Mental Health Status scores than the group of participants receiving treatment for depression. The researchers noted that there was great variability within the illness groups but that no particular disease was associated with more or less distress. They summarized their findings by stating,

> Although physical limitations and problems may be unique to particular illnesses, emotional status seems largely independent of [physical] diagnosis. We suggest that psychological status of chronically ill patients exhibits a distribution that reflects that of the population at large because adaptation represents not the demands of particular stress, such as a specific diagnosis, but rather the manifestations of enduring personality constructs and capacities. (Cassileth et al., 1984, p. 510)

Another point of controversy in the chronic illness literature is the amount of overlap shared between parents with chronic illnesses and those with disabilities. Similar to parents with chronic illnesses, one frequent assumption is that parenting with a physical disability leads to child maladjustment (Buck & Hohmann, 1983). Buck and Hohmann (1983) maintain that failing to treat parental illness and parental disability as distinct issues promotes confusion, overgeneralization, and methodological pitfalls. Certainly, some differences between the groups are evident. However, Peters and Esses's (1985) conclusion that there is little empirical evidence identifying major differences in family functioning or adjustment between the two groups continues to appear accurate. Further, Cassileth and associates' (1984) data emphasizes the variability within chronic illness and even within each illness group. Therefore, given the available literature, the authors of this chapter feel that embracing either uniformity myth—that all people with disabilities or chronic illnesses are alike—is a misleading fallacy. Instead, it seems more productive to focus on the dimensions of either condition that might interfere with parenting and assess those dimensions as directly as possible.

FACTORS THAT MAY INFLUENCE ADAPTATION TO PARENTAL CHRONIC ILLNESS

Several researchers have attempted to identify factors that may influence a family's adaptation to chronic illness as well as indicators that a family is possibly at risk for poor adjustment. For example, Hough and associates (1991) concluded from their review that a patient's spouse or significant other has the potential to be a leading force in the patient's adjustment. However, his or her impact may be positive or negative. Thus, single parents who are chronically ill may not necessarily be worse off than their married counterparts. Instead, whether having a spouse or significant other is a help or a hinderance may depend on his or her premorbid marital adjustment, personality characteristics, and reaction to the partner's illness.

Lewis and colleagues (1989) identified illness demands as another factor that influences a family's adaptation to chronic conditions. They define *illness demands* as the hardships or stressors that tax the family's resources and are direct effects of the parent's disease and its treatment. The extent of illness demands may have an important influence on adjustment of nonafflicted parents. For example, Lewis and colleagues (1989) found a positive association between the extent of maternal illness demands and presence of depressive symptomology in nonafflicted spouses.

Literature about the impact of acute parental illness also suggests that sex of the children, sex of affected parents, and age of the children during the acute phase may be important. In Compass and colleagues' study, adolescent girls whose mothers had received a diagnoses of cancer reported far more distress than any other group. Although one can only speculate as to the implications for living with a parent with a chronic illness or disability, this result suggests that developmental stages and sex may be important dimensions.

At present, the available literature provides only scant information about a few factors that may influence the effects of parental chronic illness. Perhaps

these preliminary investigations will serve as a catalyst for additional research aimed at detecting factors that may have an impact on children's adaptation.

CONCLUSIONS AND SUGGESTIONS FOR FUTURE RESEARCH

Demographic and life-style trends indicate that the number of children who live with a parent who has a chronic illness will probably increase in the years ahead. Unfortunately, there is very little empirically based literature to guide one's expectations about implications of these trends on children's adjustment. For the most part, the understanding of children's adaptation to parental chronic illness has come from studies that examine consequences for the family as a whole. Further, methodological limitations are evident in much of the available literature. The majority of this literature summarizes results of interviews with very small participant samples or surveys of affected parents' beliefs.

Until recently, researchers have designed most studies to detect problems and negative consequences of living with a parent with a chronic condition. In combination with subjective evaluations and poor controls, researchers often found the problems for which they searched. Even when they utilized objective outcome measures, researchers rarely obtained a control group for comparison purposes. Thus, the ability to draw conclusions or generalize to the population at large remains limited.

It seems appropriately circumspect to note a few general trends. Of particular note is the recent trend toward better designs using control groups and more objective measures as compared to early studies in this area. Use of better methodology has led to an increasing picture of similarity between children of parents with chronic illnesses or disabilities and children of healthy parents. Although coping with demands of a chronic illness may challenge most families, the available literature does not support the conclusion that a chronic illness is certain to disrupt parenting, obstruct family functioning, or adversely impact children.

Indeed, some qualitative studies suggest that possible positive effects may be present. For example, when 40 children of parents with rheumatoid arthritis participated in individual, semistructured interviews about their experiences, more than half reported feeling that living with an ill parent had brought their family closer than it had been prior to diagnosis (Gallez, 1993). Hough and colleagues (1991) also noted that coping with demands of a chronic illness seems to draw some families closer together.

In spite of the potential for positive outcomes, parental chronic illness certainly does not relate to positive consequences for all families. Clearly, more research is necessary to help identify circumstances in which outcomes for children of the chronically ill are poor. An additional domain of the parental chronic illness literature that has received little empirical attention is assessment and treatment of children and families who are having difficulties adjusting to a parent's illness.

Few assessment tools specifically for assessing parental chronic illness and children's adaptation currently exist. Typically, assessment procedures described in the literature have involved conducting semi-structured, unstandardized interviews with family members (e.g., Allaire, 1988; Gallez, 1993). Application of some of the well-standardized, norm-referenced assessment measures typically used by school and child psychologists might enhance one's understanding of children's reactions considerably. For example, use of objective assessment instruments designed to measure childhood depression or anxiety might help identify circumstances in which children of the chronically ill exhibit more of these symptoms than peers with healthy parents. Also, utilizing scales that have multiple informant versions and measure a broad array of internalizing and externalizing behaviors might enhance one's understanding of possible differences between parents' and children's views about the situation.

A few specific suggestions for conducting assessments of families with a chronically ill parent are apparent from the literature. Clearly, assuming that a disabled or chronically ill parent is having difficulty adjusting is unacceptable in light of Cassileth and colleagues' (1984) data. Similarly, assuming that a parent's disability or chronic illness has any particular impact on his or her child also appears unwarranted. From a social learning point of view, one needs to go beyond the chronic illness and assess exactly what the parent modeled or what the child vicariously learned.

Another suggestion for dealing with families of the chronically ill is to assess familys' understandings about the illness early because appropriate information can be a useful coping mechanism for family members (Power, 1985). Also, if a family has the ability to influence the eventual adjustment of an afflicted person, a treating clinician can develop an approach to assessment and intervention that emphasizes family involvement in the patient's adaptation (Power, 1985).

Few interventions designed to target needs of children of the chronically ill appear in the literature. Fortunately, there are a number of written resources developed for families with a disabled parent, and many of these may be quite applicable to parents with chronic illnesses. Of course, use of these and other treatment packages with children of the chronically ill must also undergo empirical evaluation.

REFERENCES

Achenbach, T. M. (1992). Developmental psychopathology. In M. H. Bornstein & M. E. Lamb (Eds.), *Developmental psychology: An advanced textbook.* Hillsdale, NJ: Erlbaum.

Allaire, S. (1988, January). How a chronically ill mother manages. *American Journal of Nursing,* 46–49.

Anthony, E. (1970). The mutative impact of serious mental and physical illness in a parent on family life. In E. Anthony & C. Kourpernik (Eds.), *The child in his family* (Vol. 1). New York: Wiley.

Bandura, A. (1969). Social learning theory of identificatory processes. In D. Goslin (Ed.), *Handbook of socialization theory and research.* Chicago: Rand McNally.

Beard, M. (1975). Changing family relationships. *Dialysis and Transplantation, 4,* 36–41.

Braham, S., Hauser, H. B., Cline, A., & Posner, M. (1975). Evaluation of the social needs of nonhospitalized chronically ill persons: 1. Study of 47 patients with multiple sclerosis. *Journal of Chronic Diseases, 28,* 401–419.

Bronfenbrenner, U. (1960). Freudian theories of identification and their derivatives. *Child Development, 31,* 15–40.

Buck, F. M., & Hohmann, G. W. (1981). Personality, behavior, values, and family relations of children of fathers with spinal cord injury. *Archives of Physical Medicine and Rehabilitation, 62,* 432–438.

Buck, F. M., & Hohmann, G. W. (1982). Child adjustment as related to severity of paternal disability. *Archives of Physical Medicine and Rehabilitation, 63,* 249–253.

Buck, F. M., & Hohmann, G. W. (1983). Parental disability and children's adjustment. In E. L. Pan, T. E. Backer,

& C. L. Vash (Eds.), *Annual review of rehabilitation* (Vol 3. pp. 203–241). New York: Springer.

Burish, T. G., & Bradley, L. A. (1983). Coping with chronic disease: Definitions and issues. In T. G. Burish & L. A. Bradley (Eds.), *Coping with chronic disease: Research and applications* (pp. 3–12). New York: Academic Press.

Cassileth, B. R., Lusk, E. J., Strouse, T. B., Miller, D. S., Brown, L. L., Cross, P. A., & Tenaglia, A. N. (1984). Psychosocial status in chronic illness: A comparative analysis of six diagnostic groups. *New England Journal of Medicine, 311,* 506–511.

Centers for Disease Control (CDC) and Prevention. (1993, January 1). Statistics and projections/trends. *AIDS information.* Atlanta, GA: Centers for Disease Control and Prevention. CDC document No. 320210:1.

Compass, B. E., Worsham, N. L., Epping-Jordan, J. E., Grant, K. E., Mireault, G., Howell, D. C., & Malcarne, V. L. (1994). When mom or dad has cancer: Markers of psychological distress in cancer patients, spouses, and children. *Health Psychology, 13,* 507–515.

Crist, P. (1993). Contingent interaction during work and play tasks for mothers with multiple sclerosis and their daughters. *The American Journal of Occupational Therapy, 47,* 121–131.

Department of Health and Human Services, Public Health Service. (1992). *Healthy people 2000: National health promotion and disease prevention objectives: Full report, with commentary.* Boston: Jones and Bartlett. (Also available as DHHS Publication No. (PHS) 91-50212. Washington, DC: U.S. Government Publication Office.)

Diamond, M. (1974). Sexuality and the handicapped. *Rehabilitation Literature, 35,* 34-40.

Dura, J. R., & Beck, S. J. (1988). A comparison of family functioning when mothers have chronic pain. *Pain, 35,* 79–89.

Feeney, J. A., & Ryan, S. M. (1994). Attachment style and affect regulation: Relationships with health behavior and family experiences of illness in a student sample. *Health Psychology, 13,* 334–345.

Gallez, P. le (1993). Rheumatoid arthritis: Effects on the family. *Nursing Standard, 7* (39), 30–34.

Glueck, S., & Glueck, E. (1950). *Unraveling juvenile delinquency.* New York: Commonwealth Fund.

Goldberg, W. A. (1990). Marital quality, parental personality, and spousal agreement about perceptions and expectations for children. *Merrill-Palmer Quarterly, 36,* 531–556.

Griffith, J. L., & Griffith, M. E. (1987). Structural family therapy in chronic illness. *Psychosomatics, 28* (4), 202–205.

Groce, N. E., & Zola, I. K. (1993). Multiculturalism, chronic illness, and disability. *Pediatrics, 91,* 1048–1055.

Hazan, C., & Shaver, P. R. (1987). Romantic love conceptualized as an attachment process. *Journal of Personality and Social Psychology, 52,* 511–524.

Heslinga, K., Schellen, A., & Verkuyl, A. (1974). *Not made of stone: The sexual problems of handicapped people.* Springfield, IL: Charles C. Thomas.

Hough, E. E., Lewis, F. M., & Woods, N. F. (1991). Family response to mother's chronic illness: Case studies of well- and poorly-adjusted families. *Western Journal of Nursing Research, 13,* 568–596.

Jackson, D. D. (1957). The study of the family. *Family Process, 4,* 1–20.

Klein, R. F., Dean, A., & Bogdonoff, M. D. (1967). The impact of illness upon the spouse. *Journal of Chronic Diseases, 20,* 241–248.

Koch-Hattern, A., Berolzheimer, N., & Thrower, S. M. (1988). Working with families. In P. D. Sloane, L. M. Slatt, & R. M. Baker (Eds.), *Essentials of Family Medicine* (pp. 1–13). Baltimore, MD: Williams & Wilkins.

Lewis, F. M., Ellison, E. S., & Woods, N. F. (1985). The impact of breast cancer on the family. *Seminars in Oncology Nursing, 1,* 206–213.

Lewis, F. M., Woods, N. F., Hough, E. E., & Bensley, L. S. (1989). The family's functioning with chronic illness in the mother: The spouse's perspective. *Social Science and Medicine, 29,* 1261–1269.

Lowrey, G. H. (1978). *Growth and development of children.* Chicago: Year Book Medical Publishers

Maccoby, E. E., & Mnookin, R. H. (1992). *Dividing the child: Social and legal dilemmas of custody.* Cambridge, MA: Harvard University Press.

McSweeny, J., Grant, I., Heaton, R., Adams, K., & Timms, R. (1982). Life quality of patients with chronic obstructive pulmonary disease. *Archives of Internal Medicine, 142,* 473–478.

Mechanic, D. (1972). Social psychologic factors affecting the presentation of bodily complaints. *New England Journal of Medicine, 286,* 1132–1139.

Minuchin, S. (1974). *Families and family therapy.* Cambridge, MA: Harvard University Press.

National Center for Health Statistics. (1989). Current Estimates from the National Health Interview Survey, United States, 1988. *Vital and Health Statistics.* Series 10, No. 173, DHHS Pub. No. (PHS) 89–1501. Hyattsville, MD: U.S. Department of Health and Human Services.

Olgas, M. (1974). The relationship between parents' health status and body image of their children. *Nursing Research, 23,* 319–324.

Peters, L. C., & Esses, L. M. (1985). Family environment as perceived by children with a chronically ill parent. *Journal of Chronic Diseases, 38,* 301–308.

Power, P. W. (1985). Family coping behaviors in chronic illness: A rehabilitation perspective. *Rehabilitation Literature, 46* (3–4), 78–83.

Pratt, L. (1976). *Family structure and effective health behavior. The energized family.* Boston: Houghton Mifflin.

Rustad, L. C. (1984). Family adjustment to chronic illness and disability in mid-life. In M. G. Eisenberg, L. C. Sutkin, & M. A. Jansen (Eds.), *Chronic illness and disability through the life span: Effects on self and family.* New York: Springer.

Rutter, M. (1966). *Children of sick parents: An environmental and psychiatric study.* London: Oxford University Press.

Sirles, A. T., & Selleck, C. S. (1989). Cardiac disease and the family: Impact, assessment, and implications. *The Journal of Cardiovascular Nursing, 3,* 23–32.

Stuifbergen, A. K. (1990). Patterns of functioning in families with a chronically ill parent: An exploratory study. *Research in Nursing and Health, 13,* 35–44.

Thomason, B., & Clifford, K. (1972). The disabled person and family dynamics. *Accent on Living, 17,* 20–35.

Thorne, S. E. (1990). Mothers with chronic illness: A predicament of social construction. *Health Care for Women International, 11,* 209–221.

Turkat, I. D. (1982). An investigation of parental modeling in the etiology of diabetic illness behavior. *Behavior Research and Therapy, 20,* 547–522.

Turkat, I. D., & Noskin, D. E. (1983). Vicarious and operant experiences in the etiology of illness behavior: A replication with healthy individuals. *Behavior Research and Therapy, 201,* 169–172.

Whitehead, W. E., Busch, C. M., Heller, B. R., & Costa, P. T., Jr. (1986). Social learning influences on menstrual symptoms and illness behavior. *Health Psychology, 5,* 13–23.

Whitehead, W. E., Winget, C., Fedoravicius, A. S., Wooley, S., & Blackwell, B. (1982). Learned illness behavior in patients with irritable bowel syndrome and peptic ulcer. *Digestive Diseases and Sciences, 27,* 202–208.

CHAPTER 25

MENTAL RETARDATION AND PHYSICAL HEALTH

James H. Rimmer, UNIVERSITY OF ILLINOIS AT CHICAGO

This chapter will focus on a significant microcosm of the pediatric and adolescent population—those with mental retardation. These children live and function in society, but often become isolated from their peers because of their mental deficiency. The chapter addresses health care issues and recommendations for future directions pertaining to this population.

EVOLUTION OF MENTAL RETARDATION

It wasn't long ago that children with mental retardation became labeled *idiots, morons,* and *imbeciles.* Each label referred to a specific level of function. Over the years, these labels became offensive and subsequently got changed to *severely retarded, moderately retarded,* and *mildly retarded.* But these terms also took on an air of disparagement, and in the 1990s, the new term became *developmental disability,* which is a generic label that includes other conditions, such as cerebral palsy and autism. Today, many professionals are opting to "de-label" children with mental retardation and are instead classifying them under the broad heading of *developmentally disabled.*

Person-first terminology has also become vogue in the 1990s. The phrase, *mentally retarded children* has become *children with mental retardation* so that the focus is on common traits with other humans first

before perceiving the impairment. The intent of this new language is to create a feeling among society that persons with disabilities have more in common with the norm than they have differences.

As a result of the stereotypes associated with persons who have mental retardation, many in this group have become identified as social outcasts (Epstein, Polloway, Patton, & Foley, 1989). The subnormal intelligence and deficits in adaptive skills in areas such as self-care and communication have left these individuals isolated from their peers. Despite these deficits, however, there is a strong movement in the United States to integrate children with mental retardation into school and other community-based programs (Saint-Laurent, Fournier, & Lessard, 1993).

In 1975, the passage of Public Law 94-142, The Education for All Handicapped Children Act, entitled all children with disabilities, including those with mental retardation, to a free and appropriate public education. The revision of this legislation in 1990, Public Law 101-476, included a name change to the Individuals with Disabilities Education Act (IDEA) and sent a strong message to members of the education community that they are not to separate children with disabilities from their peers in school programming. Today, the majority of children and adolescents with mental retardation receive their education in regular schools in their own communities.

DEFINITION

The definition of mental retardation has gone through several changes over the last three decades. In 1960, the American Association on Mental Deficiency adopted the definition that "mental retardation refers to subaverage intellectual functioning which originates during the developmental period and is associated with impairment of adaptive behavior" (Heber, 1961, p. 499). The Association defined subaverage intelligence as more than 1 standard deviation below the mean in IQ, or below 85. Over the years, experts in the field thought that too many persons met this criterion and became labeled *mentally retarded,* and in 1973 the Association changed the definition to "significantly subaverage intellectual functioning," which referred to 2 standard deviations below the mean, or an IQ below 70 (Grossman, 1973).

In 1983, the American Association on Mental Deficiency (AAMD) restructured the definition once again to state that "mental retardation refers to significantly subaverage general intellectual functioning existing concurrently with deficits in adaptive behavior and manifested during the developmental period" (Grossman, 1983, p. 11).

This definition of mental retardation once again underwent revision, and was recently replaced by a newer version. In 1992, a consensus panel organized by the American Association on Mental Retardation (AAMR; Luckasson et al., 1992) revised the definition to elucidate some of the obscure components of the older version. In the new definition, the AAMR Terminology and Classification Committee stated that:

> Mental retardation refers to substantial limitations in present functioning. It is characterized by significantly subaverage intellectual functioning, existing concurrently with related limitations in two or more of the following applicable adaptive skill areas: communication, self-care, home living, social skills, community use, self-direction, health and safety, functional academics, leisure, and work. Mental retardation manifests before age 18. (Luckasson et al., 1992, p. 5)

The authors of the new definition listed four assumptions that one must meet before classifying an individual as having mental retardation:

1. Valid assessment considers cultural and linguistic diversity as well as differences in communication and behavioral factors.
2. The existence of limitations in adaptive skills occurs within the context of community environments typical of the individual's age peers and is indexed to the person's individualized needs for supports.
3. Specific adaptive limitations often coexist with strengths in other adaptive skills or other personal capabilities.
4. With appropriate supports over a sustained period, the life functioning of the person with mental retardation will generally improve. (Luckasson et al., 1992, p. 5)

IQ Criteria

One thing that remained consistent throughout the changes in the definition of mental retardation was that it referred to a condition that resulted in subnormal intellectual functioning. However, recent revisions raised the upper boundary for classifying someone as having mental retardation to an IQ of 75 in order to reflect statistical variance seen in all intelligence tests (Luckasson et al., 1992). Similarly, raising the score 5 points will allow professionals greater flexibility in classifying individuals who really need special services but who may otherwise not have qualified for those services because they did not meet the IQ criteria.

The AAMR Terminology and Classification Committee also noted that mental retardation affects three forms of intelligence—conceptual, practical, and social intelligence—but that the inner capability most pertinent to the definition is "conceptual intelligence," which refers to cognition and learning (Luckasson et al., 1992).

Adaptive Skills Criteria

The new AAMR definition of mental retardation also expanded the concept of adaptive behavior (Reiss, 1994). In the new definition, the older term *adaptive behavior* became changed to *adaptive skills* to reflect specific function in the following 10 areas: communication, self-care, home living, social skills, community use, self-direction, health and safety, functional academics, leisure, and work. A child must be deficient in two or more of these areas to meet classification criteria for having mental retardation. Furthermore, the AAMR Terminology and Classification Committee noted that because adaptive skills may vary with chronological age, evaluation of these skills must include reference to the person's chronological age (Luckasson et al., 1992).

The difficulties that children and adolescents with mental retardation have in terms of adaptive skills results from limitations in two forms of intelligence—*practical intelligence* (ability to maintain and sustain oneself as an independent person in managing the ordinary activities of daily living) and *social intelligence* (ability to understand social expectations and the behavior of other persons and to judge appropriately how to conduct oneself in social situations) (Luckasson et al., 1992). For example, many children and adolescents with mental retardation have an extremely difficult time interacting with their peers (social intelligence) or are not able to perform activities of daily living, such as bathing and toileting effectively (practical intelligence).

By citing specific categories of adaptive skills, the authors of this new definition wanted to make it very clear that mental retardation "refers to a specific pattern of intellectual limitation and is not a state of global incompetence" (p. 12). Reiss (1994) noted that mental retardation must be viewed as a "disabling condition" based on an individual's ability to interact in his or her own environment, which can obviously be quite different among persons with mental retardation. Thus, a major emphasis of the new definition is to link individuals' capabilities (intelligence and adaptive skills) with their environments (home, work/school, community).

The AAMR included the "adaptive skill" criterion for classification of mental retardation primarily to prevent individuals raised in socially disadvantaged conditions from becoming categorized as having mental retardation based solely on the IQ criterion. Some individuals raised in socially disadvantaged conditions may have IQ scores below 70 but in other areas of function (adaptive skills) perform much like their peers and are able to meet the demands of everyday life (Baroff, 1991). In other words, they may be poor academic students, but they are still able to interact in their environments; such interactions

may involve playing basketball with peers or taking care of smaller siblings.

Age Criteria

The one aspect of the definition that has remained consistent over the years is that mental retardation itself must present before age 18. This component of the definition precludes a person who is in a car accident and sustains a closed head injury after age 18 from getting classified as having mental retardation. Nonetheless, individuals who develop normally in every capacity other than mental function (no physical injury), but meet the three criteria (deficits in intelligence, deficits in adaptive skills, and diagnosis before age 18) may still become classified as having mental retardation.

PREVALENCE OF MENTAL RETARDATION

The prevalence of mental retardation is based on a deviation from the norm on a standardized intelligence test. The average IQ is approximately 100 (Hallahan & Kauffman, 1991). Children with mental retardation fall at least two standard deviations below this value, which results in a score of 70 to 75 or below. Based on a "normal curve," approximately 2.27 percent of the population will have an IQ between 0 and 70. However, this figure includes children as well as adults. Sherrill (1993) reported that among children aged 6 to 21 years receiving special education services, mental retardation ranks as the third most common condition after specific learning disabilities and speech and language impairments.

In the last 10 years, there has been a major effort to decategorize children with disabilities. Today, many children with mental retardation enter into classes based on learning styles rather than specific diagnoses, making it difficult to estimate the number of children and adolescents who have this condition.

Classification of Mental Retardation

Although most professionals in the field of mental retardation would prefer not to categorize children with mental retardation, it is helpful from the standpoint of understanding this condition to classify children according to severity. Grossman (1983) used the following categories to describe children with mental retardation: mild, moderate, severe, and profound. However, the new guidelines developed by Luckasson and colleagues (1992) collapsed mild and moderate mental retardation into the category labeled *mild,* and severe and profound mental retardation into the category labeled *severe.*

CHARACTERISTICS OF CHILDREN BY LEVEL OF MENTAL RETARDATION

The majority of persons classified as having mental retardation fall into Grossman's (1983) category of mild mental retardation (Lubetsky, 1993). Crocker (1989) noted that this category constitutes 85 percent of the total population of individuals who have mental retardation. Some authors classify these children as having *educable mental retardation* (EMR). Their IQs are between 50 and 70 to 75, depending on the criteria used. Often, this level of retardation is not present during the preschool years. However, once a child begins school, the difficulty in learning becomes quite noticeable. A teenager with mild mental retardation will have an approximate mental age of an intellectually average child in grade school (Eichstaedt & Kalakian, 1993). As adults, however, many of these individuals blend into society and can usually maintain menial-type jobs and start their own family.

Children with moderate mental retardation, sometimes referred to as *trainable mental retardation (TMR),* have IQs between 35 and 55. At this level, delays are evident in early childhood. These children have trouble with abstract reasoning and need constant training to attain such skills as feeding, dressing, bathing, and toileting. The vast majority of children with moderate mental retardation will have problems with speech, language, and social interactions. Russell and Forness (1985) also noted that there is a higher incidence of behavioral and psychiatric disorders among this group and most individuals with Down syndrome fall into this category (Pitetti, Rimmer, & Fernhall, 1993). The majority of individuals classified as having moderate mental retardation are able to lead semi-independent life-styles.

The last two categories often get collapsed into one category under the rubric of *severe mental retardation.* IQs of these individuals are below 40, and learning even the slightest task is extremely difficult. It often takes years for these children to acquire a minimum level of competency in daily living skills, such as bathing and toileting. Many will never attain these skills and will need full-time custodial care. The vast majority of persons with mental retardation still residing in institutions are those classified as having severe mental retardation.

CAUSES OF MENTAL RETARDATION

There are a multitude of causes of mental retardation. However, approximately 30 to 40 percent present no clear etiology. It is easier to identify the causes of mental retardation for children classified in the moderate to profound range of mental retardation than for those having mild mental retardation. Genetic factors account for approximately 5 percent of the causes of moderate to profound mental retardation. Early alterations of embryonic development make up approximately 30 percent, pregnancy and perinatal problems occur in approximately 10 percent of the cases, and environmental influences and mental disorders comprise approximately 15 to 20 percent (American Psychiatric Association, 1987).

The major causes of mental retardation appear listed in the new classification system for mental retardation, *Mental Retardation. Definition, Classification, and Systems of Supports* (Luckasson et al., 1992). This system divides the causes into prenatal, perinatal, and postnatal causes. Some of the common conditions appear in Figure 25.1.

Figure 25.1 Common Causes of Mental Retardation

Prenatal
Genetic: phenylketonuria, tuberous sclerosis, Tay-sachs
Chromosomal anomalies: Down syndrome, Fragile-X syndrome
Maternal diseases: rubella, syphilis, HIV
Substance abuse: fetal alcohol syndrome

Perinatal
Brain injury: anoxia, brain trauma

Postnatal
Psychosocial factors: deprivation, malnutrition
Diseases: encephalitis, meningitis

GENETIC FACTORS

Fragile X syndrome is the most common genetic cause of mental retardation (Kerby & Dawson, 1994). It affects up to 1 in 1,360 males (Lachiewicz, Spiridigliozzi, Gullion, Ransford, & Rao, 1994). Fragile X received its name from the fragility of a specific region of the distal end of the long arm of the X chromosome, where there is constriction or breaking off (Batshaw & Perret, 1992).

The physical symptoms of this disorder in prepubescent children include low-set protruding ears, high arched palate, flattened nasal bridge, macrocephaly, poor coordination, and hyperflexible joints. In postpubescent children, other physical characteristics include an elongated face and prominent jaw, long ears, macroorchidism, and mitral valve prolapse (Batshaw & Perret, 1992). IQs of children with fragile X average around 40, and the disorder affects more males than females (Kessler, 1988). Males with fragile X often have autistic-like behaviors (Kerby & Dawson, 1994; Lachiewicz et al., 1994).

Down syndrome is another common cause of mental retardation. Approximately 10 percent of all moderate and severe cases of mental retardation are the result of this condition (Hallahan & Kauffman, 1991). Another name for this disorder is trisomy 21 because these children have three, rather than two, copies of chromosome 21. It remains the most common cause of mental retardation in persons with IQs below 50 (Kessler, 1988).

Phenylketonuria (PKU) is characterized by the inability to convert a common dietary substance, phenylalanine, to tyrosine, another genetic cause of mental retardation. Pregnant women who have PKU expose their fetuses to high levels of phenylalanine, causing damage to the developing nervous system (Gelfand, Jenson, & Drew, 1982). However, if a mother does not have PKU but is a carrier, her child will develop symptoms after birth, upon intake of dietary phenylalanine. The accumulation of phenylalanine results in abnormal brain development. Fortunately, early detection leads directly to prevention by use of a special diet that involves eliminating phenylalanine. For instance, the sides of soft-drink cans displays the warning:

"Phenylketonurics: contains phenylalanine."

Tay-Sachs disease is similar to PKU in the sense that either fathers or mothers can be carriers of the disease. It results in progressive brain damage and eventually leads to death. It occurs almost exclusively in Ashkenazi Jews (Hallahan & Kauffman, 1991).

BRAIN DAMAGE

Mental retardation caused by brain damage falls under two separate categories: infections and environmental hazards.

Infections

If a mother contracts rubella (German measles), syphilis, or herpes simplex, any of these can cause mental retardation in her offspring. Children can also incur infections that lead to mental retardation. The most common infections that cause this condition are meningitis, encephalitis, and AIDS, the latter of which is the fastest growing infectious cause of mental retardation (Hallahan & Kauffman, 1991). Some experts have projected that pediatric AIDS may soon be the leading cause of mental retardation and brain damage (Hallahan & Kauffman, 1991).

Environmental Hazards

Environmental hazards that can cause mental retardation include trauma to the skull, poisons, radiation, malnutrition, prematurity or postmaturity, and birth injury. Under "poisons," fetal alcohol syndrome (FAS) is a significant health problem in women who consume large amounts of alcohol during pregnancy.

MOTOR CHARACTERISTICS OF CHILDREN WITH MENTAL RETARDATION

Although many children and adolescents with mental retardation do not have any medical limitations, they often have difficulty performing motor skills and are therefore unable to effectively participate in many community-based sports programs.

In 1959, Frances and Rarick published a paper titled, "Motor Characteristics of the Mentally Retarded." In this study, which is a seminal study still widely quoted today, the investigators found that children with educable mental retardation were 2 to 4 years behind their peers on most measures of motor performance (Francis & Rarick, 1959). In a later study, Rarick (1980) also found that boys with mild mental retardation were inferior on motor performance tests and that girls with this same condition were even worse than boys. It appears that with increasing age, the motor performance gap between children with and without mental retardation gets wider.

The majority of children with mental retardation have serious motor delays. The greater their intellectual dysfunction, the more serious their motor deficits. Sherrill (1993) noted that this delayed motor development appears related to a disturbance in the development of postural reactions. However, part of this delay may also be due to body composition characteristics. Dobbins, Garron, and Rarick (1981) found that boys with mental retardation were shorter and had wider hips and more body fat than children without mental retardation, and Rarick, Dobbins, and Broadhead (1976) noted that skinfold measurements were significantly greater in children with mental retardation compared to children without mental retardation.

Physical Fitness Characteristics

Physical fitness in an important parameter of good health. The small number of studies that have looked at fitness levels of children with mental retardation have confirmed that they are less fit than children without mental retardation (Dichter, Darbee, Effgen, & Palisano, 1993; Eichstaedt & Lavay, 1992; Halle, Silverman, & Regan, 1983; Rarick et al., 1976). Nonetheless, Halle and colleagues (1983) noted that this lower level of fitness is not an outcome of their condition, but rather a lack of opportunity. Many children and adolescents with mental retardation become viewed as outcasts by other children and therefore become socially ostracized from playgrounds and neighborhood recreational outlets. Rarely does a child with mental retardation participate in sports programs offered by local park districts unless the district has a special recreation program.

Professionals have noted that improvements in physical fitness must not be limited to the nondisabled population (Pommering et al., 1994). Because individuals with mental retardation often have a variety of other medical needs that ostensibly seem to be more important than fitness, this health parameter often gets overlooked because of these other concerns (Crocker, 1988). This is unfortunate because several studies have reported that persons with mental retardation have extremely poor cardiovascular fitness levels and are in need of a structured exercise program (Fernhall & Tymeson, 1987; Pitetti & Tan, 1990; Pitetti, Climstein, Campbell, Barrett, & Jackson, 1992).

In a report published in 1987 in the journal *Pediatrics,* the Committee on Sports Medicine and the Committee on Children with Disabilities made a statement concerning exercise needs of children with mental retardation. In their report, the Committees noted that recreation and physical activity programs are important for all children, including children with mental impairments. However, the Committee also emphasized that because of the mental impairment, physicians when suggesting participation in athletic programs must take into consideration "the child's size, coordination, degree of physical fitness, physical maturity, physical health, and motivation" (Committee on Sports Medicine, 1987, p. 447).

For example, children with Down syndrome may have a condition known as atlantoaxial instability, defined as a laxity of the ligaments between the C_1 and C_2 vertebra. Presence of this condition contraindicates physical activities that cause excessive bending of the neck (i.e., diving, wrestling, gymnastics).

HEALTH CHARACTERISTICS OF CHILDREN WITH MENTAL RETARDATION

There has been very little research on the physical health of children with mental retardation. However, several studies conducted on adults with mental retardation have shown that as a group, adults with this condition have several predisposing health risks, including extremely high obesity levels and sedentary living habits (Pitetti & Campbell, 1991; Rimmer, Braddock, & Fujiura, 1993; Rimmer, 1994). It is plausible to assume that what appears to be a problem in adulthood would be, at least in part, a consequence of poor health habits in childhood and adolescence.

Because there are various causes of mental retardation, it is difficult to pigeonhole this group into any one category of health. Persons with mental retardation are a heterogeneous group and therefore present a diverse clinical picture in terms of physical health. Part of this diversity stems from where they reside, their socioeconomic status, and their level of mental retardation.

Luckasson and associates (1992) noted that persons with mental retardation evidence a varied range of health. For example, children with conscientious parents who place a premium on good health will probably have better health profiles than children who live at the poverty level with parents who have little or no understanding about the importance of good health. However, one must assume that because many children with mental retardation live at or below the poverty line, they are likely to have a multitude of health problems (Epstein et al., 1989).

The investigators also noted that the majority of persons with mental retardation present a diverse picture. Individuals may have problems with hearing, vision, mobility, strength, muscle tone, and coordination. Health problems include obesity, hypertension, scoliosis, chronic ear infections, or seizures. The authors of this widely publicized book also noted that these health problems are not unusually different from people who do not have mental retardation; however, because of their living arrangements, coping limitations, and poor access to health care, these problems may manifest themselves more so than in nonretarded persons (Luckasson et al., 1992). They concluded with the following statement:

> If there is a different effect on functioning for people with mental retardation, it may be partly because of the environments in which they live, work, play, socialize, and interact with others. Their environments may create unique dangers or fail to provide appropriate protection and treatment. In addition, the intellectual limitations of people with mental retardation may make it more difficult for them to cope with these associated physical problems. These coping problems may be manifested as difficulty in negotiating the health services system, poor understanding of treatment needs, difficulty with communication, and use of alternative and misinterpreted symptoms, such as self- injurious behavior. (Luckasson et al., 1992, p. 62)

Nevertheless, it would appear that physical health is not a major concern among children and adolescents with mental retardation, and despite not suffering from any specific illnesses related to their sedentary life-styles during their early years, it is likely that their health will become a major problem in adulthood.

There is also a subgroup of children and adolescents with mental retardation who will suffer afflictions from other disorders, beyond the mental impairment, that may compromise their health. For example, children with severe mental retardation may also have cerebral palsy and epilepsy. These individuals would be more likely than not to have poorer health profiles when compared to children with mental retardation who do not have any physical symptoms.

Epstein and associates (1989) reported that 11.5 percent of children with mild mental retardation have seizure disorders, and the incidence is 33 to 45 percent for individuals with severe/profound mental retardation. In general terms, the more severe the retardation, the greater the likelihood that a child will have accommodating chronic medical conditions, such as cerebral palsy and seizure disorders (Rubin, 1987).

Medication usage among persons with mental retardation is greatest in those with moderate to severe mental retardation (Epstein et al., 1989; Tanguay, 1990). A recent study by Rimmer, Braddock, and Marks (1994) corroborated this concern; the authors found that medication usage among adults with mental retardation was highest in those living in institutional settings. This probably relates to the fact that the majority of persons with mental retardation still residing in institutions are those persons classified as having severe mental retardation. In general, the major medications taken included Dilantin, Mellaril, Phenobarbital, Tegretol, and Depakote. Aside from Mellaril, used to manage psychotic behavior, the other four medications were to control seizures.

In an ongoing investigation by Rimmer and Pitetti (1994), the investigators measured body fat levels of children with mental retardation, including those with Down syndrome. In a preliminary report presented at a conference on nutrition and mental retardation, they noted that body fat levels for the boys ranged from 3 to 47 percent, and for girls, from 18 to 45 percent. Overall, girls had higher levels of obesity than boys, and the children with Down syndrome had higher levels of obesity than the children who did not have Down syndrome. If one can assume that body fat levels will increase as these individuals enter adulthood, the incidence of obesity will rise exponentially in this population.

Health Characteristics of Children with Down Syndrome

Because of the high incidence of Down syndrome and the unique characteristics presented by this group, a special emphasis on their health characteristics appears warranted. The incidence of Down syndrome is approximately 1 in 1,000 births (Crocker, 1989). Women over 35 years of age have a higher frequency of having children with Down syndrome than younger women, and women between 40 and 44 years of age have a 20.5 times higher incidence than women between 20 and 24 years of age (Batshaw & Perret, 1992).

Children with Down syndrome have atypical physical features. These features include a small skull with flattening at the back of the head and a flattened face with a recessed bridge of the nose. The eyes have a slanting appearance. The ears and mouth are small, and the tongue is large and often protrudes from the mouth. The fingers and toes are short and stubby. There is an extra flap of skin, called the epicanthial fold, located at the inner corner of the eye. These children have maloccluded teeth and their hair is coarse.

Children with Down syndrome have several health problems. In the newborn period, the most common problem is congenital heart disease, which affects almost 50 percent of infants with Down syndrome (Kolata, 1989). Many children require heart surgery at birth to correct the defect. Another common problem is congenital gastrointestinal malformations, which lead to a blockage in 12 percent of the population. Symptoms include vomiting, poor feeding, and aspiration pneumonia (Batshaw & Perret, 1992). Surgery can correct these conditions. In addition, however, children with Down syndrome have a 1 percent chance of developing leukemia, 20 times the normal risk (Kolata, 1989).

In early childhood, motor delays are the hallmark symptom in children with Down syndrome. Most do not walk before the age of 3 years, and their balance is extremely poor for much of their lives. This may re-

late to their visual problems, which include refractive errors (70 percent), strabismus (50 percent), nystagmus (35 percent), and cataracts (3 percent) (Pueschel, 1990). Middle-ear infections are also quite common, which may also affect their balance.

Hypotonia is another hallmark symptom of Down syndrome. Most children and adolescents have postural problems due to the laxity of their ligaments. They often walk with a forward head, round shoulders, and lordotic spine. Activities requiring strength or endurance are very difficult for this population.

In later childhood, additional health problems include obesity, short stature, hypothyroidism, seizures, joint dislocations, and depression. Most of these children will never reach 5 feet in height, yet their weight will be excessive relative to their height.

Approximately 17 percent of all persons with Down syndrome have a condition known as *atlantoaxial instability* (Sherrill, 1993). The vast majority of these persons, however, are asymptomatic (Pueschel, 1988). As noted earlier in the chapter, atlanto-axial instability causes a laxity of the ligaments between the C_1 and C_2 vertebrae. Therefore, this condition is a contraindication for neck exercises, and it is very important that these patients obtain cervical x-rays before participating in physical education activities (Rimmer, 1994).

FUTURE DIRECTIONS

There is much that we have yet to learn about the health characteristics of children with mental retardation. As professionals continue to emphasize the noncategorical approach, it will certainly be more difficult in the future to identify children with this condition. However, there is currently a very small amount of literature on the physical health of children with mental retardation, and based on the data published on adults with mental retardation, we definitely need to learn more about the physical health of children and adolescents with mental retardation.

The research completed on adults with mental retardation clearly shows that, as a group, this population has several health problems. Kelly, Rimmer, and Ness (1986) and Rimmer and colleagues (1993) have found very high levels of obesity in adults with mental retardation. In a later article, these authors also reported that a significant number of adults with mental retardation also had lipid profiles that place them at risk for coronary heart disease (Rimmer, Braddock & Fujiura, 1994). In a recent study, Frey and Rimmer (in press) found significantly higher levels of obesity among American adults with mental retardation compared to their German counterparts and higher levels for subjects living in community-based settings versus those living in institutions.

In a review paper, Pitetti and Campbell (1991) noted that adults with mental retardation are considered a population at risk for premature onset of cardiovascular diseases. They made several important points:

1. Adults with mental retardation have lower limits for the onset of old age and higher mortality rates than adults in the general population.
2. Young adults with mental retardation living in community-based residences have cardiovascular fitness levels representative of sedentary lifestyles.
3. Significantly more cardiovascular disorders were evident among elderly individuals with mental retardation living in the community compared to those residing in institutions.

Pitetti and Campbell (1991) concluded with the following statement:

> The seriousness of this issue cannot be overstated. To link congenitally low IQ levels to inherently inferior cardiovascular capacities would mean not only lower expectations for MR individuals but the acceptance of the consequences—that is, the acceptance of earlier onset and higher incidence of cardiovascular mortality and morbidity among the MR population. (p. 591)

Children with mental retardation appear to be a group that will sustain a greater number of health problems than the general population as they grow older. In a recent study by Rimmer and Pitetti (1994), investigators measured the body mass index (BMI) of 16 children and adolescents (10 to 18 years) with mental retardation. Preliminary results indicated that 50 percent of the sample was either at risk for becoming overweight or were already overweight according to recently developed standards by the Expert Committee on Clinical Guidelines for Overweight in Adolescent Preventive Services (Himes & Dietz, 1994).

It is logical to assume that if adults with mental retardation are at risk for coronary heart disease, then children and adolescents with mental retardation may also be leading life-styles that predispose them to a higher incidence of disease as they grow older. It is surprising that there has been such a paucity of research on health issues pertaining to a significant microcosm of the pediatric and adolescent population. Nonetheless, we need to study this population as a separate entity from children who do not have mental retardation in order to isolate characteristics of their physical health.

Many children and adolescents with mental retardation live below the poverty line and have the lowest educational levels. In a study that confirms this observation, Epstein and associates (1989) found that children and adolescents classified as having mild mental retardation were predominantly male, were from racial or ethnic minority groups, and were from socially broken homes. It is reasonable to assume that the health behaviors, such as smoking, excessive alcohol consumption, sedentary life-style, poor eating habits, and environmental hazards (i.e., lead poisoning, violence), often manifest in socioeconomically lower class groups may also be a problem among the subgroup of individuals with mental retardation. Clearly, more research is necessary to determine the health status of children and adolescents with mental retardation.

Researchers must take into consideration the cause of mental retardation (i.e., Down syndrome, fragile X, fetal alcohol syndrome) when studying this population, along with their socioeconomic status, living arrangement (i.e., institution versus community-based dwellings), and level of retardation (mild to severe). Children and adolescents classified as having moderate or severe mental retardation will have a greater number of associated chronic medical conditions than children with mild mental retardation. Understanding the physical and psychological traits at each level of retardation will be helpful in developing health education programs that would best fit the needs of each child.

SUMMARY

The area of health care for children and adolescents with mental retardation will be a major concern during the turn of the century. This significant microcosm of the pediatric population will place an increasing burden on the U.S. health care system because many of these individuals live below the poverty line and require public aid or have accompanying medical conditions.

We must emphasize the role of community support with regard to the health care of children and adolescents with mental retardation. As institutions continue to close, more and more individuals with mental retardation will live and work in the community. However, most individuals with mental retardation will not respond to media awareness on the dangers of substance abuse or lack of exercise and will therefore need professional support to help them understand the importance of good health.

Finally, we must educate parents and caregivers of children with mental retardation in such areas as nutrition, weight control, exercise, posture, sleep habits, and personal stress management techniques. They are the linchpin to enhancing the physical health of children and adolescents with mental retardation. Without their support, there is little hope of impacting this population.

REFERENCES

American Psychiatric Association. (1987). *Diagnostic and statistical manual of mental disorders* (3rd ed.). Washington, DC: Author.

Baroff, G. S. (1991). *Developmental disabilities: psychosocial aspects.* Austin, TX: Pro-Ed.

Batshaw, M. L., & Perret, Y. M. (1992). *Children with disabilities. A medical primer.* Baltimore, MD: Paul H. Brookes.

Committee on Sports Medicine. (1987). Exercise for children who are mentally retarded. *Pediatrics, 80,* 447–448.

Crocker, A. C. (1988). Medical care for adults with developmental disabilities. *Journal of the American Medical Association, 260,* 1455–1459.

Crocker, A. C. (1989). Systems of health care delivery. In I. L. Rubin & A. C. Crocker (Eds.), *Developmental disabilities: Delivery of medical care for children and adults* (pp. 30–71). Philadelphia: Lea & Febiger.

Dichter, C. G., Darbee, J. C., Effgen, S. K., & Palisano, R. J. (1993). Assessment of pulmonary function and physical fitness in children with Down syndrome. *Pediatric Physical Therapy, 5,* 3–8.

Dobbins, D. A., Garron, R., & Rarick, G. L. (1981). The motor performance of educable mentally retarded and intellectually normal boys after covariate control for dif-

ferences in body size. *Research Quarterly for Exercise and Sport, 52,* 1–8.

Eichstaedt, C. B., & Kalakian, L. H. (1993). *Developmental/adapted physical education.* New York: Macmillan.

Eichstaedt, C. B., & Lavay, B. (1992). *Physical activity for individuals with mental retardation: Infant to adult.* Champaign, IL: Human Kinetics.

Epstein, M. H., Polloway, E. A., Patton, J. R., & Foley, R. (1989). Mild retardation: Student characteristics and services. *Education and Training of the Mentally Retarded, 24,* 7–16.

Fernhall, B., & Tymeson, G. T. (1987). Graded exercise testing of mentally retarded adults: a study of feasibility. *Archives of Physical Medicine and Rehabilitation, 68,* 363–365.

Francis, R. J., & Rarick, G. L. (1959). Motor characteristics of the mentally retarded. *American Journal of Mental Deficiency, 63,* 792–811.

Frey, B., & Rimmer, J. H. (in press). Comparison of body composition between German and American adults with mental retardation. *Medicine and Science in Sports and Exercise.*

Gelfand, D. M., Jenson, W. R., & Drew, C. J. (1982). *Understanding child behavior's disorders.* New York: Holt, Rinehart and Winston.

Grossman, H. (Ed.). (1973). *Manual on terminology and classification in mental retardation.* Washington, DC: American Association on Mental Deficiency.

Grossman, H. (Ed.). (1983). *Classification in mental retardation.* Washington, DC: American Association on Mental Deficiency.

Hallahan, D. P., & Kauffman, J. M. (1991). *Exceptional children. Introduction to special education.* Englewood Cliffs, NJ: Prentice-Hall.

Halle, J. W., Silverman, N. A., & Regan, L. (1983). The effects of a data-based exercise program on physical fitness of retarded children. *Education and Training of the Mentally Retarded, 18,* 221–225.

Heber, R. F. (1961). Modifications in the manual on terminology and classification in mental retardation. *American Journal of Mental Deficiency, 65,* 499–500.

Himes, J. H., & Dietz, W. H. (1994). Guidelines for overweight in adolescent preventive services: recommendations from an expert committee. *American Journal of Clinical Nutrition, 59,* 307–316.

Kelly, L. E., Rimmer, J. H., & Ness, R. A. (1986). Obesity levels in institutionalized mentally retarded adults. *Adapted Physical Activity Quarterly, 3,* 167–176.

Kerby, D. S., & Dawson, B. L. (1994). Autistic features, personality, and adaptive behavior in males with the Fragile x syndrome and no autism. *American Journal of Mental Retardation, 98,* 455–462.

Kessler, J. W. (1988). *Psychopathology of childhood.* Englewood Cliffs, NJ: Prentice-Hall.

Kolata, G. (1989). Understanding Down syndrome: A chromosome holds the key. *New York Times,* December 5, p. C3.

Lachiewicz, A. M., Spiridigliozzi, G. A., Gullion, C. M., Ransford, S. N., & Rao, K. (1994). Aberrant behaviors of young boys with Fragile x syndrome. *American Journal of Mental Retardation, 98,* 567–579.

Lubetsky, M. J. (1993). Mental retardation. In R. T. Ammerman, C. G. Last, and M. Hersen (Eds.), *Handbook of prescriptive treatments for children and adolescents* (pp. 28–46). Boston: Allyn and Bacon.

Luckasson, R., Coulter, D. L., Polloway, E. A., Reiss, S., Schalock, R. L., Snell, M., Spitalnik, D., & Stark, J. (Eds.) (1992). *Mental retardation: Definition, classification, and systems of supports.* Washington, DC: American Association on Mental Retardation.

Pitetti, K. H., & Campbell, K. D. (1991). Mentally retarded individuals: A population at risk? *Medicine and Science in Sports and Exercise, 23,* 586–593.

Pitetti, K. H., Climstein, M., Campbell, K. D., Barrett, P. J., & Jackson, J. A. (1992). The cardiovascular capacities of adults with Down syndrome: A comparative study. *Medicine and Science in Sports and Exercise, 24,* 13–19.

Pitetti, K. H., Rimmer, J. H., & Fernhall, B. (1993). Physical fitness and adults with mental retardation. An overview of current research and future directions. *Sports Medicine, 16,* 23–56.

Pitetti, K. H., & Tan, D. M. (1990). Effects of a minimally supervised exercise program for mentally retarded adults. *Medicine and Science in Sports and Exercise, 23,* 594–601.

Pommering, T. L., Brose, J. A., Randolph, E., Murray, T. F., Purdy, R. W., Cadamagnani, P. E., & Foglesong, J. E. (1994). Effects of an aerobic exercise program on community-based adults with mental retardation. *Mental Retardation, 32,* 218–226.

Pueschel, S. M. (1988). Atlantoaxial instability in children with Down syndrome. *Down Syndrome News, 12,* 129–130.

Pueschel, S. M. (1990). Clinical aspects of Down syndrome from infancy to adulthood. *American Journal of Medical Genetics, 7 (suppl),* 52–56.

Rarick, G. L. (1980). Cognitive-motor relationships in the growing years. *Research Quarterly for Exercise and Sport, 51,* 174–192.

Rarick, G. L., Dobbins, D. A., & Broadhead, G. D. (1976). *The motor domain and its correlates in educationally handicapped children.* Englewood Cliffs, NJ: Prentice-Hall.

Reiss, S. (1994). Issues in defining mental retardation. *American Journal of Mental Retardation, 99,* 1–7.

Rimmer, J. H. (1994). *Fitness and rehabilitation programs for special populations.* Dubuque, IA: WCB Brown & Benchmark.

Rimmer, J. H., Braddock, D., & Fujiura, G. (1993). Prevalence of obesity in adults with mental retardation: implications for health promotion and disease prevention. *Mental Retardation, 31,* 105–110.

Rimmer, J. H., Braddock, D., & Fujiura, G. (1994). Cardiovascular risk factor levels in adults with mental retardation. *American Journal of Mental Retardation, 98,* 510–518.

Rimmer, J. H., Braddock, D., & Marks, B. (1994). *Health characteristics and behaviors of adults with mental retardation residing in three living arrangements.* Manuscript submitted for publication.

Rimmer, J. H., & Pitetti, K. H. (1994). *Obesity levels of children with mental retardation.* Unpublished manuscript.

Rubin, I. L. (1987). Health care needs of adults with mental retardation. *Mental Retardation, 25,* 201–206.

Russell, A. T., & Forness, S. R. (1985). Behavioral disturbance in mentally retarded children in TMR and EMR classrooms. *American Journal of Mental Deficiency, 89,* 338–344.

Saint-Laurent, L., Fournier, A., & Lessard, J. (1993). Efficacy of three programs for elementary school students with moderate mental retardation. *Education and Training in Mental Retardation, 28.*

Sherrill, C. (1993). *Adapted physical activity, recreation and sport.* Dubuque, IA: WCB Brown & Benchmark.

Tanguay, P. E. (1990). Mental retardation. In B. D. Garfinkel, G. A. Carlson, & E. B. Weller (Eds.), *Psychiatric disorders in children and adolescents* (pp. 291–305). Philadelphia: W. B. Saunders.

CHAPTER 26

SUICIDE ATTEMPTS AND COMPLETION DURING ADOLESCENCE: A BIOPSYCHOSOCIAL PERSPECTIVE

James C. Overholser, CASE WESTERN RESERVE UNIVERSITY

Anthony Spirito, BROWN UNIVERSITY SCHOOL OF MEDICINE

Dalia Adams, CASE WESTERN RESERVE UNIVERSITY

Suicidal behavior during adolescence includes a wide range of thoughts and actions. Suicidal thoughts can vary in frequency, intensity, and duration. Suicidal actions can vary across several dimensions, such as intentionality, impulsivity, and medical lethality of attempt. Even factors surrounding death by suicide can vary across individuals. Some suicides occur in adolescents who genuinely want to die, while others occur in individuals who make impulsive attempts using lethal methods. Thus, suicide ideators, attempters, and completers appear to consist of separate but overlapping populations (Linehan, 1986). In a corresponding way, suicidal adolescents can vary in their underlying psychological characteristics.

Given the diversity among suicidal adolescents, researchers and clinicians need to develop and test a comprehensive model of adolescent suicidal behavior. Clearly, no single factor, whether biological or psychological, can explain suicidal behavior among adolescents. Simple cause-effect models are inade-

quate. Instead, a biopsychosocial model (Engel, 1980) is necessary to understand the relative importance of many different factors. A biopsychosocial model acknowledges multiple pathways of causation, multiple systems (e.g., biological, psychological, and social factors), and interactions among variables and across systems.

This chapter reviews many factors that contribute to adolescent suicidal behavior. The goal of this review is to sensitize pediatric psychologists to factors that may interact to contribute to vulnerability in a particular adolescent. The biopsychosocial model may be of value in helping clinicians determine who is at risk for developing suicidal behavior, whether suicidal ideation or attempts are most likely seen, and develop a comprehensive understanding and synthesis of the many potential factors affecting outcome. At the same time, a multifactor, multilevel model helps determine treatment plans and assists clinicians in understanding how different treatments interact with each other and, with factors from the adolescent's environment, how to best promote behavior change (Schwartz, 1982).

EPIDEMIOLOGY OF ADOLESCENT SUICIDE

Suicide is the third leading cause of death in adolescents and young adults (aged 15 to 24). The suicide rate has steadily increased in this age group up to the 1980s (Rosenberg, Smith, Davidson, & Conn, 1987) and has remained high in the 1980s and 1990s. In a typical year, more than 2,000 adolescents in the United States die by suicide (National Center for Health Statistics, 1990). Suicide accounts for 14 percent of all deaths occurring to adolescents aged 15 to 19. Moreover, for every completed suicide, there are eight unsuccessful suicide attempts (Rosenberg et al., 1987); for example, in 1988, there were approximately 16,000 adolescents who received medical treatment following unsuccessful suicide attempts (Holinger, 1990). However, many more adolescents attempt suicide but never receive treatment or never become identified as suicidal. Thus, the actual number of adolescents who attempt suicide each year in the United States ranges between 200,000 and 4,000,000 (McGinnis, 1987).

One study found 7.1 percent of community adolescents had attempted suicide and 36 percent of depressed adolescents had attempted suicide at least once (Lewinsohn & Rohde, 1993). Furthermore, when high school students have completed surveys, approximately half of the students have reported that they have considered a suicide attempt (Adams, Overholser, & Lehnert, 1994; Smith & Crawford, 1986). Thus, it is important for professionals working with adolescents to be aware of the risk for suicidal behavior (both attempts and completion) because even an unsuccessful suicide attempt can change forever the life of the adolescent. Friends and family members may begin to respond differently to the adolescent, and the adolescent who has attempted suicide remains vulnerable to future suicide attempts (Lewinsohn, Rohde, & Seeley, 1994) and is at higher risk for eventual completed suicide.

A variety of demographic variables correlate with higher rates of suicide. For example, suicide rates differ by age, race, and gender of the individual. Although suicide rates are quite low for children younger than 14 years old (rate = 0.8/100,000), the rates climb substantially higher for adolescents (rate = 13.2/100,000; National Center for Health Statistics [NCHS], 1990).

Racial differences are prominent in suicide research. Whites have substantially higher rates of suicide than African Americans. Although the suicide rate for whites has been three times as high as the rate for African Americans, the suicide rate for African Americans has been increasing over recent years (NCHS, 1989). Also, Hispanic youth have a lower rate of suicide than white adolescents (NCHS, 1990). The suicide rate among Native Americans varies but is extremely high in some regions (McIntosh, 1983–1984).

Suicide rates also differ greatly across gender. In all age groups, females attempt suicide more often than males, but males complete suicide more often than females. In the United States during 1987, the suicide rate for adolescent males was 16.2 per 100,000 as compared to the rate for adolescent females of 4.2 per 100,000 (NCHS, 1989). However, in a large survey of high school students (Center for Disease Control, 1991), females were significantly more likely than males to report suicidal ideation, suicide plans, and suicide attempts.

At least part of the gender difference in suicide rates is because of the use of different suicide methods. Males are more likely to use highly lethal methods (e.g., gunshot wound to a vital organ), whereas females are more likely to use less violent and less lethal methods (e.g., drug overdose) (NCHS, 1989). Although some drugs can be lethal in high quantities, most suicide attempts by drug overdose act fairly slowly and are usually reversible if noticed and brought for medical attention. In contrast, the morbidity associated with most lethal methods (gunshot wound, jumping from a high place) occurs quickly and is often irreversible.

Demographic differences provide only a crude differentiation of suicidal versus nonsuicidal adolescents. In order to understand which adolescents are at highest risk for suicidal behavior, professionals need to examine a variety of biological, psychological, and social risk factors.

RISK FACTORS

Biological Factors

Research to date has identified very little about the biological basis of suicide among adolescents. Because of various methodological and procedural issues, almost all research on biological factors in suicide has occurred with adults. However, we can assume that the findings would generalize to adolescent samples.

Research on the biological correlates of suicide has examined the functioning of the endocrine system and neurotransmitter systems. Research has consistently linked abnormal activity of the hypothalamic-pituitary-adrenocortical (HPA) axis to depression. Although there has been some evidence of HPA hyperactivity in suicide victims (Nemeroff, Owens, Bissette, Andorn, & Stanley, 1988; Asberg, Nordstrom, & Traskman-Bendz, 1986), findings remain mixed (Mann, 1987), and abnormal HPA function may more closely relate to depressive illness than to suicidal behavior. However, the HPA axis has a functional connection to the neurotransmitter, serotonin (Meltzer, Perline, Tricou, Lowy, & Robertson, 1984), which has clearly established links to suicide.

Extensive research has occurred examining the role of monoamine neurotransmitters (dopamine, norepinephrine, and serotonin) in completed and attempted suicide. Investigators have assessed neurotransmitter levels and their activity through a variety of methods, including neurotransmitter metabolite levels in the cerebrospinal fluid (CSF) and receptor binding properties in postmortem brain tissue. Increased CSF metabolite levels indicate increased neurotransmitter activity. Decreased receptor binding and decreased binding site densities reflect a self-regulatory process and generally indicate increased levels of the neurotransmitter.

Although decreased noradrenergic activity may relate to suicidal behavior, the relationship between norepinephrine (noradrenaline) and suicide is not clear. Studies have shown that CSF levels of the norepinephrine metabolite, MHPG, both positively and negatively correlate with suicidal tendencies (Asberg et al., 1986). Other studies have found B-adrenergic binding in frontal cortex samples from suicide victims to be increased (Biegon & Israeli, 1988), unaltered

(Stockmeier & Meltzer, 1991), and decreased (Little, Clark, Ranc, & Duncan, 1993).

Decreased dopaminergic activity relates to depression and possibly to suicidal behavior. Several studies have reported that suicidal behavior correlates with low CSF concentrations of the dopamine metabolite, HVA (Mann, 1987). However, these findings are applicable to depressed patients only. Thus, low levels of dopaminergic activity may relate to an aspect of depression that increases the risk of suicide. A 5-year follow-up study (Roy, DeJong, & Linnoila, 1989) revealed that decreased dopaminergic activity related to repeated suicide attempts among depressed patients. Furthermore, low dopamine levels may more closely relate to violent rather than nonviolent suicides (Banki, Arato, Papp, & Kurcz, 1984).

The primary neurotransmitter implicated in suicide risk is serotonin. Research has found serotonin (5-HT), a serotonin precursor (5-HTP), and a serotonin metabolite (5-HIAA) to be at reduced levels in samples of suicide attempters. Low CSF 5-HIAA appears to relate to suicidal behavior regardless of psychiatric diagnosis (Asberg et al., 1986). However, postmortem serotonin receptor studies have not always yielded consistent results, but this may be due to the existence of two types (5-HT^1 & 5-HT^2) and several subtypes of serotonin receptors. The number of 5-HT^2 receptor sites tends to remain unchanged or become increased in suicide victims (Arora & Meltzer, 1989; Arranz, Eriksson, Mellerup, Plenge, & Marcusson, 1994), and the greatest increase in 5-HT^2 receptor sites occurs in violent suicides. A decreased number of 5-HT^{1D} receptor sites occurs in nondepressed suicide victims (Arranz et al., 1994). Further research is necessary to clarify differential activity of the various receptor sites and how they relate to suicide.

In general, reduced serotonin levels relate to repeated suicide attempts, impulse dyscontrol, and aggression in depressed and nondepressed samples (Roy, 1994; Roy et al., 1989; Traskman-Bendz, Alling, Alsen, Regnell, Simonsson, & Ohman, 1993). Low CSF levels of 5-HIAA can predict short-range suicide risk after attempted suicide in depressed patients (Nordstrom et al., 1994). Both low CSF 5-HIAA and low CSF HVA correlate with further suicidal behavior among depressed patients who have previously attempted suicide (Roy et al., 1989). Thus, reduced activity of serotonin and dopamine may relate to higher risk of death by suicide following an unsuccessful suicide attempt.

Although studies examining serotonin and dopamine levels have important implications for understanding the biochemical basis of suicide risk, clinically the assessment procedures are quite invasive, requiring a lumbar puncture to gather a specimen of CSF. However, we can measure serotonin metabolite levels in urine samples, which may ultimately provide a clinically useful method for assessing an individual patient's suicide risk. At present, clinical assessments of an individual's suicide risk rely on psychosocial factors.

Psychological Factors

Psychological risk factors for suicide include all aspects of the individual's psychological functioning at or before the time of the suicide attempt. It is interesting to speculate on psychological factors that were present long before the suicidal urges developed and therefore played a causal role in the suicide process. However, most psychological factors that have an empirically supported relationship with suicide risk focus on the cognitions and emotions that were present around the time of the suicidal act. Psychological risk factors focus on several main areas: psychiatric disorder, cognitive biases, impulsive tendencies, and previous life experiences.

Certain psychiatric disorders occur with some regularity in adolescents who attempt or complete suicide. Major depression closely relates to the presence of suicidal ideation and attempts among adolescents (Garrison, Jackson, Addy, McKeown, & Waller, 1991). Furthermore, a study conducted in Finland found depression is the most common diagnosis among adolescents who commit suicide (Marttunen et al., 1991). In the United States, the coexistence of antisocial and depressive symptoms correlates with a high risk for completed suicide (Blumenthal & Kupfer, 1986). Thus, depression sets the stage for many adolescents to begin thinking about death and suicide and to move closer toward their own self-destruction. Depression by itself is insufficient for suicide to occur, but it may be a common, if not necessary, antecedent for the onset of the suicide process. In addition to depression, the diagnosis of bipo-

lar disorder occurs in a substantial percentage of adolescents who have died by suicide (Brent et al., 1988).

Substance abuse may play an important role in many cases of suicide. A diagnosis of alcohol abuse significantly relates to suicidal behavior among both adolescent male and female psychiatric inpatients (Pfeffer, Newcorn, Kaplan, Mizruchi, & Plutchik, 1988). Alcohol abuse may lower a person's inhibitions, increasing the probability of acting in a reckless or aggressive manner. However, substance abuse plays a more prominent role in adolescent suicide when it occurs in the presence of a depressive disorder than when depression is absent (Brent et al., 1993). The comorbid presence of depression and substance abuse relates to increased suicidal intent (Brent et al., 1990) and increased risk of death by suicide (Brent et al., 1993). Thus, it becomes important to evaluate other suicide risk factors whenever an adolescent displays signs of either depression or substance abuse and most importantly when both problems are present.

Personality disorders relate to an increased risk of suicidal behavior. In a study from Finland on adolescents who died by suicide (Marttunen et al., 1991), 32 percent of the adolescents could have received personality disorder diagnoses. The two most common personality disorder diagnoses were antisocial personality (diagnosed in males) and borderline personality (diagnosed in both males and females). In many cases where suicidal adolescents receive a borderline personality disorder diagnosis, they also meet criteria for a diagnosis of substance abuse (Runeson, 1989).

Most adolescents who have died by suicide meet the diagnostic criteria for more than one psychiatric diagnosis (Shafii, Steltz-Lenarsky, Derrick, Beckner, & Whittinghill, 1988). For example, depression coexisting with substance abuse problems or a personality disorder suggests a substantially elevated risk beyond that accounted for by depression alone. Similarly, comorbid conduct problems in depressed adolescents relates to increased risk of suicidal behavior (Meyers et al., 1991). Thus, those adolescents at highest risk for death by suicide meet criteria for multiple psychiatric problems, often displaying tendencies for both internalizing and externalizing disorders.

It can be helpful to go beyond psychiatric diagnosis and examine psychological processes that underlie the problems that precipitate suicidal acts. Cognitive biases can play an important role in depression and suicidality. Aaron Beck (Beck, Rush, Shaw, & Emery, 1979) described the cognitive triad of depressive cognitions: a negative view of the self, one's world, and the future. A negative view of the self often involves low self-esteem and feelings of worthlessness. A negative view of one's world can involve feelings of helplessness, reactions to uncontrollable stressful events, feeling unable to cope with problems, and being unable to stop them. A negative view of the future, often described as hopelessness, seems most directly related to suicidal tendencies. Each of these cognitive factors will be described here.

Low self-esteem may be an important aspect of depression and increases the risk of suicidal ideation and suicide attempts (Overholser, Adams, Lehnert, & Brinkman, 1994). However, one study found self-esteem did not significantly differ between suicide attempters and nonsuicidal depressed adolescents (deWilde, Kienhorst, Diekstra, & Wolters, 1993). Thus, self-esteem may strongly correlate with depression, thoughts of death, suicidal ideation, and a desire to die but may not carry with it the active component that pushes an adolescent to act on these feelings.

A negative view of one's future, or hopelessness, refers to a pessimistic attitude about future events, including widespread negative expectation for the future. In many cases, suicidal patients perceive their current problems as severe and unlikely to improve even with treatment. Although depression and hopelessness closely relate to one another, hopelessness contributes unique variance to suicidal ideation beyond that explained by depression alone (Steer, Kumar, & Beck, 1993). Suicidal adolescents report more negative thoughts about the future and fewer positive thoughts about the future than do nonsuicidal adolescents (Lehnert, Overholser, & Adams, 1993). Among adolescent psychiatric inpatients, hopelessness increases with the number of suicidal gestures, seriousness of intent, and medical lethality of attempts (Robbins & Alessi, 1985; Topol & Reznikoff, 1982). However, in several studies (Brent, Kolko, Allan, & Brown, 1990; deWilde et al., 1993), adolescent suicide attempters did not report higher levels of hopelessness than did nonsuicidal depressed adolescents. Thus, hopelessness does relate to adolescent suicidal behavior, but mixed findings exist indicating the need

for further research examining the role of hopelessness in suicide risk among adolescents.

Some research has characterized adolescent suicide attempters as impulsive individuals (Kashden, Fremouw, Callahan, & Franzen, 1993; Withers & Kaplan, 1987). However, impulsiveness as a stable personality trait has been difficult to assess in a reliable and valid manner. It may be more useful to examine impulsiveness of the suicide attempt. In one study (Brown, Overholser, Spirito, & Fritz, 1991), the investigators classified adolescent suicide attempters as impulsive or reflective based on the amount of time and planning that preceded their suicide attempt. Group comparisons showed the nonimpulsive attempters felt more depressed and more hopeless and reported more frequent suicidal thoughts than their impulsive counterparts. Thus, adolescents who take time to plan their suicide attempts appear to be a particularly high-risk group.

Poor problem solving may play a role in suicidal behavior and seems related to impulsivity and hopelessness. Individuals who act impulsively often jump to conclusions without taking adequate time to think through problems and reflect on different options. Also, difficulties solving daily problems may engender feelings of pessimism and hopelessness. One recent study (Sadowski & Kelley, 1993) examined the social problem-solving abilities in 30 adolescent suicide attempters compared to 30 adolescent psychiatric control patients and 30 high school students. Suicide attempters reported less adequate problem solving and poorer problem-solving orientation than seen in either psychiatric controls or high school students. Furthermore, relative to the two other groups, the suicide attempters reported more emotional responding and less cognitive responding when confronted with problem situations. Thus, adolescent suicide attempters may have added difficulties responding to various life problems in a rational and reflective way. They may choose to deal with problems through avoidance and withdrawal instead of through active, constructive coping attempts.

In one study (Spirito, Overholser, & Stark, 1989) on adolescent coping strategies, social isolation and avoidance coping were common maladaptive strategies reported by suicide attempters. Compared to distressed and nondistressed high school control groups, adolescent suicide attempters were more likely to report using social withdrawal when faced with a problem. However, when adolescent suicide attempters were compared to nonsuicidal psychiatrically hospitalized adolescents, both groups reported using social withdrawal as a maladaptive coping strategy (Spirito, Francis, Overholser, & Frank, 1994). Thus, social isolation appears characteristic of adolescent psychopathology in general and is not specific to suicide attempters.

A potential risk factor for suicide is previous exposure to suicidal behavior. This can include having a friend or relative who attempted or died by suicide. In one study, adolescents who died by suicide were significantly more likely to have had some exposure to suicidal behavior in parents, relatives, or friends (Shafii, Carrigan, Whittinghill, & Derrick, 1985). Adolescents who had a friend attempt or die by suicide display higher levels of depression and more frequent suicidal behavior themselves than do adolescents without such experiences (Hazell & Lewin, 1993). The depression that follows the suicidal death of a friend tends to persist for at least six months (Brent et al., 1992). However, not all studies have found a relationship between adolescent suicide attempts and suicidal behavior among family members (Lewinsohn et al., 1994).

Exposure to suicide does relate to a history of previous suicide attempts by the patient. A past history of suicidal behavior significantly relates to recent suicide attempts in both male and female adolescent psychiatric inpatients (Pfeffer et al., 1988). After controlling for level of depression, adolescents who have attempted suicide once before are eight times more likely to attempt suicide again as compared to peers who have never attempted suicide (Lewinsohn et al., 1994). It appears that once an adolescent has attempted suicide, that adolescent has come to see suicide as an acceptable solution to life's problems. After an adolescent has broken the taboo against suicide, the possibility of future suicide attempts increases.

Social Factors

A lack of social support from family and friends may relate to psychopathology and suicidal behavior on the part of adolescents. Poor social skills also relate to depression (Spirito, Hart, Overholser, & Halverson,

1990). Furthermore, social withdrawal as a coping strategy relates to adolescent psychopathology and suicidal behavior (Spirito et al., 1994). Finally, compared to high school students, hospitalized adolescent suicide attempters are more likely to report the loss of a close friend or family member due to death, divorce, or the break-up of a relationship (Adams, Overholser, & Spirito, 1994). Thus, inadequate levels of social support available to an adolescent resulting from poor social skills, a tendency to isolate, or the loss of a close relationship, may play a role in the suicide process. The results of one study (King, Raskin, Gdowski, Butkus, & Opipari, 1990) indicate that adolescent suicide attempters do indeed report few supportive people in their lives.

Conversely, adolescents who report having close confiding relationships may be at reduced risk for suicidal behavior (King et al., 1990). Supportive and close relationships within the family may be particularly relevant to reducing the risk of suicidal behavior among adolescents. Suicide risk in adolescents positively correlates with levels of stressful events (Gispert, Wheeler, Marsh, & Davis, 1985), but a high degree of family cohesion reduces this effect of stressful events (Rubenstein, Heeren, Housman, Rubin, & Stechler, 1989). Furthermore, nonsuicidal high school students are more likely to report confiding relationships with parents than are suicidal students (Pronovost, Cote, & Ross, 1990). Thus, close relationships, especially within the family, seem to have a protective effect against suicide risk among adolescents.

Family relationships are an important consideration in understanding suicide risk among adolescents. Developmentally, adolescents are more independent than children, and an increasing proportion of the adolescent's significant life experiences occur outside of the family (Scarr & McCartney, 1983). However, compared with adults, adolescents are still more dependent on their families and possibly more vulnerable than adults to the stressful processes within the family (Swearingen & Cohen, 1985). An increased risk of adolescent suicidal behavior given family problems has been noted in research studies, case studies, and clinical observations. Both family-related stressful events (e.g., arguments, separations) and ongoing family dysfunction (e.g., poor communication, emotional disengagement) relate to adolescent suicidal behavior.

Family-related stressful events act as precipitants for adolescent suicidal behavior. According to the self-report of a large sample of community adolescents, thoughts of suicide primarily get triggered by family problems (Pronovost et al., 1990). Among adolescent suicide attempters presenting at emergency rooms, the most frequently reported precipitant of suicide attempts is parental problems (Tishler, McKenry, & Morgan, 1981). Thus, both adolescent suicidal ideation and suicide attempts can become triggered by family-related stressful events.

Child physical and sexual abuse, conceptualized as traumatic stressors, are important family-related stressors to consider in the study of adolescent suicidal behavior. One study (Deykin, Alpert, & McNamara, 1985) compared adolescent suicide attempters admitted to an emergency room to nonsuicidal adolescents admitted for medical reasons. The adolescent suicide attempters were three to six times more likely to have a case file with the local department of social services that responded to child abuse allegations. A relationship exists between child abuse and adolescent suicide risk (Hoberman & Garfinkel, 1988). Furthermore, a history of abuse relates to a greater number of suicide attempts and more serious attempts on the part of psychiatrically hospitalized adolescents relative to those who report no abuse history (Shaunesey, Cohen, Plummer, & Berman, 1993). Although a history of child abuse does relate to adolescent suicidal behavior, abuse may also be important in a wide spectrum of adolescent psychopathology (Kazdin, 1992). Furthermore, child abuse tends to occur in families characterized by chronic dysfunction (Alexander, 1993; Briere & Elliott, 1993), and research is essential to determine differential effects of family functioning and abuse on adolescent suicidal behavior.

In addition to family-related stressful events and traumatic events, chronic stress resulting from ongoing family dysfunction also contributes to the risk of adolescent suicidal behavior. Most studies examining the role of family functioning in adolescent suicide risk have relied on adolescents' perceptions of their families (Adams, Overholser, & Lehnert, 1994; Brent et al., 1990; King, Segal, & Naylor, 1992; Meneese &

Yutrzenka, 1990; Rubenstein et al., 1989). Suicidal adolescents report problematic parent-adolescent relationships and family dysfunction on a variety of dimensions.

Suicidal ideation in adolescents relates to poor communication (Stivers, 1988) and emotional disparity (Deykin et al., 1985) between parents and adolescents. When one considers the entire family system, adolescent suicidal ideation relates to family functioning characterized by conflict, poor communication, lack or organization, and lack of support for independence and personal achievement (Meneese & Yutrzenka, 1990). Thus, suicidal ideation among adolescents relates to several dimensions of family functioning and parent-adolescent relationships.

Family functioning variables also relate to adolescent suicide attempts. Research (Adams, Overholser, & Lehnert, 1994) shows that specific dimensions of family functioning relate to both adolescent suicide ideation and suicide attempts. Adolescent psychiatric inpatients who had attempted suicide and high school students who reported suicidal ideation perceived their families as having power struggles, poor communication, and inadequate problem-solving skills. The suicidal adolescents also reported that emotional involvement and communication of feelings among family members was problematic. In other studies (Paluszny, Davenport, & Kim, 1991; Topol & Reznikoff, 1982), adolescent suicide attempters have described their families as chaotic and poorly adjusted. Furthermore, the seriousness of suicidal intent among adolescent suicide attempters appears related to the degree of family dysfunction as perceived by the adolescents (Brent et al., 1990).

TEMPORAL FACTORS

Temporal factors provide important information often neglected in suicide risk and prevention. Suicidal adolescents report higher levels of stress during the 12 months prior to their hospitalization than do nonsuicidal depressed inpatients (Brent, Kolko, Allan, & Brown, 1990). Suicides are more likely to occur during certain stressful times than nonstressful times. Thus, evaluation of stressful life events can play an important role in understanding suicide. In a study of adolescents hospitalized following a suicide attempt (Adams, Overholser, & Spirito, 1994), the most common precipitants included major life events (e.g., legal trouble) and exit events (e.g., death of a loved one). Chronic strains (e.g., ongoing conflict with others) and stress from family and friends related to higher levels of depression and suicidal ideation.

Perhaps the most important high-risk time period occurs immediately following discharge from a psychiatric hospital. Becoming hospitalized for psychiatric problems is very stressful for most adolescents and can forever change their self-images. Furthermore, discharge from the hospital necessitates explaining their absence to teachers and peers. The stigma surrounding mental illness may further aggravate an adolescent's adjustment back into life in the community. Suicidal adolescents are at high risk for a second attempt within six months after their discharge from a psychiatric hospital (Brent et al., 1993). In one study of psychiatrically hospitalized adolescent suicide attempters, 23 percent reattempted suicide within one month and an additional 14 percent reattempted suicide within three months (Spirito et al., 1992). With the current standard of care emphasizing short-term hospital stays, it is likely that many depressed and suicidal patients will get discharged back into the same emotional environment that triggered the initial crisis, increasing the likelihood of another suicide attempt.

The sustained risk for reattempting suicide following discharge from a psychiatric hospital may be due to an improvement in depression that mobilizes the individual toward suicide. However, one longitudinal study identified cognitive factors that may underlie the tendency to reattempt suicide. Overholser, Miller, and Norman (1987) evaluated depressed and suicidal adult psychiatric inpatients at the time of their admission to a psychiatric hospital during a suicidal crisis and compared these patients to depressed, nonsuicidal inpatients. At the time of admission, both groups were similar in terms of depression severity and depressive cognitions. The investigation then reassessed both groups at the time of discharge from the hospital and again 4 months, 10 months, and 16 months post-discharge. By the time of the 16-month follow-up, both groups had recovered to an equivalent degree. However, the suicidal patients typically took much longer to recover, displayed negative cognitions that remained elevated well past the time of discharge from the hospital, and showed persistently high levels of hopelessness and suicidal ideation. Thus, the suicidal patients remained at risk for a sudden resurgence of suicidal feelings even after their depressive symptoms had begun to improve. Cognitive factors may be resistant to treatment and may underlie relapse following discharge from the hospital.

TREATMENT OF SUICIDAL PATIENTS

It is important for psychologists working with suicidal adolescents to be familiar with treatment options that are available. Unfortunately, very little research has examined utility of different treatment strategies for reducing suicide risk. Therefore, psychologists need to rely on two different areas that address treatment issues: theoretical reviews offering guidelines for treatment of suicide risk and empirically based guidelines that focus on treatment of depression but do not directly address suicide. In general, treatment of suicidal adolescents must address biological, psychological, and social factors related to the risk of suicide.

Biological factors related to treatment emphasize use of antidepressant medications. Many adolescents who become suicidal are suffering from a significant degree of depression that may be amenable to pharmacological treatment. Although antidepressant medications are quite useful with many adult patients, they are much less effective in treating depression in children and adolescents (Ambrosini, Bianchi, Rabinovich, & Elia, 1993). Therefore, clinicians may enhance treatment strategies by focusing on psychotherapy and family therapy.

Psychological factors that one can address in treatment cover a wide range of issues. Cognitive therapy can be helpful for reducing depressive thoughts and attitudes and for confronting feelings of pessimism and hopelessness. Depressed and suicidal adolescents often benefit from cognitive therapy designed to help them become aware of the relationship between thoughts, emotions, and behaviors; begin to monitor thoughts that increase the likelihood of depression; and begin to challenge the validity of certain negative thought patterns (Bedrosian & Epstein, 1984). Clients learn to monitor their automatic thoughts and evaluate evidence supporting their beliefs. Therapists encourage an attitude of collaborative empiricism in which clients perform specific activities designed to test evidence behind their beliefs. If the tests do not support their beliefs, then the clients need to consider revising these beliefs accordingly. As clients begin to make small but systematic changes in their behavior, they may be able to learn to identify and change cognitive biases that occur throughout their weekly activities (Freeman & Reinecke, 1993).

Problem-solving therapy can be helpful for many suicidal adolescents. Therapy with adolescents must often involve active teaching of new coping skills (Trautman, 1989). Feelings of hopelessness and pessimism often underlie suicidal feelings. When individuals become confronted with stressful life events, especially events for which they feel unable to cope, they may start to feel hopeless about their future. Problem-solving therapy can help teach adolescents new ways of conceptualizing problems in their lives and begin to see additional coping options that are available.

Effective use of cognitive therapy and problem-solving therapy requires establishment of a sound therapeutic alliance. The therapist must establish his or her role as a collaborator with the adolescent so that the adolescent does not perceive therapy as punishment or an extension of parental control (Wilkes & Rush, 1988). Even in short-term therapy, it is essential for therapists to develop a sound working alliance with clients so the clients feel the aim of therapy is to make changes they desire. Without this relationship, therapy is unlikely to succeed and clients may drop out of therapy prematurely.

Social factors relevant to treatment include improving the quality of relationships with one's peers and reducing conflict within the family. Social skills training can be useful to help adolescents improve their interpersonal functioning. Because depression often involves maladaptive interpersonal functioning, social skills training can help depressed adolescents learn new ways of relating to their peers (Becker, Heimberg, & Bellack, 1987). Clinicians might want to consider group therapy for treating depressed and suicidal adolescents. Group therapy can be helpful in teaching social skills and in reducing the isolation and stigma experienced by many depressed and suicidal adolescents. As their social relations improve and they develop additional close friendships,

problems in any one area become less disruptive to their overall social functioning. Thus, group therapy can help to reduce, prevent, or minimize two important factors associated with suicide attempts among adolescents: social isolation and lack of support. When working with depressed and suicidal adolescents, social skills training can be an important component of a broader treatment plan.

Family therapy can be helpful in reducing the frequency of destructive interactions between family members and in starting an adaptive process of change (Richman, 1979). Interventions that target both adolescents and their parents tend to be more effective than interventions that only target adolescents (Lewinsohn, Clarke, Hops, & Andrews, 1990). Family problems can play an important role precipitating suicidal behavior among adolescents. Family conflict tends to escalate as adolescents begin to assert their independence, and therapy can serve an important function by helping adolescents and their parents learn effective ways to communicate with each other (Lewinsohn & Rohde, 1993). Even when used as a short-term therapy approach, family therapy may help different family members begin to accept their responsibility for various problems within the family and begin to see suicidal adolescents as someone in need of assistance. Therapy can help dysfunctional families begin to move toward positive means of growth among the family members (Richman, 1986). Therapists can help increase positive feelings among family members and can promote adaptive skills in solving conflict (Rotheram-Borus et al., 1994). Many times, the progress initiated during family therapy sessions can continue after formal therapy has ended (Richman, 1986).

Clinicians must tailor the process of therapy to the needs and abilities of each adolescent. Some adolescents benefit most from action-oriented techniques, while others prefer more of a cognitive focus using the Socratic method (Wilkes & Rush, 1988). Adapting the style of therapy to an adolescent's level of cognitive development can help promote a better response to therapy (Schrodt & Fitzgerald, 1987).

The focus of therapy must vary at different stages of treatment (Overholser & Spirito, 1990). Suicidal adolescents pass through several distinct stages over the course of their recovery. It is important for therapists to plan treatment approaches that adapt to the needs of patients at particular times. For example, during an acute crisis, it is best to focus on concrete issues, such as removing access to guns, knives, or alcohol. An acute crisis episode is not the best time to attempt intensive psychotherapy. Instead, once a crisis has passed but suicidal feelings are still fairly recent, an adolescent may be willing to discuss feelings of depression and hopelessness and may begin working toward new solutions.

Even after suicidal adolescents have begun to show progress, therapy must continue to help clients develop new and effective ways of coping with suicidal feelings. It is important for therapists to be aware of the possibility of relapse in which a sudden resurgence of suicidal feelings may suddenly prompt a second suicide attempt. Adolescents must learn how to prepare themselves for high-risk situations that may elicit suicidal feelings and must practice their modified coping strategies. In this way, the long-term risk of suicidal behavior may diminish.

Adolescent suicide attempters are at high risk for dropping out of treatment after a few sessions (Trautman, Stewart, & Morishima, 1993). In an unpublished study of adolescent suicide attempters treated in an emergency room (cited in Trautman, 1989), 23 percent of the attempters failed to keep any follow-up appointments, another 19 percent kept only one appointment, and another 27 percent completed two evaluation sessions but refused to continue with treatment. Clearly, adolescent suicide attempters are at risk for noncompliance with continued treatment following their suicide attempts. Even more important is the continued risk for suicide displayed by these adolescents. Estimates indicate that 10 percent of adolescent suicide attempters will reattempt during the 12 months following their initial attempt (Hawton, Osborn, O'Grady, & Cole, 1982). In most cases, second attempts occur within 3 months after initial attempts (Hawton & Osborn, 1984).

Thus, relapse prevention guidelines (Brownell, Marlatt, Lichtenstein, & Wilson, 1986) can be helpful when treating suicidal adolescents. Even after treatment has been successful in reducing acute symptomatology, therapists must view their adolescent clients as remaining at risk for a sudden resurgence of suicidal feelings. Therapists may be able to help their adolescent clients anticipate difficult situations and practice new ways of coping. It can be helpful for adolescents to develop an emergency plan that outlines concrete steps to take if and when depression or suicidal feelings return (Lewinsohn & Rohde, 1993). Also, adolescents must learn to view progress as an ongoing activity, with occasional set-backs expected.

After a client has made adequate progress, treatment must not end abruptly. For many depressed and suicidal adolescents, it can be helpful to have occasional "booster sessions" every few months in order to allow the adolescents to stay in touch with their therapists, reassess the clients' moods and suicidal thoughts, and review material covered during the regular therapy sessions (Lewinsohn & Rohde, 1993). Because adolescent suicide attempters are at high risk for future suicide attempts, booster sessions can be an important means of adolescent suicide prevention.

SUICIDE PREVENTION STRATEGIES

The prevention of suicide is an important goal for all mental health professionals. Primary prevention strategies attempt to make changes at the societal level in order to reduce the frequency of suicide in a given population. Three general primary prevention strategies exist: restricting access to methods used when attempting suicide, educational programs designed to increase awareness of suicide risk factors and prevention resources, and establishing services in the community to help people deal with their emotional crises. Each of these three strategies will be discussed as related to the work of a pediatric psychologist.

Efforts designed to restrict access to methods used in suicide attempts usually focus on gas asphyxiation, drug overdose, and availability of handguns (see Spirito & Overholser, in press). Most relevant to prevention of adolescent suicide is reducing access to relatively lethal drugs that adolescents could use in their suicide attempts. Many adolescent suicide attempts are impulsive acts (Brown et al., 1991), and drug overdose is the most common method of suicide attempt among adolescents. Limiting access to drugs can make it difficult for adolescents to attempt suicide. Availability of a particular suicide method, such as drugs, plays a prominent role in determining lethality of the attempt (Brent, 1987). Thus, physicians and nurses must learn about suicide risk factors and the possibility of suicide by drug overdose, and they must also become more conservative in their prescription practices than they currently are.

Schools can play an important role in adolescent suicide prevention. Pediatric psychologists can play an important role as liaisons with schools, before, during, or after a student attempts suicide. Established educational programs can inform teachers and students about suicide risk factors and suicide prevention resources available in the community. Most suicide awareness programs attempt to heighten awareness of suicide as a problem among adolescents, educate participants about warning signs suggesting a person is at risk for suicidal feelings, and provide teachers and students with information about community resources to help with mental health problems (Shaffer, Garland, Gould, Fisher, & Trautman, 1988). In addition, some programs try to improve students' abilities to cope with various problems.

One suicide prevention program (Spirito, Overholser, Ashworth, Morgan, & Benedict-Drew, 1988) first assessed 473 adolescents using measures of knowledge, attitudes, and behaviors pertaining to suicide. Then, half the students participated in a 6-week suicide awareness curriculum led by their teachers. All students then completed the assessment measures again 10 weeks after the initial testing. Results showed that students who participated in the suicide awareness program increased their knowledge about suicide and were more aware of risk factors for suicide than they were prior to the program. Also, students showed attitude changes, becoming less likely to view suicidal individuals as weak or disturbed. Also, female students started the program with better understanding of suicide and fewer negative attitudes than did male students. Nonetheless, females were more likely than males to benefit from the suicide prevention program.

In a related study (Overholser, Hemstreet, Spirito, & Vyse, 1989) 471 high school students completed assessment measures regarding their knowledge and attitudes toward suicide. Approximately half of these students then participated in a suicide awareness program. Results again showed that females began the program with better knowledge and attitudes about suicide than did males, and females still benefited from the program more than did the male students. Also, students who knew a peer that had attempted suicide were more responsive to the in-formation presented in the program. Personal exposure to suicidal behavior in a peer helped these students learn factual material and change their negative attitudes toward suicidal individuals.

Despite apparent utility of educational programs, controversy exists over the risks and benefits of suicide educational programs. Some studies have failed to show educational programs have a substantial short-term (Shaffer et al., 1990) or long-term (Vieland, Whittle, Garland, Hicks, & Shaffer, 1991) impact on adolescents and their ability to deal with suicidal urges in themselves or their classmates. Furthermore, Shaffer and colleagues (1988) asserted that educational programs lack adequate utility to warrant the costs. Because suicide is a low base rate problem, effectively educating 100,000 adolescents may prevent nine suicides. Although this may not reflect a high number of adolescents, it still seems worthwhile. One suicide attempt can greatly affect the life of an adolescent as well as the lives of the adolescent's friends and family. If programs can increase the sensitivety of students, teachers, and other school personnel to suicide risk factors, warning signs, and high-risk times, it becomes easier to identify adolescents at risk for suicide. If we can then identify adolescents at risk and make appropriate resources available to these adolescents, we can subsequently prevent some suicides.

Establishing community services to help people cope with emotional crises has been the main focus of suicide prevention centers. Suicide prevention centers provide immediate, anonymous counseling free or at very low cost to individuals. Despite the logic behind suicide prevention centers, research suggests their impact in reducing the rate of suicide is weak (Dew, Bromet, Brent, & Greenhouse, 1987; Lester, 1993) or limited to certain subgroups of the population (Miller, Coombs, Leeper, & Barton, 1984). Thus, educational programs may hold the most potential for prevention of suicidal behavior among adolescents.

SUMMARY

Suicide is a complex problem reflecting the culmination of numerous biological, psychological, and social risk factors. Adolescents who attempt or die by suicide typically have a history of multiple risk factors. No single risk factor alone seems capable of pushing an individual toward suicide. Therefore, in order to understand suicide, multiple perspectives are necessary. An integration of views helps mental health professionals look beyond the limitations of any one orientation. Pediatric psychologists working with suicidal patients need to retain a focus on the synthesis of biopsychosocial factors.

Approaches to treatment and prevention of suicide among adolescents must incorporate elements from several different perspectives. Overreliance on a single approach may limit effectiveness of these techniques. Perhaps most importantly, pediatric psychologists can play a vital role in identification of suicidal adolescents and education of other professionals. Pediatric psychologists may be able to educate physicians, nurses, and secondary school teachers about suicide risk factors and effective prevention strategies. In this way, pediatric psychologists may be able to have a broad, albeit indirect, impact on numerous adolescents and their families.

REFERENCES

Adams, D., Overholser, J., & Lehnert, K. (1994). Perceived family functioning and adolescent suicidal behavior. *Journal of the American Academy of Child and Adolescent Psychiatry, 33,* 498–507.

Adams, D., Overholser, J., & Spirito, A. (1994). Stressful life events related to adolescent suicide attempts. *Canadian Journal of Psychiatry, 39,* 43–48.

Alexander, P. C. (1993). The differential effects of abuse characteristics and attachment in the prediction of long-term effects of sexual abuse. *Journal of Interpersonal Violence, 8,* 346–362.

Ambrosini, P., Bianchi, M., Rabinovich, H., & Elia, J. (1993). Antidepressant treatments in adolescents: I. Affective disorders. *Journal of the American Academy of Child and Adolescent Psychiatry, 32,* 1–6.

Arora, R. C., & Meltzer, H. Y. (1989). Serotonergic measures in the brains of suicide victims: 5-HT_2 binding sites in the frontal cortex of suicide victims and control subjects. *American Journal of Psychiatry, 146,* 730–736.

Arranz, B., Eriksson, A., Mellerup, E., Plenge, P., & Marcusson, J. (1994). Brain 5-HT_{1A}, 5-HT_{1D}, and 5-HT_2 receptors in suicide victims. *Biological Psychiatry, 35,* 457–463.

Asberg, M., Nordstrom, P., & Traskman-Bendz, L. (1986). Cerebrospinal fluid studies in suicide: An overview. *Annals New York Academy of the Sciences, 487,* 243–255.

Balon, R. (1987). Suicide: Can we predict it? *Comprehensive Psychiatry, 28,* 236–241.

Banki, C. M., Arato, M., Papp, Z., & Kurcz, M. (1984). Biochemical markers in suicidal patients. Investigations with cerebrospinal fluid amine metabolites and neuroendocrine tests. *Journal of Affective Disorders, 6,* 341–350.

Beck, A. T., Brown, G., Berchick, R. J., Stewart, B. L., & Steer, R. A. (1990). Relationship between hopelessness and ultimate suicide: A replication with psychiatric outpatients. *American Journal of Psychiatry, 147,* 190–195.

Beck, A. T., Brown, G., & Steer, R. A. (1989). Prediction of eventual suicide in psychiatric inpatients by clinical rating of hopelessness. *Journal of Consulting and Clinical Psychology, 57,* 309–310.

Beck, A. T., Rush, A. J., Shaw, B., & Emery, G. (1979). *Cognitive therapy of depression.* New York: Guilford.

Beck, A. T., & Steer, R. (1989). Clinical predictors of eventual suicide: A 5- to 10-year prospective study of suicide attempters. *Journal of Affective Disorders, 17,* 203–209.

Beck, A. T., Steer, R. A., Kovacs, M., & Garrison, B. (1985). Hopelessness and eventual suicide: A 10-year prospective study of patients hospitalized with suicidal ideation. *American Journal of Psychiatry, 142,* 559–563.

Becker, R., Heimberg, R., & Bellack, A. (1987). *Social skills training treatment for depression.* New York: Pergamon.

Bedrosian, R., & Epstein, N. (1984). Cognitive therapy of depressed and suicidal adolescents. In H. Sudak, A. Ford, & N. Rushforth (Eds.), *Suicide in the young* (pp. 345–366). Boston: John Wright.

Biegon, A., & Israeli, M. (1988). Regionally selective increases in B-adrenergic receptor density in the brains of suicide victims. *Brain Research, 42,* 199–203.

Blumenthal, S. J., & Kupfer, D. J. (1986). Generalizable treatment strategies for suicidal behavior. *Annals of the New York Academy of Science, 487,* 327–340.

Blumenthal, S. J., & Kupfer, D. J. (Eds.). (1988). *Suicide over the life cycle: Risk factors, assessment, and treatment of suicidal patients.* Washington, DC: American Psychiatric Press.

Brent, D. (1987). Correlates of the medical lethality of suicide attempts in children and adolescents. *Journal of the American Academy of Child and Adolescent Psychiatry, 26,* 87–89.

Brent, D., Kolko, D., Allan, M., & Brown, R. (1990). Suicidality in affectively disordered adolescent inpatients. *Journal of the American Academy of Child and Adolescent Psychiatry, 29,* 586–593.

Brent, D., Perper, J., & Allman, C. (1987). Alcohol, firearms, and suicide among youth: Temporal trends in Allegheny County, Pennsylvania, 1960 to 1983. *Journal of the American Medical Association, 257,* 3369–3372.

Brent, D., Perper, J., Allman, C., Moritz, G., Wartella, M., & Zelenar, J. (1991). The presence and availability of firearms in the homes of adolescent suicides: A case-control study. *Journal of the American Medical Association, 266,* 2989–2995.

Brent, D., Perper, T., Goldstein, C., Kolko, D., Allan, M., Allman, C., & Zelanek, J. (1988). Risk factors for adolescent suicide: A comparison of adolescent suicide victims with suicidal inpatients. *Archives of General Psychiatry, 45,* 581–588.

Brent, D., Perper, J., Moritz, G., Allman, C., Friend, A., Roth, C., Schweers, J., Balach, L., & Baugher, M. (1993). Psychiatric risk factors for adolescent suicide: A case-control study. *Journal of the American Academy of Child and Adolescent Psychiatry, 32,* 521–529.

Brent, D., Perper, J., Moritz, G., Allman, C., Friend, A., Schweers, J., Roth, C., Balanch, L., & Harrington, K. (1992). Psychiatric effects of exposure to suicide among the friends and acquaintances of adolescent suicide victims. *Journal of the American Academy of Child and Adolescent Psychiatry, 31,* 629–640.

Briere, J., & Elliott, D. (1993). Sexual abuse, family environment, and psychological symptoms: On the validity of statistical control. *Journal of Consulting and Clinical Psychology, 61,* 284–288.

Brown, L., Overholser, J., Spirito, A., & Fritz, G. (1991). The correlates of planning in adolescent suicide attempts. *Journal of the American Academy of Child and Adolescent Psychiatry, 30,* 95–99.

Brownell, K., Marlatt, G. A., Lichtenstein, H., & Wilson, G. T. (1986). Understanding and preventing relapse. *American Psychologist, 41,* 765–782.

Center for Disease Control. (1991). Attempted suicide among high school students—United States, 1990. *Morbidity and Mortality Weekly Report, 40,* 633–635.

Christoffel, K., Marcus, D., Sagerman, S., & Bennett, S. (1988). Adolescent suicide and suicide attempts: A population study. *Pediatric Emergency Care, 4,* 32–40.

Dew, M. A., Bromet, E. T., Brent, D., & Greenhouse, J. B. (1987). A quantitative literature review of the effectiveness of suicide prevention centers. *Journal of Consulting and Clinical Psychology, 55,* 239–244.

deWilde, E., Kienhorst, I., Diekstra, R., & Wolters, W. (1993). The specificity of psychological characteristics of adolescent suicide attempters. *Journal of the American Academy of Child and Adolescent Psychiatry, 32,* 51–59.

Deykin, E. Y., Alpert, J. J., & McNamara, J. J. (1985). A pilot study of the effect of exposure to child abuse or neglect on adolescent suicidal behavior. *American Journal of Psychiatry, 142,* 1299–1303.

Engel, G. L. (1980). The clinical application of the biopsychosocial model. *American Journal of Psychiatry, 137,* 535–544.

Freeman, A., & Reinecke, M. (1993). *Cognitive therapy of suicidal behavior: A manual for treatment.* New York: Springer.

Garrison, C., Jackson, K., Addy, C., McKeown, R., &

Waller, J. (1991). Suicidal behaviors in young adolescents. *American Journal of Epidemiology, 133,* 1005–1014.

Gibbs, J. T. (1988). Conceptual, methodological and sociocultural issues in black youth suicide: Indications for assessment and early intervention. *Suicide and Life Threatening Behavior, 18,* 73–89.

Gispert, M., Wheeler, K., Marsh, L., & Davis, M. S. (1985). Suicidal adolescents: Factors in evaluation. *Adolescence, 20,* 753–762.

Harkavy-Friedman, T. M., Asnis, G. M., Boeck, M., & DiFiore, J. (1987). Prevalence of specific suicidal behavior in a high school sample. *American Journal of Psychiatry, 144,* 1203–1206.

Hawton, K., & Catalan, J. (1987). *Attempted suicide: A practical guide to its nature and management.* New York: Oxford.

Hawton, K., & Osborn, M. (1984). Suicide and attempted suicide in children and adolescents. In B. Lahey & A. Kazdin (Eds.), *Advances in clinical child psychiatry* (Vol. 7). New York: Plenum.

Hawton, K., Osborn, M., O'Grady, J., & Cole, D. (1982). Classification of adolescents who take overdoses. *British Journal of Psychiatry, 140,* 124–131.

Hazell, P., & Lewin, T. (1993). Friends of adolescent suicide attempters and completers. *Journal of the American Academy of Child and Adolescent Psychiatry, 32,* 76–81.

Hoberman, H. M., & Garfinkel, B. D. (1988). Completed suicide in youth. *Canadian Journal of Psychiatry, 33,* 494–504.

Holinger, P. C. (1989). Epidemiologic issues in youth suicide. In C. Pfeffer (Ed.), *Suicide among youth: Perspectives on risk and prevention* (pp. 41–62). Washington, DC: American Psychiatric Press.

Holinger, P. C. (1990). The causes, impact, and preventability of childhood injuries in the United States. Childhood suicide in the United States. *American Journal of Diseases of Children, 144,* 670–676.

Kashden, J., Fremouw, W., Callahan, T., & Franzen, M. (1993). Impulsivity in suicidal and nonsuicidal adolescents. *Journal of Abnormal Child Psychology, 21,* 339.

Kazdin, A. E. (1992). Child and adolescent dysfunction and paths toward maladjustment: Targets for intervention. *Clinical Psychology Review, 12,* 795–817.

King, C., Raskin, A., Gdowski, C., Butkus, M., & Opipari, L. (1990). Psychosocial factors associated with urban adolescent female suicide attempts. *Journal of the American Academy of Child and Adolescent Psychiatry, 29,* 289–294.

King, C. A., Segal, H. G., & Naylor, M. W. (June 1992). *Family system factors and suicidality among adolescent inpatients.* Paper presented at the International Conference on Suicidal Behavior, Pittsburgh.

Kuperman, S., Black, D. W., & Burns, T. L. (1988). Excess suicide among formerly hospitalized child psychiatry patients. *Journal of Clinical Psychiatry, 49,* 88–93.

Lehnert, K. L., Overholser, J. C., & Adams, D. M. (November 1993). *Assessment of cognitions in adolescent psychiatric inpatients using the Rotter Incomplete Sentences Blank.* Presented at the Association for the Advancement of Behavioral Therapy (AABT) Convention, Atlanta.

Lester, D. (1993). The effectiveness of suicide prevention centers. *Suicide and Life Threatening Behavior, 23,* 263–267.

Lester D., & Murrell, M. E. (1980). The influence of gun control laws on suicidal behavior. *American Journal of Psychiatry, 137,* 121–122.

Lewinsohn, P., Clarke, G., Hops, H., & Andrews, J. (1990). Cognitive-behavioral treatment for depressed adolescents. *Behavior Therapy, 21,* 385–401.

Lewinsohn, P., & Rohde, P. (1993). The cognitive-behavioral treatment of depression in adolescents: Research and suggestions. *The Clinical Psychologist, 46,* 177–183.

Lewinsohn, P., Rohde, P., & Seeley, J. (1994). Psychosocial risk factors for future adolescent suicide attempts. *Journal of Consulting and Clinical Psychology, 62,* 297–305.

Linehan, M. (1986). Suicidal people: One population or two? *Annals of the New York Academy of Science, 487,* 16–33.

Little, K. Y., Clark, T. B., Ranc, J., & Duncan, G. E. (1993). B-adrenergic receptor binding in frontal cortex from suicide victims. *Biological Psychiatry, 34,* 596–605.

Mann, J. J. (1987). Psychobiologic predictors of suicide. *Journal of Clinical Psychiatry, 48,* 39–43.

Marttunen, M., Aro, H., Henriksson, M., & Lonnqvist, J. (1991). Mental disorders in adolescent suicide: DSM-III-R Axes I and II diagnoses in suicides among 13- to 19-year-olds in Finland. *Archives of General Psychiatry, 48,* 834–839.

McGinnis, J. M. (1987). Suicide in America—Moving up the public health agenda. *Suicide and Life Threatening Behavior, 17,* 18–32.

McIntosh, J. (1983–84). Suicide among Native Americans: Further tribal data and considerations. *Journal of Death and Dying, 14,* 215–229.

Meltzer, H., Perline, R., Tricou, B., Lowy, M., & Robertson, A. (1984). Effect of 5-hydroxytryptophan on serum cortisol levels in major affective disorders. II: Relation to suicide, psychosis, and depressive symptoms. *Archives of General Psychiatry, 41,* 379–387.

Meneese, W. B., & Yutrzenka, B. A. (1990). Correlates of suicidal ideation among rural adolescents. *Suicide and Life Threatening Behavior, 20*(3), 206–212.

Meyers, K., McCauley, E., Calderon, R., Mitchell, J., Burke, P., & Schloredt, K. (1991). Risks for suicidality in major depressive disorder. *Journal of the American Academy of Child and Adolescent Psychiatry, 30,* 86–94.

Miller, H. L., Coombs, D. W., Leeper, J. D., & Barton, S. N. (1984). An analysis of the effects of suicide prevention facilities on suicide rates in the United States. *American Journal of Public Health, 74,* 340–343.

National Center for Health Statistics. (1989). Annual summary of births, marriages, divorces, and deaths: United States, 1988. *Monthly Vital Statistics Report, 37*(13), 21.

National Center for Health Statistics. (1990). *Final mortality statistics, 1987.* Washington, DC: U.S. Government Printing Office.

Nemeroff, C., Owens, M., Bissette, G., Andorn, A., & Stanley, M. (1988). Reduced corticotropin releasing factor binding sites in the frontal cortex of suicide victims. *Archives of General Psychiatry, 45,* 577–579.

Nordstrom, P., Samuelsson, M., Asberg, M., Traskman-Bendz, L., Aberg-Wistedt, A., Nordin, C., & Bertilsson, L. (1994). CSF 5-HIAA predicts suicide risk after attempted suicide. *Suicide and Life Threatening Behavior, 24,* 1–9.

Overholser, J., Adams, D., Lehnert, K., & Brinkman, D. (1994). Self-esteem deficits in adolescent psychiatric inpatients. Manuscript submitted for publication.

Overholser, J., Evans, S., & Spirito, A. (1990). Sex differences and their relevance to the primary prevention of adolescent suicide. *Death Studies, 14,* 391–402.

Overholser, J. C., Hemstreet, A., Spirito, A., & Vyse, S. (1989). Suicide awareness programs in the schools: Effects of gender and personal experience. *Journal of the American Academy of Child and Adolescent Psychiatry, 28,* 925–930.

Overholser, J., Miller, I., & Norman, W. (1987). The course of depressive symptoms in suicidal versus nonsuicidal depressed inpatients. *Journal of Nervous and Mental Disease, 175,* 450–456.

Overholser, J. C., & Spirito, A. (1990). Cognitive-behavioral treatment of suicidal depression. In E. Feindler & G. Kalfus (Eds.), *Adolescent behavior therapy handbook* (pp. 211–231). New York: Springer.

Paluszny, M., Davenport, C., & Kim, W. J. (1991). Suicide attempts and ideation: Adolescents evaluated on a pediatric ward. *Adolescence, 26*(101), 209–215.

Pfeffer, C., Newcorn, J., Kaplan, G., Mizruchi, M., & Plutchik, R. (1988). Suicidal behavior in adolescent psychiatric inpatients. *Journal of the American Academy of Child Psychiatry, 27,* 357–361.

Pronovost, J., Cote, L., & Ross, C. (1990). Epidemiological study of suicidal behavior among secondary-school students. *Canada's Mental Health, 38*(1), 9–14.

Rich, C. L., Warsradt, G., Nemiroff, R., Fowler, R., & Young, D. (1991). Suicide, stressors, and the life cycle. *American Journal of Psychiatry, 148,* 524–527.

Richman, J. (1979). The family therapy of attempted suicide. *Family Process, 18,* 131–142.

Richman, J. (1986). *Family therapy for suicidal people.* New York: Springer.

Robbins, D., & Alessi, N. (1985). Depressive symptoms and suicidal behavior in adolescents. *American Journal of Psychiatry, 142,* 588–592.

Rotheram-Borus, M., Piacentini, J., Miller, S., Graae, F., & Castro-Blanco, D. (1994). Brief cognitive-behavioral treatment for adolescent suicide attempters and their families. *Journal of the American Academy of Child and Adolescent Psychiatry, 33,* 508–517.

Rosenberg, M., Smith, J., Davidson, L., & Conn, J. (1987). The emergence of youth suicide: An epidemiologic analysis and public health perspective. *Annual Review of Public Health, 8,* 417–440.

Roy, A. (1994). Recent biological studies on suicide. *Suicide and Life-Threatening Behavior, 24,* 10–14.

Roy, A., DeJong, J., & Linnoila, M. (1989). Cerebrospinal fluid monoamine metabolites and suicidal behavior in depressed patients. *Archives of General Psychiatry, 46,* 609–612.

Roy, A., & Linnoila, M. (1986). Alcoholism and suicide. In R. Maris (Ed.), *Biology of suicide.* New York: Guilford.

Rubenstein, J. L., Heeren, T., Housman, D., Rubin, C., & Stechler, G. (1989). Suicidal behavior in "normal" adolescents: Risk and protective factors. *American Journal of Orthopsychiatry, 59*(1), 59–71.

Runeson, B. (1989). Mental disorder in youth suicide: DSM-III-R Axes I and II. *Acta Psychiatrica Scandinavica, 79,* 490–497.

Sadowski, C., & Kelley, M. L. (1993). Social problem solving in suicidal adolescents. *Journal of Consulting and Clinical Psychology, 61,* 121–127.

Saltzman, L. E., Levenson, A., & Smith, J. C. (1988). Suicides among persons 15–24 years of age, 1970–1984. *Morbidity and Mortality Weekly Reports, 37,* 61–68.

Scarr, S., & McCartney, K. (1983). How people make their own environments: A theory of genotype → environment effects. *Child Development, 54,* 424–435.

Schrodt, G. R., & Fitzgerald, B. (1987). Cognitive therapy with adolescents. *American Journal of Psychotherapy, 41,* 402–408.

Schwartz, G. E. (1982). Testing the biopsychosocial model: The ultimate challenge facing behavioral medicine? *Journal of Consulting and Clinical Psychology, 50,* 1040–1053.

Shaffer, D., Garland, A., Gould, M., Fisher, P., & Trautman, P. (1988). Preventing teenage suicide: A critical review. *Journal of American Academy of Child and Adolescent Psychiatry, 27,* 675–687.

Shaffer, D., Vieland, V., Garland, A., Rojas, M., Underwood, M., & Busner, C. (1990). Adolescent suicide attempters: Response to suicide-prevention programs. *Journal of the American Medical Association, 264,* 3151–3155.

Shafii, M., Carrigan, T., Whittinghill, T. R., & Derrick, A. (1985). Psychological autopsy of completed suicide in children and adolescents. *American Journal of Psychiatry, 142,* 1061–1064.

Shafii, M., Steltz-Lenarsky, J., Derrick, A., Beckner, C., & Whittinghill, J. (1988). Comorbidity of mental disorders in the post-mortem diagnosis of completed suicide in children and adolescents. *Journal of Affective Disorders, 15,* 227–233.

Shaunesey, M., Cohen, J., Plummer, B., & Berman, A. (1993). Suicidality in hospitalized adolescents: Relationship to prior abuse. *American Journal of Orthopsychiatry, 63,* 113–119.

Smith, K., & Crawford, S. (1986). Suicidal behavior among normal high school students. *Suicide and Life Threatening Behavior, 16,* 313–325.

Spirito, A., Francis, G., Overholser, J., & Frank, N. (1994). Coping, depression, and adolescent suicide attempts. Manuscript submitted for publication.

Spirito, A., Hart, K., Overholser, J., & Halverson, J. (1990). Social skills and depression in adolescent suicide attempters. *Adolescence, 25,* 543–552.

Spirito, A., & Overholser, J. (in press). Primary and secondary prevention strategies for reducing suicide among youth. *Child and Adolescent Mental Health Care.*

Spirito, A., Overholser, J., Ashworth, S., Morgan, J., & Benedict-Drew, C. (1988). Evaluation of a suicide awareness curriculum for high school students. *Journal of the American Academy of Child and Adolescent Psychiatry, 27,* 705–711.

Spirito, A., Overholser, J., & Stark, L. (1989). Common problems and coping strategies, II: Findings with adolescent suicide attempters. *Journal of Abnormal Child Psychology, 17,* 213–221.

Spirito, A., Plummer, B., Gispert, M., Levy, S., Kurkijian, J., Lewander, W., Hagberg, S., & Devost, L. (1992). Adolescent suicide attempts: Outcomes at follow-up. *American Journal of Orthopsychiatry, 62,* 464–468.

Stafford, M., & Weishert, R. (1988). Changing age patterns of U.S. male and female suicide rates, 1934–1983. *Suicide and Life Threatening Behavior, 18,* 149–163.

Stanley, M., & Stanley, B. (1989). Biochemical studies in suicide victims: Current findings and future implications. *Suicide and Life Threatening Behavior, 19,* 30–42.

Steer, R., Kumar, G., & Beck, A. T. (1993). Self-reported suicidal ideation in adolescent psychiatric inpatients. *Journal of Consulting and Clinical Psychology, 61,* 1096–1099.

Stivers, C. (1988). Parent-adolescent communication and its relationship to adolescent depression and suicide proneness. *Adolescence, 23*(90), 291–295.

Stockmeier, C. A., & Meltzer, H. Y. (1991). *B*-adrenergic receptor binding in frontal cortex of suicide victims. *Biological Psychiatry, 29,* 183–191.

Swearingen, E. M., & Cohen, L. H. (1985). Life events and psychological distress: A prospective study of young adolescents. *Developmental Psychology, 21,* 1045–1054.

Tishler, C. L., McKenry, P. C., & Morgan, K. C. (1981). Adolescent suicide attempts: Some significant factors. *Suicide and Life Threatening Behavior, 11*(1), 86–92.

Topol, P., & Reznikoff, M., (1982). Perceived peer and family relationships, hopelessness and locus of control as factors in adolescent suicide attempts. *Suicide and Life Threatening Behavior, 12*(3), 141–150.

Traskman-Bendz, L., Alling, C., Alsen, M., Regnell, G., Simonsson, P., & Ohman, R. (1993). The role of monoamines in suicidal behavior. *Acta Psychiatrica Scandinavica, 371*, 45–47.

Trautman, P. (1989). Specific treatment modalities for adolescent suicide attempters. In Report of the Secretary's Task Force on Youth Suicide, *Vol. 3: Prevention and interventions on youth suicide.* DHHS Pub. No. 89-1623. Washington, DC: U.S. Government Printing Office.

Trautman, P., Stewart, N., & Morishima, A. (1993). Are adolescent suicide attempters noncompliant with outpatient care? *Journal of the American Academy of Child and Adolescent Psychiatry, 32,* 89–94.

Vieland, V., Whittle, B., Garland, A., Hicks, R., & Shaffer, D. (1991). The impact of curriculum-based suicide prevention programs for teenagers: An 18-month follow-up. *Journal of the American Academy of Child and Adolescent Psychiatry, 30,* 811–815.

Wilkes, T. C., & Rush, A. J. (1988). Adaptations of cognitive therapy for depressed adolescents. *Journal of the American Academy of Child and Adolescent Psychiatry, 27,* 381–386.

Withers, L., & Kaplan, D. (1987). Adolescents who attempt suicide: A retrospective clinical chart review of hospitalized patients. *Professional Psychology: Research and Practice, 18,* 391–393.

CHAPTER 27

DETERMINANTS OF ABUSE AND THE EFFECTS OF VIOLENCE ON CHILDREN AND ADOLESCENTS

Suzanne Salzinger, NEW YORK STATE PSYCHIATRIC INSTITUTE AND COLUMBIA UNIVERSITY

Parental abuse of children serves as the primary focus of this chapter, although other types of family and community violence are also addressed because of their profound effects on children and adolescents. The chapter begins with presentation of some recent information on the extent of abuse and violence and a short discussion of the phenomenology of abuse. Following is a section discussing theoretical approaches to the field—first a description of some of the major models of the etiology of abuse and then some models describing the behavioral processes giving rise to abusive acts.

The empirical research on etiological factors leading to abuse is organized in terms of an ecological framework consisting of the individual characteristics of parents and children, the interaction among family members, and the community context for maltreatment. Empirical research on the effects of abuse is presented separately for children and adolescents. With respect to children, the effects of being a victim are discussed first, then the effects of witnessing spouse abuse and domestic violence, and finally the effects of community violence. The effects of abuse on adolescents are presented first in terms of the ef-

fects of childhood victimization and then in terms of the effects of adolescent victimization.

SCOPE OF THE PROBLEM

Recent summaries (Finkelhor & Dziuba-Leatherman, 1994; Wolfner & Gelles, 1993) of the data from official statistics on crime and child abuse and national family violence surveys demonstrate dramatically that although the rates of all types of severe family violence are high, children are much more likely to be victims than parents (107 to 58 per 1000); that adolescents are two to three times more likely than adults to be victims of assault (58 to 18 per 1,000), robbery (12 to 5 per 1,000), and rape (2 to 1 per 1,000); and that they are just as likely to be victims of homicide (0.1 to 0.1 per 1,000). Differences in the rates and types of victimization at different ages are believed to be due in large measure to the dependency status of children, with younger children being subject to abuse by family members and adolescents being subject to abuse more often by acquaintances and strangers (Christofel, 1990; Crittenden & Craig, 1990). The pattern of victimization also becomes more gender specific with age, the rate of physical abuse and homicide for boys increasing over that of girls with increasing age.

Complicating the estimation of the rate of abuse is a lack of consensus on definition. Despite a fair degree of consistency in what is perceived as maltreatment among both professionals and laypersons, the factors used in defining abuse vary according to locality and the purpose for which the definitions are to be used (Giovanni, 1989). They include the commission of particular acts (Straus, 1979), the intentionality of the acts, endangerment to the child, the effect of particular acts in terms of injury and impairment, and the cultural context in which the acts are committed (Korbin, 1980).

Subclassification is also important because different dimensions of maltreatment have different negative effects on children's functioning. Manly, Barnett, and Cicchetti (1993), for example, found that children classified as both abused and neglected fared most poorly, physically neglected children next most, and physically abused children least poorly on child- and counselor-rated behavior problems, social competence, and peer behavior.

More recent conceptualization of maltreatment as part of the continuum of caregiving behavior (Burgess, 1979; Wolfe, 1987) has enabled behavioral research on child abuse to draw on the general literature on childrearing in the attempt to understand abusive practices.

THEORETICAL APPROACHES

Organizational Models of the Etiology of Abuse

Early models of the etiology of child abuse were derived from almost totally divergent perspectives. The *psychiatric model,* based on pediatric clinical case studies of battered infants and children (Kempe, Silverman, Steele, Droegmueller, & Silver, 1962) assigned the cause for abuse to characteristics of the individual perpetrator, stating that parents who committed abusive acts suffered from some form of mental illness. Although early clinical studies tended to show that abusive parents were disturbed, the question remained in dispute until recently when better controlled studies demonstrated a higher degree of psychopathology in parents of abused children (Ka-

plan, Pelcovitz, Salzinger, & Ganeles, 1983; Kaplan, 1994).

However, social scientists, taking note of the economic and social conditions associated with increased rates of abuse, took issue with a theory that placed responsibility for abuse entirely on the psychopathology of the individual parent. The *sociological model* (Gil, 1970) focused on economic conditions, societal values, and the structure of the modern family as a social institution. Support for the model came from the fact that the risk for family violence has always been found to be greater for children and the elderly, as well as for the poor, the unemployed, and people holding low-prestige jobs (Pelton, 1978; Wolfner & Gelles, 1993). Child abuse was seen as the result of family stress derived from the burden of raising children in the context of economic hardship (Garbarino, 1976).

However, neither of these models was adequate for capturing the multiplexity of the problem of child abuse. Based on the seminal work of Bronfenbrenner (1979), who conceptualized human development within an ecological context, Belsky (1980, 1993) organized the contexts giving rise to physical child abuse and neglect into a *developmental-ecological model.* It includes four ecological levels: the ontogenic level, in which the individual characteristics of the parent and child provide the "developmental context"; the microsystem level, in which the family serves as the "immediate interactional context"; the exosystem level, in which community processes provide the conditions that alter the risk for abuse; and the macrosystem level, in which cultural and even evolutionary factors provide the broader context for the occurrence of abuse.

Cicchetti and Rizley (1981), also making use of three comparable ecological levels—individual, family, and societal—incorporate the transactional view of recent developmental theory into a *transactional model.* Two types of factors are held to determine the likelihood of abuse at each level. The first consists of potentiating or compensatory factors and the second of transient or enduring factors. Combinations of these factors give rise to challengers (potentiating factors that are transient), vulnerability factors (potentiating factors that are enduring), buffers (compensatory factors that are transient), and protective factors (compensatory factors that are enduring). The model is a probabilistic one; when potentiating conditions supercede compensatory conditions, maltreatment is predicted to occur.

Models that Describe the Process of Abuse

Enough empirical data have been accumulated to enable us to develop models that describe the process of abuse. Wolfe (1987) proposes a *transitional model* of how severe physical abuse comes about within the family context. It includes multiple destabilizing and compensatory factors that operate on the family over the course of three stages. In the first stage, stressful life events and poor parenting skills combine to override social support and economic stability, reducing parents' resistance to stress and their ability to inhibit aggression. In the second stage, parents, becoming increasingly more susceptible to stressful events, begin to ascribe responsibility for misbehavior to their children and view them as being deliberately oppositional. Their parenting becomes intermittently abusive, although intervention aimed at teaching better parenting skills can be compensatory at this stage. In the third stage, parents, failing to cope effectively with increasing stressful life events, begin to feel hopeless, become easily emotionally aroused, and develop an entrenched "habitual pattern of stress, arousal, and overgeneralized responses to the child" (p. 66). Community intervention becomes necessary to reverse the abusive behavior.

Twentyman, Rohrbeck, and Amish (1984) propose a *cognitive-behavioral model* to account for child abuse. This, too, is a stage model. In stage one, parents set unrealistic expectations for their children's behavior; in stage two, children behave in ways that do not accord with parental expectations; in stage three, parents tend to attribute negative intent to the children's misbehavior; and in stage four, parents react with severe discipline and abusive behavior. Azar and Siegal (1990), elaborating on the cognitive-behavioral model, point out that the impact of various types of parental cognitive deficits depends on the child's developmental stage. Researchers working with the cognitive-behavioral model have tied their model intimately and explicitly to behavioral interventions with parents (Azar, 1989) and families (Morton, Twentyman, & Azar, 1988).

Milner (in press), focusing exclusively on the social cognition of parents, proposes a traditional *social information-processing model* to explain abuse. This four-stage model shares a number of features with the transitional and cognitive-behavioral models. In its application to abuse, the model specifically proposes that abusive, more so than nonabusive, parents tend to view their children's behavior in accordance with their own perceptual biases and distortions because they are less attentive to social events in their environment. This leads them to misinterpret their children's behavior as being motivated by hostile intent. Their information-processing style limits the array of response choices available to them, causing them to utilize more automatic power-assertive control strategies with their children. Finally, they are unable to implement parental strategies with consistency and to monitor accurately the outcome of their use of specific strategies on their children's behavior. Child noncompliance, as a result of poor parenting skill, tends to reconfirm parental misconceptions of child behavior and to result in increasingly more abusive parenting practices. In support of this model, Chilamkurti and Milner (1993) have shown that high-risk mothers differ from low-risk mothers in their perception and evaluations of child transgressions and disciplinary techniques.

The last process model to be discussed is a *social learning model* (Patterson, 1982) that accounts for occurrence of aggressive behavior among family members. Although it does not pertain exclusively to abusive behavior, it has been described in great detail and supported by a wealth of observational data on family interaction. The model states that family members negatively reinforce each others' aversive behavior. Specifically, the aversive behavior of the parent and child each ceases contingent upon the other person's coercive response. The process tends to escalate as increases in duration and intensity of aversive interchanges are selectively reinforced (Snyder, Edwards, McGraw, Kilgore, & Holton, 1994).

Because coercive behavior cycles are predicated on aversive behavior in the child as well as the parent, they may not apply in all cases of child abuse, since not all abused children are aggressive. There are, however, data showing that abused infants may be temperamentally difficult babies (Crittenden, 1981) and that abused children tend to develop aggressive behavior. The model's applicability to child abuse was shown in a study of the verbal interchanges between maltreated and nonmaltreated mother-child dyads (Salzinger, Wondolowski, Kaplan, & Kaplan, 1987). Results indicated that bouts of aggravated discourse tended to escalate in length for maltreating pairs, whereas they were attenuated for control pairs. However, all the differences were more pronounced for mothers than for their children.

Missing from these process models is an important focus on the role of affect in parenting. MacKinnon, Lamb, Belsky, and Baum (1990) propose incorporating the affective dimension in a model they put forth to explain the development of mother-child aggression. Gottman (1991) suggests that during parent-child conflict, excessive arousal may result in emotional flooding, which tends to inhibit use of constructive cognitive problem-solving strategies and to foster the use of automatic responses which are not readily susceptible to modification by environmental input. And Dix (1991) reports that maternal anger serves to give rise to coercive control strategies that maintain rather than reduce the child's emotional arousal.

No single one of the process models reviewed here accounts fully for occurrence of abusive parenting, although each highlights some significant aspects of the process. Considered together, the models complement each other and may well contribute to a unified model. Although it is not expected that the paths leading to abuse in all families will be alike, a unified process model should be able to capture and account for the more likely alternative routes.

ETIOLOGICAL FACTORS LEADING TO ABUSIVE AND PUNITIVE PARENTING

The empirical research on etiological factors associated with abuse will be organized in terms of an ecological framework (Belsky, 1980), which includes characteristics of the individual, characteristics of the interaction among family members, and community characteristics.

Although many of the etiological factors are presented as if they were single main effects, child maltreatment is, in fact, multiply determined, and each of these factors should be viewed as potentially interacting with other factors in giving rise to maltreatment. The studies on which the information on etiological factors is based vary widely in design and methodology. Factors that emerge as significantly associated with increased risk for abuse should be accepted conservatively and primarily as contributory to a process that is still largely undiscovered.

Individual Factors: Parent Characteristics

Parental History of Abusive Childhood

One of the most widely discussed features of the child abuse literature has been the claim that abusive parents were themselves abused as children. Early case history studies gave rise to highly inflated intergenerational transmission rates because they did not take account of parents who had been abused but who had not been identified later as abusive. Subsequent studies, although based on large community samples that included nonabusive parents as well, generally relied on retrospective self-report data, with all the problems of accuracy and bias that such methodologies entail. Few prospective studies have been available, and their rates vary widely as a function of differences in design (Egeland & Brunquell, 1979; Hunter & Kilstrom, 1979; Widom, 1989a).

Kaufman and Zigler (1987) concluded, after a critical review of the literature, that the case for intergenerational transmission has generally been overstated, and they estimated the rate at about 30 percent plus or minus 5 percent. Some researchers still withhold judgment about the size of the intergenerational effect, based on the inadequacies of the research base (Widom, 1989b). Others (Belsky, 1993), pointing to the long-term stability of aggression (Huesmann, Eron, Lefkowitz, & Walder, 1984) and to studies showing that "antisocial behavior patterns are passed from one generation to the next at a rate well beyond chance" (Wahler & Dumas, 1986, p. 50), are inclined to attribute part of the etiology of child abuse to parents' abuse as children.

Kaufman and Zigler (1987) have stated, "Being maltreated as a child puts one at risk for becoming abusive but the path between these two points is far from direct or inevitable" (p. 190). Compensatory factors that interrupt the cycle of abuse (Egeland, Jacobvitz, & Sroufe, 1988) include, among other things, better social support, including a supportive spouse and a relationship with a significant adult in childhood. Salzinger, Feldman, Hammer, and Rosario (1992) tested a path model that included a mother's victimization early in her own life and the likelihood that her children would be abused. They found that severe family discord and substance abuse as well as partner abuse in the mother's current family served to mediate the effect of early parental abuse on the risk for child abuse. Burgess and Youngblade (1988) suggest that general social incompetence, learned as a child in an abusive home and expressed in coercive interactions with peers, functions as an important causal pathway to adult behavior and thereby to abusive parenting.

General Psychological, Emotional, and Behavioral Characteristics of Parents

Early studies of child maltreating parents gave rise to the idea that abusive parents would be found to show a consistent pattern of personality traits and psychological disturbance—low frustration-tolerance, impulsiveness, emotional immaturity, inappropriate anger, feelings of inadequacy, and low self-esteem (Steele & Pollock, 1968). Researchers have never been able to isolate such a pattern. Instead, as Wolfe points out (1987), typologies of abusive parents are better based on parental characteristics and behavior related to their role as parents, which take into account such variables as child behavior and the other contextual contraints that affect parenting.

Parental Psychopathology

Nonetheless, there continue to be both clinical and research reports (Lahey, Conger, Atkeson, & Treiber, 1984) of affective disturbance and somatic problems among abusive parents. Utilizing standardized semistructured and structured diagnostic instruments and research diagnostic criteria, Kaplan and colleagues (1983) found a significantly higher percentage of depressive disorder and alcoholism among suburban mothers of maltreated children and adolescents than among controls. Perpetrators, compared to their

spouses, were significantly more often diagnosed as depressed, alcoholic, as having an antisocial personality disorder, and as having labile personality.

Comparisons of white middle-class suburban families of confirmed cases of physically abused adolescents with matched community sample controls (Kaplan, 1994) found that a significantly higher percentage of both mothers and fathers were diagnosed with both lifetime and current psychiatric disorders and substance abuse. Major depression and dysthymia showed the most elevated rates for mothers, and major depression, depression, and antisocial disorder showed the most elevated rates for fathers. Although rates may not differ from those of other high-risk groups, given certain predisposing conditions such as parental stress and conduct-disordered children, parents who receive such diagnoses may well be at increased risk for engaging in abusive behavior with their children (Whipple & Webster-Stratton, 1991).

Consistent with the idea that depression may be a potentiating factor in abusive parenting are results of a study by Sussman, Trickett, Iannotti, Hollenbeck, and Zahn-Waxler (1985) comparing depressed, abusive, and normal mothers in terms of childrearing practices and values. Both abusive and depressed mothers shared a number of beliefs about child responsibility for misbehavior and punishment that differed from normal mothers, although only abusive mothers coupled these beliefs with harsh, authoritarian practices.

Emotional Arousal

Some of the process models previously discussed hypothesize that a state of negative hyperarousal, which is linked closely in time with abusive behavior, is characteristic of abusive parents. It expresses itself in increased reactivity to the behavior of children and tends to block utilization of cognitive skills requisite for appropriate parenting, resulting instead in increasing impulsive automatic responses to children's perceived misbehavior. Empirical support for such a parental characteristic was found in a comparison of abusive and matched control subjects responses to videotaped scenes showing infants crying and smiling (Frodi & Lamb, 1980). Abusive subjects showed greater physiological arousal (increased skin resistance, blood pressure, and heart rate) and reported more annoyance, more indifference, and less sympathy to the babies' behavior. In a similar study, in which older children's interactions with their parents were shown to abusive and nonabusive parents (Wolfe, Fairbank, Kelly, & Bradlyn, 1983), abusive parents responded with greater negative psychophysiological arousal than nonabusive parents to the more stressful scenes.

Whether such excessive arousal is generalized hyperresponsivity to all aversive stimuli or is specific only to child-related stressors, was addressed in a more recent study in which mothers at risk for child abuse and matched low-risk mothers were compared for their physiological reactions to four types of stressful stimuli unrelated to child stressors. At-risk mothers showed greater and more prolonged sympathetic activation to the two most stressful stimuli, suggesting that " generalized sympathetic activation to both child and non-child related stressors may serve as a mediator of physical child abuse" (Casanova, Domanic, McCanne, & Milner, 1992).

Parental Cognitive Attributions to Children's Behavior

Previously it was thought that abusive parents had a more limited understanding of child development. That point of view has not been supported in the literature (see Starr, 1988, p. 130). Instead, abusive parents have been found to have unrealistic expectations for their children's behavior and poor problem-solving ability in childrearing situations (Azar, Robinson, Hekimian, & Twentyman, 1984). They tend to express a negative bias in evaluation of their children's problem behavior, considering these children to be more intentionally disobedient (Bauer & Twentyman, 1985), and they find the children's behavior to be more annoying than do other observers (Mash, Johnston, & Kovitz, 1983; Reid, Kavenagh, & Baldwin, 1987). There also is evidence that suggests abusive parents consider their children's negative behavior to be a stable internal characteristic of the child, whereas they consider positive behavior to be more the result of unstable chance external circumstances (Larrance & Twentyman, 1983). This becomes an important potentiating factor in light of findings that child-abusing parents justify their own abusive care

giving when they believe children to be deliberately defiant (Dietrich, Berkowitz, Kadushin, & McGloin, 1990).

Child Characteristics

Several child characteristics have been mentioned as being contributory to abuse—prematurity, low birthweight, difficult temperament, and illness or handicap, among others. These characteristics have been hypothesized to lead to interference in early bonding or to inadequate attachment (Lynch & Roberts, 1977). A transactional model would suggest, alternatively, that child characteristics increase the likelihood of abuse only in the presence of other parental and societal risk factors, such as social isolation, low levels of social support, and poverty, for example. It is now generally believed, based on evidence from both prospective studies (e.g., Egeland, 1988; Hunter, Kilstrom, Kraybill, & Loda, 1978) and retrospective studies (Leventhal, 1981), that if these other risk factors are controlled for, individual child characteristics disappear as risk factors, at least as independent causes for abuse (National Research Council, 1993).

Nevertheless, it is likely that some child characteristics, particularly behavior problems that may in fact have developed in response to being victimized, can contribute to the maintenance of abuse or to re-abuse (Ammerman, 1991). The fact that various forms of abuse peak at certain ages (National Research Council, 1993) and are more prevalent among children of one gender than the other suggests also that particular behaviors and characteristics associated with developmental level may interact with parent characteristics and give rise to abusive parenting.

Interaction among Family Members as an Etiological Factor

Families of maltreated children show a pervasive pattern of negative interactions and a paucity of positive interactions among their members. Because high rates of negative behavior can quickly escalate to the point of violence through a process of coercion described by Patterson (1982), negative family interaction can become an etiological risk factor for child maltreatment.

Between Parents and Children

Negativity in parent-child relationships was first documented by Burgess and Conger (1978) in detailed day-to-day behavioral observations conducted in homes of maltreated and nonmaltreated children. Not only did fewer interactions take place between maltreated children and parents, especially mothers, but the ratio of negative to positive interactions was much higher than in control families.

Other observational studies have found that abusing parents are less supportive, affectionate (Lahey et al, 1984), playful, and responsive (Kavenagh, Youngblade, Reid, & Fagot, 1988) with their children and direct fewer positive behaviors toward them (Bousha & Twentyman, 1984). They are also less emotionally responsive and more intrusive and controlling with their infants (Crittenden, 1981, 1985a; Crittenden & Bonvillian, 1984; Dietrich, Starr, & Kaplan, 1980; Dietrich, Starr, & Weisfeld, 1983; Egeland, Breitenbucher, & Rosenberg, 1980; Wasserman, Green, & Allen, 1983) and children (Mash et al., 1983; Oldershaw, Walters, & Hall, 1986). A process of escalation of reciprocated aversive interchanges has been found that is typical of maltreating but not of nonmaltreating parent-child interactions (Loeber, Felton, & Reid, 1984), especially in the context of mild disagreement (Salzinger et al., 1987) or stress (Mash et al., 1983).

Aside from the negative quality of ordinary exchanges between parents and children, maltreating parents have been found to employ different parenting strategies for purposes of control and discipline than nonmaltreating parents. They are more likely to use punishment, coercion, and threats, and less likely to use positive social reinforcers and reasoning (Loeber et al., 1984; Oldershaw et al., 1986; Trickett & Susman, 1988; Trickett & Kuczynski, 1986). Parenting strategies are also found to be less frequently contingent on the children's (Mash et al., 1983; Trickett & Kuczynski, 1986) and infants' (Crittenden, 1981) behavior. This may reflect an insensitivity to social cues as suggested by results obtained by Kropp and Haynes (1987), who found that abusive parents showed an inability to successfully identify infants' emotional signals; or it may result from a negative bias in their perception of their children's behavior; or it may reflect a belief in the effectiveness of power-assertive control strategies (Milner & Chilamkurti, 1991).

Between Parents

Although it is widely held by clinicians, laypersons, and researchers that abuse between partners or parents is a risk factor for abuse of children, there is relatively little research on the issue. Prevalence rates for partner assaults during a single year, based on the 1985 National Family Violence Resurvey, are very high—161 out of 1,000 couples—as are the rates for serious child abuse—110 per 1,000 children (Straus & Gelles, 1988). Co-occurrence of child abuse and partner abuse is seldom estimated, however most of the research on child and spouse abuse being conducted along two separate strands. A few studies speak to their joint occurrence.

Bowker, Arbitell, and McFerron (1988) found that 70 percent of wifebeaters also physically abused their children and that severity of wife beating predicted severity of child abuse. Stark and Flitcraft (1985), in a review of medical records, found that children of battered mothers were twice as likely to be physically abused as were children whose mothers were not battered. Salzinger and colleagues (1992) found that partner abuse in the child's household increased risk for child physical abuse, with a significantly higher rate of partner abuse, 54 percent, found in their low socioeconomic-status (SES) urban child physical abuse sample than in their closely demographically matched control sample, 33 percent.

Between Siblings

There is more prevalence in child-maltreating families of negative verbal and physical interactions between siblings (Burgess & Conger, 1978). Incidence rates for severe violence by children and adolescents combined, aged 3 to 17, against siblings is extremely high—530 per 1,000— as is the rate for severe violence by adolescents only, aged 15 to 17—360 per 1,000 (Straus & Gelles, 1988). Importance of these figures lies in the fact that fights between siblings have been found to be significantly associated with physical abuse of children (Herrenkohl, Herrenkohl, & Egolf, 1983).

Community Context for Maltreatment

The act of abuse is private, screened from public view, and not easily subject to potentially corrective feedback from outside the immediate family. As early as the late 1960s, abusive parents were being described in clinical studies as being isolated from their family and friends. Childrearing is not, however, a private act; community norms are reflected in styles of childrearing, and learning to parent is in large measure a process of social learning, with feedback not only from the child but from family, friends, acquaintances, and the wider community.

Garbarino and colleagues have related rates of maltreatment to the ecologies of various communities and found that economic (Garbarino, 1976) and other demographic factors likely to be disruptive or stressful to families account for a substantial portion of the variance for maltreatment (Garbarino & Crouter, 1978). Even more revealing is their finding (Garbarino & Sherman, 1980) that neighborhood residents' perceptions of "sources of help, social networks, quality of the neighborhood, and use of formal family support systems" (p. 189) differentiate high- from low-risk neighborhoods with respect to maltreatment, despite similarities in sociodemographic level.

Although the literature consistently reports a positive relationship between poverty and punitive parenting (Garbarino, 1976; Gelles, 1989; Gelles & Straus, 1979; Gil, 1970; Pelton, 1978; Steinberg, Catalano, & Dooley, 1981; U.S. Advisory Board on Child Abuse and Neglect, 1990; Wolock & Horowitz, 1979), the relationship has been found to be moderated by perceived social support. A large recent study, utilizing the National Survey of Families and Households, of the association among poverty, social support and punitive and unsupportive parenting behavior (Hashima & Amato, 1994) found that perceived social support acts as a buffer under conditions of high levels of stress generated by scarce economic resources and that actual support tends to reduce incidence of nonsupportive parenting regardless of income.

Personal social networks serve to mediate the effects of community-level variables and institutions on families. Two studies compared the networks of mothers of maltreated children to those of control mothers. Crittenden (1985b), in a study of low-income mothers of 2- to 4-year-old children, found that unstable open networks were associated with maltreatment and consisted of short-term friends, frequent contact with friends and relatives, moderate

levels of help from relatives, either very little or excessive help from friends, and moderate dissatisfaction with the dependability of relationships. Salzinger, Kaplan, and Artemyeff (1983) hypothesized that social norms for appropriate parenting are carried by distal portions of the network consisting of acquaintances and community ties, and that local deviations from these norms are more likely to be carried by less distal portions consisting of close family and close friends whose behavior is likely to be subject to similar social constraints.

Comparison of the networks of suburban mothers referred for maltreatment by Child Protective Services with those of a demographically matched control sample revealed that maltreating mothers had smaller networks, less contact with network members, and less contact especially with the extended network. Their networks showed more insularity, (i.e., the various parts of their network lacked contact with each other). Especially lacking were connections between household members and extended parts of the network, supporting the notion that feedback from the broader community was not sufficient to counter the deviant parenting found in the maltreating families. Parent insularity has also been found to obviate follow-up treatment gains of mothers trained in the behavioral management of their problem children (Wahler, 1980), suggesting that network insularity is a factor that must be addressed if parent training programs in maltreating families are to be successful.

EFFECTS OF ABUSE AND VIOLENCE ON CHILDREN

Effects on Children of Child Abuse

Abuse affects practically all aspects of a child's development. It occurs within a complicated context of mediating factors that can either mitigate or exacerbate its effects and it is often difficult to disentangle its specific effect from effects due to the contextual factors that tend to co-occur with it. Effects of abuse also depend on when in the child's life it occurs. Vulnerabilities and capabilities are different throughout a child's life and the coping responses a child makes to protect against abuse may be adaptive at one developmental stage but eventually prove to be maladaptive as the child gets older and utilizes these same strategies in a different context.

Physical Injury

Neurological impairment resulting from physical abuse (Dykes, 1986; Frank, Zimmerman, & Leeds, 1985; Martin, 1976) has direct lifelong effects on everyday functioning and has been implicated in the violent behavioral outcomes of delinquents who have been severely abused (Lewis, Mallouh, & Webb, 1989; Lewis, Shanok, Pincus, & Glaser, 1979; Shanok & Lewis, 1981). However, the effect of the infliction of less severe physical injury on long-term functioning of children is usually indirect. That is, it operates through psychological effects on the child.

Social Relationships
with Caregivers

Development of early secure attachment to caregivers provides infants and young children with working models of relationships with other people that can be drawn on to establish a psychological safe base from which to explore the environment and learn to master it. Studies using the Strange Situation Procedure (Ainsworth, Blehar, Waters, & Wall, 1978) to assess the quality of attachment in children aged 1 to 4 have found that abused children are anxiously attached to their mothers (Egeland & Sroufe, 1981; Gaensbauer & Harmon, 1982, Schneider-Rosen, Braunwald, Carlson, & Cicchetti, 1985) and reveal a pattern of anxious/avoidant behavior. By the age of 2 years, abused children, compelled by the need to adapt to maternal anger and punishment, are likely to have developed two strategies for living with an abusive parent: a negative resistant one and a compulsively compliant one (Crittenden & Ainsworth, 1989).

Lynch and Cicchetti (1991) explored expected differences in patterns of attachment to various relationship figures for somewhat older maltreated and nonmaltreated children. In general, although all children showed that the more positive and secure they felt in their relationships with other people, the less they needed to seek greater psychological proximity, maltreated children showed a weaker correlation between these two dimensions.

Other controlled observational studies have focused on the quality of the ongoing interaction between parents and maltreated children and infants, on the assumption that these interactions contribute as importantly as the less frequent acts of abuse in determining how children learn to socialize.

Although observations of the behavior of abused infants and toddlers with caregivers reveal more consistently disturbed behavior (Egeland et al., 1979; Gaensbauer & Sands, 1978; George & Main, 1979) (i.e., problems in attachment, social avoidance, and aggression), results related to behavior of older children are less consistent. Some investigations (Oldershaw et al., 1986; Reid, Taplan, & Loeber, 1981) have found the children's behavior to be more aversive and noncompliant; others (Burgess & Conger, 1978; Mash et al., 1983) have not, even though abusive mothers' behavior was found to be more directive and controlling than that of nonabusive mothers. Comparison of the verbal discourse between maltreating mothers and their children with that of control pairs (Salzinger et al., 1987) revealed that maltreating families' use of more aggravated and fewer mitigated utterances than controls was attenuated for the children.

The coercive behavior process that characterizes the interaction between mothers and aggressive children, and that depends on increased rates of aversive behavior on the part of children as well as parents (Patterson, 1982), has been suggested to account for the style of interaction that abused children learn at home and generalize to their behavior with other people. However, given the number of studies that did not find increased aversive behavior in abused children during interactions with their parents, it is unlikely that this coercive behavioral process accounts for all disturbed social interactions of abused children. Other learning processes, such as direct positive reinforcement of aggressive behavior and observational learning of aggressive and other incompetent interactional strategies between other family members, provide alternative routes to the disturbed social relationships found in abused children.

Peer Relations

Many models predict that the peer relations of abused children will be different from those of nonabused children. A recent study of 87 physically abused urban schoolchildren and 87 matched nonmaltreated classmates (Salzinger, Feldman, Hammer, & Rosario, 1993) found that abused children were less popular, involved in fewer reciprocal relationships, and their behavior was rated by peers as more aggressive and less cooperative.

Several other controlled studies of the behavior of abused children with their peers and siblings—utilizing direct observations and behavior ratings by parents, teachers, and peers—have also found that abused children are more aggressive than their non-abused nondisturbed peers (Dodge, Bates, & Pettit, 1990; Feldman et al., 1995; George & Main, 1979; Hoffman-Plotkin & Twentyman, 1984; Kaufman & Cicchetti, 1989; Kinard, 1980; Kravic, 1987; Reid et al., 1987).

Aside from aggression, other types of social incompetence, especially internalizing problem behaviors, that predispose toward social avoidance or withdrawal, have been found in these children (Feldman et al., 1995; Kravic, 1987; Salzinger et al., 1984; Wolfe & Mosk, 1983).

Whether the incompetent social behavior exhibited by abused children can be modified by giving them guided experience interacting with other children was tested by Howes and Espinosa (1985) in a study of young abused infants and toddlers. They found that rate of aggressive behavior in abused children was no different than that of normal children when their behavior was observed in well-established groups in a day-care setting. This intervention, however, may be developmentally stage specific, since older abused children engage in non-competent aggressive social behavior well into their school years when they are associating with other children on a daily basis.

Social Cognition

There is reason to believe that abused children's upbringing gives rise to distortions in the way the children appraise their own and others' behavior, intentions, and feelings (Smetana & Kelly, 1989; Smetana, Kelly, & Twentyman, 1984). Dean, Malik, Richards, and Stringer (1986) reported that abused children described the reciprocal behavior between children and between adults and children differently than nonabused children. Although partly accounted for by differences in IQ, Barahal, Waterman, and Martin (1981) also found that abused children had difficulty in role-taking or perspective-taking skills and in appropriately identifying emotions in other

people. This was borne out by Main and George's (1985) observations of abused toddlers, who were found to display different behaviors in response to agemates' distress than control children in the same day-care setting, and by Straker and Jacobson (1981), who found abused children to be less empathic than nonabused children.

Dodge and colleagues (1990) hypothesized that deviant social information processing patterns are responsible for maintaining aggressive behavior in young abused children. They examined maladaptive social information processing patterns as a possible mediating link between early harsh parental discipline and the development of later aggressive behavior (Weiss, Dodge, Bates, & Pettit, 1992) in a well-controlled longitudinal study that ruled out SES and marital violence as confounding variables. Children exposed to harsh punitive discipline were found to be poorer in encoding cues about a social event, in making correct attributions about another individual's motivation, in generating response alternatives, and in evaluating the consequences of response alternatives.

Intellectual Functioning

It is no longer believed to be the case that abused children have lower IQs than nonabused children (see Starr, 1988, p. 137). However, many abused children do show problems in learning, often reflected in poor school performance. If learning is construed as an active process, then abused children who fail to seek to achieve intellectual mastery because they are poorly motivated may develop problems meeting age-appropriate intellectual demands. The work of a number of investigators is consistent with the idea that abusive parenting slows development by punishing or discouraging curiosity, autonomy, and independent behavior (Aber, Allen, Carlson, & Cicchetti, 1989; Azar, Barnes, & Twentyman, 1988; Crittenden, 1981, 1985a), thereby contributing to passivity, fearfulness, and compliance (Crittenden 1988; Crittenden & DiLalla, 1988; Ericksen, Egeland, & Pianta, 1989; Oates & Peacock, 1984). Such behavior has been observed in maltreated children during learning tasks with their mothers and has been found to be associated with lower cognitive maturity (Aber et al., 1989). Vondra, Barnett, and Cicchetti (1989) suggest a causal chain from parent-child relationships to distorted self-perception of competence, and thence to school functioning, to explain differences between maltreated and control children's school performance.

Emotional Problems

Studies contrasting broad-band ratings of problem behavior of abused children with controls have found more problem behavior in the abused children, including more internalizing types of disturbance (Feldman et al.,1995; Reid et al., 1987; Salzinger et al., 1984; Sternberg et al., 1993) and lower self-esteem (Erickson, 1989). Cicchetti suggests that the continuing disapproval by maltreating mothers results in "overcontrol" of their children's emotions. In support of this, Cicchetti and Beeghly (1987) found that maltreated toddlers used fewer internal-state words. In older children and adolescents, significantly higher rates of psychopathology, especially depression, were diagnosed in maltreated than control children (Kaplan, Montero, Pelcovitz, & Kaplan, 1988; Toth, Manly, & Cicchetti, 1992).

Effects on Children of Spouse Abuse and Domestic Violence

The long-term effects on children of witnessing domestic violence may be as far-reaching and serious as being personally victimized (Rosenbaum & O'Leary, 1981), although children who are both victims and witnesses respond more fearfully to interadult anger than witnesses alone (Hennessy, Rabideau, & Cicchetti, 1994). In general, children of battered women have been found to show internalizing disorders (Christopoulos et al., 1987; Holden & Ritchie, 1991; Sternberg et al., 1993), but findings of more externalizing problems in older children (Wolfe et al., 1985) and of more behavior problems and aggressive behavior in boys than girls (Hilberman & Munson, 1977/1978) have not always been replicated.

Jaffe, Wolfe, and Wilson (1990) present a model for the affect of wife abuse on children's development that posits two routes to child disorder. One is direct, through exposure of the child to violent behavior, and the other is indirect, through increased stress on the mother. In the latter situation, spouse abuse produces a decline in effective child management, which re-

sults in an increase in negative child coping behaviors, which in turn add to maternal stress. In support of the indirect model, Jaffe, Wolfe, Wilson, and Zak (1986) found that women in shelters compared to matched control women were extremely elevated on scales of physical and psychological symptomatology, such as somatic complaints, anxiety, insomnia, and depression. Wolfe, Zak, Wilson, and Jaffe (1986) reported that the level of self-reported stress added significantly to severity of domestic violence in the prediction of children's adjustment. Holden and Ritchie's (1991) findings are only partially consistent with this model. Although they found maternal stress to be predictive of children's behavior problems in both child witness and control samples, no other differences in parenting were found aside from the fact that the battered women attended less and experienced more conflict with their children.

The observational social learning paradigm predicts that being a witness of parental violence and other nonconstructive means of resolving interpersonal conflicts teaches children to acquire similar social problem-solving strategies. Rosenberg (1987) found that young children from violent homes tended to endorse use of nonassertive social problem-solving techniques in dealing with peer situations and performed poorly on a measure of social sensitivity. Another study utilizing more dramatic and absorbing videotaped stimuli of parental conflict (Groisser, 1986) found that child witnesses responded in a hypervigilant fashion. Wolfe and colleagues (1986) found that children of battered women living in shelters showed less social competence than children of a nonviolent control group. However, having fewer interests and engaging in fewer social activities may not be due entirely to family violence, but may instead be a function of disruption caused by moving to a shelter. This would be consistent with the fact that *former* shelter residents' children were not rated as being socially less competent.

Views of child witnesses/child victims of their parents were studied by Sternberg and colleagues (Sternberg et al., in press). She found that as long as children were not also victims of abuse, they were able to evaluate their parents' parental, rather than spousal, roles. This represents a fairly high level of social competence or sensitivity to social cues and suggests that the picture of the social cognition of child witnesses is far from complete.

Effects on Children of Community Violence

Community violence has been called "epidemic" by a group of researchers (Reiss, Richters, Radke-Yarrow, & Scharff, 1993; Richters, 1993) who have studied the adaptational success and failure of children living in violent communities (Richters & Martinez, 1993). Exposure to violence tends to be associated with distress symptoms, such as fear, anxiety, depression, and post-traumatic stress disorder (Bell & Jenkins, 1993; Fitzpatrick & Boldizar, 1993; Martinez & Richters, 1993; Pynoos et al., 1987; Richters & Martinez, 1993). Richters and Martinez (1993) point out, however, that far from all children living in violent neighborhoods are equally exposed, and far from all such children suffer their negative consequences. In an attempt to identify factors that enable some children to achieve successful adaptation (as defined by school performance and parental ratings of social and emotional behavior) in the face of relatively high levels of community violence while others succumb to adaptational failure, these investigators found that family stability and family safety status, rather than children's level of exposure to violence in the community, determined their outcome. These results are consistent with two ecological transactional models: one proposed to account for the etiology and effects of community violence on children and the other to account for child maltreatment (Cicchetti & Lynch, 1993; Cicchetti & Rizley, 1981). Both models suggest that there are very few inevitable paths from early exposure to violence to poor outcome.

EFFECTS OF ABUSE ON ADOLESCENTS

In considering the effects of abuse on adolescents, two separate developmental trajectories may be posited: one for the effects of child victimization and the other for adolescent victimization. Even when the same outcomes are under scrutiny, the mediating variables for the effects of abuse are different, and identification of the protective and exacerbating factors mediating outcome for each has important impli-

cations for intervention. Among these mediating variables are the developmental stage of the victim when abused, duration and severity of abuse, quality of the relationship between the child and both parents, structure and developmental stage of the family, caregiving arrangements, family and child social network resources (including community resources), and family stress.

Effects in Adolescence of Childhood Victimization

Criminality, Delinquency, and Violence

A 40-year follow-up (McCord, 1983) of 232 boys whose treatment as children was classified on the basis of extensive home social worker evaluations as "Neglected," "Abused," "Rejected," or "Loved," revealed that juvenile delinquency was more common among abused (and rejected and neglected) boys than boys raised by loving parents. No differences were found among the four groups for rates of alcoholism, divorce, and occupational success. Some 45 percent of the abused or rejected boys were convicted of serious crimes, became alcoholics or mentally ill, or died young. These boys tended to have aggressive, alcoholic, or criminal parents and to be aggressive themselves. An important point to be made is that over half of the abused children did not show long-term damage, and McCords commented that maternal self-confidence and education apparently contributed to their relative invulnerability.

Widom (1989a) also followed up a large sample ($n = 908$) of substantiated child abuse and neglect cases and a demographically matched control group ($n = 667$) 20 years later in order to determine whether the maltreated groups displayed higher rates of criminal behavior. Using juvenile probation records and adult local, state, and federal records, she found significantly higher rates of adult criminality for the maltreated group (28.6 percent) than for the control group (21.1 percent) and higher rates of adult violent criminal behavior for maltreated males (15.6 percent) than controls (10.2 percent).

Demographic factors, such as age, sex, and race also contributed independently to the rate of adult criminality. Widom (1989b) estimated on the basis of a review of prospective research that about 20 to 30 percent of maltreated children become delinquent, although retrospective studies lead to estimates of approximately 8 to 26 percent. Widom (1989c) also reports that abused and neglected children begin their delinquency one year earlier than controls (16.5 vs. 17.3 years) and that they are arrested twice as often, with more being arrested as juveniles. Here, too, note that a majority of victimized children do not become delinquent. Further research is needed to better understand how family and community responses to parents' abusive behavior influence eventual adolescent outcome.

Lewis and colleagues (Lewis & Shanok, 1977; Lewis et al., 1979, 1989) believe that severity of abuse is related to the violence of adolescents' delinquent acts, but whether early victimization leads to especially violent crimes is still unresolved.

Runaway Behavior

Although only 1 percent of runaways in the 1988 National Survey of Missing, Abducted, Runaway, and Thrownaway Children in America are reported as having been physically abused at home (Finkelhor et al., 1990), two prospective studies (McCord, 1983; Widom, 1991) found a positive relationship between early victimization and adolescent running away. A comparison of 223 maltreated and nonmaltreated adolescents (Powers, Eckenrode, & Jaklitsch, 1990) who sought services from runaway and homeless youth programs in New York State during 1986–1987 revealed that maltreated youth, who comprised 60 percent of the sample, were more likely to be female and to have engaged in suicidal behavior. In all other respects they were similar to other samples of homeless youth in being poor and coming from broken homes.

Emotional Problems and Self-Destructive Behavior

Although emotional problems and suicidal behavior are believed to be adolescent sequel of early victimization, there is no work that specifically tests this for physical abuse independent of work on sexually abused adolescents.

Substance Use

Substance use has been hypothesized to be a functional adaptive response to early victimization (Cavaiola & Schiff, 1988). Studies of youth in chemical dependency and detention programs (Cavaiola et al., 1988; Dembo, Williams, Schmeidler et al., 1992; Dembo, Williams, Wothke et al., 1992) show an association between early victimization and substance use. However, it has not been possible to attribute an independent component of the association specifically to physical abuse, since most of the research has been concerned with sexual abuse or with physical and sexual abuse combined. Nor have suitable controls been utilized to rule out additional early circumstances as explanatory variables, such as family factors.

Placement

Long-term effects of abuse must include consideration of placement outside the home (Runyan & Gould, 1985; Runyon, Gould, Trost, & Loda, 1982), because that is often the societal response to severe abuse. More research is clearly needed both as to its protective effect as well as its possible contribution to an increase in risk for poor outcome. In general, although some increased risks are noted, most findings seem to suggest that placement is not detrimental, that it does not lead to greater reabuse (Bolton, Lanier, & Gia, 1981) or to an increase in delinquency (Runyan & Gould, 1985) and may improve on the results of parent treatment programs (Cohn & Collignon, 1979; Herrenkohl et al., 1980; Magura, 1981).

Adolescent Victimization

Incidence of adolescent maltreatment is almost equal to that of child maltreatment, with estimates ranging from 23 to 47 percent (Burgdorff, 1980) of all reported cases of maltreatment. The National Incidence study (Burgdorff, 1980) reports relatively smaller proportions of physical assault for adolescents than children (42 vs. 52 percent) and relatively higher proportions of psychological abuse (32 vs. 25 percent). Risk for maltreatment of females increases in adolescence and declines for males, with twice as many females as males being maltreated. At present, estimates of the proportion of cases that begin during adolescence range so widely that we are unable to establish the incidence of adolescent abuse onset.

Families of maltreated adolescents differ from those of maltreated children. The difference in socioeconomic status found between high- and low-risk cases in childhood is largely absent or at least attenuated for adolescent abuse. The National Incidence Study reporting on Olsen and Holmes' 1983 analysis, shows the families to have higher incomes (National Center of Child Abuse and Neglect, 1988), as do Garbarino and colleagues (Garbarino & Gilliam, 1980; Garbarino et al., 1986), and the parents to have more education (National Center of Child Abuse and Neglect, 1988). Families are also more likely to contain stepparents, even after taking into account that stepparents are more likely in older families. Some investigators point out that the relationship between adolescents and their stepparents is especially difficult in the case where adolescents show any sort of developmental pathology (Burgess & Garbarino, 1983; Daly & Wilson, 1981), thus adding to the risk for maltreatment.

Many of the outcomes cited as a result of early victimization are found as a result of later victimization as well. Preliminary results of a recent study (Kaplan, 1994) of 100 white suburban physically abused adolescents and 100 community controls revealed that abused youth show a significantly higher rate of systematically diagnosed psychopathology after controlling for parental psychopathology, family structure, and gender. Utilizing a semistructured diagnostic interview and research diagnostic criteria, abused adolescents were found to show significantly higher rates of major depression, dysthymia, conduct disorder, drug use/abuse, and cigarette use. Garbarino and colleagues (1986), using the Achenbach Child Behavior Checklist and Youth Self-Report Form, also found more behavior problems, especially externalizing problems, in maltreated than in nonmaltreated youth.

However, processes leading to these outcomes are generally different. Garbarino (1989) mentions a number of factors that would be expected to operate differentially in adolescent maltreatment. Adolescents have greater power than children; they have broader intimate social networks with which parents must deal; their cognitive abilities are more advanced; and they are likely to be more of a financial drain on family resources. The family system is especially important in dealing with the adolescent's desire for autonomy. Frequent conflict is most likely to be engendered in authoritarian or permissive homes and is less likely to be found in authoritative homes, which are better suited for dealing with adolescents who have reached the level of formal operational thought.

In contrast to nonabusive families, the family system of abusive families (Garbarino et al, 1986), judged in terms of adaptability and cohesion, was found to be more "chaotic" and "enmeshed" and less "flexible" and "connected." In an assessment of attitudes and values concerning punishment, using the Adolescent Abuse Inventory which measures risk for abuse (Sebes, 1983), it was found that abusive parents endorse a commitment to abusive as opposed to nonabusive responses to adolescent behavior problems.

SUMMARY

Although the effects of being a victim or a witness of abuse and violence have pervasive developmental effects throughout childhood and adolescence, it is clear that many children who are exposed to violence avoid its most devastating outcomes. In order to account for these divergent findings, it is necessary to adopt theoretical models that include interaction of both risk and protective factors at all stages of child and family development and at all significant ecological levels. Models with these characteristics have been designed primarily to account for etiology and have been useful in identifying and testing the strength of etiological and contextual factors in the prediction of abuse. Such models need to be further developed for assessing the effects of variables that mediate between abuse and child outcome. Because the phenomenology of abuse is so complex, the same models can be used heuristically as clinical guides for targeting factors for intervention with maltreating families and for designing public policy at the community level for the prevention of violence and remediation of its negative consequences.

Current findings on etiology implicate parental behavior more strongly than child behavior, although difficult child behavior, often learned as a consequence of abuse, is likely to be involved in its maintenance. Despite the fact that there seems to be no general psychological profile of abusive parents, the literature suggests that their parenting suffers from a tendency to ascribe negative intent to children's behavior, which is further exacerbated by heightened emotional arousal in response to stress. Depression and antisocial disorder are seen as possible contributing factors leading to overcontrolling, inconsistent, and harsh parenting. The current literature further suggests that there is some increased risk of parents becoming abusive if they have been abused themselves in childhood, although the risk has often been exaggerated because inadequate attention has been paid to factors that can interrupt the cycle of abuse. Interactions among family members in abusive families are characterized by a pervasive negativity that tends to escalate into abusive behavior. Because of the relative social isolation and insularity of caregivers in maltreating families, abusive behavior is inadequately constrained by community norms that ordinarily regulate behavior in nonabusive families.

The negative effects of abuse on children are found in all areas of child functioning—their physical/neurological development, their understanding of social relationships and their social interaction, especially with peers, their ability to learn, and their emotional development. Children who witness violence in either their homes or communities are also more likely to develop emotional and behavioral problems, although these effects have not yet been documented as fully as the effects of child victimization. Nor has the interaction between being a witness to or a victim of violence. Early results of studies of the effects of community violence suggest that its effects on children are mitigated by family stability and family safety.

The negative effects in adolescence of childhood victimization are found in increased rates of delinquency, with severity of abuse seemingly related to excessively violent behavior later on. Abused adolescents show increased rates of affective disorders and substance use. Research is still inadequate for understanding how society's response to early maltreatment, such as placement, mediates youths' outcome. The characteristics of families who first abuse their children in adolescence are different from those who abuse young children, and, as yet, adequate models have not yet developed for accounting for these differences in etiology and effects.

The very complexity of the phenomenon of abuse, with respect to etiology and outcome, suggests that there are many alternative levels and points of entry into the process that might be available for interventions that would be effective in preventing abuse and altering its negative outcome in abused children.

REFERENCES

Aber, J. L., Allen, J. P., Carlson, V., & Cicchetti, D. (1989). The effects of maltreatment on development during early childhood: Recent studies and their theoretical, clinical, and policy implications. In D. Cicchetti & V. Carlson (Eds.), *Child maltreatment: Theory and research on the causes and consequences of child abuse and neglect* (pp. 579–619). New York: Cambridge University Press.

Ainsworth, M. D., Blehar, M. C., Waters, E., & Wall, S. (1978). *Patterns of attachment: A psychological study of the strange situation.* Hillsdale, NJ: Erlbaum.

American Humane Association. (1982). *Annual report of the National Study of Child Abuse and Neglect Reporting.* Denver, CO: Author.

Ammerman, R. T. (1991). The role of the child in physical abuse: A reappraisal. *Violence and Victims, 6,* 87–100.

Azar, S. T. (1989). Training parents of abused children. In C. E. Schaefer & J. M. Briesmeister (Eds.), *Handbook of parent training* (pp. 414–441). New York: John Wiley.

Azar, S. T., Barnes, K. T., & Twentyman, C. T. (1988). Developmental outcomes in physically abused children: Consequences of parental abuse or the effects of a more general breakdown in caregiving behaviors? *The Behavior Therapist, 11,* 27–32.

Azar, S. T., Robinson, D. R., Hekimian, E., & Twentyman, C. T. (1984). Unrealistic expectations and problem-solving ability in maltreating and comparison mothers. *Journal of Consulting and Clinical Psychology, 52,* 687–691.

Azar, S. T., & Siegal, B. R. (1990). Behavioral treatment of child abuse: A developmental perspective. *Behavior Modification, 14,* 279–300.

Barahal, R., Waterman, J., & Martin, A. L. (1981). The social cognitive development of abused children. *Journal of Consulting and Clinical Psychology, 49,* 508–516.

Bauer, W. D., & Twentyman, C. T. (1985). The social cognitive development of abused children. *Journal of Consulting and Clinical Psychology, 49,* 508–516.

Bell, C. C., & Jenkins, E. J. (1993). Community violence and children on Chicago's Southside. *Psychiatry, 56,* 46–54.

Belsky, J. (1990). Child maltreatment: An ecological integration. *American Psychologist, 35,* 320–335.

Belsky, J. (1993). Etiology of child maltreatment: A developmental-ecological analysis. *Psychological Bulletin, 114,* 413–434.

Bolton, F. G., Lanier, R. H., & Gia, D. S. (1981). For better or worse? Foster parents and foster children in an officially reported child maltreatment population. *Children and Youth Services Review, 3,* 37–53.

Bousha, D., & Twentyman, C. (1984). Mother-child interactional style in abuse, neglect, and control groups. *Journal of Abnormal Psychology, 93,* 106–114.

Bowker, L. H., Arbitell, M., & McFerron, J. R. (1988). On the relationship between wife beating and child abuse. In K. Yllo & M. Bograd (Eds.), *Feminist perspectives on wife abuse* (pp. 158–174). Newbury Park, CA: Sage.

Bronfenbrenner, U. (1979). *The ecology of human development: Experiments by nature and design.* Cambridge, MA: Harvard University Press.

Burgdorff, K. (1980, December). *Recognition and reporting of child maltreatment: Findings from the National Incidence and Severity of Child Abuse and Neglect.* Prepared for the National Center on Child Abuse and Neglect, Washington, DC.

Burgess, R. L. (1979). Child abuse: A social interactional analysis. In B. B. Lahey & E. Kazdin (Eds.), *Advances in clinical child psychology* (pp. 142–172). New York: Plenum.

Burgess, R. L., & Conger, R. D. (1978). Family interaction in abusive, neglectful, and normal families. *Child Development, 49,* 1163–1173.

Burgess, R. L., & Garbarino, J. (1983). Doing what comes naturally? An evolutionary perspective on child abuse. In D. Finkelhor, R. Gelles, G. Hotaling, & M. Straus (Eds.), *The dark side of families.* Beverly Hills, CA: Sage.

Burgess, R. L., & Youngblade, L. (1988). Social incompetence and the intergenerational transmission of abusive parental practices. In G. T. Hotaling, D. Finkelhor, J. T. Kirkpatrick, & M. A. Straus (Eds.), *Family abuse and its consequences: New directions in research* (pp. 38–60). Newbury Park, CA: Sage.

Casanova, G. M., Domanic, J., McCanne, T. R., & Milner, J. S. (1992). Physiological responses to non-child-related stressors in mothers at risk for child abuse. *Child Abuse & Neglect, 16,* 31–44.

Cavaiola, A. A., & Schiff, M. D. (1988). Behavioral sequelae of physical and/or sexual abuse in adolescents. *Child Abuse & Neglect, 12,* 181—188.

Chilamkurti, C., & Milner, J. S. (1993). Perceptions and evaluations of child transgressions and disciplinary techniques in high- and low-risk mothers and their children. *Child Development, 64,* 1801–1814.

Christoffel, K. K. (1990). Violent death and injury in U.S. children and adolescents. *American Journal of Diseases of Children, 144,* 697–706.

Christopoulos, C., Cohn, D. A., Shaw, D. S., Joyce, S., Sullivan- Hanson, J., Kraft, S. P., & Emery, R. E. (1987). Children of abused women: I. Adjustment at time of shelter residence. *Journal of Marriage and the Family, 49,* 611–619.

Cicchetti, D., & Beeghly, M. (1987). Symbolic development in maltreated youngsters: An organizational perspective. In D. Cicchetti & M. Beeghly (Eds.), *Atypical symbolic development.* San Francisco: Jossey-Bass.

Cicchetti, D., & Lynch, M. (1993). Toward an ecological/transactional model of community violence and child maltreatment: Consequences for children's development. *Psychiatry, 56,* 96–118.

Cicchetti, D., & Rizley, R. (1981). Developmental perspectives on etiology, intergenerational transmission and sequelae of child maltreatment. *New Directions for Child Development: Developmental Perspectives on Child Maltreatment, 11,* 31–56.

Cohn, A. A., & Collignon, F. C. (1979). *NCHSR. Research Report Series. Vols. I and II: Evaluation of Child Abuse and Neglect Demonstration Projects, 1974–1977.* DHEW Publication Number PHS 79–3217.1.

Crittenden, P. M. (1981). Abusing, neglecting, and adequate dyads: Differentiating by patterns of interaction. *Merrill-Palmer Quarterly, 27,* 1–18.

Crittenden, P. M. (1985a). Maltreated infants: Vulnerability and resilience. *Journal of Child Psychology and Psychiatry, 26,* 85–96.

Crittenden, P. M. (1985b). Social networks, quality of child rearing, and child development. *Child Development, 56,* 1299–1313.

Crittenden, P. M. (1988). Relationships at risk. In J. Belsky & T. Nezworski (Eds.), *Clinical implications of attachment* (pp. 136–174). Hillsdale, NJ: Erlbaum.

Crittenden, P. M., & Ainsworth, M. D. S. (1989). Child maltreatment and attachment theory. In D. Cicchetti & V. Carlson (Eds.), *Child maltreatment: Theory and research on the causes and consequences of child abuse and neglect.* New York: Cambridge University Press.

Crittenden, P. M., & Bonvillian, J. (1984). The effect of maternal risk status on maternal sensitivity to infant cues. *American Journal of Orthopsychiatry, 54,* 250–262.

Crittenden, P. M., & Craig, S. E. (1990). Developmental trends in the nature of child homicide. *Journal of Interpersonal Violence, 5,* 202–216.

Crittenden, P. M., & DiLalla, D. L. (1988). Compulsive compliance: The development of an inhibitory coping strategy in infancy. *Journal of Abnormal Child Psychology, 16,* 585–599.

Daly, M., & Wilson, M. (1981). Child maltreatment from a sociobiological perspective. *New Directions for Child Development, 11,* 93–112.

Dean, A. L., Malik, M. M., Richards, W., & Stringer, S. A. (1986). Effects of parental maltreatment on children's conceptions of interpersonal relationships. *Developmental Psychology, 22,* 617–626.

Dembo, R., Williams, L., Schmeidler, J., & Berry, E. (1992). A structural model examining the relationship between physical child abuse, sexual victimization, and marijuana/hashish use in delinquent youth: A longitudinal study. *Violence and Victims, 7,* 41–62.

Dembo, R., Williams, L., Wothke, W., Schmeidler, J. (1992). The role of family factors, physical abuse, and sexual victimization experiences in high-risk youths' alcohol and other drug use and delinquency: A longitudinal model. *Violence and Victims, 7,* 245–266.

Dietrich, D., Berkowitz, L., Kadushin, A., & McGloin, J. (1990). Some factors influencing abusers' justification of their child abuse. *Child Abuse & Neglect, 14,* 337–345.

Dietrich, K. N., Starr, R. H., & Kaplan, M. G. (1980). Maternal stimulation and care of abused infants. In T. Field, S. Goldberg, D. Stern, & A. Sostek (Eds.), *High-risk infants and children: Adult and peer interactions.* New York: Academic Press.

Dietrich, K. N., Starr, R., & Weisfeld, G. E. (1983). Infant maltreatment: Caretaker-infant interaction and developmental consequences at different levels of parenting failure. *Pediatrics, 72,* 532–540.

Dix, T. (1991). The affective organization of parenting. *Psychological Bulletin, 110,* 3–25.

Dodge, K. A., Bates, J. E., & Pettit, G. S. (1990). Mechanisms in the cycle of violence. *Science, 250,* 1678–1683.

Dykes, L. (1986). The whiplash shaken infant syndrome: What has been learned? *Child Abuse & Neglect, 10,* 211–221.

Egeland, B. (1988). Breaking the cycle of abuse. Implications for prediction and intervention. In K. D. Browne, C. Davies, & P. Stratton (Eds.), *Early prediction and prevention of child abuse* (pp. 87–99). New York: John Wiley.

Egeland, B., Breitenbucher, M., & Rosenberg, D. (1980). Prospective study of the significance of life stress in the etiology of child abuse. *Journal of Consulting and Clinical Psychology, 48,* 195–205.

Egeland, B., & Brunquell, D. (1979). An at-risk approach to the study of child abuse: Some preliminary findings. *Journal of the American Academy of Child Psychiatry, 18,* 219–235.

Egeland, B., Jacobvitz, D., & Sroufe, L. A. (1988). Breaking the cycle of abuse. *Child Development, 59,* 1080–1088.

Egeland, B., & Sroufe, A. (1981). Developmental sequelae of maltreatment in infancy. *New Directions for Child Development: Developmental Perspectives on Child Maltreatment, 11,* 77–92.

Erickson, M. F., Egeland, B., & Pianta, R. (1989). The effects of maltreatment on the development of young children. In D. Ciccetti & V. Carlson (Eds.), *Child maltreatment: theory and research in the causes and consequences of child abuse and neglect* (pp. 647–684). New York: Cambridge University Press.

Feldman, R. S., Salzinger, S., Rosario, M., Alvarado, L., Caraballo, L., & Hammer, M. (1995). Parent, teacher, and peer ratings of physically abused and non-maltreated children's behavior. *Journal of Abnormal Child Psychology, 23,* 317–333.

Finkelhor, D., & Dziuba-Leatherman, J. (1994). Victimization of children. *American Psychologist, 49,* 173–183.

Finkelhor, D., Hotaling, G., & Sedlak, A. (1990). *Missing, abducted, runaway, and thrownaway children in America.* First Report: Numbers and Characteristics, National Incidence Studies, Executive Summary. Washington, DC: U.S. Department of Justice.

Fitzpatrick, K. M., & Boldizar, J. P. (1993). The prevalence and consequences of exposure to violence among African-American youth. *Journal of the American Academy of Child Psychiatry, 32,* 424–430.

Frank, Y., Zimmerman, R., & Leeds, M. D. (1985). Neurological manifestations in abused children who have been shaken. *Developmental Medicine and Child Neurology, 27,* 312–316.

Frodi, A. M., & Lamb, M. E. (1980). Child abusers' responses to infant smiles and cries. *Child Development, 51,* 238–241.

Gaensbauer, T. J., & Harmon, R. J. (1982). Attachment behavior in abused/neglected and premature infants: Implications for the concept of attachment. In R. N. Emde & R. J. Harmon (Eds.), *The development of attachment and affiliative systems* (pp. 263–280). New York: Plenum.

Gaensbauer, T., & Sands, S. (1979). Distorted affective communications in abused/neglected infants and their potential impact on caretakers. *Journal of the American Academy of Child Psychiatry, 18,* 236–250.

Garbarino, J. (1976). A preliminary study of some ecological correlates of child abuse: The impact of socioeconomic status on mothers. *Child Development, 47,* 178–185.

Garbarino, J. (1989). Troubled youth, troubled families: The dynamics of adolescent maltreatment. In D. Ciccetti & V. Carlson (Eds.), *Child maltreatment: Theory and research on the causes and consequences of child abuse and neglect* (pp. 685–706). New York: Cambridge University Press.

Garbarino, J., & Crouter, A. (1978). Defining the community context for parent-child relations: The correlates of child maltreatment. *Child Development, 49,* 604–616.

Garbarino, J., & Gilliam, G. (1980). *Understanding abusive families.* Lexington, MA: Lexington Books.

Garbarino, J., Schellenbach, C., Sebes, J., & Associates (1986). *Troubled youth, troubled families.* New York: Aldine.

Garbarino, J., & Sherman, D. (1980). High-risk neighborhoods and high-risk families: The human ecology of child maltreatment. *Child Development, 51,* 188–198.

Gelles, R. J. (1989). Child abuse and violence in single-parent families. Parent absence and economic deprivation. *American Journal of Orthopsychiatry, 59,* 492–501.

Gelles, R. J., & Straus, M. A. (1979). Violence in the American family. *Journal of Social Issues, 35,* 15–39.

Gelles, R. J., & Straus, M. (1988). *Intimate violence.* New York: Simon and Schuster.

George, C., & Main, M. (1979). Social interactions of young abused children: Approach, avoidance, and aggression. *Child Development, 50,* 306–318.

Gil, D. G. (1970). *Violence against children.* Cambridge, MA: Harvard University Press.

Giovanni, J. (1989). Definitional issues in child maltreatment. In D. Ciccetti & V. Carlson (Eds.), *Child maltreatment: Theory and research on the causes and consequences of child abuse and neglect* (pp. 3–37). New York: Cambridge University Press.

Gottman, J. M. (1991). Chaos and regulated change in families: A metaphor for the study of transitions. In P. A. Cowan & E. M. Hetherington (Eds.), *Family transitions* (pp. 247–272). Hillsdale, NJ: Erlbaum.

Groisser, D. (1986). Child witness to interparental violence: Social problem solving skills and behavioral adjustment. Unpublished master's thesis. University of Denver.

Hashima, P. Y., & Amato, P. R. (1994). Poverty, social support, and parent behavior. *Child Development, 65,* 394–403.

Hennessy, K. D., Rabideau, G. J., & Cicchetti, D. (1994). Responses of physically abused and nonabused children to different forms of interadult anger. *Child Development, 65,* 815–828.

Herrenkohl, R. C., Herrenkohl, E. C., & Egolf, B. P. (1983). Circumstances surrounding the occurrence of child maltreatment. *Journal of Consulting and Clinical Psychology, 51,* 424–431.

Herrenkohl, R. C., Herrenkohl, E. C., Seech, M., & Egolf, B. (1980). The repetition of child abuse: How frequently does it occur? *Child Abuse & Neglect, 3,* 67–72.

Hilberman, E., & Munson, K. (1977/1978). Sixty battered women. *Victimology, 2,* 460–470.

Hoffman-Plotkin, D., & Twentyman, C. T. (1984). A multimodal assessment of behavioral and cognitive deficits in abused and neglected preschoolers. *Child Development, 55,* 794–802.

Holden, G. W., & Ritchie, K. L. (1991). Linking extreme marital discord, child rearing, and child behavior problems: Evidence from battered women. *Child Development, 62,* 311–327.

Howes, C., & Espinosa, M. P. (1985). The consequences of child abuse for the formation of relationships with peers. *Child Abuse & Neglect, 9,* 397–404.

Huesmann, L. R., Eron, L. D., Lefkowitz, M. M., & Walder, L. O. (1984). Stability of aggression over time and generations. *Journal of Abnormal Psychology, 20,* 1120–1134.

Hunter, R. S., & Kilstrom, N. (1979). Breaking the cycle in abusive families. *American Journal of Psychiatry, 136,* 1320–1322.

Hunter, R. S., Kilstrom, N., Kraybill, E. N., & Loda, F. (1978). Antecedents of child abuse and neglect in premature infants: A prospective study in a newborn intensive care unit. *Pediatrics, 61,* 629–635.

Jaffe, P. G., Wolfe, D. A., & Wilson, S. K. (1990). *Children of battered women.* Newbury Park, CA: Sage.

Jaffe, P., Wolfe, D. A., Wilson, S., & Zak, L. (1986). Emotional and physical health problems of battered women. *Canadian Journal of Psychiatry, 31,* 625–629.

Kaplan, S. J. (1994). *Adolescent abuse: Overview of recent research findings.* Paper presented at the meetings of the American Psychiatric Association, Washington, DC.

Kaplan, S., Montero, J., Pelcovitz, D., & Kaplan, T. (1988). *Psychopathology of abused and neglected children.* Paper presented at the meetings of the American Academy of Child and Adolescent Psychiatry, Seattle, WA.

Kaplan, S. J., Pelcovitz, D., Salzinger, S., & Ganeles, D. (1983). Psychopathology of parents of abused and neglected children and adolescents. *Journal of the American Academy of Child Psychiatry, 22,* 238–244.

Kaufman, J., & Cicchetti, D. (1989). Effects of maltreatment of school-age children's socioemotional development: Assessments in a day-camp setting. *Developmental Psychology, 25,* 516–524.

Kaufman, J., & Zigler, E. (1987). Do abused children become abusive parents? *American Journal of Orthopsychiatry, 57,* 186–192.

Kavenagh, K., Youngblade, L., Reid, J., & Fagot, B. (1988). Interactions between children and abusive versus control parents. *Journal of Clinical Child Psychology, 17,* 137–142.

Kempe, C. H., Silverman, F. N., Steele, B. F., Droegmueller, W., & Silver, H. K. (1962). The battered child syndrome. *Journal of the American Medical Association, 181,* 105–112.

Kinard, E. M. (1980). Emotional development in physically abused children. *American Journal of Orthopsychiatry, 50,* 686–696.

Korbin, J. E. (1980). The cultural context of child abuse and neglect. *Child Abuse & Neglect, 4,* 3–13.

Kravic, J. N. (1987). Behavior problems and social competence of clinic-referred abused children. *Journal of Family Violence, 2,* 111–120.

Kropp, J. P., & Haynes, O. M. (1987). Abusive and nonabusive mothers: Ability to identify general and specific emotion signals of infants. *Child Development, 58,* 187–190.

Lahey, B. B., Conger, R. D., Atkeson, B. M., & Treiber, F. A., (1984). Parenting behavior and emotional status of physically abusive mothers. *Journal of Consulting and Clinical Psychology, 52,* 1062–1071.

Larrance, D. T., & Twentyman, C. T. (1983). Maternal attribution and child abuse. *Journal of Abnormal Psychology, 92,* 449–457.

Leventhal, J. M. (1981). Risk factors for child abuse: Methodologic standards in case-control studies. *Pediatrics, 68,* 684–690.

Lewis, D. O., Mallouh, C., & Webb, V. (1989). Child abuse, delinquency, and violent criminality. In D. Cicchetti & V. Carlson (Eds.), *Child maltreatment: Theory and research on the causes and consequences of child abuse and neglect* (pp. 707–721). New York: Cambridge University Press.

Lewis, D. O., & Shanok, S. S. (1977). Medical histories of delinquent and nondelinquent children: An epidemiological study. *American Journal of Psychiatry, 134,* 1020–1025.

Lewis, D. O., Shanok, S. S., Pincus, J. H., & Glaser, G. H. (1979). Violent juvenile delinquents: Psychiatric, neurological, psychological, and abuse factors. *Journal of the American Academy of Child Psychiatry, 18,* 307–319.

Loeber, R., Felton, D. K., & Reid, J. B. (1984). A social learning approach to the reduction of coercive processes in child abusive families: A molecular analysis. *Advances in Behavior Research and Therapy, 6,* 29–45.

Lynch, M., & Cicchetti, D. (1991). Patterns of relatedness in maltreated and non-maltreated children: Connections among multiple representational models. *Development and Psychopathology, 3,* 207–226.

Lynch, M. A., & Roberts, J. (1977). Predicting child abuse: Signs of bonding failure in the maternity hospital. *British Medical Journal, 1,* 624–626.

MacKinnon, C. E., Lamb, M. E., Belsky, J., & Baum, C. (1990). An affective-cognitive model of mother-child aggression. *Development and Psychopathology, 2,* 1–13.

Magura, S. (1981). Are services to prevent foster care effective? *Child and Youth Services Review, 3,* 193–212.

Main, M., & George, C. (1985). Responses of abused and disadvantaged toddlers to distress in agemates: A study in the daycare setting. *Developmental Psychology, 21,* 407–412.

Manly, J. T., Barnett, D., & Cicchetti, D. (1993, March). *The impact of severity, chronicity, subtype of maltreatment and home environment on children's socio-emotional development.* Paper presented at the meetings of the Society for Research in Child Development, New Orleans.

Martin, H. P. (1976). *The abused child: A multidisciplinary approach to developmental issues and treatment.* Cambridge, MA: Ballinger.

Martinez, P. E., & Richters, J. E. (1993). The NIMH Community Violence Project: II. Children's distress symptoms associated with violent exposure. *Psychiatry, 56,* 22–35.

Mash, E. J., Johnston, C., & Kovitz, K. (1983). A comparison of the mother-child interactions of physically abused and nonabused children during play and task situations. *Journal of Clinical Child Psychology, 12,* 337–346.

McCord, J. (1983). A forty year perspective on effects of child abuse and neglect. *Child Abuse & Neglect, 7,* 265–270.

Milner, J. S. (in press). Social information processing and physical child abuse. *Clincial Psychology Review.*

Milner, J. S., & Chilamkurti, C. (1991). Physical child abuse perpetrator characteristics: A review of the literature. *Journal of Interpersonal Violence, 6,* 345–366.

Morton, T. L., Twentyman, C. T., & Azar, S. T. (1988). Cognitive-behavioral assessment and treatment of child abuse. In N. Epstein, S. E. Schlesinger, & W. Dryden (Eds.), *Cognitive-behavioral therapy with families* (pp. 87–117). New York: Brunner/Mazel.

National Center of Child Abuse and Neglect. (1988). *Study findings: Study of national incidence and prevalence of child abuse and neglect.* Washington, DC: U.S. Department of Health and Human Services.

National Research Council. (1993). *Understanding child abuse and neglect.* Washington, DC: National Academy Press.

Oates, R. K., & Peacock, A. (1984). Intellectual development of battered children. *Australia and New Zealand Journal of Developmental Disabilities, 10,* 27–29.

Oldershaw, L., Walters, G. G., & Hall, D. K. (1986). Control strategies and noncompliance in abusive mother-child dyads: An observational study. *Child Development, 57,* 722–732.

Patterson, G. R. (1982). *Coercive family processes.* Eugene, OR: Castilia.

Pelton, L. (1978). Child abuse and neglect: The myth of classlessness. *American Journal of Orthopsychiatry, 48,* 608–617.

Powers, J. L., Eckenrode, J., & Jaklitsch, B. (1990). Maltreatment among runaway youth. *Child Abuse & Neglect, 14,* 87–98.

Pynoos, R. S., Frederick, C., Nader, K., Arroyo, W., Steinberg, A., Eth, S., Nunez, F., & Fairbanks, I. (1987). Life threat and posttraumatic stress in school-age children. *Archives of Psychiatry, 44,* 1057–1063.

Reid, J. B., Kavanagh, K., & Baldwin, D. V. (1987). Abusive parents' perceptions of child problem behaviors: An example of parental bias. *Journal of Abnormal Child Psychology, 15,* 457–466.

Reid, J. B., Taplin, P. S., & Loeber, R. (1981). A social interactional approach to the treatment of abusive families. In R. Stuart (Ed.), *Violent behavior: Social learning approaches to prediction, management, and treatment* (pp. 83–101). New York: Brunner/Mazel.

Reiss, D., Richters, J. E., Radke-Yarrow, M., & Scharff, D. (Eds.). (1993). *Violence and children.* New York: Erlbaum.

Richters, J. E. (1993). Community violence and children's development: Toward a research agenda for the 1990's. *Psychiatry, 56,* 3–6.

Richters, J. E., & Martinez, P. E. (1993). Violent communities, family choices, and children's chances: An algorithm for improving the odds. *Development and Psychopathology, 5,* 609–627.

Rosenbaum, A., & O'Leary, K. D. (1981). Children: The unintended victims of marital violence. *American Journal of Orthopsychiatry, 51,* 692–699.

Rosenberg, M. S. (1987). Children of battered women: The effects of witnessing violence on their social problem-solving abilities. *The Behavior Therapist, 4,* 85–89.

Runyon, D. K., & Gould, C. L. (1985). Foster care and child maltreatment: Impact on delinquent behavior. *Pediatrics, 75,* 562–568.

Runyon, D. K., Gould, C. L., Trost, C. C., & Loda, F. A. (1982). Determinants of foster care placement for the maltreated child. *Child Abuse & Neglect, 6,* 343–350.

Salzinger, S., Feldman, R. S., Hammer, M., & Rosario, M. (1992). Constellations of family violence and their differential effects on children's behavioral disturbance. *Child & Family Behavior Therapy, 14,* 23–41.

Salzinger, S., Feldman, R. S., Hammer, M., & Rosario, M. (1993). The effects of physical abuse on children's social relationships. *Child Development, 64,* 169–187.

Salzinger, S., Kaplan, S., & Artemyeff, C. (1983). Mothers' personal social networks and child maltreatment. *Journal of Abnormal Psychology, 92,* 68–76.

Salzinger, S., Kaplan, S., Pelcovitz, D., Samit, C., & Krieger, R. (1984). Parent and teacher assessment of children's behavior in child maltreating families. *Journal of the American Academy of Child Psychiatry, 23,* 458–464.

Salzinger, S., Wondolowski, S., Kaplan, S., & Kaplan, T. (1987). *A discourse analysis of the conversations between maltreated children and their mothers.* Paper presented at the meeting of the Society for Research in Child Development, Baltimore.

Schneider-Rosen, K., Braunwald, K. G., Carlson, V., & Cicchetti, D. (1985). Current perspectives in attachment theory: Illustrations from the study of maltreated infants. *Monographs of the Society for Research In Child Development* (serial no. 209).

Sebes, J. M. (1983). Determining the risk for abuse in families with adolescents: The development of a criterion measure. Unpublished doctoral dissertation, Pennsylvania State University.

Shanok, S. S., & Lewis, D. O. (1981). Medical histories of abused delinquents. *Child Psychiatry and Human Development, 11,* 222–231.

Smetana, J. G., & Kelly, M. (1989). Social cognition in maltreated children. In D. Cicchetti & V. Carlson (Eds.), *Child maltreatment: Theory and research on the causes and consequences of child abuse and neglect* (pp. 620–646). New York: Cambridge University Press.

Smetana, J. G., Kelly, M., & Twentyman, C. (1984). Abused neglected and nonmaltreated children's conceptions of moral and social-conventional transgressions. *Child Development, 55,* 277–287.

Snyder, J., Edwards, P., McGraw, K., Kilgore, K., & Holton, A. (1994). Escalation and reinforcement in mother-child conflict: Social processes associated with the development of physical aggression. *Development and Psychopathology, 6,* 305–321.

Stark, E., & Flitcraft, A. (1985). Women-battering, child abuse and social heredity: What is the relationship? In N. Johnson (Ed.), *Marital violence* (pp. 147–171). London: Routledge and Kegan Paul.

Starr, R. H., Jr. (1988). Physical abuse of children. In V. B. Van Hasselt, R. L. Morrison, A. S. Bellack, & M.

Hersen (Eds.), *Handbook of family violence* (pp. 119–155). New York: Plenum.

Steele, B. F., & Pollock, C. B. (1968). A psychiatric study of parents who abuse infants and small children. In R. E. Helfer & C. H. Kempe (Eds.), *The battered child.* Chicago: University of Chicago Press.

Steinberg, L. D., Catalano, R., & Dooley, D. (1981). Economic antecedents of child abuse and neglect. *Child Development, 52,* 975–985.

Sternberg, K. J., Lamb, M. E., Greenbaum, C., Cicchetti, D., Dawud, S., Cortes, R. M., Krispin, O., & Lorey, F. (1993). Effects of domestic violence on children's behavior problems and depression. *Developmental Psychology, 29,* 44–52.

Sternberg, K. J., Lamb, M. E., Greenbaum, C., Dawud, D., Cortes, R. M., & Lorey, F. (1994). The effects of domestic violence on children's perceptions of their perpetrating and nonperpetrating parents. *International Journal of Behavioral Development, 17,* 779–795.

Straker, G., & Jacobson, R. S. (1981). Aggression, emotional maladjustment, and empathy in the abused child. *Developmental Psychology, 17,* 762–765.

Straus, M. A. (1979). Measuring intrafamily conflict and violence: The conflict tactics (CT) scales. *Journal of Marriage and the Family, 41,* 75-88.

Straus, M. A., & Gelles, R. J. (1988). How violent are American families? Estimates from the national family violence resurvey and other studies. In G. T. Hotaling, D. Finkelhor, J. T. Kirkpatrick, & M. A. Straus (Eds.), *Family abuse and its consequences* (pp. 14–36). Newbury Park, CA: Sage.

Susman, E. J., Trickett, P. K., Iannotti, R. J., Hollenbeck, B. E., & Zahn-Waxler, C. (1985). Child-rearing patterns in depressed, abusive, and normal mothers. *American Journal of Orthopsychiatry, 55,* 237–251.

Toth, S. L., Manly, J. T., & Cicchetti, D. (1992). Child maltreatment and vulnerability to depression. *Development and Psychopathology, 4,* 97–112.

Trickett, P. K., & Kuczynski, L. (1986). Children's misbehaviors and parental discipline strategies in abusive and nonabusive families. *Developmental Psychology, 22,* 115–123.

Trickett, P. K., & Susman, E. J. (1988). Parental perceptions of childrearing practices in physically abusive and nonabusive families. *Developmental Psychology, 24,* 270–276.

Twentyman, C. T., Rohrbeck, C. A., & Amish, P. L. (1984). A cognitive-behavioral model of child abuse. In S. Saunders, A. M. Anderson, C. A. Hart, & G. M. Rubenstein (Eds.), *Violent individuals and families: A handbook for practitioners* (pp. 87–111). Springfield, IL: Charles C. Thomas.

U.S. Advisory Board on Child Abuse and Neglect. (1990). *Child abuse and neglect: Critical steps in response to a national emergency.* Washington, DC: Government Printing Office.

Vondra, J., Barnett, D., & Cicchetti, D. (1989). Perceived and actual competence among maltreated and comparison school children. *Development and Psychopathology, 1,* 237–255.

Wahler, R. G. (1980). Parent insularity as a determinant of generalization success in family treatment. In S. Salzinger, J. Antrobus, & J. Glick (Eds.), *The ecosystem of the "sick" child* (pp. 187–199). New York: Academic Press.

Wahler, R. G., & Dumas, J. E. (1986). "A chip off the old block": Some characteristics of coercive children across generations. In P. Strain, M. Guralnick, & H. Walkee (Eds.), *Children's social behavior: Development, assessment, and modification* (pp. 49–86). San Diego, CA: Academic Press.

Wasserman, G. A., Green, A., & Allen, R. (1983). Going beyond abuse: Maladaptive patterns of interaction in abusing mother-infant pairs. *Journal of the American Academy of Child Psychiatry, 22,* 245–252.

Weiss, B., Dodge, K. A., Bates, J. E., & Pettit, G. S. (1992). Some consequences of early harsh discipline: Child aggression and a maladaptive social information processing style. *Child Development, 63,* 1321–1335.

Whipple, E. E., & Webster-Stratton, C. (1991). The role of parental stress in physically abused families. *Child Abuse & Neglect, 15,* 279–291.

Widom, C. S. (1989a). Child abuse, neglect, and adult behavior: Research design and findings on criminality, violence, and child abuse. *American Journal of Orthopsychiatry, 59,* 355–367.

Widom, C. S. (1989b). Does violence beget violence? A critical examination of the literature. *Psychological Bulletin, 106,* 3–28.

Widom, C. S. (1989c). Child abuse, neglect, and violent criminal behavior. *Criminology, 27,* 251–271.

Widom, C. S. (1991). Childhood victimization and adolescent problem behaviors. In M. E. Lamb & R. Ketterlinus (Eds.), *Adolescent problem behaviors.* Hillsdale, NJ: Erlbaum.

Wolfe, D. A. (1987). *Child abuse: Implications for child development and psychopathology.* Newbury Park, CA: Sage.

Wolfe, D. A., Fairbank, J., Kelly, J. A., & Bradlyn, A. S. (1983). Child abusive parents' physiological responses to stressful and nonstressful behavior in children. *Behavioral Assessment, 5,* 363–371.

Wolfe, D. A., Jaffe, P., Wilson, S. K., & Zak, L. (1985). Children of battered women: The relation of child behavior to family violence and maternal stress. *Journal of Consulting and Clinical Psychology, 53,* 657–665.

Wolfe, D. A., & Mosk, M. D. (1983). Behavioral comparisons of children from abusive and distressed families. *Journal of Consulting and Clinical Psychology, 51,* 702–708.

Wolfe, D. A., Zak, L., Wilson, S., & Jaffe, P. (1986). Child witnesses to violence between parents: Critical issues in behavioral and social adjustment. *Journal of Abnormal Child Psychology, 14,* 95–104.

Wolfner, G. D., & Gelles, R. J. (1993). A profile of violence toward children: A national study. *Child Abuse & Neglect, 17,* 197–212.

Wolock, I., & Horowitz, B. (1979). Child maltreatment and material deprivation among AFDC-recipient families. *Social Service Review, 53,* 175–194.

CHAPTER 28

ETHICAL AND LEGAL ISSUES IN PEDIATRIC AND ADOLESCENT HEALTH PSYCHOLOGY

Gerard T. Barron, HEALTHSOUTH LAKE ERIE INSTITUTE OF REHABILITATION

Michael Schwabenbauer, HEALTHSOUTH LAKE ERIE INSTITUTE OF REHABILITATION

Health psychology is rapidly becoming a leading forte in American psychology today. Since creation of the division of Health Psychology (Division 38) by the APA, membership has continued to grow and now surpasses 3,000 (American Psychological Association, 1993). This continued growth has led to substantial integration for psychologists in the health care profession (Taylor, 1990), as well as to increasing exposure to several ethical concerns (Knapp & Vandecreek, 1981).

In addition, pediatric psychology has become a major focus for treatment of health-related issues within the field of clinical child psychology (Kaufman, Holden, & Walker, 1989). Thus, the broad scope of health psychology raises several pertinent ethical concerns for pediatric and adolescent practitioners. This chapter reviews several ethical and legal issues, as they relate to child and adolescent health care practitioners.

ETHICAL AND LEGAL CONSTRAINTS SHAPING CLINICAL PRACTICE

Various forces have emerged over the years to ensure ethical decision making on the part of psychologists. This ever-increasing regulation of psychology has developed due to the tremendous growth in the profession and the need for clearly defined standards of psychological practice. Psychologists must currently contend with ethical and legal standards in maintaining sound practice of the science.

The beginning of the ethical code of the American Psychological Association dates to 1938 with the formulation of a committee that examined the need for establishing ethical standards (Pryzwansky & Wendt, 1987). Over the years, several revisions have occurred and culminated in the most recent set of standards published in 1992 (American Psychological Association, 1992). Evolution of the code has been necessary due to increasing complexity and sophistication of society and the profession. In spite of this complexity, these ethical standards tend to operate through several basic underlying principles that are particularly relevant to pediatric practice and sound clinical decision making. As described by Levine, Anderson, Ferretti, and Steinberg (1993), these basic principles are the principles of autonomy, beneficence, and justice. *Autonomy* refers to the freedom to choose as well as taking responsibility for one's views (Battle, Kreisberg, O'Mahoney, & Chitwood, 1989). *Beneficence* refers to the obligation of professionals to protect the welfare of clients and do no harm, and *justice* reflects application of a sense of fairness (Battle et al., 1989).

Some authors, such as Geraty, Hendren, and Flaa (1992), argue that managed care, though reflecting a shift in societal values toward limiting spending on health care, represents an additional value that practitioners must consider when making ethical decisions; that additional value is justice to society. Important ethical decisions involving children and adolescents often involve these basic principles. Because the circumstances of an individual situation often involve competing claims based on different principles, some type of "balancing" of these claims must occur in favor of the value judged as more important in a given situation (Levine et al., 1993).

In addition to the ethical code, other established standards include the Specialty Guidelines for the Delivery of Services (American Psychological Association, 1981) and the standards for Hospital Practice (American Psychological Association, 1985, 1993). These have evolved to assist practitioners toward responsible decision making.

Further standards have also evolved from the legal profession. The existence of licensing laws in all 50 states speaks to the recognition of psychologists as independent service providers (Pryzwansky & Wendt, 1987). In contrast to private professional organizations that emphasize more stringent criteria to practice, licensure laws generally reflect minimum standards of competence. Further legal regulation has occurred through laws that recognize psychologist-client privilege, definition of the title "psychologist," and recent government regulations (Levine et al., 1993). Thus, both professional and legal standards

have emerged to regulate the practice of psychology and assist with ethical decisions. Furthermore, it is important to consider case law because the courts assert a wide range of rights and duties that have considerable impact on the host of interventions used in clinical practice (Frohboese & Overcast, 1987).

SOME SELECTED AREAS OF ETHICAL CONCERN IN PEDIATRIC AND ADOLESCENT HEALTH PSYCHOLOGY PRACTICE

Ethical dilemmas often arise from characteristics of the field and the population it serves. Others stem from the settings in which clinical services take place. It is to the former that the focus of this chapter now turns.

Competency

A basic ethical principle is that of competency to practice within the limitations of one's expertise (American Psychological Association, 1992). Recommendations for establishing competency in the field of health psychology have existed for some time and continue to-evolve. These recommendations generally include completion of training at the doctoral level according to the practitioner model, followed by two years of postdoctoral experience in health psychology (Jones, 1987; Richards, 1992). Most recently, the American Board of Professional Psychology (ABPP) has begun to award diplomas in Health Psychology. A summary of ABPP requirements includes completion of training at the doctoral level; an internship of at least 1,500 hours in an organized health care setting; five years of acceptable qualifying experience, of which four must be postdoctoral; present engagement in professional work in health psychology; evidence of continuing education; demonstration of professional commitment, as evidenced by membership in APA: and state licensure (American Board of Professional Psychology, 1993).

A variety of perspectives currently exists on training health psychologists. Provision of health psychology training can occur as a component of clinical psychology, as a Ph.D. minor, or as a free-standing doctoral program (Richards, 1992). Nonetheless, a majority of Division 38 members report backgrounds in clinical psychology (American Psychological Association, 1993). No formal standards currently exist for the training of pediatric health psychologist, although standards would dictate that individuals receive in-depth training in child clinical, pediatric, and developmental psychology. Belar (1990) listed general training to include clinical assessment and treatment skills, biological and social bases of health and disease, ethics, research methods, health policy systems and organizations, health assessment, consultation, and intervention. Readers can consult Belar (1990) for an in-depth discussion of recommended training for health psychologists.

Although self-identification was formerly the primary means of credentialing necessary in these areas, the preceding recommendations discussed above (or similar ones) will ultimately provide the standards that credentialing bodies will use to identify such specialists. Adams (1989) cautioned that the fact that specialty areas in psychology, such as neuropsychology or health psychology, are new or that one's interest in the area is longstanding provides no exemption from such legitimate requirements as standards for training.

Those trained in clinical psychology now working in these areas must be constantly vigilant of the limits of their expertise pursuant to both ethical standards and specialty guidelines for the provision of services (American Psychological Association, 1981, 1992) and resist the temptation to become "one-workshop wonders." Differences in approaches between clinical psychologists and health psychologists arise, which may have an impact on issues of competency. Clinical psychologists may not have experience with a specific disease process and thus may overdiagnose psychopathology. For example, health psychologists may see denial in an adolescent diagnosed with a chronic medical condition, such as diabetes, as an expected adaptive mechanism to reduce anxiety, but clinical psychologists without experience with this population may view denial as pathological and target it for immediate intervention (Swencionis & Hall, 1987).

The issue of competence also extends to the use of psychological devices. Examples include biofeedback equipment and devices used in the treatment of enuresis or sexual dysfunction. Lack of knowledge about how a device functions or its possible effects on clients may place some psychologists outside of the boundaries of their competence from an ethical point of view, although legal liability would depend on the degree of harm to patients and the extent to which a psychologist violated the standards of care attendant to such devices (Schwitzgebel, 1978). Merely taking a workshop or course on the use of such devices may be insufficient and, depending on skill and background, ongoing supervision may be necessary.

Clinicians utilizing such devices must ensure that treatment is appropriate, that they have obtained informed consent, that physicians have ruled out other medical problems, that referring physicians are aware of the treatment plans, and that medical consultation is ongoing. Such minimum steps are necessary, as in other interventions with medical patients, to avoid the potential charge of practicing medicine without a license (Frohboese & Overcast, 1987; Knapp & Vandecreek, 1981). Practitioners also need to be aware of any restrictions imposed on the use of a proposed instrument or device by Food and Drug Administration regulations. These regulations are subject to change by professional pressure, and it is ironic that 30 years ago, some professionals considered phonograph records medical devices because they contained instructions on how to treat insomnia (Schwitzgebel, 1978).

Informed Consent

Ethical concerns about working with common chronic health problems of children and adolescents are receiving increasing amounts of attention. An ethical principle of major concern to health practitioners is that of informed consent to treatment. As stated in the revised Ethical Principles of Psychologists,

> Psychologists obtain appropriate informed consent to therapy or related procedures, using language that is reasonably understandable to participants.... When persons are legally incapable of giving informed consent, psychologists obtain informed permission from a legally authorized person, if such substituted consent is permitted by law. (American Psychological Association, 1992, p. 1605)

Generally, adults have the right to consent to treatment, assuming they are competent to do so, following a discussion of the nature of treatment and its likely risks and benefits (Moreno, 1989). Informed consent for minors is not nearly as clear-cut because legal and health care professionals have generally considered individuals below the age of majority to be incompetent to give truly informed consent. There do not exist any clearly defined policies about seeking consent to treat from minors (Levine et al., 1993). Though guidelines continue to evolve, much controversy remains. From a legal standpoint, psychologists must acquire consent of a minor's parents or some other individual authorized to give consent (e.g., in loco parentis in most settings). Exceptions do exist, however. For example, adolescents seeking treatment for birth control, substance abuse, and other concerns may do so in some states without parental consent (Corey, Corey, & Callanan, 1993). In addition, some professionals have given increasing recognition to the "mature minor" concept, which represents individuals

who can appreciate and understand the nature of a proposed procedure and its consequences. Usually, a minor will not be deemed mature until the age of at least 15 years. The likelihood that a health professional may successfully invoke this exception increases where the proposed procedure is clearly beneficial and uncomplicated, where obtaining parental consent is impractical, where the risk of harm, to the minor is insubstantial, and where the information provided by the physician to the child is sufficiently detailed and couched in language sufficiently simple for the minor to grant consent that may be deemed to be informed. (McMenamin, 1991, p. 285)

The doctrine of informed consent consists of three components: competence, knowledge, and voluntariness (Schwitzgebel & Schwitzgebel, 1980). *Competence* refers to the ability to understand information one is receiving and to make an autonomous decision (Levine et al., 1993). *Knowledge* requires sufficient understanding of the risks and benefits involved, and *voluntariness* refers to freely given consent (Schwitzgebel & Schwitzgebel, 1980).

These components seem to emerge at varying stages in childhood and adolescent development. For example, Moreno (1989) reported that children alter their cognitive perspective of voluntariness during mid-adolescence as the prior reluctance to resist authority figures begins to give way. This seems to occur somewhat later than the conceptual development of understanding illness, which occurs around age twelve. Kaser-Boyd, Adelman, and Taylor (1985) identified the ability to think about the risks and benefits of therapy as an important factor in giving informed consent and found that most minors were able to identify at least one risk or benefit. Clearly, trends toward granting minors further privacy and autonomy beyond what they currently have continue. A growing body of evidence supports the notion that, when using usual standards of competence, fifteen-year-olds are as competent as adults (Gustafson & McNamara, 1987). Thus, a greater degree of adolescent involvement is consistent with the underlying spirit of the principle of autonomy, which forms the basis for the concept of informed consent (Marian. 1989). Incorporating adolescents into the consent process appears to be a growing trend in the profession. A recent survey of psychologists treating adolescents indicated that 70 percent of respondents attempt to obtain adolescent informed consent. The average age at which therapists ask patients for informed consent to treat is 12.8 years (Beeman & Scott, 1991).

In reference to anyone giving consent to treatment, Koocher and DeMaso (1990) emphasized the following factors: a) access to information that may influence the decision to consent; b) voluntariness to choose or refuse to participate; c) one's decision-making ability; and d) competence to consent to treatment. Kooher and DeMaso (1990) went on to define competence as "the capacity to understand, to weigh potential outcomes, and also the foresight to anticipate the future consequences of a decision" (p. 69). It is evident that an increase in understanding of cognitive and social development in children has led to further questioning of the requirement of parental consent to treatment. Forming the basis of the longstanding need for parental consent are several factors, including alleged immaturity of minors, family privacy, and the notion of parents acting to further the 'best interests' of their children (Guyer, 1991). Although these factors continue to exert a primary influence in treatment decisions, pediatric practitioners must attempt to balance parental rights and concerns with those of the children.

It is also important to consider that provision of treatment varies according to geographic location, setting (inpatient versus outpatient), and type of facility. For example, Pennsylvania has attempted to balance the rights of parents and children through implementation of the Mental Health Services Act of 1976. Adolescents age fourteen or older may receive voluntary inpatient mental health treatment, though admitting facilities must notify a minor's parents of such treatment. Parents may then challenge the need for such inpatient treatment. In contrast, involuntary inpatient treatment does not require parental or minor consent (Knapp, 1994).

Confidentiality with Minors

Closely related to the issue of informed consent is that of confidentiality. This is a quite complex issue due to the particularly sensitive nature of the therapeutic relationship through childhood and adolescence. As stated in the APA Ethical Principles (American Psychological Associations, 1992),

> Psychologists discuss with persons and organizations with whom they establish a scientific or professional relationship (including to the extent feasible minors and their legal representatives) (1) the relevant limitations on confidentiality, including limitations where applicable in group, marital, and family therapy or in organizational consulting, and (2) the foreseeable uses of the information generated through their services. (p. 1606)

As is the case with other clinical fields, there are no clearly defined standards regarding confidentiality and its limitations in relation to the ethical practice of pediatric and adolescent health psychology. Problems may stem from the fact that clinicians are attempting to balance the rights of their dual clients, parents, and children. It is important for practitioners to consider communicating to minors at the onset of treatment that parents (or the responsible adult) have legal access to therapeutic communications as holder of the privilege (Brewer & Faitak, 1989). Although this is certainly ethically and legally necessary, a conflict quickly emerges with regard to the need to develop a sense of rapport and trust within the context of a therapeutic relationship versus a child's or adolescent's concerns

regarding parental access. Research investigating the degree of self-disclosure that occurs with confidentiality assured clearly supports its value in work with adolescents (Kobocow, McGuire, & Blau, 1983).

As with informed consent, a conceptual understanding of confidentiality develops and matures through early adolescence (Messenger & McGuire, 1981). Gustafson and McNamara (1987) provided an excellent overview of varying practices in addressing the limits of confidentiality with children and adolescents. Practices range from requiring children to give consent before parents can see records to the other extreme of having therapists determine likely use of records and subsequently deciding to release records only if in a child's best interest (Glenn, 1980). Gustafson and McNamara (1987) suggested means of resolving this dilemma by recommending consideration of age and an assessment of cognitive functioning in formulating a decision regarding degree of confidentiality. These authors stated:

> Adolescents 14–15 years of age generally are as capable as adults in making well informed treatment decisions. Adolescents of this age, who demonstrate an adequate understanding of confidentiality and its limits, should be afforded the same degree of confidentiality as adults. (Gustafson & McNamara, 1987, p. 505)

Several strategies toward resolving this dilemma exist. Taylor and Adelman (1989) reported they encourage children to take the lead in sharing confidential information as appropriate with third parties. This allows children to participate actively in the decision-making process of what precisely to reveal and how to present information they shared. The authors encouraged therapists to assist children in this process and to minimize the emotional costs of disclosure.

A related issue is that of release of information to third parties. One may conclude that parents have legal access to information regarding the content of treatment sessions. Although some parents may insist on receiving such sensitive information, psychologists must work toward establishing a clear sense of privacy at the onset of treatment by requesting that parents withhold their need for information (Knapp. 1994). This approach will serve the best interests of children in most situations.

THE PRACTICE SETTING IN PEDIATRIC AND ADOLESCENT HEALTH PSYCHOLOGY

Integration of psychology into the medical care environment has resulted in development of diverse roles for practitioners in the psychosocial management of illness and health. The previous chapters in this book attest to the expanding involvement of psychologists in this area. Along with exciting opportunities for practice, however, come new quandaries and dilemmas. Health care settings are frequently fertile ground for role and task conflicts and ambiguities because of the control held by medicine and the organizational characteristics of these settings, which are increasingly stressing their "corporate" nature (Elfant, 1985; Kastenbaum, 1982). When psychologists become part of the health care team, a question of professional power relationships may become a paramount and complex issue (Miller & Swartz, 1990), and complications may adversely affect patient care. Although ethical behavior is important for psychologists in every professional activity, the health care setting, because of such factors, may pose unique problems.

In addition, the potential legal issues for psychologists who work in health care settings may be quite numerous because of the context in which they operate. A host of external restraints—such as federal, state, local, and institutional legislation, regulations, standards, policies, and case law—all come to bear in guiding the conduct of practitioners. Given the nascent state of health psychology as an area of specialization, there do not yet exist proper legal precedents to define areas of involvement (Task Force on Legal Issues, 1983). Because of the potential for overlap between psychology and other health-related professions, a clear understanding of what activities constitute legally permissible practice in this area is essential.

AREAS OF ETHICAL CONCERN

Professional Relationships

Paradigms

An important point to recognize as psychologists enter health care settings is that vast differences exist in the models into which physicians and psychologists have traditionally been socialized. In attempting to work collaboratively on a case, a physician and a psychologist may discover these paradigms clash, with the result that they do not speak the same language in conceptualizing the case or recommending treatment (Russo & Tarbell, 1984). Pragmatic issues also arise related to physician expectations and pressures for cost containment (Halgin, 1987).

In Western medicine, the dominant paradigm is the biomedical model. It attempts to explain health and sickness in terms of physical, chemical, and physiological changes in bodily systems, divorced from the psychosocial aspects of illness (Miller & Swartz, 1990). A distinction often made is that of disease versus illness, where illness is the component of discomfort arising from the perception of disease and the interaction of individuals with the environment (Krantz & Glass, 1984). Such a distinction seems to allow roles to be equitably split between psychology and medicine. A more integrated perspective, and one in keeping with the training of psychologists for this setting, is the biopsychosocial model (Engel, 1977). The traditional, reductionistic biomedical approach, argued Miller and Swartz (1990), has maintained its dominance through responses to such challenges by ignoring or attempting to diminish their importance or by attempting to incorporate aspects of those challenges while asserting the primacy of the biomedical perspective. As a result, psychosocial issues retain a devalued position.

Institutional Factors

Some authors (Kastenbaum, 1982) have viewed hospitals as ponderous city-states, in which sharp distinctions exist among classes, clashes frequently arise over power, and realities of institutions may take precedence over health care skills and judgment. In this context, according to Kastenbaum (1982), "The impulse to act on one's best knowledge and highest values is opposed by perceived constraints. The crucial question is not What should I do? It is Can I act on my judgment and principles?" (p. 1357). Elfant (1985) wrote of the intense pressure in hospital settings to act, fix, and do, referring to the medical-heroic posture as one that ultimately promotes the very behaviors it seems to eliminate—the sick patient role, the sense of helplessness about self in times of stress, and addiction to rescuers.

Conflicts of Interest and Dual Relationship Problems

Psychologists often function in hospital settings in the consultation-liaison role, one which psychiatry has occupied for years (Stabler & Mesibov, 1984). Consultants typically are specialists who briefly interact with patients, attending physicians, and other specialists and provide recommendations for dealing with specific patient problems. In contrast, when performing liaison activities, health care professionals participate as active members of treatment teams on specific services with delineated clinical responsibilities, which may include rounds, provision of psychotherapy services of patients of families, inservice training, and research (Miller & Swartz, 1990).

Consultants have greater autonomy but limited access to units and authority—they must often accept limitations for their involvement based on the specific request, and their recommendations are not binding. Because of their ongoing relationships with other team members, those in liaison roles may have greater efficacy. When functioning in the consultation-liaison role, psychologists must constantly be aware of the possibility that a conflict of interest may arise between needs of the patient and needs of the institution or other staff members.

Tancredi and Edlund (1983) questioned whether such conflicts might not be universally present in the role of psychological consultant. Physicians have typically assumed a patriarchal role, assuming responsibility for acting in patients' best interests. In meeting patients' needs, psychiatrists or psychologists in that role will generally focus on creating the necessary environment that will allow patients to make their own decisions. Consultants usually receive referrals when problems arise in the relationship between physician and patient—problems that may have important political or moral overtones. Instead of permitting psychologists to provide specific clinical services, referral sources are often (implicitly or explicitly) requesting the appearance of a persuader, a moral arbitrator, or someone with conflict-resolution skills. In answering such a referral, a psychologist may unwittingly settle into that role and ignore the issue of client welfare. In such a situation, psychologists must answer the question: To whom do they owe ultimate responsibility? To the Physician? To the patient? To the

institution? Psychologists must not overlook or ignore the interests of each of these parties.

Tancredi and Edlund (1983) outlined four types of conflict of interest situations. The dual clients (parents and child) that psychologists serve may only complicate already ethically charged situations:

1. Desires of institutional administrations may conflict with those of patients or family members. Institutions may feel pressure to discharge patients because of reimbursement issues, whereas patients may resist. In such circumstances, referrals made to psychologists often implicitly convey the message that they are to act as persuaders. When answering such referrals through a standard evaluation, both parties are likely to feel displeased.

2. Disagreements may exist between patients and family members over issues related to care. Physicians may choose to avoid the issue, thus abrogating their responsibility to mediate the conflict. Physicians making referrals under these circumstances are often implicitly requesting a communication link between the parties. Answering this referral without careful consideration has the potential for infringing on the decision-making abilities of clients through subtle manipulation while ignoring the lack of communication between the parties involved.

3. Conflict may exist between patients and treating physicians. These situations, according to Tancredi and Edlund (1983), have the greatest potential for moral ambiguity. In these circumstances, physicians often make vague requests for consultation—requests that professionals other than psychologists would generally not tolerate and that may reveal the referral as an act of hostility toward a patient (Elfant, 1985), such as "the patient is crazy." The request here may be for someone to take over responsibility for a significant portion of care, if not to build a case for a "dump" or transfer to another service. Often, patients are not even aware of the request for consultation, and they may react to the implicit message of their physicians—a message embedded in the act of referring to a "head doctor."

4. Conflict may exist between patients, physicians, and staff members. Clashes may occur between

different professional members of patients' health care teams, often over issues of power, and patient care becomes the battleground in which staff members enact these issues. In theory, a truly functional interdisciplinary team would share equal amounts of responsibility for patient care, thus addressing issues of power in such a way that allowed all team members to participate fully in patient care (Miller & Swartz, 1990). However, the issue of ultimate responsibility for patient care is difficult to overlook and resolve, and institutions and the law often vest this power in the hands of medical providers (i.e., physicians). Some psychologists in hospital settings may assume the responsibility for coordination of team efforts and see this as a natural role because they have training in group process. This also seems to provide a situation ripe for conflict of interest because psychologists may function as group therapists to their teams in addition to serving the role as team member (Miller & Swartz, 1990). This situation raises informed consent issues unless the other members of the treatment team understand and assent to this expansion of role.

Miller and Swartz (1990) asserted that psychologists in health care settings have a responsibility to make explicit these issues of power and, over time, to negotiate ways of working with other professionals, especially physicians, that minimize the likelihood of such binds and the attendant risks, thereby promoting the best interests of their clients. Psychologists must give careful consideration to all referrals, and the burden is on psychologists to seek additional information or clarification if necessary of what the physician is requesting.

Other Ethical Issues

Marketing of Services and Self-Monitoring

Because health psychology is a rapidly growing area and the public is becoming increasingly concerned about health, the potential exists for zealous practitioners to oversell techniques and make unsubstantiated claims (Swencionis & Hall, 1987). Self-help materials abound in the areas of stress reduction, relaxation, and other risk-factor modification techniques, and it is important for those marketed to the public to show proven efficacy (American Psychological Association, 1992). Swencionis and Hall (1987) also noted that health psychologists have an obligation to criticize unsubstantiated claims made by psychologists and nonpsychologists alike, such as those made by dubious "hynotherapists" to cure smoking in one session or by weight-loss programs offering a similar "quick fix" for problems related to life-style. Such claims undermine overall credibility, frequently alienate physicians, and endanger support for proper research.

Adequate Consideration of Values and Cultural Differences

In the health care area, as in others, it is important for psychologists to consider the cultural background of patients and realize that treatment must be acceptable to standards inherent in the patients' cultural affiliations. What is appropriate for a well-educated, upper-middle-class American (which most psychologists are) may not be healthy for all patients (Swencionis & Hall, 1987). Issues of patient noncompliance may then arise, which have their bases in these subtle and often implicit value differences (Elfant, 1985). When treating patients with self-control procedures, one must ensure that patients do not interpret the treatment as a promise of cure for a condition such as headaches or diabetes and that patients understand their responsibility in the treatment.

Confidentiality in the Health Care Setting

The nature of team treatment complicates issues of confidentiality and makes it difficult to guarantee privileged communication. As Pope (1990) noted, maintaining appropriate confidentiality is often difficult in hospital settings where discussion of a patient's condition may often result in inappropriate audiences hearing some of the information. It is important to discuss these issues with patients routinely, as a part of clarifying one's role, in order to set ground rules for what information one may share with the team. Patients' hospital records are likely to be available to many staff, some of whom may relate to the case only peripherally. In addition, hospital staff may release information to patients' insurance carriers, to other professionals, or to patients themselves without knowledge or review of consulting psychologists. Therefore, psychologists must take special care in documentation to include only information necessary in order to protect the privacy of patients and family members (Soisson, Vandecreek, & Knapp, 1987).

LEGAL ISSUES

Knapp and Vandecreek (1981) noted that psychologists operating in health care settings may be at increased risk for malpractice suits relative to psychologists performing in more traditional settings, because factors operating to mitigate against malpractice suits in psychotherapy are not operative in health care settings. These authors described factors that might actually lead to increased risk, including lack of a close, ongoing relationship and the fact that medical patients often have better ego strength than psychiatric patients and will not feel deterred by the rigors of a court battle. Also, because physical illness is generally not stigmatizing, patients would presumably not feel embarrassed by potential courtroom revelations. In addition, these authors noted that physical harm that might ensue from negligent acts is easier to prove and that it is easier to determine its cause than in the case of harm alleged in other areas of psychological practice.

Courts may be more likely to view well-defined behavioral interventions, the basis for behavioral medicine, as constituting a higher standard of care than exists for emotional disorders. As national standards for credentialing continue to develop, they could begin to have implications for perceived standards of care as well, and courts are less likely to rely on the locality rule in any suits that may arise (Knapp & VandeCreek, 1981).

The primary issue of liability is overstepping competency and running the risk of practicing medicine without a license. State statutes are the source of law governing the scope of practice of medicine as well as psychology and other health care professions, and administrative boards oversee their implementation and license-qualified individuals (Fish, 1984). Such statutes typically cover who has the qualifications to engage in the diagnosis and treatment of medical illness. In Pennsylvania, for example, it is unlawful for any individual to diagnose diseases,

"pretend to a knowledge of any branch or branches of medicine and surgery," or treat diseases by the use of medicine or surgery or *any other means* unless one has become licensed or received an exemption from the Pennsylvania Medical Board (Post et al., 1984, p. 549).

Although psychologists are not liable for performing within the scope of practice granted by their license, the practice of medicine can be less than obvious. Are psychologists practicing medicine when treating patients with chronic diseases or providing rehabilitation for head-injured patients? Are psychologists diagnosing disease when they offer opinions regarding the cause of patients' headaches? Medical consultation and referral and close coordination of treatment with primary physicians avoid this problem, but without it, psychologists are practicing in a gray area.

Uncertainties in the scope of practice of any profession must await statutory resolution or court decision, and because of the often protracted time lines involved, practitioners must deal with uncertainty and risk in the intervening period (Fish, 1984). A recent review of malpractice claims filed against psychologists, however, offers some consolation (Dorken, 1990). This review found that in the 13-year history of the APA insurance trust, there has been no court award for failure to identify a medical problem, failure to refer to a physician, or failure to provide appropriate psychological care to a patient with medical complications. Litigants have settled some of these claims out of court, however, and it is important to remember that decisions to settle malpractice claims are business decisions (Lentz, 1989).

If the courts perceive a health care provider as practicing medicine, case law has determined that the courts can hold that health care provider to the standard of the field of medicine he or she may have inadvertently entered (*Pitre* v. *Opelousas General Hospital,* 1988). Failure to refer and negligent diagnosis are two obvious issues that place psychologists at risk for malpractice suits (*Ehlinger* v. *Sipes,* 1988). For example, in a recent court decision (*Account Adjustment Bureau* v. *Cooperman,* 1984), the court allowed a suit to proceed against a psychologist for emotional distress allegedly suffered by parents of a child when the psychologist allegedly misdiagnosed the child as having nonpsychotic organic brain syndrome.

The courts may also find psychologists negligent when psychologists appear to be contributing to patients' decisions to terminate standard medical treatment. Even if a psychologist has coordinated a treatment program with services provided by a physician, that psychologist may be negligent if he or she does not keep the physician informed of treatment progress at least to the extent necessary to modify the treatment when indicated. This is especially true in cases involving medication and, hence, where there is the potential to reduce risks of developing side effects. For example, physicians may need to reduce medication dosage if psychologically based interventions are effective. In a recent federal court decision (*Chambers* v. *Ingram,* 1988), the court found a psychologist employed in a prison negligent, under Illinois law, for failing to provide accurate information about an inmate's condition to the prison psychiatrist, who had prescribed Haldol, which caused the inmate to experience seizures.

Psychologists must also take great care when obtaining informed consent, especially if a treatment is unproven or experimental. Discussions must include what the average reasonable patient would want to know before starting treatment. This discussion must cover the nature of the proposed treatment, risks, likelihood of success, and available alternative treatments. A case discussed by Malcolm (1986) involved the charge that a psychiatrist chose to treat his patient's major depressive disorder and narcissistic personality disorder with long-term psychodynamic psychotherapy rather than psychotropic medications or a combination of drugs and therapy. The basis of the lawsuit was, in part, the psychiatrist's failure to provide the patient with information regarding alternative treatments and relative efficacy.

SUMMARY

Although the preceding discussion is by no means an exhaustive guide to the pitfalls of practice at the interface of psychology and medicine, practitioners must be aware that, in some respects, issues of ethically and legally sound practice in pediatric and adolescent health psychology become more complex, depending on setting, roles, population served, and dynamics of the relationships involved. Because current laws do

not often define this interface clearly, the potential exists for clients to seek such clarification through the courts, thus placing those who practice in this area at potentially increased risk for tort action.

REFERENCES

Accounts Adjustment Bureau v. *Cooperman,* 204 Cal. Rptr. 881 (Cal. App. 2 Dist. 1984).

Adams, K. A. (1989). Neuropsychology is not just in the eye of the beholder. *Professional Psychology: Research and Practice, 20*(12), 488–489.

American Board of Professional Psychology. (1983). *Policies and procedures for the creation of diplomates in health psychology.* Columbia, MO: Author.

American Psychological Association. (1981). Specialty guidelines for the delivery of services by clinical psychologists. *American Psychologist, 36*(6), 640–651.

American Psychological Association. (1985). *A hospital primer for psychologists.* Committee on Professional Practice of the Board of Professional Affairs. Washington, DC: Author.

American Psychological Association. (1992). Ethical principles of psychologists and code of conduct. *American Psychologist, 47*(12), 1597–1611.

American Psychological Association. (1993). *Profile of Division 38 members: 1993.* Washington, DC: Author. (APA Education Directorate.)

Battle, C. U., Kreisberg, R. V., O'Mahoney, C., & Chitwood, D. L. (1989). Ethical and developmental considerations in caring for hospitalized adolescents. *Journal of Adolescent Health Care, 10,* 479–489.

Beeman, D. G., & Scott, N. A. (1991). Therapists' attitudes toward psychotherapy informed consent with adolescents. *Professional Psychology: Research and Practice, 20*(3), 230–234.

Belar, C. D. (1990). Issues in training clinical health psychologists. *Psychology and Health, 4,* 31–37.

Brewer, T., & Faitak, M. T. (1989). Ethical guidelines for the inpatient psychiatric care of children. *Professional Psychology: Research and Practice, 20*(3), 142–147.

Chambers v. *Ingram,* 858 F.2d 351 (7th Cir. 1988).

Corey, G., Corey, M., & Callanan, P. (1993). *Issues and ethics in the helping professions* (4th ed.). Pacific Grove, CA: Brooks Cole.

Dorken, H. (1990). Malpractice claims experience of psychologists: Policy issues, cost comparisons with psychiatrists, and prescription privilege implications. *Professional Psychology: Research and Practice, 21*(2), 150–152.

Ehunger v. *Sipes,* 434 N.W. 2d 825 (1988).

Elfant, A. B. (1985). Psychotherapy and assessment in hospital settings: Ideological and professional conflicts. *Professional Psychology: Research and Practice, 16*(1), 55–63.

Engel, G. L. (1977). The need for a new medical model: A challenge for biomedicine. *Science, 196,* 129–136.

Fish, M. S. (1984). Scope of practice. In C. H. Wecht (Ed.), *Legal Medicine Annual, 1984* (pp. 267–274). New York: Appleton-Century-Crofts.

Frohboeses, R., & Overcast, T. D. (1987). An overview of health psychology and the law. In G. C. Stone, S. M. Weiss, J. D. Matarazzo, N. E. Miller, J. Rodin, C. D. Belar, M. J. Follock, & J. E. Singer (Eds.), *Health psychology: A discipline and a profession* (pp. 217–230). Chicago: University of Chicago Press.

Geraty, R. D., Hendren, R. L., & Flaa, C. J. (1992). Ethical perspectives on managed care as it relates to child and adolescent psychiatry. *Journal of the American Academy of Child and Adolescent Psychiatry, 31* (3). 398–402.

Glenn, C. M. (1980). Ethical issues in the practice of child psychotherapy. *Professional Psychology, 4,* 613–619.

Gustafson, K. E., & McNamara, J. R. (1987). Confidentiality with minor clients: Issues and guidelines for therapists. *Professional Psychology: Research and Practice, 18* (5), 503–508.

Guyer, M. J. (1991). Informed consent to medication of hospitalized minors. *Psychotherapy in Private Practice, 9,* 166–161.

Halgin, R. P. (1987). Preparing psychologists-in-training for the medical model. *Psychotherapy in Private Practice, 5* (l), 99–103.

Jones, N. F. (1987). Credentials for health psychologists. In N. F. Jones (Ed.), *Health psychology: A discipline and a profession* (pp. 191–201). Chicago: University of Chicago Press.

Kaser-Boyd, N., Adelman, H. S., & Taylor, L. (1985). Minors' ability to identify risks and benefits of therapy. *Professional Psychology: Research and Practice, 16,* 411–417.

Kastenbaum, R. (1982). The psychologist and public policy: A report from the real world. *Professional Psychology: Research and Practice, 16*(l), 55–63.

Kaufman, K. L., Holden, E. W., & Walker, C. E. (1989). Future directions in pediatric and clinical child psychology. *Professional Psychology: Research and Practice, 20* (3), 148–152.

Knapp, S. (1994, Spring). Treatment of minors. *PSCP Times,* p. 2.

Knapp, S., & Vandecreek, L. (1981). Behavioral medicine: Its malpractice risks for psychologists. *Professional Psychology, 12* (6), 677–683.

Kobocow, B., McGuire, J. M., & Blau, B. (1982). Influences of confidentiality conditions on self disclosure of early adolescents. *Professional Psychology: Research and Practice, 14,* 435–443.

Koocher, G. P., & DeMason, D. R. (1990). Children's competence to consent to medical procedures. *Pediatrician, 17,* 68–73.

Krantz, D. S., & Glass, D. C. (1984). Personality, behavior patterns and physical illness: Conceptual and methodological issues. In W. D. Gentry (Ed.), *Handbook of behavioral medicine* (pp. 38–86). New York: Guilford.

Lentz, R. D. (1989). Malpractice: Examining the presumption of wrongdoing. *Hospital and Community Psychiatry, 40* (10), 1074–1075.

Levine, M., Anderson, E., Ferretti, L., & Steinberg, K. (1993). Legal and ethical issues affecting clinical child psychology. In T. H. Ollendick & R. J. Prinz (Eds.), *Advances in clinical child psychology* (pp. 81–120). New York: Plenum.

Malcolm, J. G. (1986). Treatment choices and informed consent in psychiatry: Implications of the Oshcroft case for the profession. *Journal of Psychiatry and Law,* Spring-Summer, 9–103.

McMenamin, J. (1991). Children as patients. William B. Tiller, Contributor. In American College of Legal Medicine, *Legal medicine: Legal dynamics of medical encounters* (2nd ed., pp. 282–317). St. Louis: Mosby Yearbook.

Messenger, C., & McGuire, J. (1981). Child's conception of confidentiality in the therapeutic relationship. *Psychotherapy: Theory, Research and Practice, 18,* 123–130.

Miller, T., & Swartz, L. (1990). Clinical psychology in general hospital settings: Issues in interprofessional relationships. *Professional Psychology: Research and Practice, 21* (l), 48–53.

Moreno, J. D. (1989). Treating the adolescent patient: An ethical analysis. *Journal of Adolescent Health Care, 10,* 454–459.

Pitre v. *Opelousas General Hospital,* 530 So. 2d 1151 (1988).

Pope, K. S. (1990). Ethical and malpractice issues in hospital practice. *American Psychologist, 45* (9), 1066–1070.

Post, B. L., Peters, B. M., Stahl, S. P., Peters, J. D., Fineberg, K. S., & Kroll, D. A. (1984). *The law of medical practice in Pennsylvania and New Jersey.* Rochester, NY: Lawyers Cooperative Publishing.

Pryzwansky, W. B., & Wendt, R. N. (1987). *Psychology as a profession: Foundations of practice.* New York: Pergammon.

Richards, J. C. (1992). Training health psychologists: A model for the future. *Australian Psychologist, 27* (2), 87–90.

Russo, D. C., & Tarbell, S. E. (1984). Child health psychology: Emerging responsibilities of the pediatric health psychologist. *Clinical Psychology Review, 4,* 495–502.

Schwitzgebel, R. K. (1978). Suggestions for the uses of psychological devices in accord with legal and ethical standards. *Professional Psychology, 2,* 478–488.

Schwitzgebel, R. L., & Schwitzgebel, R. K. (1980). *Law and psychological practice.* New York: Wiley and Sons.

Soisson, E. L., Vandecreek, L., & Knapp, S. (1987). Thorough record-keeping: A good defense in a litigious era. *Professional Psychology: Research and Practice, 18* (5), 498–502.

Stabler, B., & Mesibov, G. B. (1984). Role functions of pediatric and health psychologists in health care settings. *Professional Psychology: Research and Practice, 15,* 142–151.

Swencionis, C., & Hall, J. E. (1987). Ethical concerns in health psychology. In G. C. Stone, S. M. Weiss, J. D. Matarazzo, N. E. Miller, J. Rodin, C. D. Belar, M. J. Follick, & J. E. Singer (Eds.), *Health psychology: A discipline and a profession* (pp. 203–215). Chicago: University of Chicago Press.

Tancredi, L. R., & Edlund, M. (1983). Are conflicts of interest endemic to psychiatric consultation? *International Journal of Law and Psychiatry, 6,* 293–316.

Task Force on Legal Issues. (1983). The report on the national working conference on education and training in health psychology. *Health Psychology, 2* (5), 98–102.

Taylor, L., & Adelman, H. S. (1989). Reframing the confidentiality dilemma to work in children's best interests. *Professional Psychology: Research and Practice, 20* (2), 79–83.

Taylor, S. E. (1990). Health psychology: The science and the field. *American Psychologist 45* (l), 40–50.

AUTHOR INDEX

SUBJECT INDEX

Abuse, 429–443
  adolescent victimization, 440–442
    effects, 440–441
    prevalence, 441–442
  community context, 435–436
  effects of abuse, 436–439
    emotional problems, 439
    intellectual functioning, 438–439
    peer relations, 437–438
    physical injury, 437
    social cognition, 438
    social relationships with caregivers, 437
  effects on children of community violence, 440
  effects on children of domestic violence, 439
  etiologic factors, 432–435
    child characteristics, 434
    interactional factors, 434–435
    parent characteristics, 432–434
  prevalence, 429–430
  theoretical models, 430–432
    organizational, 430–431
    process, 431–432
Academy of Pediatrics, 17
Achenbach Child Behavior Checklist and Youth Self-Report Form, 442
Activities of Daily Living Questionnaire (ADLQ), 34, 35, 37, 39, 41
Addiction Severity Index (ASI), 212
Adolescent Drug Abuse Diagnosis (ADAD), 212
AIDS, 4, 366, 388, 405 (see also HIV)
Alcohol abuse, 203–215
  assessment of alcohol abuse in adolescents, 211–214
    drugs and alcohol interviews, 212
    psychiatric interviews, 212
    self-administered instruments, 212–214
  epidemiology of alcohol use, 203–205
  etiology of alcoholism, 206–211
    affiliation with nonnormative peers, 211
    child abuse, 210
    cognitive misattributions, 210–211
    determinants of liability, 207–211

developmental perspective, 206–207
    factors that reduce liability, 211
    family dysfunction, 209–210
    intelligence, 209
    parental discipline practices, 210
  prevention, 214
  subtypes of alcoholism, 205–206
    essential alcoholism, 205
    reactive alcoholism, 205
    type I (milieu limited), 205
    type II (male limited), 205
  treatment, 214–215
Alcohol Dependence Scale (ADS), 172
Alcoholics Anonymous (AA), 173
American Alliance for Health, Physical Education, and Recreation, 277
American Association on Mental Deficiency, 402, 403
American Burn Association, 116
American Psychological Association Task Force Report on Children's Responses to Disasters, 333
Assessment of childhood disability in a Third World country, 29–44
  assessment, 33–39
    of disability and handicap, 34–39
    purposes and scope, 33–34
  community assessment of childhood disability, 39–43
    data management, 43
    identification strategies, 42–43
    methodological issues of epidemiology, 40
    purposes of surveys, 40–41
    risk factors, 41–42
    sampling, 42
    study design, 41
  community-based rehabilitation, 30, 31, 32, 41
  screening for and identifying childhood disability, 30–33
    choice of diseases for screening, 31
    criteria for effective screening tests, 31–33
    hearing screening, 33
    purposes of screening, 30–31
    vision screening, 33

Assessment of Disabled Children in Care (ADCC), 40, 41, 43
Asthma, 141–155
  medical domain, 142–144
    clinical symptomatology, 142–143
    definition of asthma, 142
    etiology, 142
    treatment approaches, 143–144
  psychological domain, 144–154
    medical adaptation, 150–154
    psychological adaptation, 144–150
    school adaptation, 147–150, 154
Asthma Care Training (A.C.T.) for Kids, 151
Asthma Command, 151
Attention-Deficit Hyperactivity Disorder (ADHD), 144, 145, 347, 348
Avon study of smoking, 189

Baby Your Baby Program, 14–15, 25
Behavior Avoidance Test (BAT), 334
Bender-Gestalt Test, 279
Body image assessment, 79
Bogalusa heart study, 187
Budget Enforcement Act of 1990, 16
Bulimia Test-Revised (BULIT-R), 78
Burn injuries, 115–124
  epidemiology, 115–116
    developmental aspects, 116
    overview of burn injuries, 116–117
  prevention, 123–124
  psychological aspects, 117–123
    acute phase, 119–122
    behavioral problems, 122
    body image, 121–122
    challenges posed to children and families, 118
    compliance, 121
    developmental factors, 119
    family coping, 122
    mental status, 119–120
    onset, 118–119
    pain, 120–121
    premorbid psychopathology, 119
    self-excoriation, 122
    sleep disturbances and nutritional intake, 121
  rehabilitation phase, 122–123